HEART
A Physiologic and Clinical Study
of Cardio-vascular Diseases

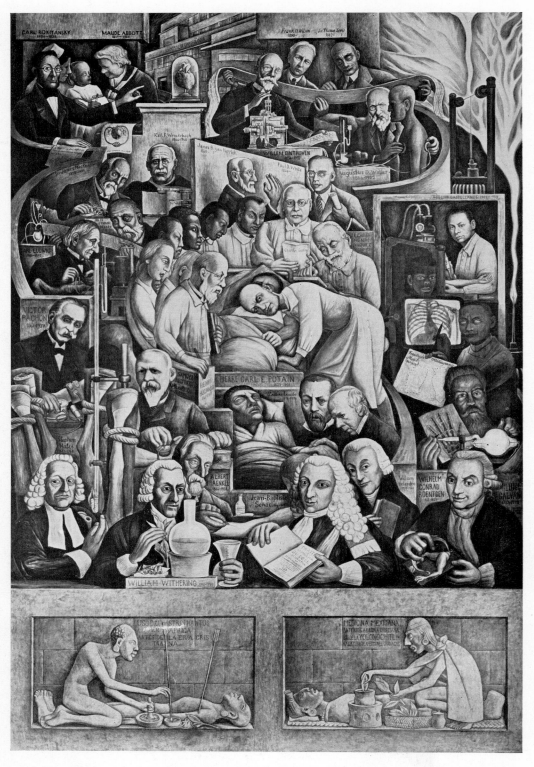

One of the murals painted by Diego Rivera for the National Institute of Cardiology of Mexico City. Some of the contemporary cardiologists can be recognized.

(Through the courtesy of Prof. I. Chavez, Director of the Institute.)

HEART

A Physiologic and Clinical Study
of Cardio-vascular Diseases

By
ALDO A. LUISADA, M.D.

Associate Professor of Medicine and Director, Division of Cardiology
at The Chicago Medical School, under a Teaching Grant of the
National Heart Institute, U. S. Public Health Service
Associate Attending Physician (Acad. Staff) and Chief of Cardiac Clinics,
The Mount Sinai Hospital of Chicago
Chief of Service and Cardiologist,
La Rabida Jackson Park Sanitarium

With a Foreword by
HERRMAN L. BLUMGART

Physician-in-Chief, Beth Israel Hospital
Professor of Medicine, Harvard Medical School

SECOND EDITION

BALTIMORE
THE WILLIAMS & WILKINS COMPANY
1954

*T*o my son *Claude*

FOREWORD

The advance in our knowledge of the heart and the vast accumulation of literature render surveys of the entire field, such as the present text, of great value. The task is Herculean for there is practically no medical discipline or field of biological science which has not contributed materially to our comprehension of the cardiovascular system in health and disease. The author brings to this undertaking unusual qualifications. He is a brilliant investigator in the pathologic physiological mechanism of cardiac disorders, such as the pathogenesis of pulmonary edema. Extensive research in clinical pharmacology and many clinical studies including graphic registration of cardiac phenomena illustrate his wide interest and experience.

In cardiology, as with medicine in general, many issues are still sub judice. It is well that from time to time the current status of these problems be reviewed and individual opinions be expressed fearlessly though they may encounter doubt, debate or even disapproval. Progress will be accelerated; by thus defining more vividly the gaps in our knowledge further speculation, clinical observation, and research will be promoted. The excellent survey of European as well as American thought made available in this text, the description of mechanical registration of cardiac action and heart sounds, and the reviews of many diseased states with the aid of diagrammatic illustrations are exceptional and heighten the usefulness of this book.

H. L. BLUMGART

Preface to the Second Edition

Medical progress advances at a fast pace and nowhere is this so clearly evident as in *cardiology*. Eight years have elapsed between the first preparation of *Heart* and that of the present edition and each chapter had to be completed, modified, or rearranged.

Three new chapters have been added to the book: Cardiovascular Syphilis, which briefly summarizes data presented in other parts of the book; Prognosis of Cardiovascular Diseases; and The Social and Legal Aspects of Heart Disease, which discusses several controversial and important problems of cardiology.

Chapters on the following subjects have been completely rewritten: technical examination, rheumatic fever, congenital heart diseases, chronic cor pulmonale, coronary heart disease, pulmonary edema, heart failure, drugs, management, prescriptions, and treatment of emergencies.

In other chapters, one or more sections were added or modified. Among them are: physiology of the electrocardiogram, endocardial sclerosis, Libman-Sacks disease, congenital anomalies of the large veins, superior and inferior caval syndromes, surgical treatment of valvular defects, and amyloid heart.

One hundred figures have been added while 160 have been deleted. As a result, the total number of illustrations has decreased. Among the new figures, 22 were reproduced from another book of the author, *The Heart Beat*, through the courtesy of the Paul B. Hoeber Co.

In spite of the many additions, the text is only slightly longer than in the first edition. This was obtained through deletion of paragraphs or words which seemed of lesser importance or had become obsolete. Thus, the usefulness of this book for consultation was not impaired.

The author wishes to thank his coworkers, all of whom have contributed to present changes and developments with stimulating discussions or keen observations.

It is to be hoped that this book will be useful to both undergraduate and postgraduate students and will simplify their task in mastering the various functions and dysfunctions of the *Heart*.

A. A. L.

Preface to the First Edition

This book has been written for the large group of physicians who desire to increase their knowledge of heart disease. Difficult technical terms have, therefore, been avoided, and complex technical discussion dispensed with wherever possible. It is the opinion of the author that some of the fundamentals contained in this text should also be of value to heart specialists.

The title of the book—*Heart*—is the result of the preponderance of material devoted to physiology of the heart and vessels and to the pharmacology of the drugs useful in the treatment of heart disease. Thus, material which can be gathered only by consulting numerous sources may be found in this volume. Such a compilation of material has been possible because of my clinical and experimental laboratory associations. Naturally, the practical importance of any new experimental study and the physiological approach to clinical problems have always been given due consideration.

To my knowledge, this volume is illustrated by a far larger number of engravings than any similar book. I resorted as far as possible to the use of sketches, of graphic schemes, and photographs, in order to avoid lengthy descriptions and to simplify the subject. Whenever an original graphic reproduction did not lend itself to simple interpretation, a sketch was substituted.

In spite of my desire to follow the classic description pattern, some differences will be found between this book and other books of cardiology. They are due to the following reasons:

1) The etiological classification of heart diseases, a scheme of beautiful simplicity, had the unexpected result of leading many practitioners to mental laziness in formulating an exact diagnosis. For this and for didactic reasons, I have avoided basing the description of heart disease on etiology alone. The diseases have been classified on the basis of anatomical-clinical syndromes, and correlation with the etiology has been made as often as possible. A detailed discussion of differential diagnosis has been added to each disease in order to aid the practitioner.

2) Personal studies on cardiovascular diseases gave me an outlook somewhat different from that of other authors. An attempt has been made to keep the expression of personal views within the most moderate limits. In spite of this, some chapters will show features distinctive from those of other books; this could not be avoided without disowning over twenty years of research. A more personal approach will be found in the discussion of the following problems: function and dysfunction of the peripheral arteries; peripheral signs of aortic insufficiency; murmurs of valvular diseases; low blood pressure; adhesive pericarditis; paroxysmal pulmonary edema; congestive failure; treatment of the cardiac patient; and graphic methods, particularly phonocardiography. The emphasis given to phonocardiography

is due, first to my belief that this method will have an ever increasing importance in cardiology; and, second, to the possibility of giving visual evidence to murmurs which are easily forgotten when described only by words.

Having been associated with Henri Vaquez and Paul D. White, cardiologists; with Cesare Frugoni and Giuseppe Zagari, internists; with Otto Loewi, Ernest P. Pick and David Rapport, biologists; I wish to state that their teachings have deeply influenced my work. My friendship with the late Soma Weiss and, chiefly, with Hermann L. Blumgart and his pupils, also led to a significant increase of my knowledge in different fields.

Acknowledgment is made of the patient work of Dr. E. Stanley Landy and Alba Faillace di Credico in revising the manuscript.

The publishers, Williams & Wilkins, have been very helpful and deserve a special word of thanks for their courtesy and co-operation.

I wish to acknowledge the kindness of the publisher Cappelli of Bologna for permitting the reproduction of a certain number of illustrations from my book *Cardiologia* published in 1938.

A. A. L.

Contents

CHAPTER 1

History of Cardiology

The fields of study on which modern cardiology is based are the following: anatomy, physiology, pathology, pharmacology, physics, general medicine, surgery, roentgenology, physical diagnosis, and comparative biology.

Chronological listing of important events is undoubtedly a sketchy and incomplete way of describing them. Still it has a certain importance, as it enables students of the subject to grasp at a glance the conditions of a part of medicine in any particular year, and also makes it possible to remember trends of thought and tendencies of this or that period.

As a rule, historical studies should include only the scientists of the past, since their work can be considered with a certain time perspective. However, inasmuch as cardiology has made tremendous advances in the last twenty years, some of the masters to whom we owe much are still alive. This makes it imperative that their names be mentioned, even though future workers will be able to evaluate their work better than those of the present.

The following chronological list starts from 1500, namely from the beginning of modern times. The nationality applies to the birthplace of the investigator; the country named is the place of residence where the work was done whenever this was different from the original place of birth.

The Sixteenth Century

1530—Leonardo Botallo (Italian, France). Description of the foramen ovale.

1543—Andreas Vesalius (Belgian, Italy) Anatomical description of the human heart; clinical diagnosis of the aneurysms.

1553–1559—
Miguel Servede (Servetus) (Spaniard)
Realdo Colombo (Italian)
Description of the lesser circulation.[1]

1554—Ambroise Paré (French). Aortic aneurysms ascribed to syphilis.

1571—Andrea Cesalpino (Italian). Description of the greater circulation. The heart is recognized as the center of the circulation.

The Seventeenth Century

1603—Fabrizio di Acquapendente (Italian). Description of the valves of the peripheral veins.

1628—William Harvey (English, Italy). Amplification of the theory and further demonstration of the circulation of blood without any interruption.

1661—Marcello Malpighi (Italian). Proof of the capillary circulation; description of the capillaries.

The Eighteenth Century

1708—Antonj van Leeuwenhoek (Dutch). Conception of the pulse.

1715—Raymond Vieussens (French). Description of the coronary circulation; description of mitral stenosis.

1726—Francesco I. Albertini (Italian). Use of inspection and palpation for lo-

---

[1] The lesser circulation had been previously described by *Ibn an Nafis* (Arab) but his studies, already three centuries old, had been forgotten.

cating the apex beat and for the evaluation of cardiac enlargement.

1728—Giovanni Maria Lancisi (Italian). Studies on the mechanism of sudden death. First evaluation of the importance of calcification of the coronary arteries and of cardiac enlargement (coronary heart disease). Description of functional tricuspid insufficiency in congestive failure.

1733—Stephen Hales (English). Experimental study of blood pressure.

1749—Jean Baptiste de Sénac (French). Textbook on heart diseases; quinine treatment of palpitation of the heart.

1755—Albrecht v. Haller (Swiss, Germany). Studies of physiology of the heart. Description of the calcification of the pericardium.

1761—Giovanni Battista Morgagni (Italian). Studies on the pathology of many lesions of the heart and of the vessels, including calcification of the coronary arteries. Description of the syndrome of "pulsus rarus permanens" (later called Stokes-Adams' syndrome).

1761—Leopold Auenbrugger (Austrian). Studies on percussion: cardiac dulness.

1768—William Heberden (English). Clinical description of angina pectoris.

1775—Luigi Galvani (Italian). Discovery of animal electricity.

1777—Lazzaro Spallanzani (Italian). The development of the embryonic heart. Studies on the capillary circulation. Laws of hemodynamics.

1785—William Withering (English). Introduction of digitalis in the treatment of congestive failure.

The Nineteenth Century

1806—Jean Nicolas Corvisart (French). Classical textbook of cardiology. Studies on the dilatation and hypertrophy of the heart. Separation of the organic from the functional disorders of the heart. Interpretation of thrills. Description of tricuspid stenosis.

1815—Joseph Hodgson (English). Textbook on the diseases of the arteries and veins; studies on syphilitic aortitis and syphilitic aortic insufficiency (Hodgson's disease).

1818—John Cheyne (Irish). Description of periodic respiration: Cheyne-Stokes' respiration.

1819—Réné T. H. Laënnec (French). Textbook on auscultation; invention of the stethoscope.

1822—Richard Bright (English). Studies on nephritis and repercussions of this disease on the heart.

1832—Dominic John Corrigan (Irish). Description of the clinical picture of aortic regurgitation; Corrigan's pulse.

1839—Joseph Skoda (Czechoslovakian). Studies on the apex beat. Diagnosis of the aneurysms of the abdominal aorta. Textbook on percussion and auscultation.

1839—Johannes E. Purkinje (Czechoslovakian, Germany). Studies of histology of the myocardium: the network of Purkinje. Description of toxic symptoms caused by digitalis.

1840—Jean Baptiste Bouillaud (French). Book on rheumatic fever; its importance as a cause of heart disease. Rheumatic fever was called "Bouillaud's disease".

1845—Johannes S. C. Schweigger (German). The first galvanometer.

1846—Carl F. Ludwig (German). Perfusion of the isolated mammalian heart.

1846–1856—Rudolph L. K. von Virchov (German). Thrombosis and embolism. Pulmonary embolism and infarction. Studies on aortic hypoplasia.

1854—Armand Trousseau (French). Paracentesis of the pericardium.

1854—William Stokes (Irish). Textbook of

cardiology; periodic Cheyne-Stokes respiration; the Adams-Stokes syndrome.

1854—Claude Bernard (French). The experimental method in physiology. The vasoconstrictor nerves.

1855—Karl v. Vierordt (German). The first sphygmograph.

1855—Albert v. Koelliker (German). Biological demonstration of the action currents of the heart.

1861—Paul Louis Duroziez (French)—Description of the double murmur over the femoral artery in aortic insufficiency; studies on the hemodynamics of this disease. Studies on pure mitral stenosis: "Duroziez's disease".

1861—Auguste Chauveau (French). Studies on the intracardiac pressure of the horse.

1862—Maurice Raynaud (French). Studies on the vaso-spastic syndrome of the extremities: "Raynaud's syndrome".

1862—Austin Flint (American). Description of the functional diastolic apical murmur in aortic insufficiency: the Austin Flint murmur.

1866—Thomas B. Peacock (British). Textbook of congenital heart diseases.

1867—Thomas Lauder Brunton (Scotch), England and Germany). Studies on the capillaries. Use of nitrites in angina pectoris.

1867—Pierre C. E. Potain (French). Description and study of the pulsations of the jugular veins.

1868—Heinrich Quincke (German). Study on the capillary pulse in aortic insufficiency: Quincke's pulse.

1868—Nativelle (French). Isolation of digitoxin.

1871—Ilia de Cyon (Polish, France and Russia). Description of the depressor nerve: Cyon's nerve.

1871—Henry P. Bowditch (American). Studies of physiology of the myo-

cardium: the law of "all or none"; the staircase phenomenon.

1872—Ludwig Traube (German). Description of pulsus alternans. Study on the double tone of the femoral artery in aortic insufficiency: the double tone of Traube.

1872-1877—Luigi Luciani (Italian, Italy and Germany). Study on the esophagocardiogram and on the pulse waves of the respiratory curve. Studies on the periodic activity of the frog's heart; the periods of Luciani.

1873—Adolf Kussmaul (German). Periarteritis nodosa. The paradoxical pulse in adhesive pericarditis: Kussmaul's pulse.

1875—Ercole G. Galvagni (Italian). Oral auscultation. Studies on adhesive pericarditis.

1875—Carl von Rokitansky (German). Studies on septal defects of the heart and many other congenital anomalies.

1876—Julius Cohnheim (German). The paradoxical embolism. Pulmonary edema. Experimental studies on many cardiovascular diseases. Studies on amyloid degeneration of the myocardium.

1877—Aristide Stefani (Italian). Studies on diastole of the heart and on the function of the arteries. Pericardial fistula.

1877—John W. Gordon (British). The first ballistocardiogram.

1878—William S. Oliver (English) Antonio Cardarelli (Italian) } Studies on the tracheal signs of aortic aneurysms; the signs of Oliver-Cardarelli.

1878—William H. Welch (American, Germany). Studies on paroxysmal pulmonary edema.

1879—Henri Roger (French). Study of the clinical syndrome due to interventricular septal defect: "Roger's disease".

1879—Leonard Landois (German). Physiology of the heart; textbook of physiology.

1881—Sigmund v. Basch (German). Description of the sphygmomanometer.

1881—Luigi M. Concato (Italian). Studies on polyserositis: "Concato's disease".

1883—Otto Schmiedeberg (German). Experimental studies on digitalis.

1883—Adolf Fick (German). Determination of blood flow.

1885—Augustus Désiré Waller (French). Graphic demonstration of the action currents of the heart.

1885—Étienne J. Marey (French). Textbook on the graphic method in experimental sciences and in clinical studies; the Marey tambour.

1885—Pierre C. E. Potain (French). Studies on gallop rhythms; the "opening snap" of mitral stenosis.

1885—William Osler (Canadian, Canada, U. S. A. and England). Studies on bacterial endocarditis: the Osler nodes.

1887—Jean Martin Charcot (French). Intermittent claudication.

1888—Étienne L. A. Fallot (French). Studies on "blue babies": the trilogy and the tetralogy of Fallot.

1888—Graham Steell (English). Description of the diastolic pulmonary murmur in mitral stenosis: the Graham Steell murmur.

1888—Arnaud (French). Isolation of ouabain.

1889—Léon Bouveret (French). Description of paroxysmal tachycardia: "Bouveret disease".

1891—Friedrich Trendelenburg (German). Studies on the veins: the operation of Trendelenburg for varicose veins.

1891—Scipione Riva-Rocci (Italian). Description of the mercury type of sphygmomanometer: the apparatus of Riva-Rocci.

1893—Wilhelm His, Jr. (German). Demonstration of the auriculoventricular bundle: the bundle of His.

1895—Kurt Huerthle (German). Electrical records of heart sounds.

1896—Wilhelm K. Roentgen (German). Description of the X-ray.

1896—Friedel Pick (German). Studies on adhesive pericarditis with liver cirrhosis: the "Pick syndrome".

1897—Victor Eisenmenger (German). Studies on congenital heart diseases: the Eisenmenger complex.

1897—William H. Broadbent (English). Studies on pericarditis.

1898—Edmond Delorme (French). Surgery of the heart in adhesive pericarditis.

1899—Henri Huchard (French). Textbook of cardiology. Studies on hypertension and on aortitis: the hypertensive Huchard's syndrome.

The Twentieth Century

1900—Daniel H. William (American). First successful suture of cardiac wound.

1900—Guide Pagano (Italian) / Luigi Siciliano (Italian). Description of the carotid sinus reflexes.

1901—Abel Ayerza (Argentine). Clinical description of the "black cardiacs": the syndrome of Arrillaga and Ayerza.

1901—Luis Morquio (Uruguayan). Description of congenital heart block.

1902—T. W. Engelmann (German). Studies on the properties of the myocardium: the law of "all or none".

1902—Ludolph Brauer (German). Costal resection in adhesive pericarditis.

1902—James Mackenzie (English). Monograph on the pulse.

1902—Friedrich H. L. Moritz (German). The orthodiagram of the heart.

1903—H. Ewald v. Hering (German). Description of atrial fibrillation in animals.

1903—Willem Einthoven (Dutch). Description of the string galvanometer. Different studies of electrocardiography. The first phonocardiograms.

1903—Karel F. Wenckebach (Dutch, Germany and Austria). Studies on cardiac arrhythmias: the Wenckebach periods. Quinidine in the treatment of heart disease.

1904—Max Cloetta (French). Isolation of the active principles of digitalis purpurea.

1904—Ludwig Aschoff (German). Studies on myocarditis: the Aschoff nodules. Studies on the structure of the normal heart: the node of Aschoff-Tawara.

1905—Nikolai S. Korotkow (Russian). The auscultatory method and the clinical measurement of diastolic pressure.

1905—Jakob Pal (Austrian). Studies on "vascular crises".

1905—Pietro Grocco (Italian). Studies on aortic aneurysms. Studies on percussion of the heart.

1906—August v. Wassermann (German). The Wassermann test.

1906—Albert Fraenkel (German). The first intravenous injections of strophanthin in congestive failure.

1906—Yandell Henderson (American). Measurement of volume changes of the heart in animals. The "cardiometer". Studies on cardiac output.

1907—Arthur Keith and Martin Flack (English). Description of the sinoauricular node: the node of Keith and Flack.

1907—Guido Banti (Italian). Studies on venous cirrhosis of the heart.

1907—Adolf Sahli (German). Studies on sphygmobolometry. Classic book of physical diagnosis.

1908—Federico Battistini (Italian). Clinical diagnosis of the ball thrombus of the left atrium.

1908—James Mackenzie (English). Studies on atrial fibrillation.

1908—Sunao Tawara (Japanese, Germany).

Studies on the normal heart: the node of Aschoff-Tawara.

1908—Maude Abbott (Canadian). Studies on congenital heart diseases.

1908—Leo Buerger (American). The syndrome of thromboangiitis obliterans of the young: "Buerger syndrome".

1909—Friedrich Trendelenburg (German). Embolectomy in pulmonary embolism: operation of Trendelenburg.

1909—Michel-Victor Pachon (French). The oscillometer; studies on blood pressure.

1909—Carl J. Rothberger (Austrian). Studies on atrial fibrillation and premature beats.

1909–1910—Camille Lian and Henry Vaquez (French). The theory of isolated right and left cardiac failures.

1909–1910—Thomas Lewis (English). The clinical diagnosis of atrial fibrillation. Studies on arrhythmias. Monograph on graphic registration of the heart beat.

1910—Hans v. Recklinghausen (German). Studies on the pulse: studies on blood pressure.

1910–1914—Maximilian Sternberg (Austrian). The "pericarditis epistenocardiaca." Studies on aneurysms of the heart.

1909–1910—Hugo Schottmueller (German) Emanuel Libman (American) } Studies on bacterial endocarditis.

1910—Walter Straub (German). Studies on the isolated frog's heart: the Straub heart.

1910—W. P. Obrastzow and N. D. Straschesko (Russian). Studies on coronary thrombosis.

1912—Theodore Goett and Julius Rosenthal (German). First studies of roentgenkymography.

1912—Francisco C. Arrillaga (Argentine). Arteritis of the pulmonary artery and arteriosclerosis of the pulmonary vessels: the syndrome of Arrillaga and Ayerza.

1912—Ernest H. Starling (English). Studies on the heart-lung preparation in dogs: the law of the normal heart, or Starling's law.

1912—James B. Herrick (American). Description of the clinical picture of myocardial infarction.

1913—Henri Vaquez and Émile Bordet (French). Roentgenology as an auxiliary branch of cardiology: a well-known textbook.

1914—Richard C. Cabot (American). Classification of heart diseases.

1914—Otto Frank (German). Technique of recording the heart sounds: the Frank capsule.

1914—Franz Volhard (German). Studies on nephritis and hypertension.

1915—Thomas C. Allbutt (British). Studies on hypertension.

1915—Hans Mautner and Ernst Peter Pick (Austrian). Studies on the venous sluices of the liver and the lungs.

1919—Adolf Spitzer (Austrian). Studies on the pathogenesis of congenital heart disease: the Spitzer theory.

1919—Augusto Murri (Italian). The law of the damaged heart, or Murri's laws.

1920—Peter Saxl (Austrian). Use of a mercurial diuretic.

1920—Harold E. B. Pardee (American). The coronary T-wave of the electrocardiogram: the Pardee T-wave.

1920—Louis Gallavardin (French). Monograph on blood pressure. Multiple studies of cardiology.

1921—Herbert Assmann (German). Classic textbook of roentgenology.

1921—Réné Lutembacher (French). Studies on arrhythmias of the heart. Studies on congenital heart diseases: the "Lutembacher's syndrome".

1921—Thomaso Jonnesco (Rumanian). Surgical treatment of angina pectoris by sympathectomy.

1921—Henri Vaquez (French). Classic textbook of heart diseases. Multiple works on heart diseases.

1921—Otto Loewi (Austrian). Studies on the "vagal substance" of the frog's heart.

1921—Robert Tigerstedt (Finn, Germany). Textbook of physiology of the circulation. Multiple experimental studies on the heart and vessels.

1921–1926—Charles Laubry (French) and Cesare Pezzi (Italian, France). Monograph on congenital heart disease. Monograph on gallop rhythms. Multiple studies of cardiology.

1924—August Krogh (Danish). Studies on the capillaries. Monograph on this subject.

1924—Tiburcio Padilla (Argentine). Monograph of electrocardiography.

1924—Johann G. Moenckeberg (German). Textbook of pathology of the heart. Studies on arteriosclerosis.

1925—Nikolai Anitschkow (Russian). Studies on arteriosclerosis; studies on myocarditis.

1926—Herbert Elias and Adolf Feller (Austrian). Studies on congestive failure.

1926—David Scherf (Austrian, Austria and U. S. A.). Studies on disturbances of the atrial myocardium; multiple studies of cardiology.

1927—Karel F. Wenckebach (Dutch, Germany and Austria) and H. Winterberg (Austrian). Classic textbook of arrhythmias of the heart.

1927—Henri Frédéricq (Belgian). Studies on the physiology of the myocardium.

1927—Ludolph Brauer (German). Studies on pericarditis; the Brauer's operation in adhesive pericarditis.

1927—Hans E. von Hering (German). Studies on carotid sinus reflexes.

1927—Herrmann L. Blumgart. (American) and Soma Weiss (Hungarian, U. S. A.) Studies on circulation time.

1928—Carl J. Wiggers (American). Textbook of physiology of circulation.

Studies on hemodynamics of valvular and septal defects.

1928–1929—Aldo A. Luisada (Italian, Italy, Austria, U. S. A.). Studies on acute pulmonary edema. Monograph on hypotension: the syndrome of hyposphygmia.

1929—Walter Forsmann (German). Catheterization of the human heart.

1930—Frank N. Wilson (American). Studies on bundle branch block and on precordial leads.

1931—Ernst Edens (German). Textbook of cardiology.

1931—Hermann Rein (German). Physiology of coronary circulation; description of the "Thermostromuhr".

1931—Paul D. White (American). Well-known textbook of cardiology. Multiple studies of cardiology.

1931–1934—Peter Stumpf (German). Eduard Zdansky (Austrian) Sidney Hirsch (American) Pietro Cignolini (Italian) } Studies of roentgenkymography.

1932—Luigi Condorelli (Italian, Austria and Italy) and Max Hochrein (German, working in the U. S. A. and Germany). Studies and monographs on coronary circulation and coronary heart disease.

1932—Arthur Grollman (American). Studies on cardiac output.

1933—Herrmann L. Blumgart, Samuel Levine and David Berlin (American). Thyroidectomy in heart failure and angina pectoris.

1933—Adalbert v. Bogaert (Belgian, France). Studies on chronaxia of the myocardium and of the bundle of His.

1933—Arthur Stoll (Swiss). Isolation of the glycosides of digitalis lanata.

1933—Wilhelm Dressler (Austrian, Austria and moved to U. S. A.). Studies on pulsations of the chest wall; studies on tricuspid stenosis.

1933—Corneille Heymans (Belgian). Studies on the carotid sinus.

1934—Harry Goldblatt (American). Experimental hypertension caused by renal ischemia: the Goldblatt kidney.

1935—Pedro Cossio (Argentine). Book of physical diagnosis in cardiology.

1935–1939—Claude S. Beck (American) and L. O'Shaughnessy (British). Various surgical attempts at revascularization of the myocardium.

1936–1941—Camille Lian and coworkers (French). Multiple studies and monograph of phonocardiography and collective auscultation.

1937—Hugo Roesler (Austrian). Textbook of roentgenology of the heart.

1937—Augustín Castellanos et al. (Cuban). Angiocardiography in children.

1939—Oscar Orias and Eduardo Braun–Menéndez (Argentine). Monograph of clinical phonocardiography.

1939—E. S. Orgain and M. A. Poston; P. H. Futcher and V. C. Scott (American). Successful sulfonamide treatment in acute bacterial endocarditis.

1939—Robert E. Gross (American). Surgical ligation of patent ductus arteriosus.

1939—George P. Robb and Israel Steinberg (American). Visualization of the cardiac chambers in the adult.

1939—Isaac Starr (American). Studies of ballistocardiography.

1944—Foundation of the National Institute of Cardiology in Mexico City.

1941–1948—André Cournand (French, U. S. A.) and coworkers. Studies on pulmonary circulation and cardiac output by catheterization of the right heart.

1941—Louis N. Katz (American). Textbook of electrocardiography. Multiple studies of experimental and clinical cardiology.

1942–1947—Emanual Goldberger (American). Studies of "unipolar" electro-cardiography.

1944—Leo Loewe *et al.* (American). Successful penicillin treatment of subacute bacterial endocarditis.

1945—Alfred Blalock and Helen B. Taussig (American). Surgical treatment of the tetralogy of Fallot.

1945—C. Crafoord and G. Nylin (Swedish); Robert E. Gross (American). Surgical treatment of coarctation of the aorta.

1945—George C. Henny and Bert R. Boone (American). The electrokymograph.

1946—Maurice Marchal (French). Studies of densigraphy of the lungs.

1947–1949—Aldo A. Luisada (Italian, U. S. A.), Felix G. Fleischner (Austrian, (U. S. A.) and coworkers. Studies of electrokymography of the heart, great vessels, and lungs, in normal subjects and in clinical conditions.

1947—Helen B. Taussig (American). Text-book of congenital heart diseases.

1948—Foundation of the National Heart Institute in the U. S. A.

1948—Myron Prinzmetal (American). The method of radiocardiography.

1947–1948—Maurice Lenègre *et al.* (French), Antonio Battro *et al.* (Argentine) and Hans Hecht (Swiss, U. S. A.). Intracardiac electrocardiography.

1948—Claude S. Beck (American), A. M. Vineberg (Canadian), and M. Fauteux (Canadian). Revascularization of the ischemic heart; coronary neurectomy.

1950—Robert C. Brock (British). Surgical dilatation of the stenotic pulmonic valve.

1949–1951—Charles P. Bailey (American). Commissurotomy of mitral stenosis. Various interventions in valvular defects.

1949–1952—David Scherf (Austrian, U. S. A.) and coworkers. Myron Prinzmetal (American). Experimental and clinical studies on atrial fibrillation and premature contractions. Monographs on the former (M. P.) and the latter (D. S.).

BIBLIOGRAPHY

1. CASTIGLIONI, A. *A History of Medicine.* New York, Knopf, 1941.
2. EDENS, E. *Krankheiten des Herzens.* Berlin, Springer, 1929.
3. HERRICK, J. B. *A Short History of Cardiology.* Baltimore, Thomas, 1942.
4. LUISADA, A. A. Bull. Hist. Med., 1944, suppl. 3, 152.
5. SIGERIST, H. E. *Einfuehrung in die Medizin.* Leipzig, 1931.
6. VAQUEZ, H. *Les Maladies du Coeur.* Paris, Baillière, 1928.
7. WHITE, P. D. *Heart Disease.* New York, Macmillan, 1944.
8. WILLIUS, F. A., AND KEYS, T. E. *Cardiac Classics.* St. Louis, Mosby, 1941.
9. FISCHER, I. *Biographisches Lexicon der hervorragender Aertze der letzten fuenfzig Jahre.* Wien, Urban und Schwarzenberg, 1933.
10. HUEBOTTER, F. H., AND VIERORDT, H. *Biographisches Lexicon der hervorragender. Aertze aller Zeiten und Voelker.* Wien, Urban und Schwarzenberg, 1929.
11. WILLIUS, F. A., AND DRY, T. J. *A History of the Heart and Circulation.* Philadelphia, Saunders, 1948.

CHAPTER 2

Development and Structure of the Cardiovascular System

Development of the Cardio-vascular System

In an early stage of embryonic life, the heart is represented by a simple elongated tube (the *primitive cardiac tube*). Various circular narrowings soon separate five different structures which follow each other in the direction of the blood stream. They are called the *sinus venosus*, the *atrium*, the *ventricle*, the *bulbus cordis*, and the *common arterial trunk* (figs. 1 and 2).

Elongating, the cardiac tube then bends and twists itself, forming an "S" with the venous end toward the back and the left, and the arterial end upwards and toward the front (fig. 1). Further changes occur rapidly as the venous end moves upward behind the arterial end, and at the same time undergoes a movement of torsion. At this stage, a deep *atrioventricular groove* separates the *venous part* (*primitive atrium* plus *sinus venosus*) from the *arterial part* of the heart (*primitive ventricle* plus *bulbus cordis*). Therefore, at this time, the heart fundamentally consists of only two chambers like that of the fish (*bilocular heart*) (fig. 2).

Later, on each side of the primitive atrium, a bulge appears (future atrium) and the round *atrioventricular opening* flattens into a transverse one into which the *atrioventricular valves* develop. The primitive ventricle soon shows an anterior and a posterior groove, separating the right half from the left. The right ventricle, though small, is lengthened by the bulbus cordis and looks larger than the left. The primitive atrium and ventricle, and the bulbus, are then each divided into two separate cavities by *septa*, or walls. A *vertical septum*[2] arising in the upper part of the back wall of the atrium proceeds downward toward the atrioventricular opening and fuses with *another septum*[3] which has divided the latter. By the time the fusion is complete, a *defect* has developed in the lower part of the interatrial wall.[4] However, this first opening is soon covered by a *third formation*[5] which develops to the right of the first and parallel to it. As this new wall develops upward from below and never reaches the end, a *second opening* will remain in the upper part of the septum, called the *foramen ovale*[6] (fig. 3). This is the foramen which is still open in the newborn. It is guarded on its left side by the first septum which acts like a *valve*. Thus, blood may pass through the foramen but only from the right to the left atrium and not in the opposite direction.

At this stage, we have a heart made of three chambers, two communicating atria plus one ventricle, similar to that of the amphibia (*trilocular heart*).

An *interventricular muscular septum*, growing upwards from the apex, then fuses with the interatrial septum and divides the two ventricles. Anteriorly, it fuses with the septum which has meanwhile developed in the bulbus cordis. The two ventricular chambers communicate for a time through an *interventricular foramen*.

[2] This septum is called *septum primum*.

[3] This formation is called *septum intermedium*.

[4] This is called *first oval defect* or *foramen ovale primum*.

[5] This formation is called *septum secundum*.

[6] This defect is called *foramen ovale secundum* or *foramen Botalli*.

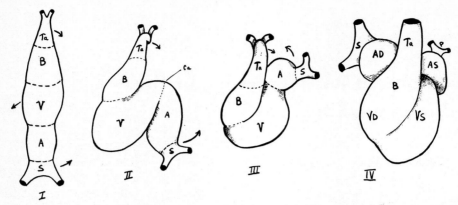

FIG. 1. Early stages of development of the heart (Adapted from Pichon). I, II, III are seen from the left; IV is a frontal view. S, sinus venosus; A, atrium; Ca, atrial canal; B, bulbus cordis; V, ventricle; Ta, arterial trunk; Vd, right ventricle; Vs, left ventricle.

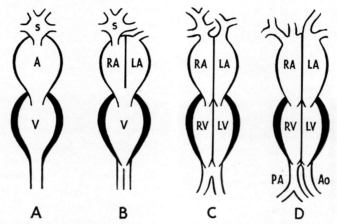

FIG. 2. The hearts of different vertebrates. A, fish (shark); B, amphibia (frog); C, reptiles (alligator); D, mammals; RA, right atrium; LA, left atrium; RV, right ventricle; LV, left ventricle. S, sinus venosus; AO, aorta; PA, pulmonary artery. (Adapted from Kingsley's *Comparative Anatomy*. Courtesy of Blakiston Co.)

Shortly afterwards, the *common arterial trunk*[7] is divided by another structure into two separate vessels: the *aorta* and the *pulmonary artery*. The division proceeds until the interarterial septum meets with the septum of the bulbus cordis on one end, and with the aorto-pulmonary septum on the other.

Four *endocardial cushions* are present at the end of the bulbus. In the process of division, the right and left cushions are also divided, so that on each side of the septum

three endocardial swellings will be left, the future *semilunar cusps* of the aorta and pulmonary artery (fig. 4).

Six *arterial arches*[8] arise from the arterial trunk, go toward the back, and open into two large vessels (*dorsal aortae*). These arches are at first symmetrical, but soon become asymmetrical owing to the early atrophy of the first, second, and fifth arch. The third arch participates to the formation of the carotid arteries; the fourth and sixth

[7] This is also called *the truncus arteriosus*.

[8] They are also called *arteries of the branchial arches*.

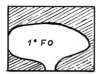

FIG. 3. Development of the interatrial septum, from the left. 1 FO, first foramen ovale; FB, second foramen ovale, or foramen Botalli. (Adapted from Arey's *Developmental Anatomy*. Courtesy of W. B. Saunders Co.)

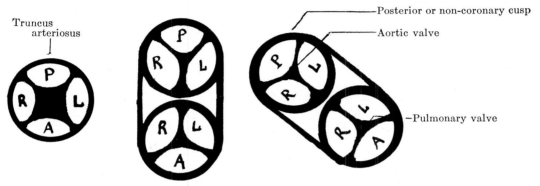

FIG. 4. Scheme explaining the development and names of the semilunar valves of the aorta and pulmonary artery. (Grant's *Method of Anatomy*, The Williams & Wilkins Co.)

also develop into vessels of primary importance. The fourth artery will form the *aortic arch* on the left side and the proximal portion of the *subclavian artery* on the right.

The sixth artery will form *the right branch of the pulmonary artery* on the right side; the left branch and *the ductus arteriosus* on the left (fig. 5).

The mammalian embryo recapitulates all stages of development which can be encountered in lower vertebrates.

The gradual increase in volume and pressure which occurs at the higher levels of the scale leads to elimination of the right ventricular aorta and leaves only two outlets, the left aorta and the pulmonary artery.

In conclusion, there are two main phases of cardiovascular development: the first concerns itself with *the formation of the atrioventricular loop;* the second, with *the absorption of the bulbus, the development of the septa*, and that of *the inflow and outflow tracts of the ventricles.*

The following processes are of paramount importance: a) formation of the bulbus cordis; b) torsion of the primitive tube; c) formation of the main septa (interatrial, interventricular, bulbar, interarterial septa); d) incorporation of the sinus venosus into the right atrium and of the bulbus cordis into the ventricles; e) evolution of the arterial arches; and f) closure of the foramen ovale, of the ductus arteriosus, and of the ductus venosus. If any of these fundamental processes is modified or incomplete, congenital heart disease occurs. The torsion of the primitive tube has a special importance for the future development of the heart.

THE FETAL CIRCULATION

The circulation of a 6-month-old fetus takes place in the following way.

Maternal blood comes from the placenta through *the umbilical vein*. This blood, saturated with oxygen, goes largely to the liver (5, 7) and partly to *the inferior cava* through a connecting vessel.[9] The opening of the inferior cava into the heart is rather

[9] This is called the *ductus venosus Arantii*.

FIG. 5. The arterial arches and the resulting arteries in man. In black, the definitive vessels; in white, the obliterated sections. C, common carotid arteries; P, pulmonary artery; S, subclavian arteries; D, ductus arteriosus; AA, abdominal aorta. (Adapted from Arey.)

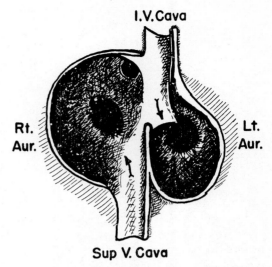

FIG. 6. Circulation of the blood in the atria of the fetus. Section of the heart seen from above (after Barron). The arrows indicate the predominant direction of the blood coming from the two venae cavae.

high and nearly median, so that its mouth is bisected by the interatrial septum near the foramen ovale. About two-thirds of the blood of the inferior vena cava go directly into the left atrium; about one-third, on the contrary, enters the right (5, 6) (fig. 6). From the left atrium, the blood (received via the inferior vena cava and the pulmonary veins) goes to the left ventricle, then to the aorta. In the latter, the blood mixes with that coming from the pulmonary artery via the ductus arteriosus and is distributed to the whole body.

The venous blood coming from the head and the upper extremities reaches the right atrium via the superior cava. Directed by a ridge,[10] this blood goes straight toward the right atrioventricular valve and, after slight admixture with that of the inferior cava, enters the right ventricle and proceeds into the pulmonary artery. Part of it goes to the lungs, and a large part to the aorta through the patent ductus arteriosus (fig. 7). The blood of the *abdominal aorta* goes not only

[10] This is called the *tubercle of Lower.*

to the lower extremities and to the viscera, but also to the umbilical arteries, and from them to the placenta.

The main features of the fetal circulation are the following:

a) *Partly oxygenated blood* circulates in the inferior vena cava and in the right heart of

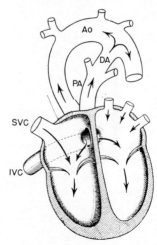

FIG. 7. Circulation in the heart and large vessels of a fetus near term. DA, ductus arteriosus; PA, pulmonary artery; AO, aorta; IVC, inferior vena cava.

the fetus. *Blood only partly oxygenated* circulates in the left heart and in the aorta.

b) There is *a double circulation within the right atrium*, with only slight mixture of the bloods coming from the two cavae.

c) There are *two shunts*, that between the atria, and that between pulmonary artery and aorta. The blood passes from the inferior cava to the left atrium via the foramen ovale; from the pulmonary artery to the aorta via the ductus.

CHANGES OCCURRING AFTER BIRTH

The main changes brought about by birth are related to the beginning of the pulmonary respiration and the end of the flow of maternal blood from the placenta.

The expansion of the lungs causes a fall of pressure and an increase of flow within the pulmonary artery. A greater amount of blood then returns to the left atrium raising the pressure in this chamber.

The following changes take place:

a) *Closure of the foramen ovale.* This is due to the apposition of the valve-like membrane on the opening of the foramen. It takes place as soon as the pressure is reduced in the inferior vena cava and in the right atrium (lack of maternal blood) (5). A rise in pressure in the left atrium due to increase in the pulmonary circulation, may also occur. The functional closure is sudden. The anatomical closure may take a few days.

b) *Closure of the ductus arteriosus.* The ductus arteriosus usually closes a few minutes after birth (5, 6) owing to the contraction of a muscular ring innervated by vagal fibers. This is possible, first, because there is a fall of pressure in the pulmonary artery due to the beginning of respiration; and second, because of the direct action of oxygen upon the musculature of the ductus (8). Among the different possibilities, that of a carotid sinus-vagal reflex caused by the higher carotid pressure has also been considered (10). The functional closure of the ductus occurs from a few minutes to a few

days after birth; anatomical closure, on the other hand, takes much longer, and is due to thrombosis of the ductus and transformation of the latter into a band of fibrous tissue.

c) The *closure of the ductus venosus* is brought about by the contraction of a muscular bundle, innervated by sympathetic fibers (5, 9).

CAUSES OF MALFORMATIONS

Malformations of the heart may be due to developmental arrest, maldevelopment, or pathology, during fetal life. *Arrest of development* may cause isolated septal defects or patency of the ductus. *Maldevelopment* may cause entry of the pulmonary veins into the right atrium, aortic hypoplasia, isolated bicuspid valve, or the transposition complexes. *Pathology* of a normally formed heart may be due to inflammation, glycogen infiltration, or abnormality of other organs.

General Outline of the Cardiovascular System

The cardiovascular system is a complex apparatus whose function is that of circulating the blood. Schematically, it is composed of *a central pump* and of an extensive *distribution system*. At the center is *the heart*, the largest and strongest organ of the system. Actually the heart is made of two separate parts, *the right* and *the left heart*, which work simultaneously, but are connected to separate distributing systems.

The *right heart* sends its blood through the pulmonary artery to the network of pulmonary vessels, a distribution system which is called *the lesser circulation.*

The *left heart* sends its blood to the rest of the body through the aorta and a second larger distribution system called *the greater circulation* (figs. 8 and 9).

The blood collected by the *general system of veins* flows to the right heart by way of the two main venous trunks, *the superior* and *the inferior vena cava.* The blood collected by the *system of the pulmonary veins*

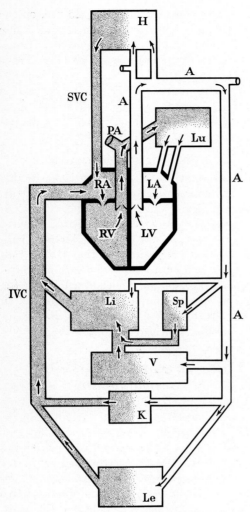

FIG. 8. General scheme of the circulation. Lu, lungs; Li, liver; Sp, spleen; K, kidneys; Le, legs; H, head; A, aorta; PA, pulmonary artery; V, visceral vessels of portal circulation; RA, right atrium; LA, left atrium; RV, right ventricle; LV, left ventricle.

Some vascular districts have special features. They are:

a) *The hepatic system*, where the blood is partly supplied by an artery (the *a. hepatica*) and in larger part is supplied by a very important venous collector (the *v. portae*) (fig. 8).

b) *The gastro-intestinal-splenic system*, where the blood flows into the vena portae and thence to the liver.

Not all organs of the abdomen are included in this latter system, as *the kidneys* and *the genital organs* are independent of it (fig. 8).

The *vessels of the brain* and *the vessels of the heart* also have special features.

All large vessels, connected to the ventricles, are called *arteries*, regardless of the type of blood which flows in them. The name is connected to their special structure. The large arteries branch successively into smaller and smaller arteries until the network is made up of minute, microscopic vessels having a different structure called *capillaries*. From the capillaries, the blood is collected into larger vessels, the smaller veins. These gradually unite into larger collecting trunks, *the veins*, which at last bring the blood back to the main venous collectors and to the heart.

THE HEART

The heart is a thoracic organ located between the two lungs and above the diaphragm. It is the largest and most important organ of the mediastinum. The average weight of the heart is shown in table 1 (17).

The *average ratio of heart weight to body weight* in the male is 0.43 per cent; in the female, 0.40 per cent. In thin persons, the ratio is somewhat higher than in fat individuals (39).

The *capacity of the cardiac chambers* in the adult is the following:

Right atrium................. 34–142 cc.
Left atrium.................. 18–64 cc.
Right ventricle. .... 25–71 cc.
Left ventricle. .... 11–70 cc.

flows to the left heart by way of *four pulmonary veins* (figs. 8 and 9).

The blood flowing to each of the two halves of the heart does not enter the main chamber, called the ventricle, directly, but first fills a reception chamber, called *the auricle or atrium*. There are, therefore, four separate chambers or cavities, the two atria and the two ventricles, and each half has an atrium and a ventricle (figs. 8 and 9).

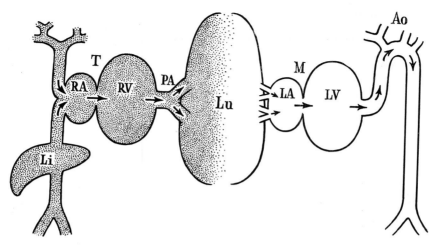

Fig. 9. The circulatory system separated into its main constituents. Symbols as in figure 8

The heart may be schematically divided into:

a) The *pericardium*, a sac which contains the heart.

b) The *myocardium*, or muscular part of the heart.

c) The *endocardium*, or internal membrane, which coats the internal surface and forms the valves.

The heart is placed obliquely in the thorax with the base toward the right and the back, and the apex toward the left and the front.

The heart is made of four sections which contain four cavities, the two atria and the two ventricles. The division of the four sections can be recognized from the outside owing to the existence of grooves where the vessels of the heart itself are located. These are: the *atrioventricular groove* and the two *interventricular grooves* (anterior and posterior).

1) *The right atrium* receives blood brought by the two main venous collectors, *the superior vena cava* and *the inferior vena cava*. It is connected to the right ventricle by means of the *right atrioventricular valve*, also called *the tricuspid valve*. It is separated from the left atrium, which is on its left, by *the interatrial septum*.

The right atrium is at the base of the heart and therefore to the right and posteriorly.

A groove separates *the sinus of the venae cavae*, which is a kind of funnel into which these veins open, from the rest of the cavity. The opening of the superior vena cava is more anterior, that of the inferior vena cava is more posterior. Both, however, open near the septum. The opening of the former has no valve; the opening of the latter has an incomplete semilunar valve (*Eustachian valve*) which may partly prevent a backflow into the vein.

The largest collecting vein of the heart, *the coronary sinus*, also opens into the right atrium, near the mouth of the superior vena cava. This is also protected by a thin valve, *the coronary valve*. A small closed funnel, the *right atrial appendage*, goes upwards and toward the front.

2) *The right atrioventricular opening* is placed along a nearly horizontal axis directed toward the front and the left, and only slightly downwards. The opening is oval and measures an average circumference of 115 mm. (15). It is made of a crescent-

TABLE 1

AGE	FEMALES	MALES
years	*gm.*	*gm.*
1	32.8	42.2
5	80.3	83.7
10	125	130.9
20	250	310

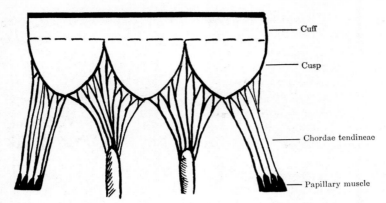

— Cuff

— Cusp

— Chordae tendineae

— Papillary muscle

FIG. 10. Diagram of the tricuspid valve and of its papillary muscles. (After Grant.)

like fibrous expansion, closed by soft connective fibers. The opening is completed by a valve composed of *three leaflets or cusps, the tricuspid valve.* Each of the leaflets is attached by means of thin tendinous fibers to strong muscles, *the papillary muscles,* which are connected with the ventricular wall. One of the cusps is *inferior* (nearer to the diaphragm), one is *medial* (nearer to the septum), and one is *anterior* (nearer to the opening of the pulmonary artery) (fig. 10). Each papillary muscle

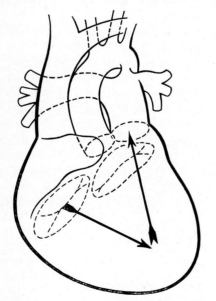

FIG. 11. The movement of the blood stream in the cavity of the right ventricle. (Adapted from Zdansky.)

controls the two adjacent halves of two leaflets.

3) *The right ventricle* receives the blood from the right atrium through the tricuspid valve and pumps it into the pulmonary artery through the semilunar valves. As both openings are at the base of the ventricle, there are two sections in its cavity. One is *the inflow chamber,* which is posterolateral; the other is the *outflow or arterial chamber* (also called *infundibulum* or *conus arteriosus*), which is anterior and nearer to the septum (fig. 11). The ventricle has a semicircular shape when observed in a transverse cut (fig. 12). The average thickness of its wall is 4.1 mm. at the base (18).

4) *The opening of the pulmonary artery* is directed obliquely upwards and towards the left. It is round and has an average diameter of 70 mm. (15). It is completed by a valve, composed of three crescent-shaped leaflets, the *semilunar cusps.* Each of them has a small nodule in the middle of its free margin (*the nodule of Morgagni*). The leaflets are not inserted into a fibrous ring but their base has a fibrous expansion which penetrates between the muscular fibers of the ventricle. Above each cusp is a slight dilatation of the artery, *the sinus of Valsalva.*

5) *The left atrium.* This chamber is smaller than the right. It receives the blood from the lungs through *four pulmonary veins,* two nearer the septum, two others toward the left (fig. 12). It is the most posterior of

all heart cavities and has, therefore, a closer contact with the descending aorta, the esophagus, and the spine. The left surface of the interatrial septum is similar to the right, already described. A small closed funnel, the *left atrial appendage*, takes a downward turn between left ventricle and pulmonary artery. The left atrium communicates with the left ventricle through the left atrioventricular opening.

6) *The left atrioventricular opening* has a rounded shape, an oblique axis toward the front, the left, and downwards, and an average circumference of 101 mm. (15). It is formed by a crescent of fibrous tissue closed in front by soft connective fibers. It is completed by the left atrioventricular valve which has two cusps or leaflets. It is called, therefore, *the bicuspid valve* or, more commonly, the *mitral valve*. The two valvular cusps are similar to those of the tricuspid except that they are more rectangular. This similarity also exists in the arrangement of both *the tendinal strings (chordae)* and *the papillary muscles*. One of the two leaflets is *anterior* and *medial* (it is also called the *aortic leaflet of the mitral valve* owing to its position); the other is *posterior and more lateral*. The two papillary muscles are also *anterior* and *posterior* but each controls the two adjacent parts of the two leaflets of the valve via the tendinal strings (*chordae*).

7) *The left ventricle* receives the blood from the left atrium through the mitral valve and pumps it into the aorta through the semilunar valves. Here again there are two sections: one is the *inflow chamber*, which is more posterior; the other is the outflow or *arterial chamber* (also called *conus arteriosus* or *infundibulum*), which is more anterior. The ventricle has a circular shape when observed in a transverse section (fig. 12). The average thickness of its wall is 10.2 mm. (17).

8) *The aortic opening* is directed obliquely upwards, and towards the right and the back. The outflow chamber, which leads to it, is between the ventricular septum, the

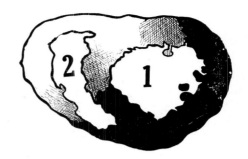

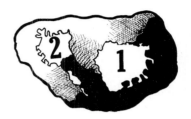

Fig. 12. Transverse sections of the ventricles at two different levels, 1, left ventricle; 2, right ventricle.

two papillary muscles, and the anteromedial leaflet of the mitral valve. The opening has an average circumference of 67 mm. (15) and is completed by *three semilunar cusps*. The structure of the valvular apparatus is similar to that of the pulmonary valve. Their names and positions are described in figure 4.

9) The *interventricular septum* is a curved formation separating the two ventricles. It has its concavity toward the left ventricle (fig. 12). Its average thickness is 10 mm. (17). It is mostly formed by muscular fibers. However, a triangular area placed at the base of the ventricles is much thinner (2 mm.) and consists of fibrous tissue.[11]

10) The *interatrial septum* is a wall separating the two atria. Its average thickness is 2.5 mm. It is mostly made of muscular tissue. However, its posterior and lower part is thinner and consists of fibrous tissue.[12]

---

[11] This is called the *pars membranacea* and represents the area where the septum closed last.

[12] It corresponds to that area where *the foramen ovale* has been occluded by its valve.

THE LARGE ARTERIES

The position and the shape of the two largest arteries, the aorta and the pulmonary artery, are demonstrated by figures 13, 14, and 15. *The pulmonary artery* has an average length of 50 mm. and an average caliber of 35 mm. (15). It soon divides into *a right and a left stem*, the left being practically the prolongation of the main artery.

The aorta is a large arterial trunk which first goes upwards (*ascending a.*), then backwards around the hilum of the left lung (*aortic arch*), and then downwards along the spine (*descending a.*). The latter is called *thoracic aorta* above the diaphragm and *abdominal aorta* below it.

The *coronary arteries* are branches of the ascending aorta. The *innominate artery* (soon dividing into *the right subclavian* and *the right carotid artery*), the *left carotid*, and the *left subclavian*, are branches of the aortic arch.

A *dilatation*, present above the aortic valves (called *aortic bulbus*), contains the *three sinuses of Valsalva* or *aortic sinuses*. These should be called *right* and *left coronary sinuses*, and *noncoronary sinus*. A slight *narrowing* exists between arch and descending aorta, *the aortic isthmus*, sometimes followed by a slight dilatation. A tubular zone of fibrous tissue, called the *annulus fibrosus*, connects the left ventricle with the aorta proper. This structure arises from the bulbus cordis and forms part of the wall of the aortic sinuses.

Average measures are given in table 2 (15, 17).

Several important considerations concerning the large arteries are the following:

a) The division of the common carotid arteries into *internal* and *external carotid*.

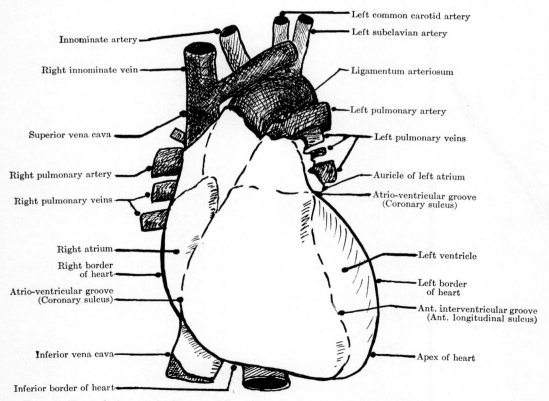

FIG. 13. Frontal view of the heart and large vessels. The pericardium is left white. (After Grant.)

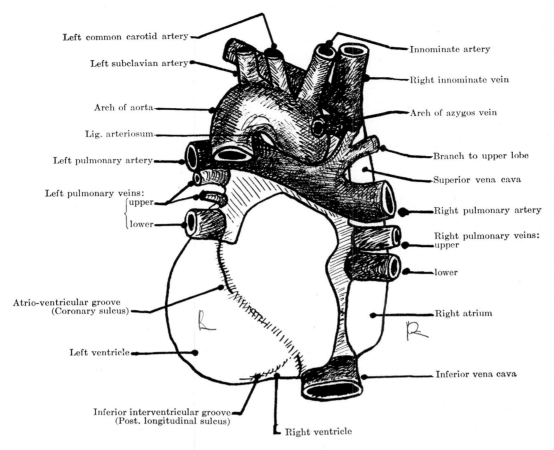

Left common carotid artery

Left subclavian artery

Arch of aorta

Lig. arteriosum

Left pulmonary artery

Left pulmonary veins:
upper
lower

Atrio-ventricular groove
(Coronary sulcus)

Left ventricle

Inferior interventricular groove
(Post. longitudinal sulcus)

Innominate artery

Right innominate vein

Arch of azygos vein

Branch to upper lobe

Superior vena cava

Right pulmonary artery

Right pulmonary veins:
upper

lower

Right atrium

Inferior vena cava

Right ventricle

Fig. 14. Posterior view of the heart and large vessels. The pericardium is left white. (After Grant.)

A dilatation is present at the point of branching, the *carotid sinus*. The carotid sinus is found in the neck at the level of the upper margin of the cricoid cartilage (fig. 17).

b) The division of the abdominal aorta into two large vessels, the *common iliac arteries*, takes place about 10 mm. above the umbilicus.

One of the peculiarities of the *venous system* is the following: the veins of the thoracic walls (*intercostal veins*) are afferent to a larger venous collector, the *vena azygos*. The latter originates in the abdomen (where it is connected with the system of the inferior vena cava), runs in the thorax to the right of the spine, and then opens into the superior cava. Effect of slow circulation in the vena azygos will be felt in the pleural cavities.

STRUCTURE OF THE PERICARDIUM

The *visceral pericardium* is a thin layer of cells, adherent to the heart (*epicardium*). The *parietal pericardium*, on the contrary, is made of a serous layer which is supported by strong fibrous tissue, thus forming a bag or sac. The mediastinal pleura coats a large part of the pericardial sac. A small amount of fluid is normally present in the *pericardial cavity*. It makes the movements of the heart easier.

The base of the pericardial sac adheres to the diaphragm over a triangular area which includes *the fibrous center* and part of the

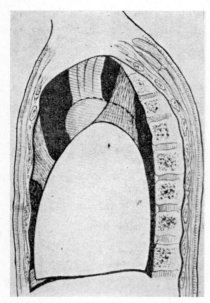

FIG. 15. Section of the mediastinum from the left. In black are those parts which are outside the heart and vessels.

TABLE 2

SECTION	DIAMETER	LENGTH
	mm.	mm.
Ascending aorta.............	28	50–70
Aortic arch.................	20–28	—
Thoracic aorta.............	20	175–200
Abdominal aorta.............	17–20	130–150

fuses gradually with the *external coat* of the vessels. On the contrary, the serous layer of the sac is continued by the epicardium. The irregular line of insertion is about 50 mm. from the beginning of the pulmonary artery, and 68 mm. from that of the aorta (15).

The superior vena cava has an extra- and an intra-pericardial section. *The inferior vena cava* has a very short intrathoracic course (10–15 mm.). The openings of the two hepatic veins into the cava are either within the diaphragm or slightly above it; in such a case the pericardium coats not only part of the inferior cava but also a small portion of the hepatic veins (fig. 19).

muscular diaphragm. A thin *hiatus* (*space of Larrey*) enables the pericardium to contact the peritoneum.

A few thickenings of the pericardium, called *ligaments*, connect the sac with the surrounding structures (fig. 18). The highest part of the pericardial sac contacts the large vessels, mainly the superior cava, the aorta, and the pulmonary artery (figs. 13 and 14). There, the fibrous tissue of the pericardium

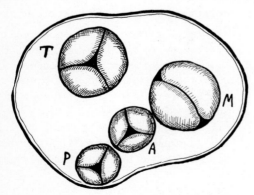

FIG. 16. The valves of the heart as seen from the base.

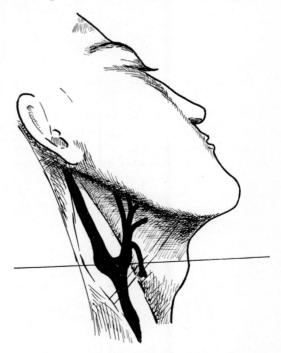

FIG. 17. The site of the carotid sinus

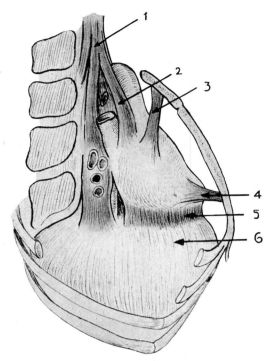

FIG. 18. The ligaments of the pericardium. 1, 2, vertebropericardial ligaments; 3, superior sternopericardial ligament; 4, inferior sterno-pericardial ligament; 5, phrenopericardial ligament; 6, diaphragm. The sternum is submitted to traction. (From Rouvière.)

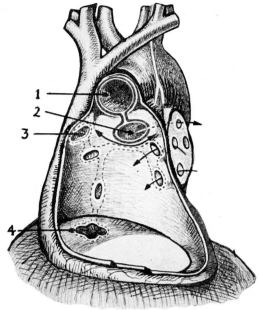

FIG. 19. The pericardial sac, open and distended. 1, aorta; 2, pulmonary artery; 3, superior vena cava; 4, inferior vena cava and hepatic veins. (Adapted from Brauer and Fischer.)

STRUCTURE OF THE MYOCARDIUM

A section of myocardium, parallel to the surface of the heart, reveals that the fibers form networks with narrow meshes stretched in one main direction.

The *cardiac muscle fiber* consists of nuclei, myofibrils, sarcoplasm, sarcolemma, and intercalated disks. The myofibrils are similar to those of ordinary striated fibers and are composed of the same types of disks. It has been shown in tissue culture that two myo-cardial cells, which are not completely separated by a membrane and seem to have a partially continuous protoplasm, may beat with independent rhythms. This favors the view that myocardial cells are *independent cells*.

Atria

The muscular fibers of the atria radiate from a central area which surrounds the opening of the superior vena cava. These fibers are rich in sarcoplasm and are surrounded by a network of thick fibrillary connective tissue. It has been stated that the atrial myocardium has more water and more collagen than the ventricular.

Ventricles

According to an old description, the ventricles are "two muscular sacs enclosed in a third." More recent studies (24, 27) show that the myocardium is formed by several muscles which can be dissociated and which possess independent blood supplies.

One of the main parts of the ventricles is made of fibers which start superficially, spiral over the external surface of the heart, twist themselves around the apex, and then form the internal part of the left ventricle along with the papillary muscles. This muscle is made of two layers called *the superficial sinospiral* and *the superficial bulbospiral muscle.*

A second main part forms the deep layers and the papillary muscles of the right ventricle, together with that part of the left ventricle which lies between the deeper and the more superficial parts of the adjacent muscle. This can be divided into three separate muscles: a) One is limited to the wall of the left ventricle and is called *the deep bulbospiral muscle.* b) One is a spiral sheet which surrounds the left ventricle, then splits in order to enclose the right ventricle and form its chief muscle layer; it is *the deep sinospiral muscle.* c) The third encircles both ventricles in a spiral scroll manner and is called *the scroll muscle.* The latter three muscles are limited to the upper three-quarters of the ventricular mass.

The myocardial fibers (*myofibrils*) are a special kind of striated muscular fibers. They are called "incompletely striated" and have,

as a special character, the property of dividing and uniting repeatedly so that they assume the pattern of a continuous network, or *syncytium.* Therefore, the isolation of each fiber, typical of the skeletal muscles, is lacking.

Automatic or Specific System of the Heart

Several formations of a more specific tissue are present in the myocardium (fig. 20). They possess to the highest degree the ability to produce periodic stimuli, a property called *automatism.* The automatic system can be divided into two parts, the sinoatrial and the atrioventricular.

a) The *sinoatrial system* consists of the *sinoatrial node* (*node of Keith and Flack; s-a node*) and of its *junctional fibers.* The *s-a node* begins at the union of the superior vena cava with the right atrium and extends, like a curved band, down to the mouth of the inferior vena cava. It is about 25 to 30 mm. long and 2 to 5 mm. thick in the adult (22, 31). The *junctional fibers* radiate out from the node in all directions and soon

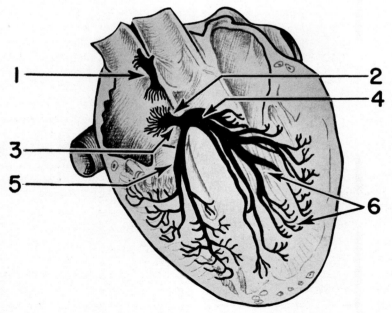

FIG. 20. The specific system of the heart. 1, sinoauricular node; 2, auriculo-ventricular node; 3, bundle of His; 4, left stem and its branches; 5, right stem; 6, left stem.

merge with the common atrial fibers (22). There are no anatomically differentiated bundles in the atria. However, certain bundles are preferred because they are shorter. One of them is *the bundle of Bachmann*, connecting the right with the left atrium (22). Other bundles, connecting the s-a node with the a-v node, have been described on the basis of functional disturbances caused in animals by their ligature (20, 21) but not on an anatomical basis. Among them is the *bundle of Wenckebach*.

b) The *atrioventricular system*, or *conducting system*, is made of the atrioventricular node with the junctional fibers, of the bundle of His, and of its ramifications. The *atrioventricular node (node of Tawara; a-v node)* is a rounded formation present in the posterior and lower part of the atrial septum. It is about 5 mm. long and 2 to 3 mm. wide (31). *Junctional fibers* connect it with the right atrium, the septum, and the left atrium (22). Gradually, this node becomes a *slender bundle, the bundle of His*, which goes through the fibrous tissue at the base of the ventricles.

The *bundle of His* is 1 to 2 mm. in diameter, and 10 to 18 mm. in length (15, 31). It runs in the interventricular septum between the aortic and the tricuspid rings and continues downwards toward the base of the septal papillary muscle (24). It is prolonged by the *right stem*, a thinner bundle which subdivides itself into multiple branches within the right ventricle. On the left side, *there actually is no main stem* (23, 24) because of a sudden splintering into multiple thin bundles going toward the left ventricle.

Each subdivision continues branching again and again into smaller branches, until individual fibers, the *Purkinje fibers*, connect the conducting system with the common fibers of the ventricles.

In *normal human beings the bundle of His represents the only muscular connection between atria and ventricles*. A variation from the normal is represented by another connection between right atrium and right ventricle, the *bundle of Kent*, which is normal in lower mammals (22), or by *isolated thin muscular bundles* connecting either atrium with the respective ventricle.

The *conductive tissue* of the heart is somewhat different from the rest of the myocardium. Its fibers are thinner, they are less clearly striated, and are mixed with a rich system of nerve cells, nerve trunks, and nerve fibrils (24).

THE ENDOCARDIUM

The endocardium is a whitish, translucent membrane which coats the whole internal surface of the heart. The usual endocardium is made of three different layers, the most superficial being an endothelium. The valves also have an endothelium, supported by connective tissue. *The leaflets of the cardiac valves normally do not possess blood vessels* (15).

THE ARTERIES OF THE HEART

Two arterial vessels supply blood to the heart itself. They are the left and right coronary arteries, branches of the ascending aorta (fig. 21).

The *left coronary artery* partly surrounds the pulmonary artery, then proceeds into the anterior interventricular groove, and is prolonged by the *anterior descending* or *interventricular branch* running toward the apex (fig. 21a). This artery gives blood to the *anterior* surface of the ventricles. A branch of the left coronary artery, the *circumflex branch*, leaves the main trunk early and surrounds the heart, passing along the atrioventricular groove (fig. 21a).

The *right coronary artery* originates from the aorta on the right, follows the anterior part of the atrioventricular groove, then reaches the posterior interventricular groove, where a *posterior descending branch* continues it, running toward the apex (fig. 21a). This artery supplies blood to the *posterior* surface of the ventricles. In 50 per cent of

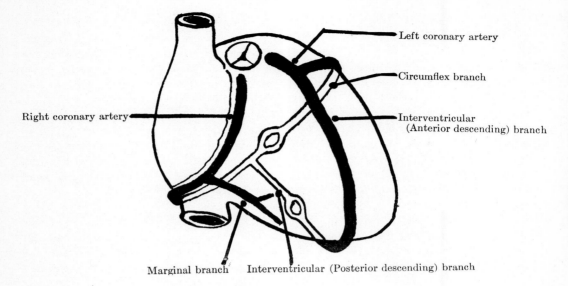

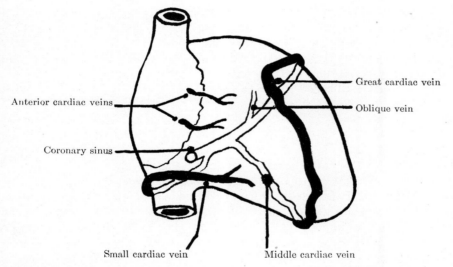

FIG. 21. A (top), the coronary arteries; B (bottom), the coronary veins. (After Grant.)

the cases, there is a third small coronary artery, the *conus artery*, which arises directly from the aorta and supplies the conus arteriosus (45).

In 80 per cent of the cases, each atrium is supplied by its respective coronary artery. On the contrary, the *interventricular septum and the adjacent part of the ventricles always have a mixed supply, partly from the right and partly from the left coronary artery.* However, the left coronary supplies chiefly

the anterior part of the septum; the right, chiefly the posterior.

The mouths of the coronary arteries are high enough so that they cannot be closed by the semilunar valves. Each of them is surrounded by a ring, or *sphincter*, of smooth muscle fibers (26).

The coronary network can be schematically divided into two sections: a) the *larger trunks*, which run over the surface of the heart, and b) the *smaller vessels*, which penetrate deeply into the myocardium and are submitted to the effects of its contraction.

A *few anastomotic branches* exist at any age between the small coronary arteries, and are not particularly developed in older people unless there is coronary heart disease (28, 29). These channels may carry blood in either direction and connect the branches of the right with those of the left coronary artery. Moreover, a free anastomosis exists between the capillaries of the two systems.

The coronary pattern is not the same in all hearts (29). In about one-half of them, the right coronary predominates (group I); in about one-third, the blood supply is balanced between the two coronaries (group II); the smaller group includes those hearts where the left coronary predominates (group III) (29).

As far as the conducting system is concerned, the blood supply to this delicate section of the myocardium has been studied in great detail. The *s-a node* receives its blood from one atrial artery only (30). This, however, is somewhat variable as it may be a branch of either the right or the left circumflex. This artery gives origin to a vascular ring which circles the mouth of the superior vena cava. The main artery of both the *a-v node* and the *bundle of His* is the *ramus septi fibrosi* (23, 28, 30), a small branch of the right coronary. However, the lowest part of the bundle is supplied by the *ramus limbi dextri* (25, 28, 30), a branch of the anterior descending artery, i.e. of the left coronary artery.

In addition to the more conventional blood supply, the myocardium can be nourished: a) through extracardiac anastomoses, b) through the Thebesian vessels, and c) through reversal of flow in the coronary veins (33) (fig. 22). The most important *normal extracardial anastomoses* are between coronary arteries and bronchial arteries through the vasa vasorum of the first part of the aorta and the pulmonary artery. Other anastomoses may occur whenever there is adhesive pericarditis. The *Thebesian vessels*

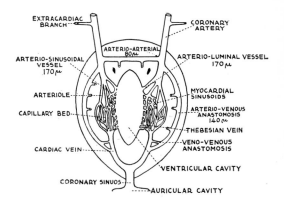

COLLATERAL CIRCULATION OF THE HEART

Fig. 22. Vessels taking part in the collateral circulation of the heart. (From Prinzmetal and co-workers, Arch. Card. Mexico. Courtesy of the authors.)

are the remnants of tortuous spaces which supply blood to the heart of the embryo. These vessels open in the endocardium and make a network which communicates with the capillaries of the myocardium and adds its supply to that of the more conventional coronary arteries. Reversal of the flow in the veins seems possible on the basis of animal experimentation (33, 34) and may contribute to the nourishment of the heart.

THE VEINS OF THE HEART

The venous blood of the heart can escape following several routes: a) through the *great cardiac vein* which ends in the *coronary sinus*, a venous dilatation opening into the right atrium (fig. 21b); b) by way of *smaller veins* which run over the surface of the heart and open into the right atrium independently from the above; c) through the *Thebesian vessels* which open directly into any of the four heart cavities; or d) through *arterio-luminal* and *arterio-sinusoidal* connections, thence into the heart chamber (33, 34).

THE LYMPHATIC VESSELS

The lymphatics of the heart form an extensive subendocardial network, better developed in the ventricles. The main collector vessels run into the superficial grooves of the heart and are connected with lymph-nodes placed at the bifurcation of the trachea.

Connections between the supradiaphragmatic and the infradiaphragmatic network of lymphatic vessels may have importance in the transmission of bacteria from the peritoneum to the pericardium and vice versa.

STRUCTURE OF THE ARTERIES

Three different layers are present in all arteries: a) the *internal coat* or *tunica intima*, b) the *middle coat* or *tunica media*, and c) the *external coat* or *tunica externa*. Marked differences existing in the structure of the middle coat facilitate the division of these vessels into *large arteries* and *small arteries*.

Large arteries. The internal coat has an *endothelium* supported by connective tissue containing different layers. The *middle layer* is made of a tremendous amount of elastic tissue with a few muscular cells. The external coat is relatively thin and made of common connective tissue.

Small arteries. The *internal coat* is made of an *endothelium* supported by an elastic layer. The *middle layer* is a thick, typically *muscular*, coat made of smooth cells arranged in a circular way. The *external coat*, also relatively thick, is made of common connective tissue, but also contains an elastic layer.

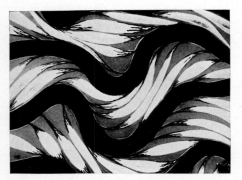

FIG. 23. Connections between muscular fibers (white) and elastic bundles (black) in a medium-sized artery. (Courtesy of Dr. Hans Elias.)

Both the large arteries and those of medium size have their own vessels in the external coat. These may penetrate the middle layer and are called *vasa vasorum*.

The connections between the muscular and the elastic structures of the arteries are of special functional importance (40, 41) (fig. 23).

The nerves supplying the small arteries form plexuses in the tunica adventitia, between this and the media, and within the media (44). The arterioles are accompanied by a small number of nerve fibers, usually two or three, while only one fiber may be found in the precapillaries.

STRUCTURE OF THE CAPILLARY SYSTEM

The small arteries, or *arterioles*, divide into smaller vessels, called *precapillaries* or *metarterioles* (32). These lead into *channels* which connect the arterioles with the venules. The *true capillaries* are side branches of the channels and are connected to each other in most organs making a network-like pattern (32).

The aspect of the different capillary systems varies, however, according to the organ in which they are contained. Among them, the *capillary networks* (different organs), the *capillary loops* (skin), and the *ansiform networks* (intestinal villi) can be recognized. In addition to the specialized capillary beds of various organs, there is *a basic nutritional type of capillary unit* (42, 43). This consists of a central channel which joins a terminal arteriole and a venule; its initial portion, called *metarteriole*, has discontinuous muscle cells; the rest is called *a-v or thoroughfare channel* and has no muscle cells. Branches which come off abruptly from a metarteriole also have some muscle cells; these branches are called *the precapillaries* and their muscles are called the *precapillary sphincters* (fig. 24).

The capillaries are accompanied by fine-beaded fibers running close to the vessels or, occasionally, at some distance from them (44).

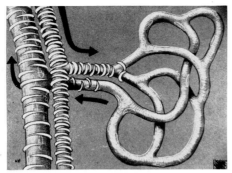

FIG. 24. Arrangement of muscular fibers (white) in the arterioles, precapillaries, and venules; the capillaries have no muscular fibers. (Courtesy of Dr. Hans Elias.)

The capillary wall is made of a thin protoplasmic membrane, with multiple nuclei, which is made of *endothelial cells* united by their margins (fig. 24). These are supported by a delicate network of reticular connective tissue with occasional perivascular cells called *Rouget cells* which should not be mistaken for muscular elements (36).

STRUCTURE OF THE VEINS

The venous wall contains three different coats or tunicae. The *internal coat* is similar to that of the arteries, having an *endothelium* and an *elastic membrane*. The *middle coat* is much thinner than that in arteries of a similar diameter. It contains *muscular* and *elastic elements* in a network of rather soft connective tissue. The *external coat* is thicker than that in the arteries and may contain muscular elements.

Membranous pockets, called *valves*, can be found in the veins. They are mainly present in the veins of medium size and in those of the limbs. They are made of a double layer of endothelium with a thin layer of connective tissue between them.

Both large and medium veins have their own vessels which run in the external coat and are called *vasa vasorum*.

BIBLIOGRAPHY

1. PICHON, A. *Les Maladies Congénitales du Coeur.* Traité de Méd. Int., Paris. Masson, 1928.
2. SPITZER, A. Virchow's Arch., 1923, **243,** 81.
3. BROWN, J. W. *Congenital Heart Disease.* London, J. Bale Med. Publ., 1939.
4. AREY, L. B. *Developmental Anatomy.* Philadelphia, Saunders, 1941.
5. BARRON, D. H. Physiol. Rev., 1944, **24,** 277.
6. BARCLAY, A. E., BARCROFT, J., BARRON, D. H., FRANKLIN, K. J., AND PRICHARD, M. M. L. Brit. J. Radiol., 1939, **12,** 505; and Am. J. Anat., 1941, **69,** 383.
7. FRANKLIN, K. J., BARCLAY, A. E., AND PRICHARD, M. M. L. J. Anat., 1940, **75,** 75.
8. KENNEDY, J. A., AND CLARK, S. L. Am. J. Physiol., 1942, **136,** 140.
9. BARRON, D. H. Anat. Rec., 1942, **82,** 398.
10. BARCROFT, J., KENNEDY, J. A., AND MASON, M. F. J. Physiol., 1938, **92,** 1P.
11. HERTWIG, I. *Elements der Entwicklungsgeschichte des Menschen und Wirbelthiere.* Jena, 1910.
12. GRAY, H. *Anatomy of the Human Body.* 24th Ed. Philadelphia, Lea & Febiger, 1942.
13. PIERSOL, G. A. *Human Anatomy.* 9th Ed. Philadelphia, Lippincott, 1930.
14. BRASH, J. C. *Cunningham's Textbook of Anatomy.* 7th Ed. New York, Oxford Univ. Press, 1937.
15. CHIARUGI, G. *Istituzioni di Anatomia dell'Uomo.* 2d Ed. Milano, S.E.L., 1926.
16. DE VECCHI, B. *Manuale di Tecnica delle Autopsie.* Milano, Vallardi, 1928.
17. VIERORDT, BIZOT. Quoted by DE VECCHI.
18. TANDLER, J. *Anatomie des Herzens.* Jena, Fisher, 1913.
19. ELIAS, H., AND FELLER, A. *Stauungstypen bei Kreislaufstoerungen.* Berlin, Springer, 1926.
20. CONDORELLI, L. Cuore e Circol. Rome, 1930, **14,** 221.
21. CONDORELLI, L. Zeitschr. exp. Med., 1929, **68,** 516.
22. SCHERF, D., AND BOYD, L. J. *Clinical Electrocardiography.* St. Louis, Mosby, 1940.
23. GÉRAUDEL, E. *Le Mécanisme du Coeur et ses Anomalies.* Paris, Masson, 1928.
24. ROBB, J. S., AND ROBB, R. C. Am. Heart J., 1942, **23,** 455.
25. GLOMSET, D. J., AND BIRGE, R. F. Am. Heart J., 1945, **29,** 526.
26. CESARIS-DEMEL, A. Atti Gruppo Cardiol. Ital., 1st Meeting, Roma, Pozzi, 1935.
27. LOWE, T. E., AND WARTMAN, W. B. Brit. Heart J., 1944, **6,** 115.
28. GROSS, L. *Blood Supply to the Heart.* Oxford Med. Publ., 1921.
29. SCHLESINGER, M. J. Publ. 13, Am. Assoc. Adv. Sci.; also: Am. Heart J., 1938, **15,** 528.

30. LASCANO, E. F. *Irrigación Normal del Nódulo de Keith y Flack, Haz de His y sus Ramas.* Buenos Aires, El Ateneo, 1942.
31. WIGGERS, C. J. *Physiology in Health and Disease.* Philadelphia, Lea & Febiger, 1944.
32. CHAMBERS. Quoted by Wiggers.
33. BELLET, S. In *Cyclopedia of Medicine, Surgery and Specialties.* Philadelphia, Davis; 1943, **3**, 769.
34. LENDRUM, B., KONDO, B., AND KATZ, L. N. Am. J. Physiol., 1945, **143**, 243.
35. WEARN, J. T., METTIER, S. R., KLUM, T. G., AND ZCHIESCHE, L. J. Am. Heart J., 1933, **9**, 143.
36. VOLTERRA, M. Sperimentale (Florence), 1927, N. 3.

37. GRANT, J. C. B. *An Atlas of Anatomy.* Baltimore, The Williams & Wilkins Co., 1951.
38. VELASQUEZ, T. Arch. Inst. Nac. Card. Mexico, 1950, **20**, 495.
39. SMITH, H. L. Am. Heart J., 1928, **4**, 79.
40. BENNINGHOFF, A. Zeit. Zellforsch. u. mikr. Anat., 1927, **6**, 348.
41. SCHULTZE JENA, B. S., Morph. Jahrb., 1939, **83**, 230.
42. CHAMBERS, R., AND ZWEIFACH, B. W. Am. J. Anat., 1944, **75**, 173.
43. CHAMBERS, R., AND ZWEIFACH, B. W. Ann. New York Acad. Sci., 1946, **46**, 683.
44. MILLEN, J. W. J. Anat., 1948, **82**, 68.
45. SCHLESINGER, M. J., ZOLL, P. M., AND WESSLER, S. Am. Heart J., 1949, **38**, 823.

CHAPTER 3

The Normal Functions of the Heart and Vessels

The chief function of the circulation is to carry blood to the tissues in order to maintain a relatively constant condition of the intercellular fluid. Carrying oxygen to, and carbon dioxide from the periphery; carrying nourishing substances from the intestine and waste products to the kidneys and liver; and carrying specific substances and heat from one organ to another, are some of the functions of the circulation.

The circulatory system maintains a constant condition of the internal environment of the cells only by constant work and continuous compensatory reactions.

The Heart

The sole function of the heart is a rhythmic mechanical contraction. This sets the blood in motion throughout the circulatory system. The different parts of the heart have specific roles in the production and utilization of this contraction.

THE MYOCARDIUM

The heart muscle has four fundamental properties (1): automatism, excitability, conductivity, and contractility.

A fifth property, *tonus*, was admitted until 20 years ago, then was denied. Studies of the author (186) indicate that the *resting length* and *the diastolic length* of the heart fibers vary with different physiological and pharmacological stimuli. This property of modifying the resting length might well be called *intrinsic tonus* and probably has importance in the determination of cardiac volume. However, accurate evaluation of this property is, so far, purely experimental.

Automatism is the property of producing rhythmic stimuli. Although present in the entire myocardium, this property is highly developed in the specific system (pacemaker and conducting system), and especially in its highest parts, as shown by the different automatic rhythms (page 34).

Excitability is the ability to react to definite stimuli. This property is common to all striated muscles, but has special features in the heart owing to greater duration of the refractory period (page 30).

Conductivity is the ability to receive and transmit stimuli. This property is influenced by the duration of the refractory period.

Contractility is the ability of a muscle to shorten itself, thus performing a definite function. It is, therefore, common to all striated and smooth muscles.

The *functional properties of the myocardium* have been studied in various experimental "preparations". The most important of these are: a) Isolated and perfused heart (frog, turtle, dog) (3). b) Open chest experiments; mechanical transmission of the heart movements (amphibia, mammals) (4, 5); volume tracings (6, 7). c) Heart-lung preparations (dog) (8, 9). d) Isolated papillary muscle (cat, dog) (185).

A series of phenomena, well known to students of physiology, led to recognition of certain "heart laws" which are described in the following paragraphs.

1) *The law of "all or none."* When the heart is stimulated, its reaction is of *maximal intensity*, whatever the intensity of the stimulus (4). The same law is true for an isolated fiber of a skeletal muscle (10) but

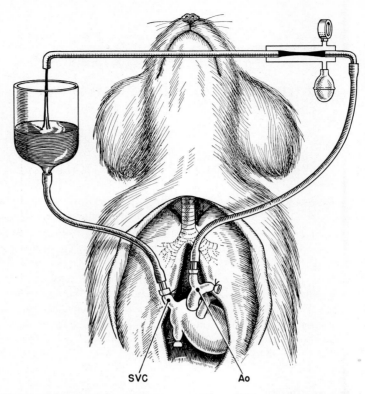

SVC   Ao

FIG. 25. Sketch of Starling's heart-lung preparation. SVC, superior vena cava; Ao, aorta

not for a complete skeletal muscle owing to the different thresholds of the various fibers; stronger stimuli cause more fibers to contract and cause, therefore, a stronger contraction. Owing to the syncytial structure of the myocardium, all normal cardiac fibers have the same threshold and they contract as a single unit.

Variations of the excitability and contractility of the heart muscle, because of mechanical (initial length of the fibers), chemical (concentration of H-ions), or physiological phenomena (changes of blood supply, fatigue), may change the intensity of reaction to a stimulus (11). This may explain apparent exceptions to the law which holds true when conditions remain constant.

2) *Refractory period.* The extreme shortness of the period during which the skeletal muscle is unexcitable (refractory period) causes gradual fusion of contractions and the occurrence of a *tetanus. This is impossible*

in the normal heart muscle (12).[13] During contraction, the heart muscle does not react to abnormal stimulation (*absolute refractory period*). After the end of contraction, the heart muscle becomes more and more excitable until the excitability becomes normal (*relative refractory period*, ref. 12). It is apparent that only exceptionally strong stimuli may induce contraction in this phase and that the stronger the stimulation, the sooner a contraction may take place.

3) *Influence of the initial length.* Distention of the heart chambers by increased inflow increases the length of the cardiac fibers and leads to proportionally stronger contractions. This property, recognized by

[13] Special experimental conditions (abnormally high content of Ca, cooling of the heart, or ouabain, in addition to rapid stimulations) may lead to occurrence of *tetanus* in the myocardium of the frog (157), and in that of mammalians (186 187).

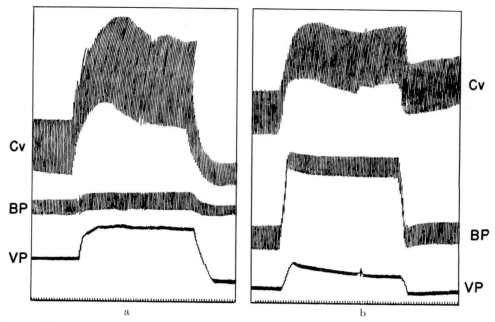

Fig. 26. Increase in volume of the heart taking place in a heart-lung preparation. a, The venous return is increased. b, The peripheral resistance is increased. Cv, cardiac volume; VP, venous pressure, Bp, arterial pressure. (Adapted from original tracings of Starling.)

Starling (13), is common to all striated muscles[14]. The following conclusions were reached on heart-lung preparations (fig. 25): a) If the venous return to the heart is increased, the diastolic volume becomes greater and cardiac output increases (fig. 26a). b) If the peripheral resistance is increased, cardiac output is mintained constant, but the diastolic volume again becomes greater (fig. 26b).

A direct relationship between oxygen consumption of the myocardium and initial length of the ventricular fibers, i.e. diastolic volume, has also been demonstrated. It should be noted that, whenever nervous, metabolic, or endocrine influences play a role, the heart does not follow strictly Starling's law. On the other hand, a failing heart may fail to respond to such influences and follow more closely such law.

4) *Cardiac "tonus."* The problem of

cardiac tonus has been discussed for a long time. Tonus is "the sustained partial contraction by virtue of which muscle fibers resist stretching more than they would on account of their inherent elastic properties alone" (14). Cardiac tonus is different from the tonus of smooth muscles (the ability to maintain a slow contraction—page 49), and from that of the skeletal muscles (a sustained, minimal tetanic contraction). Its existence in experimental cardiac preparations has been proven by the author (186). However, the possible importance of this property is still under study.

PHYSIOLOGICAL REQUIREMENTS OF THE ISOLATED HEART

The heart of a mammalian, when isolated and perfused (17a), maintains a steady and rhythmic contraction under certain conditions. The fluid reaching the heart must contain *oxygen*, must be warmed to *body temperature*, and must have a definite *pressure*.

[14] According to subsequent studies (154), *tension of the myocardial fiber*, and not length, is the important factor.

The hourly oxygen consumption of the isolated mammalian heart averages 3.24 cc. per gram of the organ in conditions similar to those taking place in the organism at rest (15).

Temperatures between 26° and 40°C. are tolerated, causing proportional variations of the heart rate (16).

The isolated heart is very sensitive to changes of the reaction (pH) because it has only a low buffering power (16). A small concentration of lactic acid (0.07 per cent) causes severe arrhythmias.

TABLE 3

	%
Sodium chloride	0.9
Potassium chloride	0.02
Calcium chloride	0.02
Magnesium chloride	0.01
Glucose	0.1
Sodium bicarbonate	0.1
Sodium phosphate	0.005

The chemical composition of the fluid, necessary for keeping the heart alive, has been studied by *Ringer*, *Locke*, and *Tyrode* (17, 32, 33, 43). The best solution, similar to that of mammalian plasma minus proteins, is shown in table 3 (17, 43).

Calcium in excess (or in normal concentration but in the absence of potassium) *increases the duration of systole*, and later stops the heart in systole (*calcium rigor*).[15] *Potassium in excess* (or in normal concentration in the absence of calcium) *increases the duration of diastole*, and later stops the heart in diastole (*potassium inhibition*). An increased alkalinity (higher pH) acts like a calcium excess; a decreased alkalinity (lower pH) acts like a potassium excess.

Since a solution not containing *sodium* is also unsuitable for the heart, it is apparent that *an exact calcium-potassium-sodium*

[15] *Calcium rigor* occurs only in the amphibian heart; either *ventricular fibrillation* or *arrest* without rigor are more common in the mammalian heart (see also note 13, page 30).

balance is essential for a good myocardial function.

Carbon dioxide has a complex action. In addition to its action on the centers of the medulla (stimulation of the respiratory, vasomotor, and vagus centers), an excess of CO_2 acts directly on the myocardium. It depresses automatism (slower rate) and conductivity (prolonged a-v conduction). On the contrary, an insufficient concentration of CO_2 leads to incomplete and shorter diastole with decreased cardiac output.

METABOLISM OF THE HEART MUSCLE

The heart utilizes glucose, fats, and, perhaps, amino acids and lactic acid. *Glucose* is partially used to restore the glycogen content and partially burned. *Lactic acid* is removed on a large scale from the blood of the coronary system but its utilization has not been demonstrated so far. *Fats* are used virtually only when carbohydrates are scarce. *Amino acids* are not used as such.

The process of muscular contraction is as follows (162). The contractile structure is based on a protein complex, *actomyosin*, and on a water-soluble nucleotide, *adenosine triphosphate* (ATP). Myosin links with ATP by binding Mg and K ions. At high salt concentration, the myosin-ATP complex remains separated from actin; at lower salt concentration, actin and myosin-ATP unite. The shift in ion concentration, necessary for these changes, is brought about by the wave of excitation which spreads into the myocardium. Separated, actin and myosin-ATP are straight filaments with high energy (dilatation). United, they dehydrate and shrink, forming a shorter, more stable, and energy-poor state (contraction). If the fibers are not allowed to shorten, tension develops.

The chemical reactions taking place in the myocardium are similar to those of the skeletal muscles (16). They can be summarized as follows: a) *Adenosine triphosphate* is broken down to adenylic acid and phosphoric acid (no oxygen required). b) *Phosphocreatin* is broken down to phosphoric acid plus creatin (no oxygen required). c) *Glycogen* is broken down to lactic acid (no oxygen required); part of the energy resulting from this reaction is utilized for the resynthesis of phosphocreatin. d) *Lactic acid* is burned with formation of carbon dioxide and water (oxygen necessary); part of the resulting energy is utilized for the resynthesis of glycogen.

The conversion of glycogen to lactic acid involves a large number of enzymatic reactions. Under physiological conditions, muscle glycogen breaks down to lactic acid and water, providing a large amount of energy. Among the different steps, one of the most important is that leading to formation of *pyruvic acid*. When there is a relative lack of oxygen, lactic acid is present in excess.

In a normal animal, both glycogen and lactic acid may be carried to the heart by the blood since their synthesis may take place in other organs. An important difference between cardiac muscle and skeletal muscle is that the former cannot withstand any major "oxygen debt". Therefore, cardiac contraction does not continue if the heart does not receive an adequate and continuous oxygen supply.

The metabolism of glucose in the body is aided by a system of co-enzymes containing some well-known vitamins. *Thiamin* is a co-enzyme which (with carboxylase) makes possible an anaerobic reaction in which pyruvic acid is oxidized to acetaldehyde and carbon dioxide. *Niacin and riboflavin* appear to be necessary in the formation of other co-enzymes which are associated with the carbohydrate metabolism. *Vitamins A* and *C* may play some part in oxidation processes *in vivo* but there is as yet no convincing evidence of this. *Vitamin E* seems related somehow to the oxidation system of the muscles.

THE PACEMAKER OF THE HEART AND THE CONDUCTING SYSTEM

Studies on the origin of the automatic impulses of the heart and on the spreading of the stimulus were first made on amphibia (*Stannius, Gaskell, Kent*). The amphibian heart contains three ganglia: *Remak's* (between sinus and right atrium), *Ludwig's* (in the interatrial septum), and *Bidder's ganglion* (in the atrioventricular groove).

Ligation of the sinoatrial junction stops contraction of the atria and ventricle (*1st Stannius ligature*) without changing the contractions of the sinus (17b). A second ligation around the atrioventricular junction (*2nd Stannius ligature*) causes reappearance of ventricular contractions (17b). The common explanation is that the first ligation interrupts the spreading of the stimulus while the second causes contractions of local origin by irritation of either Bidder's ganglion or the myocardium itself.

In higher species, as in man, the *pacemaker* lies either within the sinoatrial node (*s-a node*) or in the surrounding tissues (14). Apparently *the pacemaking activity, which is the cause of the heart beat, is the result of the spontaneous development of rhythmic oscillations of electric potential* (18). Whenever a change of potential of sufficient intensity occurs, a propagated discharge is set up, and stimulation of the surrounding myocardium takes place. The conduction follows the fibers of the myocardium, at variable rates which are directly proportional to the size of the fibers (29). *Stimuli set up by the activity of the pacemaker usually reach the rest of the heart before any other stimulus has arisen anywhere.*

The impulse spreads like a wave[16] in the wall of the right atrium with a speed of 600–1200 mm. per second (19), so that the

[16] A wave of excitation is a series of physico-chemical changes accompanied by electrical phenomena, and spreading like a wave. As contraction follows excitation, *a wave of contraction follows the wave of excitation.*

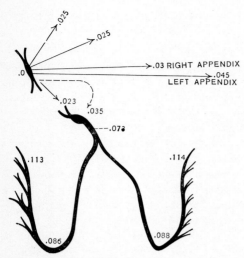

FIG. 27. The conduction system of the dog's heart and the approximate times of spread of the impulse in the atrial and ventricular conduction systems. Scheme. (From Wiggers' *Physiology in Health and Disease.* Courtesy of the author and Lea & Febiger.)

right atrial appendage receives it about 0.03 second later. As the left atrium is excited only 0.045 sec. after the beginning of the impulse, there is little difference in time between the excitations of the right and left atria. *This points to a very rapid rate of transmission in the interatrial bundles.*

While no special conduction pathways exist for transmission between *s-a node* and *a-v node*, the stimulus spreads over direct bundles of the interatrial septum.[17] Therefore, excitation of the a-v node precedes that of the right appendage and takes place 0.023 sec. after the starting of the impulse (20) (fig. 27).[18]

[17] It has been suggested that functionally specialized pathways within the atrial septum connect the *S-A node* to the *A-V node* (20, 22, 25b). It has also been stated that all fibers going to the *A-V node* unite in one point between coronary sinus and fossa ovalis (22).

[18] According to *Lewis,* the speed of transmission of the impulse is as follows:

	mm./sec.
Purkinje fibers	4000
Atrial muscle	800
Ventricular muscle	400
A-V node	200

The descending impulse is definitely delayed on reaching the a-v node. We do not know as yet whether this is due to higher resistance or to the relay of the impulse to a new center (21). Further progress of the stimulus takes place with great speed in the *bundle of His and its branches.* As a result, the endocardial surfaces of the septum are excited first, then the papillary muscles. Within 0.04 sec. after the stimulus has left the *a-v node,* the entire endocardial surface of the ventricles is reached, that of the right slightly earlier than that of the left ventricle (fig. 27).

The upper part of the interventricular septum is stimulated first, then the apex of the ventricles, later their base. Transmission from the endocardial surface to the rest of the myocardium follows fibers of the Purkinje system which penetrate almost to the epicardium (29).

Whenever the descending impulse fails to reach the different parts of the myocardium, a lower "center" becomes the pacemaker of the heart. Experimental and clinical evidence has revealed the automatism of the different centers, i.e. the frequency with which they are able to form stimuli. The different rates in man are as follows:

s-a node	40 to 150 per min.
a-v node	30 to 50 per min.
bundle of His	18 to 30 per min.

The study of the electrocardiogram has greatly increased our knowledge of the process of excitation of the heart.

THE ELECTROCARDIOGRAM (126–131)

The human body, like that of any animal, can be considered as a "volume conductor", e.g. a medium which permits the conduction of electricity in all three dimensions. Electrical currents generated in any point can reach, therefore, any other point of the body. Mention should be made, however, of the theory which admits that the resistance of different tissues of the body to transmission of cardiac currents varies considerably, so that the peripheral ECG is influenced only by "favorable spots" of the heart (28).

Bioelectrical phenomena are similar in all living tissues and are easily studied in unicellular organisms. In any living cell at rest, a difference of potential exists between the inside of the cell and the external surface. *The inside of the cell is negative; the outside, positive.* The electrical charges on the two sides of the membrane are equal in number and opposite in sign, forming *doublets* or *dipoles.* The membrane is said to be *polarized* and impermeable, so that no flow of current takes place.

When the cell is excited and becomes active, a sudden decrease in the electrical resistance of the membrane takes place; the negative ions flow outwards and the difference of potential between the inside and the outside decreases. The cell, previously polarized, becomes *depolarized* by effect of the excitation, and its outside becomes negative with respect to the surrounding cells (fig. 28). Usually, stimulation causes a local depolarization; then, since the positive external surface is connected with the nega-

tive internal surface by means of the depolarized area, an electric current is formed. This current excites and depolarizes, in turn, the adjoining regions so that *a wave of excitation and depolarization is gradually propagated.* During the spreading of the excitation, the positive ions precede the negative.

Immediately following the depolarization of the cell (and during contraction, if this is a muscle cell), *the process of repolarization* starts; it results in the restitution of the positive and negative charges to their respective positions along the surface of the membrane. This phenomenon is based on physico-chemical processes of a "reparative" nature. Repolarization of an isolated cell usually starts in those areas where depolarization first began (fig. 28).

The fundamental nature of the processes of excitation and conduction in the unicellular element is similar to that of equivalent phenomena taking place in nerve fibers or muscle cells. It has been said that, in the myocardium, impulses are conducted more rapidly in a longitudinal than in a transverse direction. However, the syncytial nature o

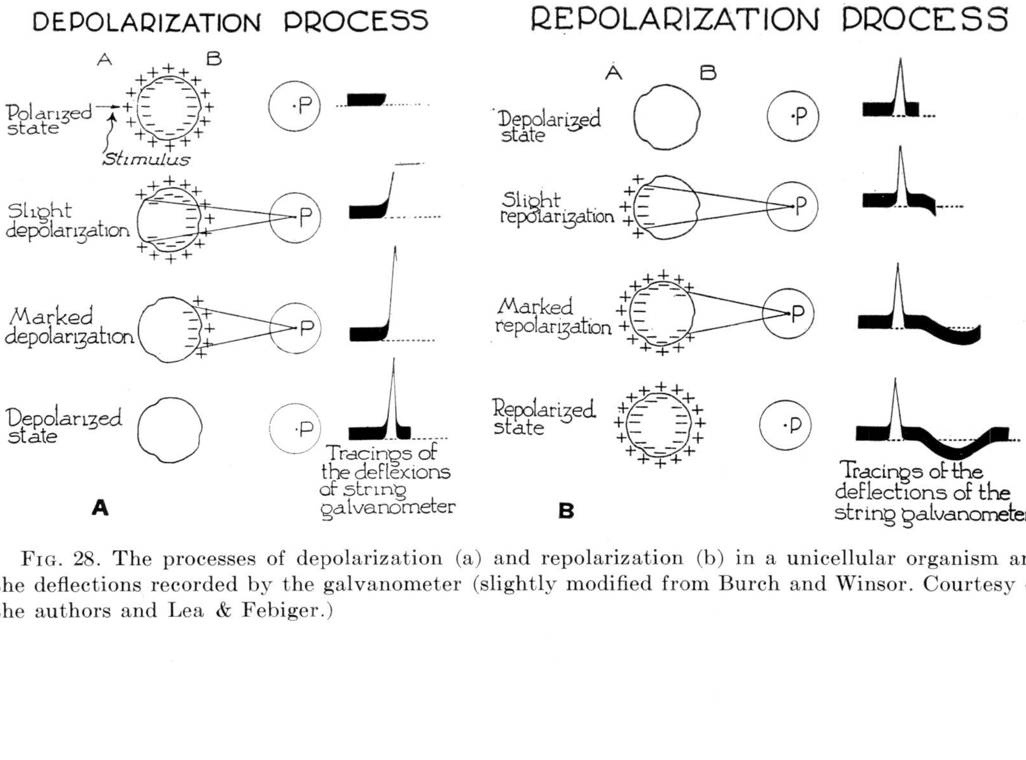

FIG. 28. The processes of depolarization (a) and repolarization (b) in a unicellular organism and the deflections recorded by the galvanometer (slightly modified from Burch and Winsor. Courtesy of the authors and Lea & Febiger.)

the heart muscle insures conduction in all directions.

The wave of depolarization reaches first the subendocardial muscle layers, then spreads toward the epicardium. The balance of electrical forces is always such that the endocardial surface of the heart is relatively negative in comparison to the epicardial surface.

A diphasic action current is observed under the following conditions: if we have a cell or a round-shaped organ and we stimulate one point, depolarization starts in a small superficial area; gradually, that area becomes larger and larger and the change of potential (positive potential) increases up to a maximum which is reached when about one-half of the cell, or organ, is depolarized while the other half is still polarized; as further conduction takes place, the tracing

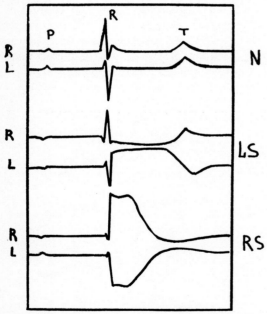

FIG. 29. The electrocardiogram of the frog after a lesion of one side of the heart. N, right (R) and left (L) chest leads before the experiment. LS, same tracings after application of KCl solution to the left side of the heart. RS, same tracing after application of KCl solution to the right side of the ventricle (From B. Kisch, Exper. Med. & Surg. Courtesy of the author.)

gradually drops to the basal line. Repolarization is a slower process, causing a wave in the opposite direction (negative potential) which continues until the process is completed. During repolarization, the negative ions precede the positive.

Cardiac repolarization starts in the subepicardial layers and from them spreads toward the endocardium. This explains the upright final wave of the electrocardiogram.

Local injury or cooling of the heart muscle prevents local depolarization and causes block of the impulse. As a result, a *monophasic*, plateau-like, wave is observed, reaching the level which was reached by R before the injury.[19]

The equivalent of an injury to the cardiac muscle is obtained by local application of potassium chloride with resulting partial depolarization: the baseline shifts to a positive or negative potential (fig. 29).

The ventricles form a kind of irregular shell, open at the base in the region of the a-v valves. This causes spreading of potentials which are different according to the area facing the heart and which are revealed by the electrocardiogram (page 124).

The *electrocardiogram* is a composite curve in which various accidents, or waves, have definite positions. These waves have been called P, Q, R, S, and T (fig. 30). The first part of the ECG, which is composed of the P wave and of minor accidents, is called the *atrial complex* because it bears a definite relationship to the activity of the atria (fig. 31). The second part of the ECG, which is composed of the more constant positive waves R and T and of the possible negative waves Q and S, is called the *ventricular complex* because it is connected with the activity of the ventricles. More exact details of nomenclature, technical details, and reading of ECG's will be given later (page 124).

[19] The difference in potential brought about by pinching the heart muscle, cooling its surface, reducing the blood supply, or applying KCl, has been termed the *current of injury*.

Atrial complex. The excitation of the sino-atrial node is not recorded in clinical tracings but may be recorded by means of an intra-atrial electrode (124, 125). As we have no way of detecting it otherwise, we may assume that it precedes the beginning of the P wave by a small fraction of a second (0.01 sec.?). The P wave is the resultant of the depolarization of both atria. It is a blunt, round deflection, lasting from 0.08 to 0.10 sec. in normal individuals. *Inactivation of the atria* is usually not revealed by the ECG. Cases with long delay (or block) of the ventricular contraction may show, however, a small dip (called the atrial T wave—or *Ta*) which is due to repolarization of the atrial myocardium.

Atrioventricular interval. The P wave is normally followed by a period of apparent inactivity during which the electrocardiogram reveals no deflection. The sinoatrial stimulus, which started its descending course at the beginning of the P wave and has reached the a-v node *during* that wave, is now performing the following functions, not revealed by the ECG: a) activating the a-v node, b) spreading through the bundle of His, and c) spreading through the branches of the bundle and Purkinje fibers. For this reason, the interval between initiation of the P wave and that of the ventricular complex (so-called *P-R interval*) represents the following phenomena: a) sino-nodal conduction, b) nodal latency, and c) nodo-

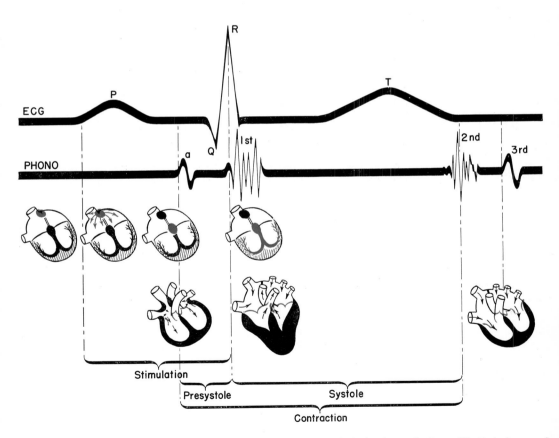

Fig. 30. The different waves of the electrocardiogram and their time relation with the phases of cardiac expansion and contraction. ECG, electrocardiogram; PHONO, sound tracing. The spread of the excitation wave is marked in red.

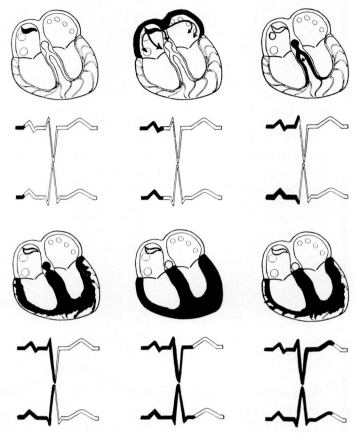

Fig. 31. The various phases of excitation compared with the electrocardiogram. Upper sketches, spreading of stimulus. Lower sketches, electrocardiogram in chest leads from the right (above) and the left side (below).

ventricular conduction. The normal duration of the P-R interval is between 0.12 and 0.20 seconds.

Ventricular complex. The ventricular complex is composed of a *rapid initial deflection* (*QRS*), a period of rest, and a slow, rounded, *final deflection* (*T-wave*). The QRS represents the period between beginning and completion of the *ventricular depolarization*; the T wave represents the period between beginning and completion of the *ventricular repolarization*.

THE MECHANICS OF CARDIAC ACTION

The phenomena of cardiac contraction and dilatation have been studied in different ways: a) by introducing manometric tubes into the different cardiac chambers and recording the pressure changes taking place in them (31a); b) by recording the activity of different parts of the heart in open chest experiments either through direct transmission of the movements (31) or through volumetric changes (6, 7, 31, 36); c) by recording the movements of the chest wall produced by the activity of the heart (animals, human beings); d) by recording the movements of the blood flowing to and from the heart (31c), and of the air in the respiratory passages (34) by effect of cardiac action; and e) by recording the heart sounds together with other manifestations of cardiac activity (14, 39, 40). Since an extensive description of the graphic tracings currently employed on patients will be given later (chapter 5), only brief reference to them will be made here.

The heart cycle starts with the *contraction of the atria*, also called *atrial systole*. A wave of contraction follows that of excitation from above downwards (14) with a very efficient propulsive wave toward the ventricles. A backflow toward the large veins is prevented by the initial contraction of the musculature at the opening of the veins, and by the venous pressure which is rather high in this phase. Atrial contraction takes place in a short phase which immediately precedes ventricular contraction and is called *presystole*. As the *a-v valves* are open throughout all stages of atrial contraction, the rise in pressure within the atria is not great and the contraction is mainly revealed by movement of blood. Still, there is a small increase of ventricular pressure (fig. 34). Atrial contraction is not indispensable because the greatest part of ventricular filling occurs in early diastole. However, it completes ventricular filling and contributes to the normal function of the a-v valves. In rapid heart action and in mitral stenosis, atrial contraction may acquire a much greater importance.

Initiation of ventricular contraction in-creases the pressure in the ventricles and *atrioventricular valves* (tricuspid valves in the right heart; mitral valve in the left heart). Immediately afterwards, the *contraction of the papillary muscles* prevents an eversion of these valves and permits a further rise of pressure, until the pressure existing in the aorta and in the pulmonary artery, respectively, is equalized, and then exceeded. In this short period, the ventricular contraction builds up pressure without causing motion of blood. This short phase is called the *period of tension* or the *period of isometric contraction* because the muscle fibers of the ventricles contract steadily but without any shortening.

As soon as the ventricular pressure exceeds that of the respective artery, the *semilunar valves open* and the outflow starts. During this *period of outflow or ejection*, the fibrous septum which supports the a-v valves is lowered by the contraction of the ventricles and a remarkable increase in size of the atria takes place, causing suction of blood from the veins (fig. 32). From beginning to end, the ventricular pressure maintains a steady course, which is revealed by a kind of *plateau* in the intraventricular tracings.

Despite their apparently delicate struc-

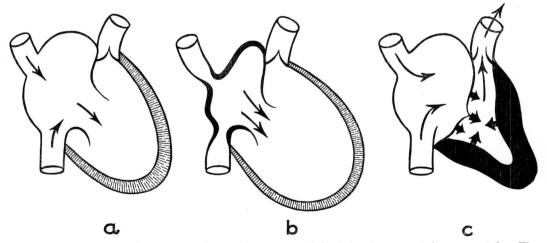

a   b   c

Fig. 32. The muscular events of the heart. a, mid-diastole; b, presystole; c, systole. The atrioventricular junction is lowered by the ventricular contraction creating an aspiration in the venoatrial reservoir.

ture, the flaps of *the a-v valves* have considerable strength and resistance. When closed, they do not merely touch, but form a surface contact without folds. Closure is started by the eddy currents (37) and increased by the ventricular contraction which immediately follows. Eversion is prevented by *the chordae tendineae*, held by *the papillary muscles*. The fact that the musculature of the septum is the first to contract together with the papillary muscles, insures a timely closure of the valves. The termination of atrial contraction contributes to the closure of the a-v valves because the *eddy currents* set up by the flow through the orifices and a *reversal of the gradient of pressure* bring the leaflets into position. This is shown by the temporary and periodic insufficiency which frequently develops in cases with incomplete a-v block. In the event of delayed a-v conduction, there may be a double closure of the a-v valves, the first at the end of atrial contraction, the second at the beginning of ventricular systole.

The *semilunar valves* of the aorta and pulmonary artery resemble pockets attached to the wall of the vessel. The blood, contained in the pockets, keeps the valves away from the wall. Both the *reversal of the gradient of pressure* created by the sudden cessation of outflow and the *eddy currents* determine closure of these valves at the end

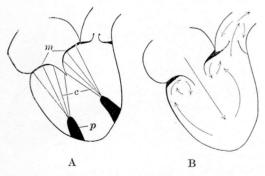

A   B

FIG. 33. The mechanism of the cardiac valves. A, The action of the chordae tendineae on the mitral valve. B, The importance of turbulent flow and eddy currents in closing the cardiac valves. (From Wiggers' *Physiology in Health and Disease*. Courtesy of the author and Lea & Febiger.)

of ventricular systole. Firm attachment of the valves, muscular support from the ventricular base, and lateral apposition, prevent any possibility of eversion, in spite of the lack of chordae tendineae (38).

Each ventricle may be visualized as a pump which keeps the stream circulating in one direction because of the existence of valves.

During *ventricular contraction*, all diameters of the heart decrease; *the base is pulled downward*, the large vessels are stretched, but the apex does not move upward. The spiral arrangement of the muscular bundles of the ventricles makes their contraction very efficient, so that the blood is virtually wrung out. It also causes the heart to rotate to the right, pressing the apex more firmly against the chest wall. This, together with the increased firmness of the ventricular mass, will cause the *apex beat*.

At the end of ventricular systole, ventricular pressure drops to zero. Following an extremely brief interval of latence (so-called *protodiastole*), the semilunar valves of the aorta and pulmonary artery close. A short time interval separates this phase from the subsequent opening of the a-v valves: the *isometric relaxation period*. Ventricular filling starts after the end of this period, e.g. following the opening of the a-v valves.

The *interventricular septum* seems to have an important dynamic role (160) and a large part of right ventricular contraction is probably due to this structure.

Filling of the ventricles has the following features:

a) *An initial phase of rapid filling (early diastole)*. This is caused by the difference in pressure between an overfilled atrium and an empty ventricle. Studies showing an *active* ventricular diastole (36) in this phase have not been supported by later evidence. At this time, the entire venoatrial reservoir experiences a drop in pressure due to acceleration of the stream upon the opening of the atrioventricular valves.

b) *A phase of slow filling (mid-diastole)*. The gradual filling of the ventricles slows

TABLE 4

PHASE	MUSCULAR ACTION	VALVULAR ACTION	HEART SOUNDS
Presystole	Auricles contract, ventricles dilate		Fourth (auricular)
Systole Tension (isometric contraction)	Ventricles contract	a-v valves close, semilunar valves open	First
Ejection	Ventricles contract, auricles dilate markedly		
Diastole Protodiastole		Semilunar valves close	Second
Isometric relaxation		a-v valves open	
Early diastole	Ventricles dilate quickly while the auricles empty		Third
Mid-diastole or slow diastole	Auricles and ventricles fill up slowly		
Late diastole or presystole	Auricles contract, ventricles dilate		Fourth (auricular)

down the inflow and a gradual pressure rise takes place in the venoatrial reservoir.

c) A *late phase of rapid filling (presystole)* caused by the atrial contraction which completes ventricular filling. The veins and the atria show a sudden increase in pressure. As soon as the atrial contraction is completed, the ventricles start contracting because the descending stimulus has already reached the ventricular myocardium.

The following time intervals in seconds may be considered typical of a normal heart with a rate of 68:

Ventricular systole
tension........................ 0.06
maximal ejection.. .... 0.12
reduced ejection................ 0.16
                               ————
                               0.34

Ventricular diastole
protodiastole................... 0.04
isometric relaxation............ 0.07
rapid filling................... 0.10
slow filling.................... 0.20
atrial dynamics
    dynamic interval............ 0.05
    atrial contraction.......... 0.06
                               ————
                               0.52

The Heart Sounds

Auscultation of the normal heart reveals *two sounds (or tones)*, occasionally three. Recording of the heart sounds by means of phonocardiography (page 88) often reveals *four sounds* (fig. 34).

The first sound takes place at the beginning of ventricular systole and lasts through the tension period and the beginning of the ejection period. The second sound is shorter; it takes place at the end of systole and during the isometric relaxation period. The name *"systolic sounds"* has been suggested by the author (146) for these two constantly heard sounds. The other two less frequently heard sounds take place during diastole. The name *"diastolic sounds"* has been suggested for them (146).

Time Relationship of the Heart Sounds

The following dynamic phenomena take place at the time of the heart sounds.

a) *Systolic sounds:*
   1st sound
      Initiation of ventricular systole, closing of the a-v valves, opening of the semilunar valves.

2nd sound
> End of ventricular systole, closing of the semilunar valves, opening of the a-v valves.

b) *Diastolic sounds:*

3rd sound
> Rapid passive filling of the ventricles.

4th sound
> Rapid active filling of the ventricles due to atrial contraction.

First sound complex. It has been proven (147) that the two main vibrations of the first sound complex coincide with those two waves of the cardiogram and of the tracing of intraventricular pressure which are caused by two valvular events (closure of the a-v values and opening of the semilunar valves). It has also been shown that the muscular vibrations of the empty heart are extremely faint and barely appreciable (147).

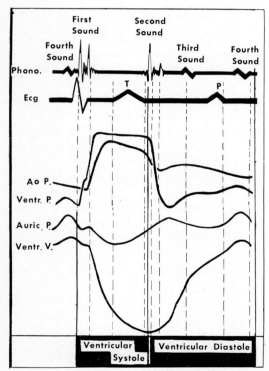

Fig. 34. Atrial, ventricular, and aortic pressures. Phono, sound tracing; Ecg, electrocardiogram; Ao. P., aortic pressure; Ventr. P., ventricular pressure; Auric. P., atrial pressure; Ventr. V., ventricular volume.

However, the first sound is the result of both muscular and valvular factors. Sudden changes in muscular tension activate, first, the a-v valves, and then the semilunar valves. This rapid succession causes a *double vibration* of the cardiac wall which is further transmitted to the chest wall including high and low frequency components. Although simultaneous with the action of the valves, these vibrations are likely to arise in both the valvular and the muscular structures as a response to rapid changes in tension and pressure. In other words, the first sound is the audible expression of that complex movement of the heart which is also revealed by the first part of the apical thrust.

Second sound complex. The second sound complex is caused mainly by the closing of the semilunar valves and the resulting vibrations of the heart and the chest wall. However, vibrations of vascular origin (40, 41) and even the opening of the a-v valves (148) contribute to its formation, at least in certain cases.

Third sound. This sound arises in the ventricular wall as the result of the vibrations caused by the onrush of blood at the moment of rapid passive filling of the ventricles (40, 41). The third sound has been attributed to valvular vibrations (a theory which now has only historical interest) or to the apical impact on the chest wall; this, however, may be only a concurrent factor (42).

Fourth sound. This sound, as clinically recorded, arises in the ventricular wall and is caused by the blood rushing into the ventricular chambers because of atrial contraction (40). Earlier vibrations can be attributed to the atrial contraction *per se* but can be recorded only from the esophagus.

Fifth sound. This sound may appear from 0.08 to 0.16 sec. after the third sound and has been attributed to an elastic rebound of the ventricular wall which would set up vibrations in the myocardium and possibly in the cardiac valves (161). However, it is possible that this sound merely represents a splitting of the third sound (146).

Further data will be given on page 90.

CARDIAC OUTPUT AND RESIDUAL BLOOD

The thoracic and abdominal large veins represent, together with the right atrium, a *systemic venous reservoir* which contains a large volume of blood under low pressure.

The amount of blood ejected into the aorta during each ventricular contraction is called *stroke volume* or *systolic discharge*. It averages between 70 and 80 cc. A similar amount of blood is removed from the systemic reservoir with only 3 to 5 mm. changes in the right atrial pressure.

The average volume of the right ventricle is probably around 50 cc. at the end of systole and around 130 cc. at the end of diastole (152). This means that, in the average subject, 50 cc. of *residual blood* are left within the right ventricle in normal conditions.[20]

The pulmonary veins and the left atrium represent a *pulmonary venous reservoir* which is integrated by that of the lungs (page 54). This reservoir is less distensible than the systemic and its pressure changes are wider.

The *left ventricle* contains about 50 cc. at the end of systole and about 130 at the end of diastole. This means again that 50 cc. of *residual blood* are left within the ventricle at the end of systole. According to *Nylin* and coworkers (136, 149, 150), from 50 to 71 per cent of the total heart volume during life is represented by residual blood.

The normal volume of the living heart is about 700 cc.; 300 cc. represent the volume of the heart muscle. If the stroke volume is 140 cc. (70 cc. from each ventricle), *the residual blood in the heart at the end of systole will be 260 cc.;* 100 cc. seem to be left within the two ventricles while the rest is within the atria.

Multiplication of systolic discharge by the heart rate per minute gives *the minute volume* or *cardiac output.*

In normal conditions the systolic discharge of each ventricle is the same; therefore, the flow of blood into the aorta and pulmonary artery is the same. However, small temporary differences may occur; the excess of blood discharged by one ventricle is then absorbed temporarily by the vessels of the systemic or pulmonary systems while a certain amount may be retained in one-half of the heart as residual blood.

It is apparent that the heart may increase its output in one of the three following ways:

a) *By increasing the systolic discharge* and maintaining a constant rate.

b) *By accelerating the rate per minute* and maintaining a constant systolic discharge.

c) *Through reflex changes of ventricular contraction* which are independent of right atrial changes. These are made possible by the existence of residual blood within the heart and by the pulmonic reservoir, and are frequently correlated with the effect of epinephrine (153, 155).

Cardiac output can be determined on the basis of oxygen consumption if we know how much oxygen is consumed by the tissues per minute and how much oxygen a definite volume of blood (100 cc.) can supply to the tissues. In order to calculate cardiac output in this way, it is necessary to measure the content of oxygen of both the arterial and the venous blood.[21] Practical

---

[20] According to other studies (156), the average residual blood of the right ventricle in man is 89 cc., or 50 cc. per square meter of body surface. This average was made between widely separated figures.

[21] The average amounts of oxygen and carbon dioxide in the blood of healthy young adults at rest, at sea level, are approximately the following:

	ARTERIAL BLOOD	VENOUS BLOOD
Oxygen		
Volumes per cent.....	20	15
Saturation..........	100	70
Carbon dioxide		
Volumes per cent.....	45	50
Tension............	40	46
pH...................	7.34	7.32

difficulties involved in obtaining these samples instigated the development of indirect methods now in use (page 155). They are based on the determination of the oxygen consumption and the carbon dioxide elimination of the tissues, and are exact only if the two following conditions exist:

a) Same output from both ventricles.

b) An exact and constant proportion between the gas exchange and the amount of blood circulating in the lungs.

The average *cardiac output in man*, under *basal conditions*,[22] is 3.2 liters per square meter of body surface in 1 minute. It is even more exactly proportional to body weight, being about 76 cc. per kilo. *An average man has a cardiac output of 5.6 liters*

TABLE 5. *Blood volume of various mammalians (percentage of body weight)*

Horse	9.7
Bullock	7.7
Sheep	8.0
Goat	6.2
Dog	7.2
Cat	6.5
Rabbit	6.2

per min. and, with an average pulse of 66, a *systolic discharge* of 84 cc. (45b).

Cardiac output is reduced when the subject stands; it is increased by the intake of foods and liquids. Physical exercise increases both the pulse rate and the systolic discharge. This is possible on account of marked increase of venous return.

BLOOD VOLUME—CIRCULATION TIME— BLOOD FLOW

The *blood volume* of mammalians can be determined approximately on the basis of a percentage of the body weight. Table 5 gives some average data (145).

In normal man, *plasma volume* is between

[22] *Basal conditions* are those excluding muscular activity, disease, extremes of environmental temperatures, and food intake, within the last 12 hours.

4 and 5 per cent of body weight and the hematocrit values for venous blood are 40 to 50 per cent (162).

Circulation time can be measured from a peripheral vein to a peripheral artery, from a vein to the lungs, or from the lungs to an artery. Average *arm-to-tongue time* is 14 sec.; average *arm-to-lung time* is 7 sec.; average *lung-to-cheek time* is 6 sec. (page 156).

Blood flow has been determined for various organs with the following results (163):

ORGAN	LITERS PER MINUTE
Kidneys	1.3
Brain	0.8
Extremities	1.8
Liver	1.3–1.5

THE HEART RATE

The rate of the heart varies with its size and weight. This general law is true not only in human beings of different ages and sizes but also in animals of different species (46). The heart rate decreases regularly with the increase in weight of the heart following the growth of the organism from childhood to maturity. The length of ventricular systole and that of the P-R interval increase at the same time (46). These facts are shown in table 6.

The *average pulse rate* in a healthy man is between 61 and 64 if taken in basal conditions. The range may extend between 50 and 100 (121), with the lower rate for trained individuals and the higher for individuals with low excitability of the vagus nerve and high metabolic rate. Women have 7 to 8 beats per minute more than men.

TABLE 6

AGE	BODY WEIGHT	HEART WEIGHT	HEART RATE PER MINUTE	P-R INTERVAL
	kg.	*gm.*		*sec.*
Newborn	3.3	23	135	0.11
1 year	9.5	42	115	0.12
2 years	12.0	50	105	0.12
5 years	16.5	65	90	0.13
10 years	26.0	103	78	0.14
15 years	44.0	163	68	0.16
20 years	60.0	250	62	0.18

TABLE 7

ANIMAL	BODY WEIGHT	OXYGEN CON-SUMPTION	CARDIAC OUTPUT	PULSE RATE PER MIN.	STROKE VOLUME
	kg.	*cc./min.*	*cc.*		*cc.*
Ox.........	500	1740	34,800	60	580
Horse......	500	1450	29,000	34	852
Man.......	70	253.5	5,070	70	72
Sheep......	50	199	3,980	75	53
Dog.......	10	72.5	1,450	100	14

Table 7 gives cardiac output and stroke volume in various species (145).

PRESSURES IN THE CHAMBERS OF THE HEART—FUNCTION OF THE ATRIA

The pressure in the right atrium is higher than intrathoracic pressure but very near to atmospheric pressure. It has been found that in an individual lying down at rest, *right atrial pressure varies between 0 and +8 mm. Hg. Left atrial pressure is slightly higher. The right ventricle has a systolic pressure of +20 to +25 Hg; the left ventricle, one of 110 to 150 mm. Hg. In both ventricles, diastolic pressure is zero, or, at most, may reach up to 5 mm. Hg* (47).

Deep inspiration affects markedly the pressures of the right heart chambers. Right atrial pressure may drop to -7 while right ventricular pressure may drop to $+20/-6$. On the contrary, *cough* may raise right atrial pressure to $+60$ mm. Hg and right ventricular pressure to $+80$ (158).

The thinness and weakness of the right atrial wall and its distensibility account for the fact that the filling volume of this chamber is about twice that of the left atrium (159).

As atrial contraction lasts but a small fraction of the total cycle (about one-tenth of a second), *the atria remain dilated during most of ventricular diastole and during all of ventricular systole, and serve as a reservoir for the blood coming to the heart.* The traction developed by the ventricular muscles on the atrioventricular junction dilates the atria and causes suction on the veins during ventricular systole (fig. 32).

The *atrial appendages* seem to have little propulsive function and serve as complementary spaces which fill the deep niches at the base of the heart during ventricular systole.

In conditions different from the normal, as in the case of a very fast heart rate, diastole shortens tremendously. In such a case, atrial contraction includes nearly all of the entire diastole and acquires a much greater importance.

Nervous and Chemical Control of Cardiac Activity

Efferent nerve fibers reach the heart from both the *vagus nerves* and the *sympathetic ganglia*. The vagal fibers terminate in ganglia which are situated in the wall of the atria. From these, postganglionic fibers carry impulses to the s-a node and the a-v node, to the atrial muscle, and to the bundle of His. The *right vagus supplies a greater number of fibers to the s-a node; the left vagus supplies a greater number to the a-v node.*

The preganglionic fibers of the *sympathetic system* leave the *thoracic section* of the spinal cord and terminate in the three cervical ganglia and in the first five thoracic ganglia (figs. 35 and 36). However, only postganglionic fibers emerging from the ganglia T2 to T5 seem to have an accelerating effect on the heart (165). As the sympathetic fibers reach only the atrial myocardium, the ventricular function is modified by the sympathetic only through the conducting system (118).

The *vagus nerve* has a persistent and predominant action on the heart, as shown by the fast heart rate which follows removal of all autonomic nerve fibers. It *slows the heart rate* by acting on the pacemaker of the heart, thus producing depression of automatism. It *weakens the atrial contraction* (depression of contractility) and *shortens the refractory period of the atria* (increase of excitability) (fig. 37). The amplitude and duration of the action currents recorded

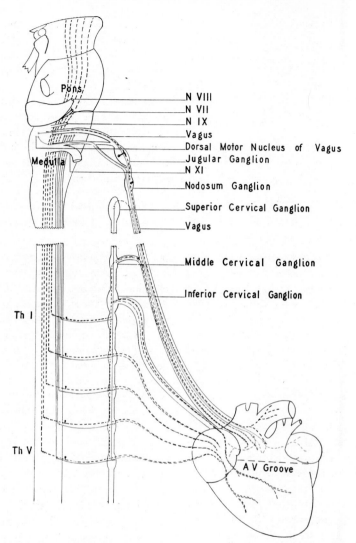

Fig. 35. Schematic diagram of the innervation of the mammalian heart. (From *Physiology in Modern Medicine*. Courtesy of Prof. Philip Bard and C. V. Mosby Co.)

The red continuous lines represent *sympathetic* (*accelerator*) *preganglionic fibers*, which end at cells in the inferior, middle, and superior cervical ganglia, and also in the ganglia of the upper thoracic chain. The continuous line running through the chain represents a series of *preganglionic fibers* connecting with various cells. The dotted red lines indicate the *sympathetic postganglionic distribution* to the heart. The green continuous lines represent *vagal preganglionic fibers* and the dotted black lines indicate *sensory fibers* coursing in the *vagus* to the medulla (aortic nerve and vagal afferents from the heart chambers) and in the *sympathetic* strands to the dorsal spinal roots (thoracic I to V). The latter mediate pain. The *afferent fibers* of the vagus arise from cells of the T-shaped unipolar type situated in both the nodose and jugular ganglia.

from the atrial muscle is severely reduced by stimulation of the vagus.

The vagus nerve *slows the impulses through the conducting system* (depression of con-

ductivity). The ventricles are affected indirectly by the increased length of diastole which increases their filling and gives a longer interval during which premature

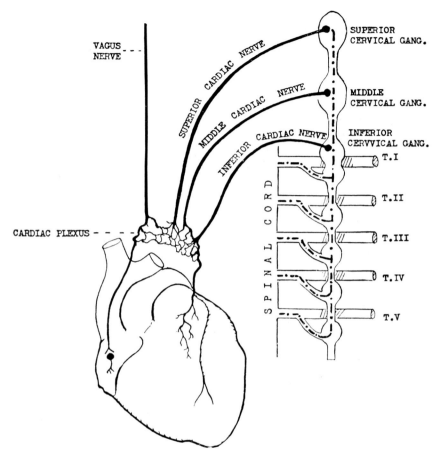

FIG. 36. Diagram of the cardiac nerves. Broken lines, preganglionic sympathetic fibers. (From Best and Taylor: *The Physiological Basis of Medical Practice*, The Williams & Wilkins Co.)

beats may occur. However, there is some evidence of direct influence of the vagus on the ventricles (165).

The response to vagal stimulation varies according to the existing rate of the atria. If there is rapid, normal, or slow atrial rate, vagus stimulation slows down that rate. On the contrary, if the atria contract *very rapidly* (400 or more contractions per second), vagal stimulation further increases the rate of discharges and causes atrial fibrillation (164).

The normal heart can be stopped temporarily by excessive vagus stimulation (page 86). However, this pause is not permanent because automatic ventricular contractions soon begin. Stimulation of the right vagus

may cause temporary arrest of the entire heart (action on the pacemaker). Stimulation of the left vagus may cause temporary arrest of the ventricles by blocking the stimuli in the conducting system (action on the a-v node and on the bundle of His).

The action of the *accelerans* (*sympathetic fibers*) is less marked. Stimulation of these nerves causes *increased heart rate* (stimulation of automatism) and *increased force of contraction of both atria and ventricles* (stimulation of contractility). The efficiency of the heart muscle increases, probably through decrease of the pH.

Both the actions of the cardiac vagi and the cardiac sympathetic nerves result from the liberation of chemical substances, as

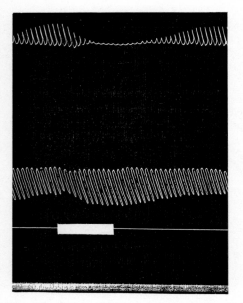

Fig. 37. Action of the vagus on the turtle's heart. Electrical stimulation of the right vagus depresses the contractility of the atrium without impairing the conductivity. A-V block takes place on further increasing the intensity of the current. Upper tracing, atrial contractions. Lower tracing, ventricular contractions.

shown by *Loewi* in 1921 (48). Coupling two isolated frog hearts so that perfusion fluid of the first would circulate in the second showed that stimulation of the cardiac nerves of the first heart was followed by similar effects in the second (fig. 38). This result was called "humoral transmission of the nerve effect." Since then, it has been demonstrated, and is universally accepted, that all autonomic and skeletal nerves act by liberating chemical substances. The cardiac vagus acts by liberating *acetylcholine*; the cardiac *sympathetic* acts by liberating *sympathin* (48, 49), an epinephrine-like (or adrenine-like) substance.[23] Acetylcholine

[23] It was customary to say that epinephrine and acetylcholine act like the sympathetic and the vagus, respectively. Demonstration of the humoral nature of nerve action makes it more accurate to say that *sympathetic and vagus fibers act like epinephrine and acetylcholine, respectively.*

The term *adrenine* is synonymous with epinephrine and refers to the product of the adrenal

is promptly inactivated by a *cholinesterase* present in the blood and, therefore, has only a local action at the site of production. On the contrary, sympathin diffuses into the blood stream, is carried to all parts of the body, and has prolonged effects which are added to those of epinephrine (49).

Epinephrine (*adrenine*), discharged into the blood stream, has powerful effects on the heart. Some of them are indirect, being due to peripheral effects; others are due either to direct action on the heart or to a synergistic effect with the locally liberated sympathin (49). How *acetylcholine* acts is still unknown but the most likely explanation is that it acts by modifying the electrical behavior of the cell membrane (121).

THE SENSORY NERVES OF THE HEART

Habitual stimuli applied to the myocardium do not cause pain (50). On the other hand, lesions of the coronary system are a frequent cause of pain.

Animal experimentation and surgical interventions in man demonstrate that *centripetal stimuli originated in the myocardium and coronary vessels follow sympathetic fibers* (118). They reach the central nervous system by way of two *cardiac nerves* traversing the middle cervical and the inferior cervical ganglion. The inferior cervical ganglion is often fused with the first thoracic and has the name of *stellate ganglion* (fig. 35).

Centripetal stimuli, coming from the heart, proceed along the *white rami communicantes* and the *posterior roots of the thoracic section* of the spinal cord (roots 1 to 5) (see also page 431).

A second path includes the fibers of the *depressor nerve* which predominantly supply the endocardium (118).

Functions of the Pericardium

The functions of the pericardium have been widely discussed and even completely denied. *The pericardial sac supports the*

medulla. The term *adrenalin* refers to the commercial preparations.

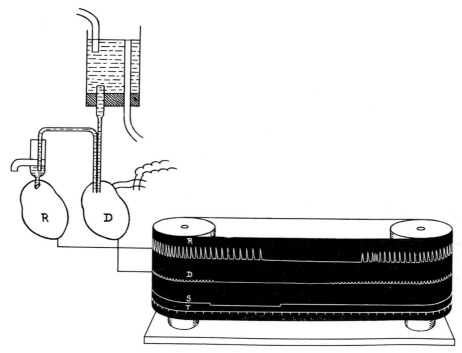

Fig. 38. *Loewi's classic experiment demonstrating the humoral transmission of nerve action.* Electrical stimulation (S) of the vagus of the heart D first slows heart D, and then heart R. The latter is slowed by acetylcholine which was produced by nerve action and passed from one heart to the other.

heart. Having a certain tension due to its connection with other structures, *it partly determines the shape of the heart* (fig. 19). The tension of the pericardium limits the possible distention of the heart. Chemoreceptors have been found in the pericardium (118). Other possible functions will be discussed later (page 60).

Functions of the Arteries

The functions of the arteries cannot be properly evaluated without a full understanding of the general properties of smooth muscles.

Smooth muscles are usually arranged in sheets or layers around hollow organs. The typical contraction of a smooth muscle is sluggish but there is great difference between the smooth muscles of various organs of the body (51).

Smooth muscles, including excised arteries, exhibit *rhythmic contractions*. These contractions are usually slow and somewhat irregular but may, on the contrary, develop more rapidly, especially as a reaction to sudden distention. One of the most typical features of smooth muscle is its peculiar tendency to exhibit a sustained, persistent contraction called *tonus.* Hollow organs are usually able to adapt themselves to the volume of their content. It has been proven that the pressure of a full organ (stomach, bladder) may be the same when a different amount of fluid is contained in it. Peristaltic contractions do not seem to be essentially influenced by different lengths of the fibers. Nevertheless, an increase in tonus will alter the distensibility of an organ whenever a sudden change of pressure is developed in its cavity.

Smooth muscles repond to a great variety of stimuli. *Distention* is one of the most effective, especially if rapid (11).

The arterial wall has the unique position of containing a fluid under a very high pressure. As the arterial wall is rhythmically

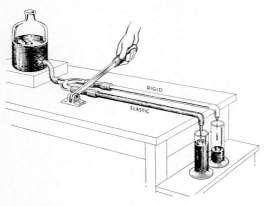

FIG. 39. *Marey's experiment on the action of elasticity of the arteries*. Mechanical interruption of the flow gives different effects in different tubes: poorer flow and interrupted stream in the rigid tube; more abundant flow and continuous stream in the elastic tube.

dilated by each pulse wave, it is apparent the the *vascular tonus* should not be considered as acting like a stopcock on the peripheral vessels. When tonus increases, the arteries are still able to dilate at the passage of the pulse wave, but the amplitude of the dilatation will be lessened. Therefore, a moderate vasoconstriction decreases the systolic dilatation and the following elastic reaction of the peripheral arteries, so that these become more similar to rigid tubes. Only in the extreme degrees of vascular contraction, as with the *vascular spasms* of minute arterial vessels caused by local irritation, does the artery become a rigid tube.

If the smooth fibers of the arterial wall are stretched by the passage of the blood wave and recoil immediately afterwards, it is possible that this recoil is not a purely passive phenomenon. However, the rapidity of the recoil is theoretically against participation of smooth fibers.

Two types of experiments seemed to prove the activity of the arterial wall: a) the recording of potentials from large or medium arteries, timed with the propagation of the pulse and not caused by electrical artifacts (57, 58); and b) the demonstration that

diameter changes are not exactly parallel to pressure changes in normal conditions (60).

The following properties should be admitted:

a) An *elastic reaction* to the dilatation caused by the pulse wave (*retractility*). This property is maximal in the large arteries so that the aorta may be considered as an elastic reservoir. A *muscular reaction* to the dilatation caused by the pulse wave (*contractility*) is, as already said, under discussion.

b) A persistent condition called *tonus*, maximal in the small arteries. The greater the tonus, the lesser the retraction.

The part played by the elasticity and by the contractility of the arteries is shown by two experiments. The first was devised by *Marey* and is based on a model in which an elastic tube carries more fluid than a rigid one (fig. 39). The second was devised by the author (55, 56) and is based on a frog preparation not including the heart. A rhythmically interrupted flow leads to greater output. The difference between the output during constant flow and that during interrupted flow is not increased by morphine but is tremendously increased by adrenalin. This was interpreted as indicating that the latter also stimulates rhythmic smooth muscle reaction while the former causes only a steady increase of tonus.

Two different types of disturbance of the arterial function have been demonstrated in cold blooded animals (60). The first is *tonic rigidity* which occurs whenever the artery is submitted to local irritation or injury and which prevents dilatation of the vessel at the passage of the pulse wave. The second is *arterial paralysis* which occurs under the action of certain drugs or after CNS injury; it causes a condition of the arterial wall which prevents vasomotor constriction.

It has been proven that, in normal small arteries, slow passive distention is effectively compensated by reactive changes of tonus (191).

Regulation of Circulation and Vasomotor Control

The central nervous system regulates the circulation through: a) changes of cardiac output, b) changes of arterial resistance, and c) changes of venous return. Cardiac output may vary independently of venous return, though only for a limited period (utilization of residual blood, page 43). Venous return may vary independently of arterial constriction through variations of the capacity of blood reservoirs (page 59) and modifications of venous tonus. The CNS regulates blood pressure through immediate reaction to stimuli of the numerous pressoreceptors (page 52) and slower adjustments to other stimuli. Blood pressure is maintained remarkably constant in the presence of frequent changes of cardiac output. This is due to a *regulating center* located in the hypothalamus.

It is possible that vasomotor impulses are mediated by a chemical agent secreted in the arterial wall (enzyme?) which, acting on the hypertensinogen of the plasma, causes formation of a hypertensive substance (176). If this is confirmed, secretion of *renin* by the kidney (page 59) would be but a particular case of a widespread phenomenon of the entire vascular system.

The existence of *vasomotor nerves* was demonstrated by *Claude Bernard* in 1852 (61). The neuro-humoral theory which has been gradually developed in the wake of *Loewi's* studies (48, 49) has altered our views on vasomotor innervation. Demonstration that a sympathetic nerve fiber may act through liberation of acetylcholine led to classification of the fibers, on a purely functional basis, into *adrenergic* and *cholinergic* (62). A fiber which acts by secreting sympathin (epinephrine-like action) is said to be adrenergic; a fiber which acts by secreting acetylcholine (acetylcholine action) is called cholinergic.

The dilatation and constriction of the peripheral arteries is controlled by two main centers on the floor of the 4th ventricle of the medulla: *the vasodilator and vasoconstrictor centers.* Secondary centers are present in the spinal cord; higher centers, in the hypothalamus.

The normal condition of the arteries is that of a balance between nervous impulses, namely between *constrictor* and *dilator tonus.* The former predominates, as shown by the fact that cutting of the splanchnic nerves doubles the blood flow in the viscera.

The vasomotor tonus is maintained: a) by centripetal stimuli coming from various organs or nerve centers, b) by the action of chemicals circulating in the blood stream, and c) by the stretching effect of arterial blood pressure (168).

Several *endocrine glands* take part in the regulation of the circulation. They are: a) the *thyroid,* b) the *parathyroids,* c) the *posterior pituitary,* and d) the *pancreas* (indirectly).

It has been proven that the interplay between *adrenalin* and *nor-adrenalin* is important in the control of heart rate and peripheral resistance; that several steroids (including those of the adrenal cortex) have a role in the regulation of blood pressure and blood volume; and that the liver exerts an important effect on circulation, revealed by a higher and more steady arterial pressure (173), an effect which seems connected with the responsiveness of the cardiovascular system to various vasoactive substances (179).

The importance of the vasomotor system lies in the fact that it is more a *blood-distributing* than a pressure-regulating system. The nervous discharges may be directed not only towards particular areas of the body but also towards arteries of a certain caliber in preference to others.

Multiple *cutaneo-visceral reflexes* occur whenever the skin is stimulated by heat or cold, and they seem to have a segmental distribution.

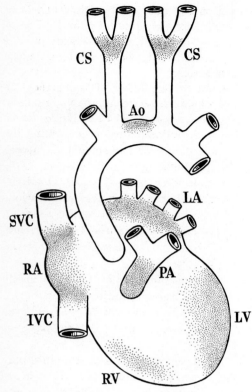

Fig. 40. Location of the specific receptors in the heart and large vessels. In blue, the venopressor system. In red, the arteriopressor system. CS, carotid sinus; IVC, inferior vena cava; SVC, superior vena cava; Ao, aortic arch; PA, pulmonary artery; RV, right ventricle; LV, left ventricle; RA, right atrium; LA, left atrium.

Pressoreceptors and Cardiovascular Reflexes

Definite areas of the large veins, of the heart, and of the large arteries, contain nervous receptors which are sensitive to changes in pressure: the *pressoreceptors*. Distention of the cardiac or vascular wall stimulates these receptors, causing cardiovascular reflexes of paramount importance in the maintenance of circulation. Decrease of the average distention, on the other hand, causes opposite reactions.

1) *System of the venae cavae and of the right atrium.* Multiple studies (63–66) led to recognition of a mechanism which adapts the heart rate and the arterial pressure to the venous return. The sensitive receptors are located in the walls of both venae cavae near their opening into the right atrium, and in the wall of the latter (fig. 40). The centripetal stimuli reach the vasomotor center and the cardio-accelerans center by means of the vagus nerve. The centrifugal fibers of the accelerans and of the vasoconstrictors complete the reflex arc. Increased venous pressure causes an increase of heart rate (*Bainbridge reflex*, ref. 63a) and blood pressure (64), and a faster respiration (66). However, stretching of the inferior cava and of the right atrium may also cause bradycardia, lowering of blood pressure and respiratory inhibition (175, 177). The venopressor reflex, acting against the depressor reflexes of the large arteries, permits the maintenance of a high blood pressure during physical exercise. A different veno-pressor reflex takes place when venous pressure drops to a very low level (64); it has a particular importance after a severe hemorrhage in preventing a vascular collapse.

In addition to the regulation of arterial pressure in the greater circulation, these venoatrial reflexes also regulate the pressure in the lesser circulation and in the venous system (67).

2) *System of the aortic arch, of the carotid sinus, and of the cerebral vessels.* This system has a fundamental importance in regulating the arterial pressure. The specific receptors are located in the aortic arch and at the bifurcation of the common carotid arteries (67, 68) (fig. 40). Similar receptors have been found in the cerebral vessels (169). Others, found in the subclavian arteries (67) and the abdominal aorta (68), have a secondary role.

Near the pressoreceptors are other receptors, sensitive to chemical changes of the blood, called *chemoreceptors*. These are located in the *aortic body*, in the *carotid bodies*, and in the *cerebral vessels* (170).[24]

[24] The *carotid body* is a glandular structure containing many sinusoidal vessels, located near the carotid sinus bilaterally. The *aortic body* is a similar structure, located in the aortic arch.

The reflex arc, based on the presso-receptors, has the following centripetal fibers:

a) For the aortic receptors, the fibers of the *depressor nerve*, or *nerve of Cyon* (71), which join the *vagus* in man.

b) For the carotid receptors, the fibers of the *nerve of Hering* (72), which soon join the *glossopharyngeal nerve*. A thin filament goes from the nerve of Hering to the superior cervical ganglion of the *sympathetic*, and another joins the *vagus*. These centripetal fibers reach the vasomotor center and the *cardio-inhibitor* center in the medulla. The centrifugal part of the reflex is based upon the *vagus* for the heart (68), upon the *sympathetic* for the peripheral arteries (73, 74).

Increased pressure in the large arteries is followed by a decrease in heart rate (brady-cardia) and a drop in blood pressure (hypo-tension) (fig. 41). Decreased pressure in the large arteries is followed by increased heart rate (tachycardia) and increased blood pressure (hypertension).

It has been shown that the state of con-traction of the arteries where the presso-receptors are located is important in the regulation of blood pressure. The greater the resistance to stretch, the less severe is the reflex. Thus the amount of adrenaline and noradrenaline contained in the blood regu-lates to some extent the arterial pressure (166).

It has been demonstrated that *action currents* are always present in the carotid nerves (75) and that they increase in in-tensity during cardiac systole, even when blood pressure is normal. When blood pres-sure is high, these currents increase in fre-quency and intensity; they are present only during systole when blood pressure is low.

The *cardiac reflex* is more sudden than the *vasomotor reflex* but is of shorter dura-tion. The vagus nerve accounts for most of the reflex at the beginning while sympa-thetic inhibition maintains cardiac slowing later (141). If the slowing of the heart is

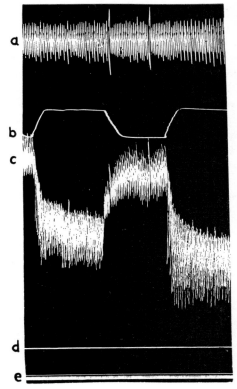

FIG. 41. Reflex changes of the respiration and blood pressure caused by prolonged distention of the carotid sinus in the dog. a, respiration; b, pressure in the sinus (balloon); c, pressure in the femoral artery; d, zero line of arterial pressure; e, time in seconds.

too prolonged, *atrial* or *ventricular escapes* arise and maintain circulation until sinus rhythm is resumed. The vagal response to carotid sinus distention occurs *mainly on the side of the stimulation* but there is also a small contralateral reaction. The vasomotor response, on the other hand, has a large *crossed* component (141).

The connection of the vasomotor center with the adrenal glands may determine a prolonged hypertensive reaction by means of epinephrine secretion whenever blood pressure drops too much in the aorta and the carotid arteries.

The changes of heart rate and blood pres-sure which take place in normal people in changing from recumbent to erect position, and vice versa, are deeply influenced by carotid sinus reflexes.

External compression of the carotid sinus in man causes a sudden drop in blood pressure through direct mechanical stimulation of the receptors. On the contrary, compression of the common carotid artery causes an increase in blood pressure by decreasing the distention of the carotid sinus.

Carotid and aortic impulses may change the respiratory rate (fig. 41); if sufficiently intense, carotid stimuli may even reach the cerebral cortex (irradiation of reflexes) (76).

The *aortic body* and the *carotid bodies* are sensitive to changes in the concentration of CO_2 and O_2 and to changes of the pH of the blood. Reflexes starting from these organs may change the heart rate, the blood pressure level, and the respiratory rate. In particular, *lack of oxygen causes a reflex vasoconstriction*. Normal regulation in man is not influenced by the carotid bodies (7). Abnormal and pathological conditions, on the other hand, are followed by reflex actions involving these bodies. Both hormones and drugs may act on them.

3) *System of the pulmonary artery and veins and of the left atrium*. Specific receptors, sensitive to pressure changes, are present in the pulmonary artery and veins and in the wall of the left atrium (78–80, 177). Distention of walls of these chambers causes bradycardia and a drop of pressure, both in the lesser and the greater circulation. The centripetal path of the reflex is the vagus; the centrifugal goes along both sympathetic and vagus.

4) *System of the ventricles and of the coronaries*. The walls of both cardiac ventricles (mainly those of the left) and the coronary vessels, are very sensitive to adequate stimuli. Distention of the cavities, chemical irritation, and lack of blood in the coronary vessels, have been shown to be particularly effective (81–86, 177), and are followed by pain and by multiple reflexes.

The complex function of these regulating mechanisms may be summarized by admitting *two fundamental systems*, one *venocardiac*, the other *cardio-pulmo-arterial*.

Injection of certain drugs (veratridine, nicotine, ATP, etc.) into the coronary arteries of the cat or the left coronary of the dog causes apnea, bradycardia, and a fall of blood pressure (*von Bezold-Jarisch reflex* (188, 189). This reflex is still obscure and does not seem to be caused by action on chemoreceptors.

Marey's law originally stated that the heart rate varies in inverse proportion with the level of the blood pressure, high blood pressure causing bradycardia and vice versa. This law is actually the result of cardiovascular reflexes and may be considered true, within limits.

Pulmonary Circulation

The blood of the right ventricle reaches the left atrium after having passed through the lungs. The amount of blood passing through the lesser circulation (lungs) should be the same as that passing through the greater circulation (all the rest of the body) in a given time. An exception to this general rule is made by the reservoir function of the pulmonary vessels (see below).

The volume of blood contained in the pulmonary vessels is modified by the relative discharge of the two sides of the heart and these are affected by dynamic changes of the systemic circulation.

The *capacity* and the *extensibility* of the pulmonary vessels are such that a severe increase in blood flow may be accommodated by them with only slight changes in pressure.

The *speed* of the pulse wave in the pulmonary circulation has been measured in man and found about one-third of that of the greater circulation (182).

The *mean pressure* in the *pulmonary artery* is approximately 18 mm. of mercury, about one-sixth that of aortic pressure. Figures taken from numerous studies in dogs give 40/10 mm. Hg as average figures of *systolic/diastolic pressure*, with a *pulse pressure* of 30. In human beings, the pressure is 25–30/10.

Pulmonary venous pressures vary between 3 and 12 mm. Hg. The pressure in the capillaries of the lungs is about one-sixth of that of the capillaries of the greater circulation.

In the course of normal breathing, the pressures of the pulmonary artery and veins fall during inspiration and rise during expiration, even when the heart rate is regular. Increased inspiratory capacity of the pulmonary bed, exceeding the increased discharge of the right ventricle, seems to be the cause for these periodic changes (87).

The capillaries of the lungs are surrounded by air and are practically in contact with the atmosphere. These minute vessels are very distensible and have a tremendous surface which may average 140 square meters. Their capacity may be influenced by:

a) Changes of the intrathoracic pressure due to respiration.

b) Changes in the output of the right ventricle due to variation of venous return and not proportional to the resistance met in the left atrium.

c) Vasomotor phenomena of the pulmonary vessels.

The pulmonary circulation is very adaptable to changes in volume of the circulating blood (85–87) owing to two different mechanisms:

a) Opening of *reserve capillaries*, usually closed.

b) Existence of large *sinusoidal veins*, able to collect blood and to empty later by contraction (88).

These mechanisms enable the lung to act as a *blood reservoir* preventing noxious effects on the left heart (86, 180). The lungs normally contain one-fifth of the blood volume.

The question of innervation of the pulmonary arteries has been the source of discussions and numerous investigations. The relatively weak contractility of these vessels and the fact that their active contraction is often prevented and opposed by changes of the heart function render definite conclusions difficult. Both the vagi and the sympathetic nerves seem to bring vasodilators and vasoconstrictors to the lungs (84). Pharmacological evidence seems to indicate that *adrenergic fibers dilate* and *cholinergic fibers constrict the pulmonary arteries* in the intact organism.

Contraction of the pulmonary veins, demonstrated in rabbits and guinea pigs (89), is still doubtful in man.

Coronary Circulation

The circulation of the coronary arteries may be schematically divided into two parts: that of the larger vessels, *running on the surface* of the heart, and that of the smaller vessels, *penetrating into the walls* of the heart.

Blood pressure tracings of the main coronary trunks are similar to aortic tracings. Their mean pressure varies with that of the general arterial pressure and averages about *one-fifth of that of the aorta*.

The *coronary blood flow* is large, averaging about 5 per cent of the total cardiac output. In the dog, the right coronary artery receives about one-fifth of the total coronary inflow; the left coronary artery, four-fifths.

The flow in the small, intramural, coronary arteries of the left ventricle is influenced by the following factors.

a) Mean aortic pressure.

b) Aortic diastolic pressure (a large part of the flow takes place during diastole).

c) Ventricular contraction itself, which opposes arterial flow (squeezing of the capillaries, however, accelerates venous flow).

d) Vasomotor actions.

e) Pressure of the right atrium, against which the coronary veins must empty.

The velocity of blood flow diminishes during ventricular contraction (91) without, however, dropping too low (14). This is due to the fact that the rise of pressure taking place in the aorta during early systole is able to overcome the greater resistance

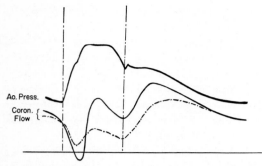

Ao. Press.

Coron. {
Flow {

FIG. 42. The flow of blood in the left coronary
artery. Double wave: the higher of the two is in
diastole. Upper tracing, pressure in the aorta.
Lower continuous tracing, flow in the main coronary artery. Lower dotted tracing, flow in the
intramural branches. (Adapted from Wiggers.)

due to muscular contraction. Even if blood
flow is greater during diastole, a substantial
flow also takes place during systole (14)
(fig. 42).

The coronary vessels are largely supplied
with afferent and efferent fibers (118). The
majority of the studies, dealing with the
problem of *coronary innervation*, indicate
that the sympathetic carries vasodilator
fibers of adrenergic type and the vagus
brings vasoconstrictor fibers of cholinergic
type. Further evidence shows that stimulation of the stellate ganglia causes an increase
in coronary flow, independent of blood pressure changes (92). Clinical evidence confirms the existence of reflex disturbances of
the coronaries, especially in the presence of
gastric or gall bladder lesions.

Reflexes of cardiac origin regulate the
coronary flow, increasing it with increased
cardiac output and, within physiological
limits, with increased cardiac rate.

Reflexes of extracardiac origin have great
importance. It has been proven that distention of the stomach, esophagus, gall
bladder or bile duct, is followed by reduction
of the coronary flow through the action of
parasympathetic fibers (135). The same
result follows distention of the carotid sinus.

Coronary blood flow increases with *exer-*

cise: this is due to increased aortic pressure,
coronary vasodilation (apparently due to
decreased action of the vagus), or both.

The rich innervation of the coronary vessels enables the nervous system to regulate
their caliber in proportion to the work of
the heart. The fact that some sensory nerve
fibers supply the coronary arteries with one
branch and the myofibrils with another
makes possible peculiar axon reflexes (118).

The effect of *heart rate* on the coronary
flow of the denervated heart is the following
(132): at slow rates, acceleration *increases*
the flow; at averate rates, changes of the
heart are *without effect*; at rapid rates, acceleration of the heart *decreases* coronary
blood flow. In spite of possible reflex regulation, a very rapid heart rate is accompanied
by impairment in the coronary flow.

The coronary arteries contain an unusually large number of longitudinal and
spiral muscle fibers in the media (167).
Contraction of these fibers dilates the vessels.
Thus, sympathetic dilatation may be obtained through a different structural arrangement and not through a different
functional reaction from that of other arteries.

The chemical composition of the blood
deeply affects the volume of coronary flow.
Anoxia increases the coronary flow with a
maximal dilatation of the vessels when
arterial saturation falls to 50 per cent of
normal (in the intact animal). *Asphyxia*
is followed by similar changes, and it seems
that the vasodilation is connected with
accumulation of products of muscular metabolism owing to incomplete oxidation
(adenosine, adenylic acid, adenine, etc.).

In the denervated heart, coronary flow is
independent of *changes of cardiac output*
as long as heart rate and mean aortic pressure are constant. However, *reflexes* modify
this in the innervated heart.

The decrease of coronary flow due to the
muscular contraction of the heart is considerably greater in the left ventricle than

in the right. However, most of the studies dealing with intramyocardial pressure were made on denervated preparations; compensatory reflexes oppose the paradoxical decrease of blood supply as the work of the heart becomes greater (132, 133). While ventricular contraction opposes the flow of blood through the capillaries, it squeezes the blood out of them and increases the flow in the coronary sinus. It is possible that coronary sinus outflow occurs only during diastole (134).

As already stated (page 25), the coronary blood flow returns to the cardiac cavities through *the coronary sinus, the superficial cardiac veins, the Thebesian veins*, and *the sinusoidal vessels*. The major portion of the blood from the left ventricle flows through the coronary sinus while the greater part of that from the right ventricle flows through the anterior cardiac veins into the right atrium. Only a small amount of blood reaches the cavities through the other vessels in normal conditions.

The pressure changes of the *coronary sinus* have been studied in man (171). Apart from respiratory variations, three positive waves have been noted in the tracing: one, presystolic, due to atrial contraction; one, systolic, due to ventricular contraction; and the third, due to increased flow in diastole.

The action of drugs on the coronary circulation is summarized in table 8 (132).

Hepatic and Portal Circulations

The liver receives blood, not only from the *hepatic artery* in which the blood flows under a high pressure, but also from the *portal system* which carries blood that has passed through the capillaries of the gastrointestinal apparatus and of the spleen. The arterial supply of the liver (about one-fourth of the total volume of blood entering the liver) insures an adequate amount of oxygen. The pressure of the arterial vessels is lowered, by resistance, to a level at which it does not interfere with the flow of portal blood into the liver. Arterial blood and portal blood meet in the peripheral part of the lobules, where they enter the *sinusoids*. The mixed blood proceeds through these large channels to the center of the lobule where it enters the branches of the *hepatic veins*. It is then collected into larger and larger veins until it reaches the inferior vena cava. The average amount of blood passing through the liver has been estimated as equivalent to over one-fifth of cardiac output (100b).

It is apparent that the portal blood is in the unique position of passing through *two capillary systems*. Therefore, the pressure in the hepatic capillaries is very low (3–4 mm. Hg). As the walls of these capillaries are permeable to plasma proteins, the effective osmotic pressure will also be about 3–4 mm. Hg. Lymph is formed with great ease and contains a percentage of protein as high as that of the blood.

Complex regulatory mechanisms exist in the hepatic vessels. They were demonstrated in dogs by *Mautner* and *Pick* (89) and confirmed in human beings (93, 94). Spiral or annular bands, acting like *sphincters*, exist at the junction of the hepatic veins with the cava, near the central veins within the liver, and in the sinusoids. Both the terminations of the portal veins and those of the hepatic artery may contract, and vasoconstriction of the mesenteric vessels may also occur; therefore, multiple changes may take place. It is not clear, as yet, whether a *sluice* or *throttle mechanism* exists in man or whether there is a diffuse contraction of the entire hepatic venous system (178).

The hepatic veins contract under the action of certain chemicals (peptone, histamine, digitalis) and relax under the action of others (epinephrine). We know little, as yet, about innervation of the hepatic veins. While most splanchnic arterioles are constricted by epinephrine, those of the small intestine seem to dilate (16).

TABLE 8

INCREASED CORONARY FLOW	DECREASED CORONARY FLOW	MECHANISM
Nitrites ++		Dilatation of the vessels (greater than blood pressure drop?)
	Digitalis glycosides in toxic doses	Vasoconstriction connected with vagus stimulation?
Digitalis glycosides in therapeutic doses		
Xanthines, especially theophylline ++ and aminophylline +++		Vasodilation (greater than blood pressure drop?)
Morphine +		Due to central action?
Papaverine +++ and khellin ++++		Direct action on smooth muscles of the coronary arteries
	Foreign proteins, pituitrin, pitressin, angiotonin	Direct action on smooth fibers of coronary arteries
Adrenalin, ephedrine		Direct dilatation of the small vessels; possible constriction of large coronary arteries (in man) compensated by increased blood pressure
Thyroxin		Action probably connected with tachycardia and increased blood pressure
Acetylcholine, mecholyl, doryl— in small dose	Acetylcholine, mecholyl, doryl— in large dose	These actions may vary from one species to another and with the dose
Atropine		Through inhibition of vagal stimuli
Coramin	Nicotine	
Nembutal, insulin, histamin	Histamin	The results are different in the various species and may vary with the dose

It has been demonstrated that, in shock, the liver becomes the seat of formation of a *vaso-depressor material* (VDM) which makes the terminal arterioles refractory to the action of epinephrine. The possibility that this substance is a normal component of the blood and takes part in the regulation of blood pressure, has been advocated (143).

Splenic Circulation

The vascular spaces of the splenic pulp have a large capacity and may contain a large percentage of the blood volume. We owe to *Barcroft* (95) the knowledge that the spleen is an organ of different size under varying conditions. The comparative size of animal spleen has been shown to differ under the influence of emotion, exercise, hemorrhage, asphyxia, pregnancy, and death. As both the capsule and the trabeculae of this organ contain smooth muscle, the conception of "spleen contractility" was soon established. However, muscle fibers are poorly distributed in the human spleen (96) and undeniable rhythmic changes of the spleen volume were attributed to variations of blood flow (97). Negative assertions (98) justify the following conservative view. There is no doubt that the volume of the spleen may vary under different conditions and a percentage of the contained blood may be mobilized; there is no question that the spleen may shrink under the effect of sympathetic stimuli or epinephrine. We do not know whether this is due to contraction of the arterial musculature or to that of other elements of the spleen.

Blood Reservoirs

We have seen that many organs of the body, containing a large amount of blood, may act as *blood reservoirs* or *blood depôts*. These are the lungs, the liver, and the spleen. The *large veins* all over the body, possibly also the large arteries, may act as reservoirs. The *subpapillary plexus* of the skin also constitutes a reservoir of considerable volume. Concurrent dilatation of large sections of the *capillary network* may alter the capacity of the vascular system completely and may have the function of blood depôt.

In addition to these more mechanical examples of reservoirs, we should keep in mind that many organs and tissues are able to store tremendous amounts of fluid, thereby preventing great changes in the composition of the blood. Among them, the liver, the peritoneal cavity, and the skin, are the most important.

Experiments based on the rapid intravenous injection of physiologic salt solution amounting to even three times the blood volume have been made in dogs without impairing the life of the animals. This would not be possible if water were not removed from the blood very rapidly (99).

Renal Circulation—Renal Pressor System

The average weight of the heart approximates that of the kidneys. More than one-fifth of the total blood volume (1200 cc.) flows through the kidneys in 1 minute (100). This tremendous blood flow is apparently due to the high degree of development of the glomerular apparatus and to the high pressure of the renal artery.

Histological studies (101) seem to indicate the existence of specialized secretory cells in the wall of the afferent glomerular arterioles. These might be the source of a proteolytic enzyme, called *renin*, which is normally present, but is excreted in greater amount if abnormal local conditions of circulation occur (102).

It was thought that *anoxia* was the cause of release of renin. It seems now that the kidney contains pressoreceptors, and that *renin is released when blood pressure drops below 80 mm. Hg in the renal arterioles* (174).

Action of renin on a fraction of blood plasma leads to formation of a new substance, called *angiotonin* or *hypertensine*. This is probably a polypeptide and exerts a powerful hypertensive action through direct stimulation of the smooth muscles of the peripheral arteries. Angiotonin is rapidly destroyed in normal conditions by the action of another enzyme present in the blood and in many organs, called *angiotonin inhibitor* or *hypertensinase*.

This hormonal action of the kidney may be important in physiological conditions associated with low blood pressure and in the clinical syndrome of hypotension and certainly is important in clinical hypertension.

In addition to the better known renal pressor system (see above), another pressor substance has been described. This was called *vasoexcitatory material* (VEM) and potentiates the action of epinephrine on the arterioles. The possibility that this substance, definitely important in shock, takes part in the normal regulation of blood pressure, has been advocated (143). This substance differs from hypertensine because it has no direct action on smooth muscles and it may be produced *in vitro* in the absence of blood plasma components (143).

Branches of both the sympathetic and the vagus nerves reach the kidneys. Stimulation of one splanchnic nerve results in reduction of urine volume on the same side. If the renal nerves are previously cut, however, stimulation of one of the splanchnic nerves causes a profuse flow of urine. This shows that sympathetic fibers constrict the renal vessels and that increased pressure in the renal artery (as obtained by nerve stimulation after cutting of the renal nerves) causes increased filtration in the glomeruli.

The kidneys have a very important rôle in maintaining a normal plasma volume and a normal osmotic balance between intravascular and extravascular fluids.

Cerebral Circulation

A feature of the cerebral circulation is the impossibility of great expansion of its vascular bed owing to the rigid walls of the skull. A greater oxygen supply to the brain is assured more through increase in the speed of blood than by dilatation of the vessels. Therefore, important variations of the intracranial flow are dependent upon the level of blood pressure in the general circulation. However, vasomotor actions have also been demonstrated (103). These have importance when localized, because changes in one vascular district may be compensated by opposite changes in another

and are not hindered by the bony structure of the skull. Sympathetic fibers are vasoconstrictor just as in the visceral districts. Vascular spasms have been demonstrated by direct experimental observation (104) and have importance in human pathology.

It should be remembered that *carbon dioxide*, independently of any general effect, is a powerful dilator of the cerebral vessels.

Functions of the Veins—Control of Venous Return

The return of blood through the venous system is due only partly to remaining force after it has passed through one or more capillary systems. Many different mechanisms have been recognized which favor the venous return:

a) Contractions of the veins (105–107).

b) Decreasing pressure in the large veins due to the action of the heart (systolic suction, page 39).

c) Aspirating effect of the low pressure existing in the thorax on the right atrium and the large veins.

d) Action of skeletal muscles on the nearest veins.

e) Action of respiration.

Respiration develops a multiple action on the heart and on the veins. During inspiration, the diaphragm contracts and exerts pressure downwards. As a result, the following changes will take place:

a) The intrathoracic pressure becomes lower and the intra-abdominal pressure higher, favoring a blood movement from the abdomen to the thorax.

b) The liver is compressed by the diaphragm and "wrung out" (108, 142).

c) The pericardial sac is distended and its complementary sinuses open favoring the filling of the atria (108). The mouths of both cavae, but mainly that of the inferior cava, are dilated.

As a result, the blood moves from the portal circulation to the heart, mainly during inspiration (108). The blood of the lower extremities and that of the head, on the contrary, shows less marked changes and a more constant course. Still, a remarkable inspiratory collapse of the superficial veins of the neck may be observed.

Central regulation controls tonus and contractility of the veins. Venous constriction leads to reduction of venous vascular volume; this temporarily increases venous return and may raise central venous pressure (if the right heart cannot elevate its output). Carotid sinus, aortic, pulmonary, and atrial reflexes, are involved in the regulation of venous tonus. Acidosis and anoxia cause venous contraction and increase venous pressure.

Venous pressure varies with the caliber of the vessels. It is about 3.3 mm. Hg (4.5 cm. H₂O) in the *venules*, about 6 mm. Hg (8 cm. H₂O) in the *large veins*, and very close to 0 before entering *the right atrium* (page 45). The normal pressure *in the veins of the arm* is about 5 mm. Hg (7 cm. H₂O) with the arm at the level of the right atrium; a pressure gradient of 3 to 4 mm. Hg exists in the normal circulation between a vein of the arm and the right atrium.

The pulsating pressure existing in the arterial system is damped out by the arterioles and it is normally *not* transmitted to the capillaries. It has been stated that, in conditions of high temperature, hyperthyroidism, or sleep, pulsations can be observed in the capillaries or veins. It is quite probable, however, that the rhythmic changes in color of the skin are due only to pulsation of the arterioles. Venous pulsations may be due to rapid flow through the a-v capillaries or to transmission from the nearest artery.

Functions of the Capillaries

The main function of the arteries and veins is to maintain an adequate blood flow through the capillaries, in order to preserve the essential aim of the circulation. This is the transfer of water, dissolved substances, and gases from the blood to the extracapillary spaces, and from these to the blood.

The arterioles, the capillaries, and the venules seem to constitute an *organic unit* having a variable capacity. The number of venules containing an active flow varies constantly but a progressive restriction of blood flow may take place without interrupting the continuous flow to the veins. This is made possible by the existence of *preferential channels* having a central position and, occasionally, an anatomical differentiation (144). Direct visualization shows a periodic constriction and dilatation of the terminal arterioles and precapillaries which is independent of the larger arteries (144). The interchange of material through the capillary wall occurs mainly *between* the cells and not through them (144).

The capillary wall is permeable to all plasma constituents of small molecular size. The plasma proteins, on the contrary, are made up of larger molecules and do not pass through this wall unless it is damaged. The smallest of the plasma proteins is the *albumin* molecule which is still 350 times heavier than that of glucose.

Dissolved oxygen is more concentrated in plasma than in tissue fluids, and therefore moves out of the blood by simple diffusion.[25]

The plasma proteins, being nondiffusible, exert *osmotic pressure* on the capillary wall, tending to retain and attract water. This avoids the possibility of too much fluid being lost with resultant emptying of the capillaries. This osmotic pressure is largely due to the albumin molecules.[26] The capillary blood pressure, on the other hand, tends to push water through the wall and is called, therefore, *filtration pressure.*

[25] As known, the largest amount of oxygen is carried by the red cells and not by the plasma. However, as soon as oxygen passes from the plasma to the tissues, the red cells rapidly "unload" their oxygen, so that the whole process is carried on uniformly and quickly.

[26] It is now recognized that the capillary wall is not completely impermeable to proteins. A restricted rate of diffusion exists for fibrinogen, albumin and globulin, so that their osmotic pressure is reduced to from 70 to 90 per cent of what it would be under conditions of free diffusion.

A *perfect balance is always present between capillary filtration pressure and osmotic pressure* unless severe changes develop.

Direct experiments have proven that in any given capillary at the level of the heart, water is lost from the plasma at the arterial end and is taken up at the venous end. In capillaries below the level of the heart, gravity adds to the filtration pressure, and there tends to be a loss of water from the capillaries.

In the capillaries of the pulmonary circulation, there is little tendency towards any outward filtration of water under normal conditions. This is because their blood pressure is less than the osmotic pressure. On the other hand, blood pressure is high in the capillary loops of the renal glomerulus, even approaching the arterial pressure, so that a large amount of water is filtered from them into the lumen of the Bowman's capsule.

The balance of fluid exchange is also maintained by *delicate vasomotor adjustments* which vary the surface over which outward filtration takes place (145). It has been maintained that *outward filtration* takes place chiefly in the preferential channels while *inward filtration* occurs in the true capillaries having marked variations of flow and pressure as a result of contraction of the precapillary sphincters (145).

The *normal pressure in the capillaries* is about 25 mm. Hg both in man and in the other mammals. The average pressure is determined by: a) the *vis a tergo* (arterial pressure), b) the resistance to outflow (venous pressure), c) the balance between filtration pressure and osmotic pressure, d) mechanical pressure of the surrounding tissues, and e) capillary contractility.

Localized effects on the feeding artery and on the vein of outflow may cause *diffuse changes*. Local contractility may influence the pressure in an *individual capillary*.

It is now known that the dynamic function of the *arteriole* is the regulation of the resistance from arteries to capillaries. The *metarterioles*, on the other hand, undergo periodic dilatations and constrictions at intervals of 15 sec. to 3 min. These may well control the patency and the filling of groups of capillaries (14, 119).

Arteriovenous anastomoses are present in the human skin. They are usually closed under normal conditions and at room temperature but open under critical conditions, rapidly shunting a certain amount of blood without its having to pass through the capillaries with loss of temperature (109). A different view admits that these *a-v capillaries* always have a vigorous circulation and offer little resistance to the blood flow in contrast to the true capillaries.

Microscopic observation of the human capillaries in the nail bed gives the opportunity to observe that a single capillary may undergo the following changes:

a) Complete disappearance, evidence of tonic contraction of its wall.

b) Complete filling, without evidence of any active influence on its content.

c) Slow progression of large bead-like dilatations, whose motion is slower than that of the red cells in the lumen (117).

The forces which determine changes of the capillaries are, on the one hand, the activity of the *reticulus* (110) (opening and closing of the capillaries) and, on the other hand, the activity of the *endothelium*. This is endowed with some kind of *tonus*, a property which is analogous to the elasticity of other structures and may be modified by poisons or drugs (184).

The term *vasomotion* has been used in reference to periodic vasomotor activity of the terminal vascular bed which is due to contractions and relaxation of the smooth muscles of the precapillary organs (184).

Evidence of innervation of the capillaries should be considered as inconclusive. Regulation of the capillary flow is obtained through arteriolar and venular changes plus direct action of products of the metabolism.

Capillary resistance to flow is regulated by

two hormones (190). *Cortisone increases capillary resistance while a somatotropic anterior pituitary hormone (STH) decreases it.* Normal capillary resistance seems to reflect a balance between the two hormones.

Whenever the skin is stimulated by physical agents (stroking, heat, cold, ultraviolet light, etc.), capillary dilatation takes place, preceded by dilatation of the arterioles. The arteriolar dilatation seems caused by a reflex (*axon reflex*); the capillary dilatation is due to formation of a *histamine-like substance* in the area of irritation. Most of the changes in capillary diameter which occur when a tissue passes from rest to an active state are the result of lack of oxygen and accumulation of metabolism products.

Blood Pressure

Blood pressure, or more correctly "arterial blood pressure", continuously oscillates between two extremes. The *maximum* corresponds to the peak of the pulse in a pressure curve and is called *systolic pressure*, because it takes place during the systolic contraction of the ventricles. The *minimum* corresponds to the foot of the pulse in a pressure curve, and is called *diastolic pressure*, because it takes place at the end of ventricular diastole, just prior to the arrival of the following wave (fig. 43).

The basic factors which influence the blood pressure can be studied on experimental models.

The two fundamental data of the blood pressure are *mean pressure* and *pulse pressure* (figs. 43 and 44).

Mean blood pressure rises when one of the following changes takes place:

a) The rate of the pump increases.

b) The systolic discharge increases.

c) The peripheral resistance increases.

It falls, on the contrary, if any of these factors decrease.

Pulse pressure is increased by any of the following changes:

a) Decreased heart rate.

b) Increased systolic discharge.

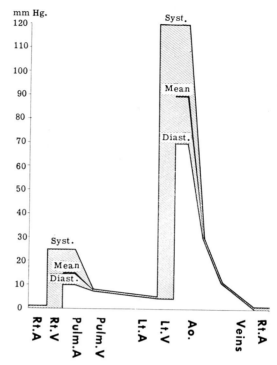

Fig. 43. The pressure in the various sections of the cardiovascular system.

c) Decreased extensibility of the aorta.

d) Decreased peripheral resistance.

It decreases, on the contrary, if any of these factors varies in the opposite sense.

It is apparent that the combination of changes of pulse pressure and mean pressure can modify the systolic and the diastolic pressure, these being only the secondary expressions of the basic pressure elements.

Studies of the changes of the pressure in an *elastic system* show that the pulse pressure gradually decreases while the mean pressure is nearly constant (113). *A system of rigid tubes,* on the contrary, shows a gradual drop of the mean pressure with barely any change of the pulse pressure (fig. 45). These facts have a certain bearing on the study of the pressure in different arteries of the same individual.

If the tubes are rigid, a rapid increase in the pressure of the fluid as it enters the tube produces a compression wave which

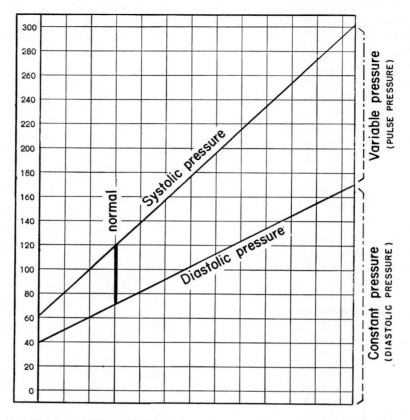

FIG. 44. The different elements of blood pressure in the normal subject and in the common deviations from norm.

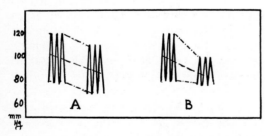

FIG. 45. Changes occurring in the oscillating pressure of a system of tubes. A, rigid tubes; B, elastic tubes.

travels with the velocity of sound to the end of the system. The increased pressure causes increased flow but the rate of increase of the latter is slower than that of the former because of inertia of the fluid (121). *If the tubes are distensible*, as are blood vessels, they present changes in caliber and

length which make up the visible "pulsation." The pressure wave is transmitted more slowly than in rigid tubes and is damped out faster by the imperfect elasticity of the system (121).

Blood pressure presents continuous *rhythmical fluctuations*. These may be due to the following causes (123):

1) Changes of cardiac activity.
2) Effect of respiratory activity:
   a) Mechanical effect of the respiratory pump mechanism.
   b) Irradiation of impulses from the respiratory to the vasomotor center (*Traube-Hering waves*).
3) Rhythmical variations of tone of the vasomotor center much slower than respiration (*S. Mayer waves*).

The blood pressure has different average

levels in the various species as shown by table 9 (145).

The *average level of blood pressure in man* is 120 mm. Hg for the systolic and 75 mm. Hg for the diastolic. Extreme ranges of *normal blood pressure* are 150 and 95 for the systolic, 90 and 60 for the diastolic (115).

Blood pressure level in the first part of life can be seen in table 10, made from *Allen's* data (115).

It is now agreed that systolic blood pressure rises until the age of 16, then drops about 10 mm. until the age of 18 (115). Diastolic pressure reaches a level of about 75 mm. between 14 and 16 and then remains constant. There is an unusual degree of lability between 17 and 20 years of age. *Then blood pressure becomes stabilized with an average of 120/75 for men and 113/70 for women, and does not change with age unless pathological processes occur.*[27] *This means that normal figures vary between 95/65 and 150/90 and that these extremes should be considered as borderline figures as long as they are recorded in basal conditions* (note 22, page 44).

The blood pressure tends to be higher in broad-built persons than in thin slender individuals (140).

Blood pressure varies physiologically under the action of emotion, physical exercise, meals, temperature changes, etc. The complex of changes due to meals and sleep usually reaches 25 mm. Hg for the systolic and 10 mm. for the diastolic in bedridden patients (116). The average minimum is found between 3 and 5 a.m.; the average maximum between 3 and 5 p.m. (116).

[27] The old rule that normal systolic pressure increases with age and that it is equivalent to 100 plus the age of the person is based on actual data and can be used as a rule of thumb (172). However, *such an increase is not caused by a physiological process but by a frequent and benign aging of the arteries.* Therefore, while no therapeutic measure is justified in a man of 60 who has a systolic pressure of 160, another 60-year-old man may have a systolic pressure of 120 *without deviating from norm.*

TABLE 9. *Mean blood pressure of various animals (carotid artery)*

ANIMAL	MEAN PRESSURE mm. Hg
Horse	150–190
Cow	125–160
Calf	160–180
Sheep	90–140
Goat	120
Pig	145–185
Dog	120–175
Cat	140–170

The mean pressure of the dog is lower than indicated by the above figures, reported from *Dukes* (145). Normal dogs have a mean pressure of 120 to 140 mm. Hg.

TABLE 10

	NEWBORN INFANTS	END OF 1ST WEEK	END OF 1ST MONTH	3–9 YEARS	10–12 YEARS	13–14 YEARS	16 YEARS
Systolic pressure	43–55	60	82	91	99	104	120
Diastolic pressure	—	—	—	—	60	65	76

The fall in blood pressure along the arterial system depends upon the relative sizes and lengths of the different vessels. Thus, while capillaries are the narrowest vessels, their great number and short length combine to make them offer less resistance to flow than the arterioles which are the site of the greatest pressure drop.

The Arterial Pulse

The left ventricle empties itself at each beat into the aorta. The aorta offers little resistance to the flow of blood. Its distensibility is such that there is a variable resistance according to the heart rate and the rapidity of pressure changes.

When the pressure rises suddenly (ventricular systole), the aortic volume has a considerable increase amounting to the creation of a new space (*aortic reservoir*). When the pressure falls (ventricular diastole) the retraction of the wall can be compared to the reinjection of blood from the reservoir into the arterial system so that the pressure tends to be maintained in spite of the lack of flow from the heart.

The *pulse wave* caused by the contraction of the heart travels through the aorta and large vessels much faster than the rate at which the blood flows toward the periphery. The difference becomes considerable in the abdominal aorta and in the large arteries of the lower extremities. The difference disappears, on the other hand, in the arterioles as the pulsating pressure is converted into steady pressure and flow.

At every point of its progress, the pulse wave is accompanied by a stretching of the arterial walls resulting in the enlargement of the vessel, and by an acceleration in the flow of blood. At the closure of the semilunar valves, the recoil of the aorta maintains the onward drive of the blood. At this time the peripheral arteries are still undergoing distention but they return to their smaller size as the excess of blood flows through the capillaries. The distention caused by the emptying of the left ventricle into the aorta spreads through the arterial system toward the periphery in the form of a wave which is felt as "the pulse."

The central pulse of the aorta is characterized by:

a) A *sudden rise* (opening of aortic valves).

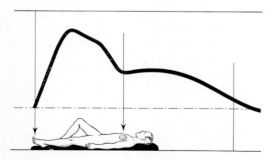

FIG. 46. When the front of the pulse wave reaches the most distant capillaries, the end of the wave is still in the left ventricle. Normal person. Duration of ejection period of systole: 0.24 seconds. Time necessary for reaching the arteria dorsalis pedis: 0.20 seconds. Speed: 6 meters per second.

b) A *systolic plateau* with an occasional peak (systolic ejection).

c) A sudden fall, called the *incisura* (closing of aortic valves).

d) A few rapid after-vibrations.

e) A slow secondary wave, called the *dicrotic wave.*

f) A slow descent until the next wave starts.

The shape of the *systolic part of the pulse* may vary according to four factors: ventricular ejection, transmission time of the pulse wave, reflected waves, and flow through the arterioles. Vasoconstriction tends to cause a steeper rise by reducing the peripheral flow while vasodilatation produces a rounded shape with slow descent before the incisura (120).

The *peripheral pulse* is different from the central pulse. The curve is more rounded, the incisura becomes like a rounded valley, and the dicrotic wave like a gently rounded hill. The distance between the peak of the main wave and the peak of the dicrotic wave increases toward the periphery showing that the latter has less speed (fig. 62).

The peripheral pulse represents *a basic pressure wave* created in the aorta and transmitted toward the periphery *plus waves reflected from the periphery.* These reflected waves are projected back into the aorta almost simultaneously and create by summation a large pressure oscillation or *standing wave* within the large arterial reservoir (183). This summated wave rises just after the foot of the basic wave has reached the femoral artery, so that the two waves merge. As a result, *the systolic peak of the femoral pulse is higher than that of the aortic pulse.*

A sudden increase in speed takes place with the passage of the pulse; then the blood flow slows down.

It should be remembered that the length and speed of the pulse wave are such that the latter includes nearly all the arterial system. When the front of the wave is in the arterial dorsalis pedis, the end of it is flowing into the aorta (fig. 46). However, an extremely rapid heart rate may lead to the existence of more than one wave in the arterial system (117).

The velocity of the pulse wave in man varies according to the type of artery. It is about 5 meters per second in the more elastic aorta, about 8 meters per second in the more muscular iliac and brachial arteries (120, 181).

Regulation of the Respiration; Correlations Between Respiratory System and Circulation

The activity of the respiratory center, which is located in the medulla, is modified by a chemical and a reflex mechanism.

Chemical regulation is based on the results of either *carbon dioxide* or *pH* changes on the respiratory center. Any increased content of CO_2 (*hypercapnia*), as well as any decreased pH (*acidosis*), leads to increased activity of the respiratory center.

The *reflex action* may be either excitatory or inhibitory. Distention of the carotid sinus and of the aorta depresses the respiration. Distention of the large veins increases the respiration. Stimuli arising in the lungs and various other organs may act in different ways upon the respiratory center. Stimulation of the chemoreceptors of the carotid and aortic bodies, on the other hand, may temporarily increase the depth and rate of respiration. It should be kept in mind that respiratory changes, induced by chemoreceptors, take place virtually only in emergencies and not as a response to physiologic phenomena. Asphyxia, high altitude flying, prolonged under-sea swimming, and intravenous drug administration, should be considered outside this range.

Inspiration increases the filling pressure of the right atrium and the amplitude of the variations of right atrial pressure due to atrial contraction. The greater filling pressure leads to greater output of the right ventricle. This, however, is largely accommodated in the pulmonary vessels, and left ventricular output may be decreased. A little later, the left ventricle receives an increased flow, so that both systolic and pulse pressure rise in the systemic circulation (138).

BIBLIOGRAPHY

1. ENGELMANN, T. W. Arch. Anat. Phys., 1902, 443; also: Pfluegers Arch., 1896, **65,** 109 and 535.
2. SCHELLONG. Deut. med. Woch., 1926, **52,** 862.
3. STRAUB, H. Bioch. Zeit., 1910, **28,** 394.
4. GASKELL, W. H. J. Physiol., 1883, **4,** 43; 1884, **5,** 46; and 1888, **7,** 1. Also in *Schaefer's Textbook of Physiology.* Edinburgh, Pentland, 1900.
5. a) LUDWIG, C. Zeit. f. rat. Med., 1849, **7,** 203.
   b) ENGELMANN, T. W. Pfluegers Arch., 1892, **52,** 357.
   c) FRANK, O. In *Tigerstedts Handbuch der physiol. Methoden;* 1913, **2,** (4), 176.
   d) STRAUB, H. In *Abderhalden Handbuch der biolog. Arbeitsmeth.;* 1923, **5,** (4), 911.
6. HENDERSON, Y. Am. J. Physiol., 1906, **16,** 325.
7. ROTHBERGER, J. Pfluegers Arch., 1907, **118,** 353.
8. STARLING, E. H., *et al.* J. Physiol., 1914, **48,** 357 and 465.
9. KATZ, L. N., *et al.* Am. J. Physiol., 1945, **143,** 507.
10. PRATT, F. H., AND EISENBERGER, J. P. Am. J. Physiol., 1919, **49,** 1.
11. BARD, P. *Macleod's Physiology in Modern Medicine.* 9th Ed. St. Louis, Mosby, 1941.
12. a) BOWDITCH, H. P. Ber. der Saechsischen Ges. der Wiss., 1871.
    b) HOFF, H. E. Yale J. Biol. & Med., 1942, **14,** 635.
13. STARLING, E. H., AND VISSCHER, M. B. J. Physiol., 1927, **62,** 243.
14. WIGGERS, C. J. *Physiology in Health and Disease.* 4th Ed. Philadelphia, Lea and Febiger, 1944.
15. EVANS, C. L., AND STARLING, E. H. J. Physiol., 1914, **49,** 67.
16. BEST, C. H., AND TAYLOR, M. B. *The Physiological Basis of Medical Practice.* Baltimore, The Williams & Wilkins Co., 1950.
17. a) LANGENDORFF, O. Pfluegers Arch., 1895, **61,** 291; and Erg. Phys., 1905, **4,** 764.
    b) STANNIUS. Arch. Anat. Phys., 1852, 85.
18. BOZLER, E. Am. J. Physiol., 1942, **136,** 543.
19. LEWIS, T., MEAKINS, J., AND WHITE, P. D. Phil. Tr., London, Ser. B., 1914, **205,** 375.
20. EYSTER, J. A. E., AND MEEK, W. G. Heart, 1914, **15,** 119; and Am. J. Physiol., 1922, **61,** 117 and 130.

21. a) GÉRAUDEL, E. *Le Mécanisme du Coeur et ses Anomalies.* Paris, Masson, 1928.
    b) VAQUEZ, H., AND DONZELOT, E. *Les Troubles du Rythme Cardiaque.* Paris, Ballière, 1926.
22. CONDORELLI, L. Zeit. exp. Med., 1929, **68,** 493.
23. ROBB, J. S., AND ROBB, R. C. Am. J. Physiol., 1936, **115,** 43.
24. LEWIS, T. *Diseases of the Heart.* London, Macmillan, 1933. Also *Clinical Disorders of the Heart Beat.* New York, Hoeber, 1916. Also *The Mechanism and Graphic Registration of the Heart Beat.* London, Shaw, 1925.
25. a) EPPINGER, H., AND ROTHBERGER, C. J. Wien. klin. Woch., 1909, **22,** 1091.
    b) ROTHBERGER, C., AND SCHERF, D. Zeit. exp. Med., 1927, **53,** 792.
26. HOFF, H. E., NAHUM, L. H., AND KISCH, B. Am. J. Physiol., 1941, **131,** 687 and 700.
27. KISCH, B., NAHUM, L. H., AND HOFF, H. E. Am. Heart J., 1940, **20,** 174.
28. KATZ, L. N. Am. Heart J., 1937, **13,** 17.
29. HOFF, H. E. New England J. Med., 1941, **225,** 28 and 1944; **231,** 529.
30. KISCH, B., Cardiol., 1940, **4,** 304. Also KISCH, B., NAHUM, L. H., AND HOFF, H. E. Am. Heart J., 1940, **20,** 174.
31. a) MAREY, E. J. *La Circulation du Sang.* Paris, Masson, 1881.
    b) LUCIANI, L. *Fisiologia dell' Uomo.* 6th Ed. Milan, S.E.L., 1923.
    c) STRAUB, H. In *Abderhalden's Handb. der biol. Arbeitsmethoden,* 1923, **5** (4), 885.
32. RINGER, S. Numerous articles published in J. Physiol. from 1882 to 1886.
33. LOCKE, F. S. Zentralbl. Phys., 1901, **14,** 670.
34. LUISADA, A. A. Am. Heart J., 1942, **23,** 676.
35. SMITH, J. R. Am. Heart J., 1944, **28,** 661.
36. STEFANI, A. *Contributi alla Fisiologia del Cuore e dei Vasi.* Reprinted by R. Acc. dei Lincei (Rome), 1916, **11,** 669.
37. CERADINI, G. Gazz. Med. Ital. Lomb. (Milan), 1871; also LUCIANI (31b).
38. TIGERSTEDT, R.: *Die Physiologie des Kreislaufs.* Berlin, Springer, 1921–1923.
39. HOUSSAY, B. A. Presse Méd., 1936, **44,** 1353.
40. ORIAS, O., AND BRAUN-MENÉNDEZ, E. *The Heart Sounds in Normal and Pathological Conditions.* New York, Oxford Univ. Press, 1939.
41. RAPPAPORT, M., AND SPRAGUE, H. B. Am. Heart J., 1941, **21,** 257 and 1942; **23,** 591.
42. BOYER, N. H. Am. Heart J., 1942, **23,** 797.
43. SOLLMANN, T. *A Laboratory Guide in Pharmacology.* Philadelphia, Saunders, 1922.
44. GROLLMAN, A. *The Cardiac Output of Man in Health and Disease.* Baltimore, Thomas, 1932.
45. a) STARR, I., RAWSON, A. J., SCHROEDER, H. A., AND JOSEPH, N. R. Am. J. Physiol., 1939, **127,** 1.
    b) COURNAND, A., AND CO-WORKERS. J. Clin. Investigation, 1942, **21,** 287; and 1945, **24,** 106.
46. LUISADA, A. A., MAUTNER, H., AND WEISZ, L., Arch. Pediatr., 1941, **58,** 562.
47. a) LENÈGRE AND MAURICE. Report to the Société Française de Cardiologie, 1944.
    b) RICHARDS, D. W., COURNAND, A., ET AL. Am. J. Physiol., 1942, **136,** 115.
    c) LAGERLÖF, H., AND WERKÖ, L. Acta Phys. Scand., 1948, **16,** 75.
48. LOEWI, O. Pfluegers Arch., 1924, **206,** 135; and 1925, **208,** 694.
49. CANNON, W. B., AND ROSENBLUETH, A. *Autonomic Neuro-Effector Systems.* New York, Macmillan, 1937.
50. HARVEY. Quoted by BEST AND TAYLOR (16).
51. FISCHER, E. Physiol. Rev., 1944, **24,** 467.
52. a) HUERTHLE, K. Pfluegers Arch., 1912, **147,** 582; also 1915, **162,** 302, 304, 359, and 413; also 1923, **200,** 49.
    b) KURSCHAKOFF. *Peripheral Arterial Circulation* (Russian). Moskow, State Medical Publ. House, 1930.
53. MAREŠ, F. Pfluegers Arch., 1916, **165,** 159.
54. FRENCKELL, G. Erg. inn. Med., 1930, **37,** 100.
55. LUISADA, A. A., AND TREMONTI, P. Lo Sperimentale (Florence), 1928, **82,** 401.
56. TREMONTI, P. Arch. Farmac. Sperim. (Rome), 1928, **46,** 119, 129 and 145.
57. LUISADA, A. A. Zeit. exp. Med., 1933, **91,** 432, 440 and 450.
58. a) DUNGERN V., M. Zeit. exp. Med., 1934, **94,** 754.
    b) UNGHVÀRY, L., AND OBÀL, F. Zeit. Kreislauff., 1940, **32,** 667.
59. HUERTHLE, K. Pfluegers Arch., 1935, **236,** 385; and Zeit. Kreislauff., 1934, **26,** 273.
60. MARCEAU, M. F. J. Phys. Path. Gen., 1938, **36,** 15 and 33, and 1939, **37,** 536. Also Exp. Med. and Surg., 1948, **6,** 13.
61. BERNARD, C. *Leçons sur la Physiologie du Système Nerveux.* Paris, 1858.
62. DALE, H. H. J. Physiol., 1933, **80,** 108.
63. a) BAINBRIDGE, F. A. J. Physiol., 1915, **50,** 65.
    b) SASSA, K., AND MIYAZAKI, H. J. Physiol., 1920, **54,** 203.
    c) NONIDEZ, J. F. Am. J. Anat., 1937, **61,** 203.
64. McDOWALL, R. J. A. J. Physiol., 1934, **85,** 5P; also Physiol. Rev., 1935, **15,** 98.

65. ANREP, G. V., AND SEGALL, H. N. Heart, 1925, **13**, 61.

66. HARRISON, T. R., AND CO-WORKERS. Am. J. Physiol., 1932, **100**, 417.

67. HEYMANS, C. New England J. Med., 1938, **219**, 147.

68. HEYMANS, C., BOUCKAERT, J. J., AND RE-GNIERS, P. Le Sinus Carotidien et la Zone Homologue Cardio-Aortique. Paris, Doin, 1933.

69. MCDOWALL, R. J. S. J. Physiol., 1934, **83**, 36P and 37P.

70. HUERTHLE, K., AND KOCH, E. Pfluegers Arch., 1935, **235**, 360.

71. CYON DE, E. Les Nerfs du Coeur. Paris, Alcan, 1906.

72. HERING, H. E. Pfluegers Arch., 1924, **206**, 721.

73. THOMAS, C. B., AND BROOKS, C. M. Am. J. Physiol., 1935, **113**, 130; and 1937, **120**, 195.

74. BACQ, Z. M., BROUHA, L., AND HEYMANS, C. Arch. int. Pharmacol. et Ther., 1934, **48**, 439.

75. BRONK, D. W., AND STELLA, G. J. Cell. & Comp. Physiol., 1932, **1**, 113.

76. KISCH, B. Lectures at the International University of Santander. Koeln, Kuschbert, 1934.

77. DRIPPS, R. D., AND COMROE, J. H. Am. J. Med. Sci., 1944, **208**, 681.

78. SCHWIEGK, H. Pfluegers Arch., 1935, **236**, 206.

79. BRUNELLI, B. Arch. Farmac. Sper., 1933, **56**, 557; and Fis. e Med. (Rome), 1933, **4**, 781, 872 and 887.

80. PARIN, V. V. Am. Rev. Soviet Med., 1944, **1**, 251; and Am. J. Med. Sci., 1947, **214**, 167.

81. DALY, DE B., I., AND VERNEY, E. B. J. Physiol., 1927, **62**, 330.

82. CATALDI, G. M. Arch. Mal. Coeur, 1935, **28**, 604.

83. RUBINO, A. Folia Med. (Naples), 1937, **23**, 1166.

84. JARISCH, A. Arch. Kreislauff, 1940, **7**, 260.

85. HOCHREIN, M. Deut. Ges. Kreislauff, 1935, **8**, 5; and Arch. Kreislauff, 1938, **14**, 24.

86. HOCHREIN, M., AND KELLER, C. J. Klin. Woch., 1934, **13**, 1383.

87. DALY DE B., I. Physiol. Rev., 1933, **13**, 149.

88. SJÖSTRAND, T. Quoted by BARD (11).

89. MAUTNER, H., AND PICK, E. P. Muench. med. Woch., 1915 (2d), **62**, 1141; and Bioch. Zeit., 1922, **127**, 72.

90. ENGEL, D. J. Physiol., 1941, **99**, 161, and 1943, **102**, 281.

91. ANREP, G. V., CRUICKSHANK, E. V., DOWN-ING, A. C., AND SUBBA RAU, A. Heart, 1927, **14**, 111.

92. GREGG, D. E., AND SHIPLEY, R. E. Am. J. Physiol., 1944, **141**, 382.

93. KATZ, L. N., AND RODBARD, S. J. Pharmacol. & Exper. Therap., 1939, **67**, 407.

94. SNYDER, C. D. Physiol. Rev., 1942, **22**, 54.

95. BARCROFT, J. Am. J. Med. Sci., 1930, **179**, 1.

96. GIUNTI, G. Arch. Ital. Anat. Ist. Pat., 1939, **10**, 123.

97. GRINDLEY, J. H., AND HERRICK, J. F. Proc. Staff Meet. Mayo Clin., 1938, **13**, 663.

98. RAVENNA, P. Arch. int. med., 1940, **66**, 879.

99. ZAK, E. Wien. Klin. Woch., 1930, **43**, 1589.

100. a) SMITH, H. W. The Physiology of the Kidney. New York, Oxford, 1937. Also J. Mt. Sinai Hosp., 1943, **10**, 41–108.
    b) BRADLEY, S. E. Bull. New England Med. Cent., 1945, **7**, 224.

101. GOORMAGHTIGH, N. Bruxelles Med. Abstr., J.A.M.A., 1939, **113**, 2457.

102. a) GOLDBLATT, H., LYNCH, J., HANZAL, R. F., AND SUMMERVILLE, W. W. J. Exp. Med., 1934, **59**, 347.
    b) BRAUN-MENÉNDEZ, E., FASCIOLO, J. C., LELOIR, L. F., MUÑOZ, J. M., AND TAQUINI, A. C. Hipertension Arterial Nefrogena. Buenos Aires, El Ateneo, 1943.

103. COBB, S. Assoc. Res. Nerv. & Ment. Dis., 1929, **9**, 458.

104. RISER, M. In Le Spasme Vasculaire, by HEYMANS AND BROUHA. Clermont Ferrand, Imprimerie de l'Avenir, 1937.

105. HOOKER, D. R. Physiol. Rev., 1921, **1**, 112.

106. GOLLWITZER-MEYER, K. Erg. der Phys., 1932, **34**, 1145.

107. MCDOWALL, R. J. S. Physiol. Rev., 1935, **15**, 98.

108. SCHUR, M. Erg. inn. Med., 1934, **47**, 348.

109. GRANT, R. T., AND VIKO, L. E. Heart, 1929, **15**, 103.

110. VOLTERRA, M. Arch. Mal. Coeur, 1927, **20**, 451.

111. KROGH, A. Anatomie und Physiologie der Capillaren. Berlin, Springer, 1924.

112. LUISADA, A. A. Zeit. exp. Med., 1929, **65**, 774.

113. LUISADA, A. A. Ipotensione e Iposfigmia. Deficienze di Circolo. Rome, Pozzi, 1929.

114. ALVAREZ, W. C., AND STANLEY, L. L. Arch. int. Med., 1930, **46**, 17.

115. ALLEN, E. V. Normal Blood Pressure. In Stroud's Cardiovascular Disease. Philadelphia, Davis, 1945 (vol. 2).

116. LUISADA, A. A. Rif. Med. (Naples), 1925, **41**, 817.

117. LUISADA, A. A. Arch. Mal. Coeur, 1927, **20**, 65.

118. a) PLECHKOVA, E. Bull. de Biol. et de Méd. Expér., 1936, **1**, 6, 402.

   b) LAVRENTIEV, B. I. Am. Rev. Soviet Med., 1946, **3**, 229.

119. a) ZWEIFACH, B. W. Am. J. Anat., 1936, 37, **60**, 473; and Cold Spring Harbor Symp. Quant. Biol., 1940, **8**, 216.

   b) PONDER, E. in Howell's *Textbook of Physiology*. Philadelphia, Saunders, 1946.

120. LAMPORT, H. In Howell's *Textbook of Physiology*. Philadelphia, Saunders, 1946.

121. HAMILTON, W. F. In Howell's *Textbook of Physiology*. Philadelphia, Saunders, 1946.

122. HOFF, H. E. In Howell's *Textbook of Physiology*. Philadelphia, Saunders, 1946.

123. SCHWEITZER, A. J. Physiol., 1945, **104**, 21.

124. LUISADA, A. A., RUBINO, A., AND CANELLA, C. Cardiol. (Basel), 1937, **1**, 280.

125. HECHT, H. Am. Heart J., 1946, **32**, 39.

126. ASHMAN, R., AND HULL, E. *Essentials of Electrocardiography*. New York, Macmillan, 1944.

127. BURCH, G., AND WINSOR, T. *A Primer of Electrocardiography*. Philadelphia, Lea and Febiger, 1945.

128. SODI PALLARES, D. *Nuevas Bases de Electrocardiografía*. Ed. del Inst. Nac. de Cardiol., Mexico, 1945.

129. ASHMAN, R., AND CO-WORKERS. Am. Heart J., 1943, **25**, 16 and 36; 1943, **26**, 473 and 495.

130. BAYLEY, H. R. Am. Heart J., 1944, **27**, 657.

131. WILSON, F. N., AND CO-WORKERS. Am. Heart J., 1931, **7**, 203, 207, and 305; 1934, **10**, 46 and 176.

132. RATNOFF, O. D., AND PLOTZ, M. Medicine, 1946, **25**, 285.

133. GREGG, D. E., AND SHIPLEY, R. E. Mo. Conc. Cardiovasc. Dis., 1944, **13**, N.4.

134. JOHNSON, J. R., AND WIGGERS, C. J. Am. J. Physiol., 1937, **118**, 38.

135. GILBERT, N. C., LE ROY, G. V., AND FENN, G. K. Am. Heart J., 1940, **20**, 519.

136. NYLIN, G. Am. Heart J., 1943, **25**, 598.

137. McMICHAEL, J., AND SHARPEY-SCHAFER, E. P. Brit. Heart J., 1944, **6**, 33.

138. LAUSON, H. D., BLOOMFIELD, R. A., AND COURNAND, A. Am. J. Med., 1946, **1**, 315.

139. COURNAND, A. Bull. New York Acad. Med., 1947, **23**, 27.

140. a) ROBINSON, S. C. AND BRUCER, M. Arch. Int. Med., 1939, **64**, 409.

   b) BRUCK, M. Cardiol. (Basel), 1940, **4**, 165.

141. WANG, S. C., AND BORISON, H. L. Am. J. Physiol., 1947, **150**, 712 and 722.

142. ECKSTEIN, R. W., GRAHAM, G. R., LIEBOW, I. M., AND WIGGERS, C. J. Am. J. Physiol., 1947, **148**, 745.

143. SHORR, E., ZWEIFACH, B. W., FURCHGOTT, R. F., AND BAEZ, S. Trans. Assoc. Am. Physicians, 1947, **60**, 28.

144. CHAMBERS, R., AND ZWEIFACH, B. W. Ann. New York Acad. Sci., 1946, **46**, 679; also Physiol. Rev., 1947, **27**, 436.

145. DUKES, H. H. *The Physiology of Domestic Animals*. 6th Ed. Ithaca, Comstock Publ. Co., 1947.

146. LUISADA, A. A. Acta Med. Scand., 1952, **142**, (Suppl. 266), 685.

147. LUISADA, A. A., ALIMURUNG, M. R., AND LEWIS, L. Am. J. Physiol., 1952, **168**, 226.

148. LUISADA, A. A., MENDOZA, F., AND ALIMURUNG, M. R. Brit. Heart J., 1949, **11**, 41.

149. NYLIN, G. Am. Heart J., 1945, **30**, 1; and Brit. Heart J., 1945, **7**, 81.

150. NYLIN, G., AND HEDLUND, S. Am. Heart J., 1949, **37**, 543.

151. FRIEDMAN, C. E. Am. Heart J., 1950, **39**, 397.

152. McMICHAEL, J., AND SHARPEY-SHAFER, E. P. Brit. Heart J., 1944, **6**, 33.

153. STEAD, E. A., AND WARREN, J. V. Arch. Int. Med., 1947, **80**, 237.

154. DI PALMA, J. R., AND REISS, R. A. Am. J. Physiol., 1948, **155**, 327.

155. HAMILTON, W. F., AND REMINGTON, J. W. Am. J. Physiol., 1948, **153**, 287.

156. BING, R. J., HEIMBECKER, R., AND FALHOLT, W. Am. Heart J., 1951, **42**, 483.

157. SPADOLINI, L. Arch. di Fis., 1949/1950, **49**, 166 and 287.

158. MALAMANI, V., BOBBA, P., AND BALDRIGHI, C. Folia Card., 1951, **9**, 229.

159. LITTLE, R. C. Am. J. Physiol., 1949, **158**, 237.

160. GUBNER, R., UNGERLEIDER, H. E., AND HIRSHLEIFER, I. Interamer. Congress of Card. Chicago, 1948.

161. SZENT-GYÖRGYI, A. Science, 1949, **110**, 411.

162. PRICE, P. B. J. A. M. A., 1951, **145**, 781.

163. FRIEDBERG, C. K. *Diseases of the Heart*. Philadelphia, Saunders, 1949.

164. a) LEWIS, TH., DRURY, A. N., AND OTHERS. Heart, 1921, **8**, 311 and 341.

   b) SCHERF, D., AND TERRANOVA, R. Am. J. Physiol., 1949, **159**, 137.

   c) PRINZMETAL, M., AND COWORKERS. *The Auricular Arrhythmias*. Springfield, Thomas, 1952.

165. PETERSON, L. H. Circ., 1950, **2**, 351.

166. HEYMANS, C., AND VAN DEN HEUVEL-HEYMANS, G. Circ., 1951, **4**, 581.

167. DUANCIC, V. Zeit. Kreslauff., 1942, **34**, 99.

168. FOLKOW, B. Acta Phys. Scand., 1949, **17**, 289.

169. RODBARD, S., AND SAIKI, H. Am. J. Physiol., 1952, **168**, 234.

170. TAYLOR, R. D., AND PAGE, I. H. Circ. 1951, **4**, 184.

171. CULBERTSON, J. W., HALPERIN, M. H., AND WILKINS, R. W. Am. Heart J., 1949, **37**, 942.

172. RUSSEK, H. I., AND ROTH, M. M. Am. Heart J., 1946, **32**, 468.

173. POLI, G. AND ROSSI, C. R. Arch. di Fis., 1949, **48**, 143.

174. DIVRY, A. Arch. Int. Phys., 1951, **59**, 211.

175. GHEORGHIU, P., AND COWORKERS. Bulet. Stint. Bucarest, 1950, 2/2, 85.

176. DE LA BARREDA, P., DE MOLINA, A. F., AND JIMENEZ DIAZ, C. Bull. Inst. Med. Res., 1948, **1**, 53.

177. AVIADO, D. M., AND COWORKERS. Am. J. Med. Sci., 1950, **220**, 707.

178. THOMAS, W. D., AND ESSEX, H. E. Am. J. Physiol., 1949, **158**, 303.

179. PAGE, I. H. Am. J. Physiol., 1950, **160**, 421.

180. LEVY, M. N., AND BERNE, R. M. Proc. Soc. Exper. Biol. & Med. 1949, **72**, 147.

181. SCHNABEL, T. G., RASHKIND, W. J., AND PETERSON, L. H. Am. J. Physiol., 1950, **163**, 748.

182. FLEISCHNER, F. G., ROMANO, F. J., AND LUISADA, A. A. Proc. Soc. Exper. Biol. & Med., 1948, **67**, 535.

183. HAMILTON, W. F., AND DOW, P. Am. J. Physiol., 1939, **125**, 48.

184. ZWEIFACH, B. W. Third Confer. on "Factors Regulating Blood Pressure". New York, J. Macy Jr. Found., 1949.

185. CATTELL, McK., AND GOLD, H. J. Pharmacol. & Exper. Therap., 1938, **62**, 116.

186. LUISADA, A. A., AND WEISS, M. Am. J. Physiol., 1954, **176**, 123.

187. WHITEHORN, W. V. XIX International Congress Physiology, Montreal, 1953.

188. VON BEZOLD, A. Untersuch. physiol. Lab. Wuerzburg, 1867, **1**, 73.

189. JARISCH, A., AND ZOTTERMANN, Y. Acta Phys. Scand., 1948, **16**, 31.

190. KRAMAR, J. XIX International Congress of Physiology, Montreal, 1953.

191. FOLKOW, B. Acta Phys. Scand., 1952, **27**, 99.

CHAPTER 4

The Clinical Study of the Cardiac Patient

The study of the cardiac patient is based upon history, physical examination and technical study.

History

The importance of the history cannot be overemphasized. However, the value of history is based on its accuracy. An adequate history is taken only by a man with clinical experience who knows how to elicit and evaluate the evidence given by the patient.

In the appraisal of the patient's complaints, two points should be kept in mind. 1) There is no symptom which is absolutely typical and can be accepted as evidence of heart disease. 2) A patient may have severe lesions of the cardiovascular apparatus without any symptoms. Therefore, not only the practitioner but also the cardiologist, to whom a "cardiac" patient has been referred, must bear in mind that the patient in question may not be a cardiac patient at all. In the following list of common complaints, different causes which may be responsible for the symptoms have been indicated.

CHIEF COMPLAINT

Palpitation is a common complaint based on the awareness of the heart beat. It often results from emotional disturbance and may not imply heart disease. It may be caused by increased force of cardiac action, rapid heart rate, or irregular heart action. Therefore, tachycardia and arrhythmias, as well as heart failure, are usually accompanied by palpitation. It may be due to abnormal increase or decrease of blood pressure. Palpitation is often related to hormonal unbalance (puberty, menopause, hyperthyroidism), fever, and even gastrointestinal disorders, or emotion.

Exertional dyspnea may be caused by early heart failure. On the other hand, it may be due to anemia, gastrointestinal disorders, emotional factors, fever, and pulmonary diseases. *Paroxysmal dyspnea* is nearly always due to heart disease but may be confused with bronchial asthma and vice versa. The possible occurrence of such attacks should be kept in mind, and adequate information requested.

Precordial pain upon exertion is frequently associated with heart disease. However, it may be caused by emotional factors, acute pericarditis or pleuritis, pleuropericardial adhesions, gastrointestinal disorders, or anemia. Even wider is the range of possible causes of *persistent procordial pain*, as intercostal neuralgia and acute lesions of abdominal viscera may be mistaken for cardiac attacks. Precordial pain due to coronary insufficiency is usually located *within the left anterior axillary* line and is seldom circumscribed to a small area. It frequently radiates to the left shoulder, the back, the left side of the neck, or the left arm and hand. In the last case, the ulnar side of the hand is typically predilected. It is frequently a deep, oppressive pain and may be felt at the base of the xiphoid process.

Fatigability (*asthenia*) is a frequent sign of cardiovascular disease. It is frequently caused, however, by anemia, lack of physical training, fever, pulmonary lesions, gall bladder and liver diseases, renal diseases, and malnutrition.

Cough is a common symptom of heart disease. It may be caused by pulmonary congestion, pulmonary edema, pulmonary infarction, aortic aneurysm or aortitis, chronic bronchitis, and other less frequent diseases (26).

Hemoptysis is not unusual in heart disease. It may be caused by pulmonary congestion or edema, aortic aneurysm, pulmonary infarction, or arteriosclerosis. It is particularly frequent in diseases with active congestion of the lungs (patent foramen ovale, patent ductus, Eisenmenger's syndrome) and in those having passive (or both active and passive) congestion of the lungs (mitral stenosis, Lutembacher's syndrome). It is favored by varices of the bronchial veins, arteriosclerosis of the pulmonary arterioles, or abnormality in the coagulation of the blood.

Nosebleeds (*epistaxis*) are common in rheumatic fever. *Hoarseness* (*disphonia*) may be evidence of cardiovascular lesions; however, it is frequently observed in pulmonary and mediastinal lesions.

Swelling of the legs (*edema*) is often due to cardiac failure. It may be caused by bilateral varicose veins; it may be favored by hepatic and renal lesions, anemia, myxedema, and vitamin deficiency, through changes in the osmotic properties of the blood.

Paroxysmal attacks of giddiness, dizziness, or fainting (*vertigo, syncope*) are frequently caused by cardiovascular lesions. On the contrary, they may be due to anemia, undernourishment, diseases of the nervous system, or changes of blood pressure (hypertension, hypotension).

Jaundice (*icterus*) is occasionally due to heart disease (through the influence that it has upon the liver) or follows pulmonary infarction. It is, however, much more frequently caused by lesions of the biliary system.

Epigastric distress or heaviness, hyperacidity, and belching, may be the result of cardiac disease. These disturbances are more often due to gastrointestinal or gallbladder disorders and to vitamin deficiencies.

Sleeplessness (*insomnia*) is a common sign of cardiovascular disease but may be due to numerous other diseases and to mental upset.

Headache (*cephalalgia*), *buzzing of the ears, or disturbances of vision* may be caused by cardiovascular disease, metabolic disorders, local conditions, or diseases of the nervous system.

PRESENT ILLNESS

In recording the details of the "present illness," the circumstances and modalities under which the different symptoms appeared and the sequence of their occurrence should be carefully recorded.

Information concerning how much exertion, above that which is customary for the patient, would cause either dyspnea or precordial pain is of value. This may supply an index about the functional efficiency of the heart when allowance is made for other conditions causing the same result (age, obesity, pulmonary emphysema, anemia, etc.). The number of pillows required for sleep may be taken as an index of the degree of orthopnea (shortness of breath relieved by upright position).

Attacks of *paroxysmal dyspnea* and *pulmonary edema* are often reported only if the physician describes their picture without, however, exerting suggestive influence on the patient.

When trying to ascertain the features of some acute attack, personal observations of the patient, and those of members of his household and of other physicians, should be requested and properly evaluated.

PAST HISTORY

This may reveal important data in evaluating the possible cause of heart disease. A history of tonsillitis, chorea, joint pains, or nosebleeds, or of long periods of malaise and weakness, may indicate the previous occurrence of *rheumatic fever*. A negative statement about any of these data does not exclude that rheumatic fever may have occurred. A history of streptococcic infections, diphtheria, or scarlet fever; of nephritis, syphilis, tuberculosis, diabetes, or bronchial asthma, is often significant.

A negative statement about venereal disease (including such family data as repeated abortions or stillbirths, and the occurrence of a single "benign" ulcer) does not exclude the possibility of *syphilis*.

The use of *drugs* (digitalis, nitroglycerine, quinidine, xanthines, barbiturates, sulfonamides, thyroid extract) and their effects, should be recorded.

A *review of the systems* at this point may elicit further symptoms which will be helpful in establishing date of onset and extent of damage.

Family and social history, marital history, occupational history, and knowledge of habits and vices, complete the clinical history and should be recorded with the customary rules of history taking.

Physical Examination

The importance of physical examination has decreased since many accurate technical methods of study have become available. It is still of great importance to the cardiologist, and even more to the practitioner who may not have the free use of such methods.

The orthodox teaching is that physical examination should include inspection, palpation, percussion, and auscultation. This may lead to a stereotyped method of examination (1). One should see which is the special objective to attain in the particular case and use any available method in reaching it. This includes both physical and technical methods.

GENERAL EXAMINATION

The general examination gives a first impression which may be of use after a more detailed examination.

In the first place, the general data of the patient will be noted. These include sex, age, build, height and weight, nutrition, decubitus, mental state, and color.

Erythema or *nodules* may be significant in rheumatic disease; *petechiae*, in subacute bacterial endocarditis.

Among the various decubitus, the *sitting* (*orthopneic*) *position*, the *bent forward* (*genupectoral*) *position*, and the *squatting position* (children), are particularly significant.

The *type of breathing*, and the presence of cough, and sputum, should be noted.

The existence of pallor, cyanosis, edema of the face, or jaundice, will be noted. As far as cyanosis is concerned, its distribution (nose, earlobes, nails, hands, feet, etc.) and its severity are of importance. In some cases, an increase in cyanosis after exertion or after exposure to cold is significant.

Cyanosis (kyanos = blue) is typical of rheumatic lesions of the mitral valve. Cyanosis is constant in the complex congenital heart diseases with shunting of the blood from the lesser to the greater circulation. Severe cyanosis is also constant in chronic lesions of the lungs with resulting *cor pulmonale*. Cyanosis may be a sign of heart failure, and is frequent in polycythemia. A local cyanosis may be due to peripheral vascular disease. If the feet are more cyanotic than the hands, this may indicate that a severe congenital malformation of the heart is present: the blood flows from the pulmonary artery into the aorta through the ductus and supplies largely the lower extremities (24). Exercise may accentuate this type of cyanosis.

Subicterus (slight jaundice) is frequent in the lesions of the tricuspid valve, in constrictive pericarditis, and in certain systemic or infectious diseases (rheumatic disease, syphilis). It is also common after pulmonary infarctions.

Hands, feet, and nose should be examined in order to ascertain the existence of *clubbing* and of *nodes* or *nodules*. *Clubbing* may be present in chronic cor pulmonale (through the pulmonary lesions), subacute bacterial endocarditis, and congenital heart disease. *Nodes* may be a sign of subacute bacterial endocarditis; *nodules*, of rheumatic disease.

Existence, distribution, and severity of *peripheral edema* should be recorded. One should observe the extension and turgidity of *collateral veins*, visible venous networks, spider angiomatas, and swollen lymph nodes.

Before starting a more detailed examination, the physician should also note temperature, respiratory rate, pulse rate, and blood pressure.[28]

Examination of the pulse has lost much of the importance it had in the past. Still, it may yield much valuable information in the hand of an experienced physician.

The following data will be noted.

a) Whether the pulse is *regular* (*rhythmic*) or *irregular* (*arrhythmic*). If irregular, the possibility that the irregularity occurs either *occasionally* or *periodically* (*allorhythmic pulse*) should be investigated. If the irregularity occurs periodically, a possible connection with the phases of respiration should be investigated. This is easily done by asking the patient first to breathe deeply and slowly (increase of the irregularity) and then to "hold his breath" (disappearance of the irregularity). The occasionally irregular pulse is called *intermittent pulse*. One of the most common types of allorhythmic pulse is the *bigeminal pulse*: a small pulse, due to a premature beat, closely follows the main pulse wave (page 349).

b) Whether the pulse is *rapid* or *slow*. The rate of the pulse (number of pulsations per minute) should be noted. A very slow pulse rate (80 in an infant, 60 in a child, 40 or less in an adult) suggests heart block.

c) Whether the pulse is *celer* (*collapsing*) or *tardus*. A *pulse celer* is that which quickly dilates the artery (typical in aortic insufficiency). A *pulsus tardus* is that which dilates the artery slowly (typical in aortic stenosis).

d) Whether the pulse is *small* or *large*, *soft* or *hard*. The first quality deals with the

volume of the pulse, the second with the ease or difficulty of compressing the artery up to the point of disappearance of the pulse, namely with the pulse pressure. A *small pulse* may be found in low blood pressure, mitral or aortic stenosis, heart failure, myocardial infarction, and occasionally in hypertension. A *large pulse* is typical of hypertension, and may also be found in the tetralogy of Fallot. A condition of *rigidity* of the arterial wall may be noted as evidence of arteriosclerosis.

e) Whether it is a *pulsus alternans*. This type of pulse is perfectly regular but shows the alternate occurrence of larger and smaller pulse waves (page 373).

f) Whether it is a *dicrotic pulse*, having a second small wave after the peak of the main wave. In some cases, the dicrotic pulse should be differentiated from the bigeminal or alternating pulse.

Comparison of the two radial pulses may reveal a smaller pulse on the left side, as in some cases of ductus arteriosus, aneurysm of the aortic arch, or atherosclerosis. In the case of aneurysm, the left pulse often is also delayed. More exceptionally, small pulse on the right side may be caused by aneurysms, complex congenital lesions, or atherosclerosis.

A *comparison of the radial with the femoral pulse* may reveal a small femoral pulse (coarctation of the aorta, embolism or thrombosis of the abdominal aorta) or, on the contrary, a large and strong femoral pulse (aortitis, aortic insufficiency). A delay of the femoral pulse may be caused by aneurysm of the abdominal aorta.

A *thrill*, either over the forearm or over the femoral artery, may be found in aortic regurgitation, patent ductus arteriosus, aortitis, fever, hyperthyroidism, or arteriovenous fistula.

Palpation of the *temporal arteries* and of the *arteria dorsalis pedis* on both sides completes the general examination and may reveal local changes of pulsation. In vascular diseases of the lower extremities, palpation of the popliteal, femoral, and posterior tibial

[28] Blood pressure measurement is actually part of the technical study of the patient. However, every physician is supposed to "take" blood pressure, and this should be done before the examination of the different systems. Details of blood pressure measurements will be given later (page 159).

arteries may give additional valuable information.

Regional examination may follow the usual rules. In the *examination of the head*, special attention should be paid to the existence of *exophthalmos* (protrusion of the eyes) and related ocular signs suggesting hyperactivity of the thyroid gland. Failure of the pupils to react to light (*Argyll-Robertson sign*) and their irregularity or inequality, may suggest syphilis. The *eye-grounds* have a special importance in hypertension. The mouth and throat may reveal chronic infections or evidence of vitamin deficiency.

The *examination of the neck*, apart from the existence of a large thyroid gland (suggesting a thyrotoxic heart) and of a *tracheal tug* (evidence of aortic aneurysm), should be devoted to the study of the vessels of the neck.

It is not always easy to distinguish the pulsations of the jugular veins from those of the carotid arteries. The *arterial pulsation* is rapid, limited, forceful, and easily palpable. The *venous pulsation*, on the contrary, is slow, undulant, and diffuse, and seems to disappear when the finger is placed on the pulsating area.

Increased pulsation of the carotid arteries is typical of aortic regurgitation, hypertension, aortitis, aortic aneurysm, atherosclerosis of the aorta, patent ductus arteriosus, and the tetralogy of Fallot. It is not uncommon in endocrine disorders (menopause), emotional states, anemia, or fever. Inequality between the right and left carotids may be found in aneurysm of the aortic arch (including dissecting aneurysm), patent ductus arteriosus, and, more rarely, atherosclerosis of the aorta. A strong pulsation above the right clavicle may be caused by aneurysm or by persistence of the right aortic arch.

The *jugular veins* may be constantly engorged, presenting only some degree of collapse during expiration. This is due to an obstacle to the passage of blood from the veins into the heart (blocked venous return) and is typical of the superior caval syndrome.

The veins may show strong pulsations. If these are of a physiological type, three for each apex beat (page 99), they are evidence of increased activity of the heart. They are common, therefore, in mitral valve defects, hypertension, anemia, and hyperthyroidism. Congestive failure is usually accompanied by strong jugular pulsations, evidence of high pressure in the right atrium.

An abnormal type of jugular pulsation, with systolic expansion, takes place in regurgitation of the tricuspid valve and is a valuable diagnostic sign (page 270).

Auscultation of the jugular veins reveals three dull sounds if the waves are high; it may reveal a confused, continuous murmur (*venous hum, bruit du diable*) in children or anemic patients.

Auscultation of the carotid arteries and of the suprasternal notch (2) is useful in differentiating various cardiac murmurs.

Examination of the thorax. Chest deformities will be noted because they may have relationship to heart disease. Abnormal *bulges* and *pulsations* of the chest outside the conventional precordial area are usually due to either an enlarged heart or aneurysms. *Arterial pulsations* in the intercostal spaces indicate the development of arterial collateral circulation, evidence of coarctation of the aorta.

Examination of the pleura and of the lungs will be made carefully. Pleural effusion, common in congestive failure; evidence of pulmonary emphysema; wheezing rales, common in cardiac asthma; and moist rales of small caliber, evidence of alveolar transudation, should be looked for and recorded.

The presence of *rales* may contribute to a correct diagnosis. Rales are common in conditions associated with a higher pressure of the pulmonary circulation (mitral valve defects, patent foramen ovale, transposition of the large vessels, Eisenmenger complex); they are uncommon in those associated with a lower pulmonary pressure (tricuspid stenosis or atresia, pulmonic stenosis or atresia, certain cases of adhesive pericarditis).

Areas of pulmonic consolidation may be evidence of pulmonary infarctions.

Examination of the abdomen may yield several important data. The most significant are:

a) Existence of *ascites*, which is more frequently seen in tricuspid valve lesions, constrictive pericarditis, and polyserositis.

b) *Enlargement of the spleen*, which is common in bacterial endocarditis as well as in acute infections and usually absent in rheumatic disease.

c) *Enlargement of the liver*. This is frequently a sign of congestive failure. It may be present, however, in tricuspid lesions and in constrictive pericarditis, even without failure. It may be caused by lues. *The liver may show active pulsations* which are appreciated by palpation (tricuspid regurgitation).

d) *Epigastric pulsations*, caused by abnormal dynamics of either the heart or the abdominal aorta.

e) Existence of *collateral veins* over the abdominal surface may have importance in the evaluation of a complex cardiohepatic syndrome.

Examination of the legs. The presence of edema, the superficial veins, and the pulsations of the femoral, popliteal, tibial, and pedal arteries, will be investigated. The study of the arteries may require the use of an *oscillometer* (page 160). Changes in the color and temperature of the skin in different positions and after exertion may have importance.

EXAMINATION OF THE HEART

Inspection

Inspection is the oldest method of examination. A first glance at the precordial area reveals whether there are *small venous*

dilatations, as frequently seen in chronic cardiac patients. These are sometimes related to anterior pericardial adhesions. It shows whether or not there is *bulging* of this area which is evidence of enlargement of the heart but is far more severe when heart disease has started at an early age (or is congenital). In infants and children, marked left-sided bulge may indicate severe enlargement of the right heart (24).

Any movement of the precordial area should be carefully observed. Among them, the following should be considered:

a) The *point of maximum impulse* (so-called *apex beat* or *apex impulse*). This is a positive pulsation which takes place during ventricular systole. It is usually located *in the 4th or 5th left interspace, on or within the midclavicular line*. Absence of this pulsation does not constitute an abnormality because an apex beat is present only in 25 per cent of normal adults (23).

The apex beat is more lateral in stocky, short individuals; it is nearer to the midline in thin, long persons. A change from the recumbent to the standing position alters the position of the apex beat by causing a moderate drop and some rotation of the heart; this tends to rest lower and more vertically.

A *systolic depression* in the area of the apex beat is a definite abnormality which may be caused by enlargement of the right ventricle or adhesive pericarditis.

b) *Multiple pulsations* in different intercostal spaces are usually the sign of an enlarged heart, animated by strong contractions. Exceptionally, they may be observed in young individuals with a thin chest, especially during excitement.

c) A small bulge, animated by *strong, expansive pulsations*, is usually a sign of aneurysm.

d) A *massive movement of the chest (see-saw movement)*. One region of the chest presents a forward thrust while another is being depressed (3). It may be caused by tricuspid insufficiency, severe dilatation of the aorta plus aortic insufficiency, or adhesive pericarditis.

e) A positive pulsation in the *2nd right interspace* is evidence of aortic dilatation; in the *2nd left interspace*, of pulmonic dilatation. A *positive pulsation at the epigastrium* is due to vertical position of the heart or right ventricular enlargement, and is frequently encountered in pulmonary emphysema.

f) *Enlargement and predominance of either ventricle* is revealed by the following movements (3). If the left ventricle predominates, the left thoracic wall moves suddenly to the left in systole, the right thoracic wall moving inwards at the same time. If the right ventricle predominates, there is a sudden forward thrust of the median area and epigastrium with a retraction of the lateral walls (page 260).

g) Dilatation of the aortic arch is often revealed by *a visible pulsation in the region of the suprasternal notch.*

Palpation

Palpation is also a long-established method of examination, well known to ancient Egyptian and Greek doctors. Its importance has been reemphasized in our time (3). Through palpation, one may localize the apex beat even when it is faint or invisible. The best procedure is the following: first the palm of the hand is applied to the precordium in order to obtain a general impression; then, search for the apical thrust will be made using the tips of the 2nd, 3rd, and 4th fingers.

Many details of the apex beat can be recognized by palpation. Among them, the existence of a *double impulse* (as in cases with a gallop rhythm) is one of the more significant.

Palpation may also reveal a *snap* in the 2nd interspace on either side of the sternum. This is caused by the closure of the semilunar valves and is present when pressure is high, either in the aorta (snap at the right of sternum) or in the pulmonary artery

(snap at the left of sternum). A distinct pulsation in the 3rd left interspace may be found whenever the conus of the right ventricle is enlarged, as in cases of mitral stenosis.

Palpation may reveal the existence of a *thrill.* This is the tactile expression of vibrations arising in the heart and causing also a murmur. The poor sensitivity of the hand in comparison with the ear is responsible for the fact that usually only the murmur of valvular stenosis is accompanied by a thrill (loud and low-pitched vibrations). A thrill seldom accompanies valvular insufficiency and this only if there is rupture or eversion of the cusps (aortic valve) or rupture of a chorda (mitral valve—4). The sensitivity of the fingers to vibrations of cardiac origin in the range of murmurs is so far below that of the ear that search for a thrill has become a matter of academic curiosity (30).

The following thrills can be palpated:

a) *A diastolic thrill, either at the apex or over the 4th left interspace,* is evidence of narrowing of the mitral valve.

b) *A systolic thrill at the apex* is usually due to a rapid undulation and vibration caused by myocardial damage.

c) *A systolic thrill over the 2nd right interspace* is caused by narrowing of the aortic valve, occasionally by an aortic aneurysm.

d) *A systolic thrill over the 2nd left interspace* is caused by narrowing of the pulmonic valve, patency of the ductus arteriosus, or extreme dilatation of the pulmonary artery.

e) *A systolic thrill in the 3rd–4th interspaces near the sternum* is evidence of communication between the two ventricles (*septal defect*).

Palpation should be also made with both hands (*bimanual palpation*). It may confirm the existence of massive movements of the chest wall.

Palpation of the precordium is completed by palpation of the epigastrium and of the

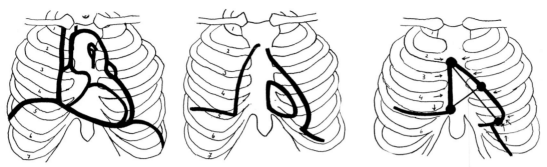

FIG. 47. Percussion of the cardiac area. a, Projection of the heart and large vessels on the surface of the chest. b, Absolute (inner profile) and relative (outer profile) cardiac dulness on percussion. c, Cardiac area and diameters with palpated percussion.

liver. If the right hand is placed over the left lobe of the liver and the left hand on the right lobe and moderate pressure is applied, one may appreciate *an expansive pulsation of the liver*, an important sign of tricuspid regurgitation. This hepatic pulsation is different from the aortic pulsation (abrupt, limited to the epigastrium) and from that of the enlarged right ventricle (limited between xiphoid process and *left* costal border (3). Details of epigastric pulsations and liver pulsations will be given later (pages 98 and 99).

Lastly, *edema of the precordial wall* may be recognized by palpation. It is a sign of purulent pericarditis, if localized.

To sum up, palpation is the method of choice in studying the character and location of the cardiac impulse and is useful in detecting abnormal pulsations.

Percussion

Percussion of the heart was introduced by *Auenbrugger* in 1761 (5) even though it is possible that it was used by the great masters of the Egyptian and Greek schools (6).

Percussion of the heart aims at the localization of *cardiac dulness* and, therefore, evaluation of the cardiac size. Training and experience are necessary but the results are valuable whenever x-ray is not available.

The area of absolute dulness is a small area of dull sound obtained by light percussion. It represents that area of the heart which is not covered by the margins of the lungs (fig. 47). It may disappear in pulmonary emphysema. *The area of relative dulness* is a much larger area than the former. It nearly coincides with the cardiac apex and is much nearer on the right to the real limit of the heart (fig. 47). The fact that there is no absolute coincidence between relative dulness and projection of the organs in the region of the base is due to the deep position of some organs (fig. 48). The area of relative dulness is obtained by strong percussion.

The *method of percussion* matters little as long as it is constantly employed, so that one becomes expert in its use. Percussion involves not only the sense of hearing but also that of touch because the finger, used as a pleximeter, feels the induced vibrations (7).

Different methods for measuring the heart dulness have been described. The author's view is that measurement of the horizontal distance between apex and midsternal line (transverse diameter) has no real value, varying too widely between normal subjects of different build. Far better is the measurement of the following two diameters:

a) *A longitudinal or oblique diameter* between the 2nd right costal cartilage (fixed point) and the apex (fig. 47).

b) *A broad diameter* between the cardiohepatic angle and the left border, perpendicular to the other (fig. 47).

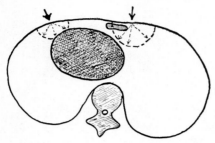

Fig. 48. Causes of error in percussion of the heart. On the left side of the chest, dulness is 1 or 2 centimeters *outwards* of the actual limits on account of the curvature of the ribs and the superficial position of the "apex". On the right side of the chest, dulness is 1 or 2 centimeters *inwards* of the actual border on account of the flat surface of the chest and the deep position of the right atrium. (After Cossio.)

The oblique diameter is normally from 8 to 9 cm. and measures chiefly the size of the left ventricle. The transverse diameter is normally from 7 to 8 cm. and measures chiefly the size of the right ventricle. Even when the transverse diameter is not measured, it will be kept in mind that the distance between right cardiac border on the 4th rib and the midline is increased by right ventricular enlargement.

The first phase of delimitation of the cardiac dulness is that of drawing *the left border* by percussing horizontally along the intercostal spaces from left to right. *The apex* will be recognized by percussion made along different rays, or spokes. *The cardiohepatic angle* will be defined by first percussing along the right midclavicular line from above downwards, then along the intercostal spaces from right to left.

In normal individuals, *the manubrium of the sternum* gives a clear resonant sound; *the cardiohepatic angle* is a right angle; *the dulness in the 3rd left interspace* does not exceed 2 cm.

Dulness in the 2nd and 3rd right interspaces may be caused by: dilatation of the ascending aorta, aneurysm of the aorta, persistence of the right aortic arch, mediastinal lesions, pericardial effusion, adhesive pericarditis, or tetralogy of Fallot.

Dulness in the 2nd and 3rd left interspace may be caused by dilatation of the left atrial appendage, the pulmonary conus, or the pulmonary artery. This sign may be found in mitral stenosis, patent ductus arteriosus, or aneurysm of the pulmonary artery.

The cardiohepatic angle becomes obtuse in the following lesions: pericardial effusion; right atrial enlargement due to tricuspid lesions, atrial septal defect, or congestive failure; pleuropericardial adhesions.

Occurrence of the apex beat *within* the area of dulness is a sign of pericardial effusion.

The presence of an area of dulness between the spine and the left scapula may be caused by left atrial enlargement, as well as by pericardial or pleural effusion.

To sum up, percussion is still a valuable method for recognition of the heart size and shape.

Auscultation

Auscultation of the heart is probably an old method of examination. We have, however, only indirect evidence of its use until *Laënnec* in 1819 (8) established it on a systematic basis and described the first stethoscope. More recent contributions (9, 10) have enhanced the value of this method by explaining the physical laws of auscultation. Also, contributions brought by phonocardiography have explained some pitfalls of auscultation.

The stethoscope. The stethoscope is an instrument which provides a closed acoustic system for transmitting the sounds originated within the thorax to the observer's ear. The transmission is effected by the air contained in the system. The stethoscope ends in a chest piece which may be an open *bell* or a *flat chamber*, closed by a membrane. When the bell is applied to the skin, the latter acts like a membrane whose acoustic properties vary according to the pressure of the bell (10).

Large bells transmit low-pitched sounds

better; small bells are used for better localization of murmurs. On the other hand, large bells collect much better the low-pitched sounds originating in the ventricles, like the third and fourth sound and the "gallop" sounds. The best tubing for a stethoscope seems to be a short one (25 cm.) with a bore of 3 mm. (31). An improvement of the stethoscope is the *electrically amplifying stethoscope*. This is useful for physicians who are hard of hearing and for adjusting the intensity to the best level of audibility.

Human ear. The human ear can be considered as the receptor end of an acoustic system. It is well known that it is an imperfect instrument. Knowledge of its limitations may explain some of the failures of auscultation and certain unavoidable discrepancies between clinical impression and objective graphic data. These limitations may be summarized as follows:

a) Pure tones of different pitch and the same intensity are heard as tones of different intensity.

b) The ear more easily detects changes of pitch than changes of intensity (except in the lower frequency range where changes of pitch may not be detected at all). As a result, a *higher-pitched* tone may be heard as a *louder* tone.

c) The ear is sensitive to vibrations between 20 and 20,000 cycles per second; however, sensitivity is poor for the lower-pitched vibrations and becomes gradually better for the higher-pitched. The heart is the source of vibrations between 5 and 800 per second (soft murmurs occasionally reach 1000). Therefore, *many cardiac vibrations are in the range of infra-sounds (nonaudible sounds)* while others are heard only if very loud or by particularly sensitive and trained observers.

d) The scale of sensitivity of the ear with regard to frequency increases very rapidly, *on a logarithmic ratio.* In the frequency band of 1,000 cycles, a given increase of intensity results in the same increase in loudness; while in higher-frequency bands, lesser increases of intensity cause the same result.

e) In the presence of certain loud or high-pitched sounds, the ear may be unable to detect weaker or lower-pitched sounds which follow immediately. This phenomenon is called "masking."

Physical characteristics of the heart sounds and murmurs. Cardiac vibrations include frequencies between 0 and 1000 per second (10). Those between 0 and 5 per second have no acoustic value. The vibrations taking place during diastole (third and fourth sound) and small vibrations at the beginning and end of the first and second sound, have frequencies between 5 and 50 per second while most of the other vibrations of these sounds are between 50 and 100 per second. The *low-pitched rumbles* are made of vibrations between 50 and 140, only occasionally including components between 140 and 400. The *friction rubs* include vibrations between 140 and 660 per second. The *high-pitched murmurs* are composed of vibrations between 140 and 660 per second, only occasionally including components between 660 and 1000. The latter are found only in some of the "soft" murmurs and have the same pitch of those vibrations which are set up by normal breathing.

Areas of auscultation. Clinical experience has shown that sounds and murmurs which originate in a definite valve are usually heard best in a specific area of the precordium.

The classic and well-known scheme should be somewhat modified. The author's view is that the following areas should be considered (fig. 49):

a) Sounds and murmurs arising in the *mitral valve* are heard best in the 4th left interspace, at the apex, or along the left cardiac border. They are well transmitted to the left axilla and, if very loud, to the left side. Murmurs due to regurgitation are transmitted much farther than those due to narrowing of the valve. They are louder in expiration.

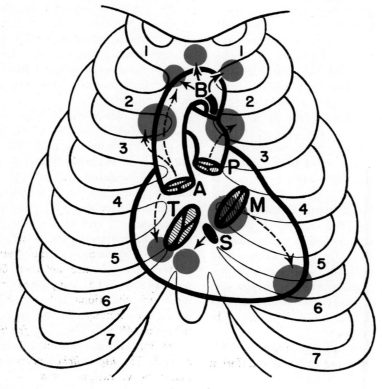

Fig. 49. Areas of auscultation (red) as compared with projection of the valves and defects (black). A, aortic valve; P, pulmonic valve; T, tricuspid valve; M, mitral valve; B, ductus arteriosus; S, ventricular septal defect.

b) Sounds and murmurs arising in the *tricuspid valve* are heard at the base of the xiphoid process or in the 4th and 5th right interspaces. They have a poor transmission. They are louder in inspiration (34).

c) Sounds and murmurs arising in the *aortic valve* are heard best over the 2nd right interspace. If due to stenosis, they radiate to the suprasternal notch (2, 33) and along the carotid arteries. If due to regurgitation, they may be heard along the sternum and even at the xiphoid process. If the murmurs are loud, they are transmitted to the spine.

d) Sounds and murmurs arising in the *pulmonic valve* can be heard in the 2nd left interspace with a narrow area of transmission. If due to stenosis, they are transmitted to the left clavicle and the back; if caused by insufficiency, to the 3rd right interspace.

e) Murmurs arising in a *ventricular septal defect* are heard best in the 3rd or 4th left interspace near the sternum; they are rarely transmitted toward the apex and are frequently transmitted toward the right side.

f) Murmurs arising in the *patent ductus arteriosus* are heard best in the 2nd left interspace with wide transmission to the 2nd right interspace, the suprasternal notch, and the carotid arteries.

g) Murmurs due to *coarctation of the aorta* are heard best in the back, between the left scapula and the spine (32).

Cardiac murmurs can be classified in the following way: *Valvular*—due to damage of the cardiac valves causing either stenosis or insufficiency (rheumatic, bacterial, arteriosclerotic, or congenital). *Myocardial*—caused by damage to heart muscle resulting in *relative* stenosis or insufficiency (myocarditis; myocardial dysfunction secondary to metabolic, anemic, avitaminic, coronary, or pericardial heart disease). *Hematic*—due to severe changes of blood composition favoring whirlpools, usually during systole. *Vascular*—due to primary or secondary dilatation of the aorta or pulmonary artery leading to either relative insufficiency or relative stenosis (luetic, hypertensive, pulmonary, or congenital dilatation; dilatation due to increased blood volume). *Abnormal structural*—due to congenital shunts or severe malformations. *Extracardiac*—(cardio-pulmonary; cardio-serous).

Murmurs apparently innocuous may be due to:

a) Initial rheumatic heart disease (dilatation or edema of mitral ring; edema of mitral leaflets or papillary muscles; structural lesion or functional distention of pulmonary artery; initial aortic stenosis).

b) Mild congenital heart disease (pulmonic stenosis, aortic stenosis, coarctation of the aorta, atrial or ventricular septal defect).

c) Anemia.

d) Pregnancy.

e) Unknown.

Special remarks should be made *concerning murmurs in infants and children* (24). A *loud systolic murmur* may be heard shortly after birth and subsequently disappear; it is probably caused by the blood passing through the ductus which is subsequently obliterated. Persistence of a loud, rasping, systolic murmur for some weeks indicates the existence of a congenital malformation but localization of the murmur is not possible on account of the small size of the heart. *Diastolic murmurs* are seldom heard under one year of life. A *continuous murmur* suggests patency of the ductus.

Whenever *the 2nd sound is split*, this indicates the existence of both the aortic and the pulmonic openings; splitting is not heard in atresia of one of them or in persistence of the truncus arteriosus.

It has been stated that from 30 to 50 per cent of children have a "functional," (frequently musical) systolic murmur over the 2nd or 3rd left interspace (38). It is the author's belief that this murmur, even though frequently benign, is not always so. It may be caused by early rheumatic heart disease, mild pulmonic stenosis, or atrial septal defect.

Further details about intracardiac murmurs will be given later (page 93). It should be added that *typical transmission of the cardiac murmurs* has been questioned and even denied (11). It is the author's view that, while very loud murmurs may be transmitted in all directions by soft and bony structures, most cardiac murmurs of average intensity are transmitted to typical areas because they follow the stream of blood which is causing them.

Murmurs may be *soft* (high-pitched), *rough* (low-pitched), and occasionally *musical*. When low-pitched, a murmur may be called a *rumble*.

The *phase* of a murmur should be noted. A murmur may be in *early systole, mid-systole*, or *late systole*, and may *continue throughout systole*. A murmur may also be in *early diastole*, in *mid-diastole*, or *in pre-systole*, and it may *continue throughout diastole*. A murmur may show an *increasing loudness* (murmur *"in crescendo"*, typical of mitral stenosis) or a *decreasing loudness* (murmur *"in decrescendo"*, typical of aortic insufficiency).

Indication of the *intensity of the systolic murmurs* can be done by dividing them in six gradations (14) as follows:

Grade 1 = the faintest audible murmur having an appreciable duration.

Grade 2 = a slight murmur.

Grade 3 = a moderate murmur.

Grade 4 = a loud murmur.

Grade 5 = a very loud murmur.

Grade 6 = the loudest possible murmur.

Grade 3 to 6 murmurs are usually caused

by organic heart disease (14). A grade 1 or 2 murmur may be connected with increased velocity of the blood flow, and the latter is often related to anemia or rapid heart action, as experimental studies have demonstrated (15).

A particular type of auscultation is that which can be effected during apnea by means of a gastric tube introduced into the esophagus and connected with the stethoscope (25). Heart sounds and murmurs are heard very clearly; the murmur of mitral regurgitation is heard with special clarity with the tip of the tube at 20 to 40 cm. from the dental arch.

Routine auscultation of the heart should proceed in the following way:

First, *the two normal heart sounds should be noted*; their absolute and relative intensity, the area where they are heard best, their timbre, and their duration, will be recorded. The *timbre* depends upon additional vibrations (extra-sounds, murmurs) which, being near, are confused with the basic sounds. The *1st sound* is normally louder at the apex; the *2nd sound*, at the base. This is easily explained, as the 1st sound is more influenced by the closure of the mitral valve; the 2nd, by the closure of the semilunar valves. In physiological conditions, the 2nd sound is slightly louder over the 2nd right interspace than over the left (except in young children and infants where the opposite is frequently true). This is due to the fact that the closure of the aortic valves gives a snapping sound better heard on the right than on the left, while closure of the pulmonic valves gives a softer sound owing to lower pressure of the pulmonary artery.

Alteration in the sounds of the heart is often as important as cardiac murmurs. However, judgment of the intensity of the 1st and 2nd sound for a given individual may be difficult. In the timing of the heart sounds and murmurs, it is customary to listen first at the base of the heart where the sharp 2nd sound is easy to detect. Then,

by moving the stethoscope toward the apex, the observer tries to retain the position of the same sound in relation to other phenomena.

Marked diminution of the intensity of the 1st sound at the apex may be evidence of myocardial weakness. *Marked accentuation of the 1st apical sound* is often found in mitral stenosis.

Accentuation of the 2nd aortic sound is found in patients with hypertension, atherosclerosis, or syphilis of the aorta. *Accentuation of the 2nd pulmonic sound* is found in patients with mitral stenosis or cor pulmonale, and may be interpreted as evidence of increased pressure in the pulmonary artery. *Decreased intensity of the 2nd sound* is found in aortic and pulmonic stenosis, respectively.

The existence of *additional sounds during diastole* (triple and quadruple rhythms) should be noted.

General Classification of the Triple and Quadruple Rhythms (29)

While the occurrence of one extra-sound in diastole is a common cause of triple rhythm (*gallop rhythm*); and that of two extra-sounds in diastole, of quadruple rhythm (*train-wheel rhythm*), other possibilities should be considered. Actually a triple rhythm can be due also to the occurrence of one of the following phenomena: a) an opening sound or snap of the mitral valve; or b) a split-second sound because of bundle branch block or high pressure in the pulmonary artery. Again, a quadruple rhythm may be due to addition of a diastolic sound plus splitting of the second sound on account of bundle branch block (37).

Therefore, the following possibilities should be considered:

I. Triple Rhythms
    A. *Diastolic* (page 370).
        a) Atrial (or 4th sound).
        b) Ventricular (or 3rd sound).
        c) Summation (3rd plus 4th).

B. *Systolic* (page 455).
   a) Apical
   b) Basal
C. *Opening snap* (or sound) of the mitral valve (page 228).
D. *Split-second sound.*

II. Quadruple Rhythms

A. Train-wheel rhythm (loud 3rd and 4th sounds).
B. Loud 3rd or 4th, and split second sound.
C. Systolic plus diastolic sound.
D. Split second sound plus opening snap of the mitral valve.

Splitting of the 2nd sound at the base is due to nonsimultaneous closure of the aortic and pulmonic valves and is more often heard over the pulmonic area. Occasional or periodic splitting may be physiological, especially in children. A definite reduplication, on the contrary, suggests increased pulmonic pressure or bundle branch block. *Splitting of the 1st sound* may be due to a loud and separate occurrence of the two valvular components of the 1st sound (35, 36) (page 91). It is never caused, as formerly believed, by bundle branch block (37).

The observer should further listen for the presence of *friction rubs* which are evidence of pericarditis.

To sum up, auscultation is an invaluable aid in the diagnosis of valvular defects (murmurs), in the recognition of lesions of the myocardium (extra-sounds, splitting of the second sound, gallop), and in the diagnosis of aneurysms.

Practical applications of phonocardiography, which in the author's view is superior to clinical auscultation, have *not* made the latter obsolete. As a matter of fact, *auscultation should always precede phonocardiography.*

Functional Tests

Functional tests aim at evaluating the reserve capacity of the heart muscle, the reactions of the cardiovascular system when placed under strain, and the reactivity of the autonomic nervous system.

Exercise test. The simplest functional test is that represented by exercise. Even though a "standard" exercise test is impossible, one should try to adapt the severity of the test to the age, weight, and training of the patient (page 129). Such a test has a real value when effected in a comparative way and on the same patient. The patient should be asked to bend 10 or 20 times on his knees.

Normal subjects show a moderate increase of the heart rate (from 70 to 100), of the respiratory rate (from 12 to 15 or 16), and of systolic pressure (from 120 to 130–135). *These changes should not last more than 2 minutes.* Heart failure is revealed by dyspnea, rapid heart rate, irregularity of the pulse, and blood pressure drop with reduced pulse pressure. Occasionally, blood pressure may rise more than in normal subjects because of accumulation of carbon dioxide in the blood. When the changes of heart rate and respiration last too long, they represent a definite abnormality even if they lie within the normal range of variation. Patients with coronary heart disease may complain of precordial pain and may reveal premature contractions. Valvular murmurs usually increase in intensity.

A special type of exercise test is the *two-step Master test* which was devised for coronary patients (page 129).

Cold-pressor test (page 161).

Valsalva and Mueller tests. The *Valsalva test* is an attempted forced expiration with closed glottis (16). The *Mueller test* is an attempted forced inspiration with closed glottis (17). The first is obtained by inviting the patient to strain as he does when straining at stools.

The Valsalva test, in normal individuals, gives a tremendous decrease in amplitude of pulse, even to the point of disappearance. The heart rate becomes slow at first (increased intrathoracic pressure), then rapid (anoxemia), then slow again after the end of the test (carotid sinus reflex). Systolic blood pressure may drop to zero during the test, but rises to 130–140 mm. Hg afterwards.

The Mueller test increases the heart rate during the test, decreases it afterwards.

X-ray studies have shown that the heart becomes smaller during the Valsalva test (decreased venous return), and larger during the Mueller test (increased venous return). In both cases, however, the change is moderate. Important changes and abnormalities occur in congenital heart diseases (patent ductus arteriosus) and in latent congestive failure.

Carotid sinus reflex—stimulation of the vagus. The study of the carotid sinus reactivity may have importance in many patients. This may be obtained in two ways:

a) By placing the patient on a *tilting bed* and studying the changes of the pulse as he passes from the horizontal to the head-down position (stimulation of the carotid sinus caused by distention). This is the most physiological stimulation and may be accomplished in an even simpler way by studying the patient first in standing and then in a recumbent position. The pulse rate decreases 10 to 20 beats per minute in the latter and further 10 to 20 in the head-down position.

b) By massaging the sinus region of one side with the fingers. Compression of the sinus from the outside is an *abnormal* stimulation of the pressoreceptors. It usually obtains remarkable results in patients with hypersensitive carotid sinus but may cause no changes in normal individuals. The compression will be tried first on one side, then on the other, never on both sides simultaneously. Slowing of 10 to 20 per minute is normal; extreme bradycardia or stoppage of the heart is abnormal.

Reflex stimulation of the vagus may be obtained by compressing the eyeballs with a steady and firm pressure (*oculocardiac reflex*). It has been shown that this test causes a stimulation of both the vagus and

the sympathetic (21), the first usually predominating. The heart rate slows down only 5 to 10 beats per minute in the average subject. Patients with hyperactivity of the vagus nerve may show cardiac arrest and disappearance of the pulse for many seconds. Ventricular escapes usually appear after a few seconds in such patients and maintain the circulation. The test will be made with the patient lying supine on a couch and the pressure will be applied with thumb and index finger of the right hand. The patient usually does not feel the suspension of the heart beat.

No dangers are involved in these tests, except in patients with severe coronary heart disease where the maneuvers are contraindicated.

Pharmacological Tests

Different tests use the action of drugs for the study of cardio-vascular functions.

Atropine sulphate—1 mg. by subcutaneous injection (heart block, bradycardia).

Amyl nitrite—1–2 drops by inhalation (angina pectoris, heart block, tachycardia) (page 129).

Quinine hydrochloride—0.5 gm. by subcutaneous or intravenous injection (a-v paroxysmal tachycardia, ventricular tachycardia, premature beats).

Mecholyl chloride—10–25 mg. by intravenous injection (paroxysmal tachycardia).

Adrenaline hydrochloride—0.5–1 mg. by subcutaneous injection (low blood pressure, bradycardia, angina pectoris).

Dosage and mode of action of these drugs will be given in chapter XXXII.

BIBLIOGRAPHY

1. BRAMWELL, C. General Cardiology. In *The Principles and Practice of Cardiology* by BRAMWELL AND KING. London, Oxford Univ. Press, 1942.
2. LUISADA, A. A. Rass. Internaz. Clin. Ter. (Naples), 1937, **18**: 733.
3. DRESSLER, W.: *Die Brustwandpulsationen.* Vienna, Maudrich, 1933. Also *Clinical Cardiology.* New York, Hoeber, 1942.

4. WHITE, P. D. *Heart Disease*. 3rd Ed. New York, Macmillan, 1944.

5. AUENBRUGGER, L. Translated and reprinted. *Cardiac Classics* by WILLIUS AND KEYS. St. Louis, Mosby, 1941.

6. MUCH, H. *Hippokrates der Grosse*. Berlin, Hippokrates, Verlag, 1926.

7. FRUGONI, C. Riv. Crit. Clin. Med., 1910, 11, n. 44, 45, 46.

8. LAËNNEC, R. Translated and reprinted. *Cardiac Classics* by WILLIUS AND KEYS. St. Louis, Mosby, 1941.

9. ORIAS, O., AND BRAUN MENENDEZ, E. B. *The Heart Sounds in Normal and Pathological Conditions*. New York, Oxford Univ. Press, 1939.

10. RAPPAPORT, M. B., AND SPRAGUE, H. B. Am. Heart J., 1941, 21, 257 and 1942; 23, 591.

11. LEVINE, S., AND LIKOFF, W. B. Arch. Int. Med., 1944, 21, 298.

12. GROCCO, P. Ann. Univ. Lib. Perugia, 1887/ 1888, 3, 131 and 161.

13. PALMIERI, G. G. In *Tratt. di Semeiotica* by VIOLA. Milan, Vallardi, 1933.

14. LEVINE, S. A. *Clinical Heart Disease*. Philadelphia, Saunders, 1937.

15. LUISADA, A. A., AND MAUTNER, H. Exper. Med. & Surg., 1943, 1, 282.

16. VALSALVA, A. M.: *Opera*. Venice, Pitteri, 1740.

17. MUELLER, J. (1838). Quoted by LUCIANI (22).

18. CROWDEN, G. P., AND HARRIS, H. A. Brit. Med. J., 1929, 1, 439.

19. ASCHER, B. Wien. Klin. Woch., 1908, 21, 1529.

20. DAGNINI. Comun. Soc. Medico-Chir. Bologna, June 17, 1908.

21. DANIELOPOLU AND CO-WORKERS. Arch. Mal. Coeur., 1923, 16, 161; and Bull. Soc. Med. Hop. de Paris, 1923, 47, 386.

22. LUCIANI, L. *Fisiologia dell' Uomo*. Milan, S. E. L., 1923.

23. NIEHAUS, F. W., AND WRIGHT, W. D. Am. Heart J., 1945, 30, 605.

24. TAUSSIG, H. V. *Congenital Malformations of the Heart*. New York, Commonwealth Fund, 1947.

25. LIAN, C. Arch. Mal. Coeur, 1945, 38, 221.

26. MACBRYDE, C. M. *Signs and Symptoms. Their Clinical Interpretation*. Philadelphia, J. B. Lippincott Co., 1947.

27. CARRAL Y DE TERESA, R. *Semiologia Cardiovascular*. Inst. Nac. de Cardiol., Mexico, 1947.

28. ORTIZ RAMIREZ, T. Arch. Lat.-Amer. Cardiol. y Hematol., 1933, 5, 115.

29. LUISADA, A. A., AND ROITMAN, M. Arch. Inst. Card. Mexico, 1948, 18, 345.

30. COUNIHAN, T. B., RAPPAPORT, M. B., AND SPRAGUE, H. B. Circ., 1951, 4, 716.

31. RAPPAPORT, M. B., AND SPRAGUE, H. B. Am. Heart J., 1951, 42, 605.

32. LIAN, C., AND DANG, VAN CHUNG. Presse Med., 1950, 58, 585.

33. LIAN, C. Acta Card., 1948, 3, 48.

34. RIVERO CARVALLO, J. M. Rev. Esp. Card., 1950, 4, 498.

35. LUISADA, A. A., MENDOZA, F., AND ALIMURUNG, M. R. Brit. Heart J., 1949, 11, 41.

36. LUISADA, A. A., ALIMURUNG, M. R., AND LEWIS, L. Am. J. Physiol, 1952, 168, 226.

37. LUISADA, A. A., AND CONTRO, S. J. Mt. Sinai Hosp. (New York), 1952, 19, 70.

38. ASH, R. Penn. Med. J., 1941, 44, 484.

Chapter 5

The Technical Study of the Cardiac Patient

The study of a cardiac patient is based upon data obtained through taking of history, physical examination, and technical examination. The technical data can be used fully only if correlated with the history and the physical findings of the patient.

Some technical methods represent an extension and completion of our senses. It could be said that fluoroscopy is inspection in depth; orthodiagraphy, a more perfect percussion; cardiography and sphygmography, a more perfect palpation; and phonocardiography, a finer and more perfect auscultation. On the other hand, electrocardiography, electrokymography, and ballistocardiography have no counterpart in the methods of physical examination and supply data which otherwise would be unavailable.

Cardiovascular dynamics causes vibrations of the chest wall which are spread over a wide frequency range, from 0 to 1000 per second. These vibrations can be detected in various ways by physical or technical examination according to the frequency.

On account of the undeniable connection existing between high and low frequency vibrations of the thoracic and abdominal walls, a common terminology should be used for the various waves. Therefore, the terms 1, 2, 3, 4, and their subdivisions (1a, 1b, 2a, 2b) which refer to the heart sounds (page 90), should be used for other graphic tracings, in order to indicate those waves which take place at the time of the heart sounds.

Tracings of the Heart Sounds (Phonocardiograms or Stethograms)

The purpose of phonocardiography is the graphic registration of the sounds and murmurs which originate in the heart and vessels, consequent to cardiac action. Therefore, the essential principles of phonocardiography cannot be dissociated from those of clinical auscultation (page 80).

Two methods were chiefly used by the pioneers of phonocardiography (1–6). The first utilized a microphone in combination with a string galvanometer (1); the second, a capsule with a small mirror attached to the vibrating membrane (2). Both systems were imperfect and, accordingly, of limited use. More recently, phonocardiography has been based on the use of a crystal microphone and an amplifying electrocardiograph (7).

THE PHONOCARDIOGRAPH

The phonocardiograph is composed of two main parts: the stethograph-amplifier and the microphone with the chest-piece.

Stethograph-amplifier. This part of the system is usually incorporated in a larger apparatus which also records electrocardiograms and sphygmograms. The stethograph-amplifier employs thermionic vacuum tubes based on a resistance-capacity coupled circuit. This is completely independent of another similar circuit which is used for electrocardiography.

The microphones. A microphone is a device which transforms sound waves into equivalent electrical pulsations.

The *piezo-electric crystal microphone* is based on the principle that stresses set up in a crystal of Rochelle salt (or quartz) by sound waves vary proportionately the output of electric potentials. The natural period of the crystal is about 10,000 cycles per second. Even if this is somewhat lowered by the diaphragm, the result is still far above the frequency of the vibrations set

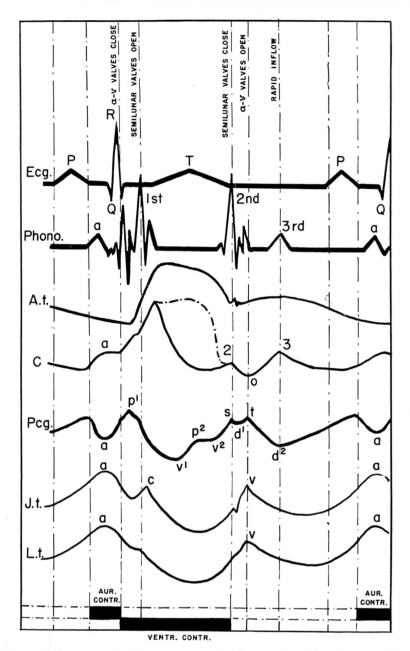

FIG. 50. Time relationship of the different waves of various tracings. Ecg, electrocardiogram; Phono., phonocardiogram; A.t., aortic tracing (carotid or subclavian tracings); C, cardiogram; Pcg., pneumo-cardiogram; J.t., jugular tracing; L.t., liver tracing; AUR. CONTR., atrial contraction; VENTR. CONTR., ventricular contraction.

up by the heart. This type of microphone has been developed into different models, one of which is used for cardiography (page 95) while the following two are used for phonocardiography (7).

a) *The stethoscopic microphone.* In this microphone, a special case contains the cartridge and an *acoustic high-pass filter.* This filter eliminates the vibrations of extremely low frequency having importance only for the mechanical cardiogram and protects the crystal from sudden high pressures. The filtering is made by a duct or channel which allows free passage of all vibrations above 30 per second while it arrests or decreases the slower vibrations. Moreover, the response of the stethoscopic microphone has a rising characteristic so that the higher the pitch of the sound, the better it is transmitted. *The resulting tracing corresponds to that auditory picture which is presented to the ear by an average stethoscope.* It is used for the study of both the relatively slow and the relatively high frequencies, and includes many vibrations which, being barely audible or not audible on account of their pitch, can be termed as "infra-sounds."

b) *The logarithmic microphone.* The overall frequency response of this microphone is equivalent to the sum of the curve of the human audiogram plus that of the average acoustic stethoscope. The resulting response is *a graphic picture of the heart sounds as they are perceived by the average observer.* A special filter attenuates the low-frequency components of the sounds or murmurs; the over-all decrease is compensated by the amplifier of the stethograph which increases the sound vibrations on a logarithmic scale (other deficiencies of the ear naturally cannot be reproduced). The resultant trac-

ing gives a good transcription of the high-pitched or soft murmurs, like the aortic diastolic murmur.

The galvanometer employed for recording these tracings has the ability to reproduce vibrations up to 600 per second in the stetho-cardiette, up to 1000 per second in the twin-beam.

In one of the latest apparatus, a *single microphone is used* and either a stethoscopic or a logarithmic record can be obtained by flipping a switch which changes the electrical characteristics of the microphone.

THE HEART SOUNDS IN THE PHONOCARDIOGRAM

The so-called heart sounds are noises, i.e., *impure tones,* composed of a number of vibrations, different in frequency and intensity. Each component imparts a distinctive quality to the whole sound. Even high-pitched sounds usually have some low-pitched component, and vice versa.

The phonocardiogram of a normal subject may record up to four heart sounds (7–10) (figs. 51, 52, 53a). It is customary to call the two loudest and most commonly heard sounds (or tones) the first and the second sound. As already said (page 41), the first of them takes place during early ventricular systole; the second, at the end of ventricular systole. For this reason,

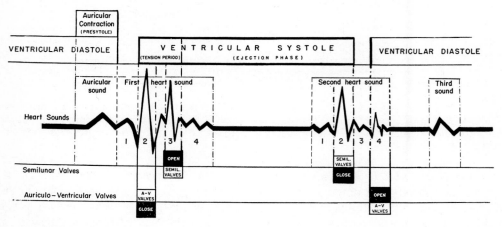

Fig. 51. The vibrations of the sound tracing (phonocardiogram) and the valvular events of the heart

they have been called *the two normal systolic sounds* (197). The other two, less constant, sounds, are the third and fourth sound which take place during diastole. According to the same classification, they should be called *the two normal diastolic sounds* (197).

Systolic Sounds

The first sound. It has been stated (7, 9) that four factors take part in the formation of this sound: the atrial, the muscular, the valvular, and the vascular. Actually, the muscular factor is revealed only indirectly, through the effect that the contraction has on the position of the valves. The atrial factor is to be taken into consideration only in children, where the fourth sound may seem to continue into the first. Therefore, only the vascular factor may occasionally cause separate vibrations. The main vibrations are due to a single, complex, musculo-valvular mechanism (page 42), even if separate elements (or components) may be frequently identified within this sound (194). Five different parts have been described. *Part I* is a small, low-pitched vibration which coincides with, or slightly follows, the R wave of the electrocardiogram. Cases with a-v block or atrial fibrillation present this vibration; therefore, it should be considered as coincident with and caused by ventricular tension (195). *Part II* consists of one or two large vibrations which are indirectly caused by *the closure of the a-v valves* (figs. 51 and 52). This part of the sound precedes the rise of the pulse in the carotid and subclavian tracings. *Part III* is made of smaller vibrations which may include vibrations of the myocardium or the chest wall. *Part IV* consists of one or two large vibrations. It is caused indirectly by *the opening of the semilunar valves* of the aorta and pulmonary artery (page 42). This part corresponds with the rise of the pulse of the subclavian and carotid arteries and the end of rise in the tracing of intraventricular pressure. *Part V* takes place during the ejection period. It is made of

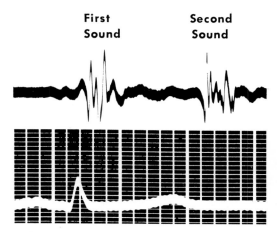

FIG. 52. Normal phonocardiogram. The first sound has a very clear splitting due to separate development of the two valvular components. The second sound also seems split on account of the large opening sound (os) of the mitral valve. Woman of 35, no heart disease.

one or two slow vibrations with superimposed rapid vibrations. It is caused by distention of the large arteries and by the whirlpools of blood flowing into them.

The second sound. It is caused by the rapid succession of the closure of the semilunar valves of the aorta and pulmonary and the subsequent opening of the a-v valves, as well as by the causes of these valvular events (page 42). Four parts or components can be distinguished within the sound (7, 9). *Part I* consists of one or two low-pitched and small vibrations which coincide with the beginning of protodiastole. This part of the sound coincides with the end of the T wave of the electrocardiogram and the incisura of the pulse in the tracings of the carotid and subclavian tracings. *Part II* consists of one diphasic or triphasic vibration of high pitch and high amplitude. It is caused by *closure of the semilunar valves.* *Part III* consists of one or two low-pitched vibrations of small amplitude due to shaking of the heart and vessels and representing aftervibrations. *Part IV* is due to *the opening of the a-v valves* and the result of this event on the ventricular wall. In most normal

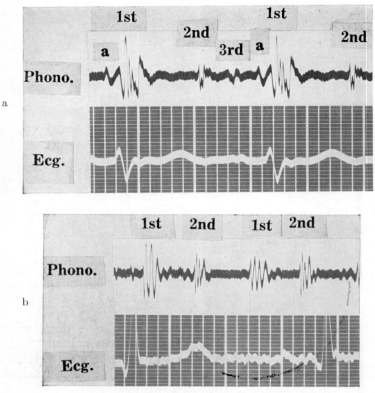

FIG. 53. Normal sound tracings compared with the electrocardiogram. a, The four heart sounds in a normal young man. b, Fetal heart sounds and maternal electrocardiogram.

subjects, this vibration is extremely small or even imperceptible. However, normal subjects can present in this phase a single, large, *low-pitched vibration*, which has been called the *opening sound of the mitral valve* (*os*) (184) (fig. 52). This part of the sound coincides with: a) the lowest point of the linear tracing of the apex or midprecordium (point *2b* of cardiogram); b) the *v* wave of the phlebogram (this wave may follow *os*); c) a notch which is often present in the electrokymogram of the left ventricle.

Diastolic Sounds

The diastolic sounds are usually two, the third and fourth sound. They may be fused in a single sound-complex whenever there is severe tachycardia (page 370). The possible existence of a *fifth sound* following the third has been advocated by *Calo* (196)

while the author admitted instead the possibility of splitting of the third sound (197).

The third sound is not always recorded. It is more common in children, adolescents, and young adults with a slender body and a flat chest. It consists of a single, slow vibration, usually not larger than one-third or one-fourth of the second sound. The third sound occurs at the peak of the phase of "rapid passive filling" (page 40) and coincides with: a) the peak of wave *3* of the apex cardiogram; b) the end of rapid relaxation in the electrokymogram of the left ventricle.

The fourth sound (*atrial sound*) is recorded frequently as a small, low-pitched vibration having a height of about one-third to one-fourth of the first sound. It may consist of a diphasic or even triphasic vibration. It may be followed by a small after-vibration. It is recorded best at the apex or midprecordium, especially in the left decubitus, but may be recorded at the epigastrium as well. It is favored by tachycardia and is more common in children and adolescents. The fourth sound is only indirectly related to the atrial contraction. A comparison between tracings recorded via the esophagus and tracings recorded at the apex has shown that the fourth sound takes place earlier in the former than in the latter. This shows that the sound recorded at the apex is only the result of an impact of the blood pushed by the atrial contraction against the ventricular wall. The fourth sound takes place at the peak of the last phase of ventricular diastole, that of "rapid active filling" due to the atrial contraction.

Fetal Sounds

The fetal sounds can be recorded by the use of a stethoscopic microphone and a large funnel (fig. 53b). A rubber strap is placed around the abdomen of the mother and the microphone is placed where auscultation reveals the fetal sounds. A simultaneous electrocardiogram of the mother is recorded in order to exclude the possibility that the sounds are caused by pulsations of the mother's arteries. The latter would present the same rate as that of the mother's heart.

Murmurs

Systolic murmurs. A systolic murmur is revealed by the phonocardiograph as a series of vibrations of different pitches. Only in certain cases does the tracing present regular vibrations of a single frequency; then, auscultation reveals a "musical" or "sea-gull" murmur. The following types of systolic murmurs can be observed:

a) A *prolongation of the second phase* of the first sound.

b) A *prolongation of the total duration* of the first sound which lasts beyond the peak of the *c* wave of the jugular tracing or even the peak of the main wave of the carotid tracing.

c) A *murmur in decrescendo*. It ends before the second sound and is composed of vibrations of different pitches. It is typical of *mitral regurgitation* and is recorded best at the apex, in the left decubitus.

d) A *diamond-shaped murmur*. The vibrations start soon after the end of the first sound, increase toward the middle of systole, decrease later. They are made of various frequencies with predominance of the medium type. The murmur is typical of *absolute* or *relative stenosis of the aorta or pulmonary artery*. The peak of the murmur corresponds to that of the pulse in the carotid tracing.

e) A *loud, all-systolic murmur*. This is typical of *severe aortic* or *pulmonic stenosis*. It covers the first sound, lasts throughout all systole, and ends with the second sound, which may not be visible.

f) A *low-grade, all-systolic murmur*. This is usually made of *high-pitched vibrations* and lasts throughout all systole. It is recorded mostly at the apex and may occur in *mitral regurgitation*, especially in children.

Basal diastolic murmurs. The following types can be recognized:

a) A *prolongation of the second aortic or pulmonic sound*. The second sound is made of three or four vibrations *in decrescendo*. It is typical of initial aortic or pulmonic insufficiency.

b) A *diastolic murmur in decrescendo*. It is typical of advanced *aortic* or *pulmonic insufficiency*. The murmur starts as a prolongation of the second sound and gradually decreases in intensity until it disappears during mid-diastole. If the vibrations are regular, there is a *sea-gull cry* type of murmur. The murmur may be separated from the second sound by a brief interval (198).

Apical diastolic murmurs. Frequently the murmurs are loudest over the midprecordium and should be called "rumbles" on account of the predominance of low frequency vibrations.

a) *Early-diastolic rumble*. Following the second phase of the second sound, there is a pause of silence, then an *opening snap of the mitral valve*. This vibration is followed immediately by a variable number of irregular vibrations, at times only three or four.

One or two louder vibrations may correspond to the peak of the wave of rapid filling. On the other hand, the vibrations may continue throughout most of diastole, increase in presystole, and continue until the following first sound.

b) *Presystolic murmur.* It corresponds to that short phase of diastole preceding the first sound during which occurs the atrial contraction. It frequently presents a type *in crescendo* and its vibrations continue with those of the first sound. However, in certain cases, the murmur decreases before the beginning of the first sound (199).

Continuous murmur. This type of murmur is typical of *fistulas* between vessels. It frequently has the auditory type of a *machinery-murmur* and is found in *patent ductus arteriosus* and *arteriovenous fistulas* (fig. 183). The duration of the murmur is such that it does not coincide exactly with the cardiac phases; it usually is loudest at the end of systole, covers the second sound, and then decreases in diastole.

TECHNIQUE OF PHONOCARDIOGRAPHIC EXAMINATION

The phonocardiogram has not become familiar to physicians because of lack of familiarity with the technique and lack of knowledge relative to the interpretation of the records.

The only requirement for the *examining room* is relative isolation from outside noises. The patient should be placed on a cot, supported by pillows, in a semi-recumbent position. Thus, other types of records can be taken at the same time. The patient should be stripped to the waist and covered by a sheet so that different parts of the precordial area may be successively exposed. He should be instructed to "hold his breath" on a signal from the observer so that any interference with respiratory sounds may be avoided. A rubber strap, tied around the chest of the patient (above the right shoulder and below the left arm), holds a microphone over any point of the chest.

Both the *choice of the microphone* and *that of the areas to be studied* require a preliminary examination on the part of the physician. *During routine examination, the latter should quickly evaluate the most outstanding features of auscultation and mark the necessary points.*

The first step in the *study of a phonocardiographic record* is the *recognition* and *localization* of the different sounds and murmurs so that each of them can be named. This is based on comparison of the time at which they occur with the time of occurrence of waves of other simultaneously recorded tracings. For each sound, one should examine: a) *location* (phase of systole or diastole); b) *duration*; c) *amplitude*; d) *frequency of the vibrations*. Further studies should be made in order to compare sounds and murmurs observed in one cycle with others observed in a following cycle (changes caused by respiration, alternation, arrhythmias), and in order to compare sounds and murmurs obtained over different areas.

The *routine phonocardiographic examination* should be done in the following way. One lead of the electrocardiogram is selected on account of the best development of the various waves and is used throughout. If the waves are small, an increased voltage (2 cm. per mv.) is used. *Five tracings are recorded:* apex, mid-precordium, pulmonary artery, aorta, tricuspid. The stethoscopic microphone with the large funnel is used (in children or persons with a bony chest, the medium or small funnel should be preferred). After each tracing, the logarithmic microphone with a similar funnel is substituted to the stethoscopic and a second record is taken. In case of soft murmurs, the diaphragm chest piece is used for the logarithmic tracing. When using a twin-beam, the switch from one to the other type of tracing can be done without changing microphone.

The *special phonocardiographic examination* includes: tracings taken outside the conventional areas; records in special phases of respiration (inspiratory or expiratory apnea); tracings in special positions (patient sitting or bent forward); functional tests; and simultaneous tracings of various kinds (phonocardiogram and low frequency tracing of the apex; phonocardiogram and carotid or jugular tracing, etc.).

Phonocardiography has been developed slowly on account of technical difficulties. Its importance is becoming greater from year to year. One should bear in mind that auscultation and phonocardiography are two inseparable approaches to the study of the same phenomena. Therefore, whenever auscultation is useful, phonocardiography also is of help for diagnosis.

Phonocardiography should not be considered merely as a way to check and confirm auscultatory findings. It is *more accurate than auscultation* because it is not hampered by various physiological and psychological limitations inherent in auscultation. Having control of subsonic and borderline bands of vibrations, *phonocardiography covers a more extensive range.*

Differential diagnosis is considerably aided by phonocardiography in patients with the following diseases: rheumatic heart diseases with valvular lesions; luetic heart disease with aortic valve damage or aortitis; calcific aortic stenosis; congenital malformations of the heart and large vessels; bacterial endocarditis; adhesive and constrictive pericarditis; conditions associated with extensive myocardial damage (myocarditis; coronary heart disease; hypertensive heart disease); and disturbances of the heart rate and rhythm.

Low Frequency Tracing of the Precordium (Cardiography)

The name *cardiogram* was given in the past only to records of the apex beat. It is now possible to obtain records from nearly every point of the precordial area; any of them may bear the same name, with added indication of the area: i.e. "apex cardiogram," "cardiogram—2nd left interspace," etc.

These tracings were studied first by means of plain *tambours* (18); then by the use of a tambour with a metal spring and a button (19); and later by a tambour or funnel connected to a Frank's capsule (22, 23). Two methods have been used recently: linear cardiography and manometric cardiography.

LINEAR CARDIOGRAPHY (21, 201)

The *linear microphone* is a crystal microphone which has the characteristics of recording all mechanical vibrations from 0 to 1000 cycles per second, set up by cardiac action without any distortion (7). The value of the electrical potential is proportional to the intensity of the vibrations. As the low frequency vibrations are even 10,000 times larger than those of the cardiac sounds, the degree of amplification needed to register the former is so small that the latter are recorded only as minute notches, or not at all.

MANOMETRIC CARDIOGRAPHY (202)

The chest piece is connected by a short piece of hard tubing to the tube of an electromanometer. The latter is provided with a high sensitivity microphone and the whole system is filled with air.

Comparative studies (201) have shown that only slight differences are present between tracings of "linear" and "manometric cardiography." They consist of slightly larger rapid waves in the former, slightly larger slow waves in the latter. For various practical reasons, "linear cardiography" is still preferable to "manometric cardiography."

The usual technique of recording is the following. The patient is placed in a supine or semirecumbent position with complete muscular relaxation. A rubber strap is placed around his chest. A low funnel of 5 cm. in diameter with a side opening is screwed onto a "stethoscopic" microphone, placed over any point of the precordium, and held in place by the rubber strap. Thus

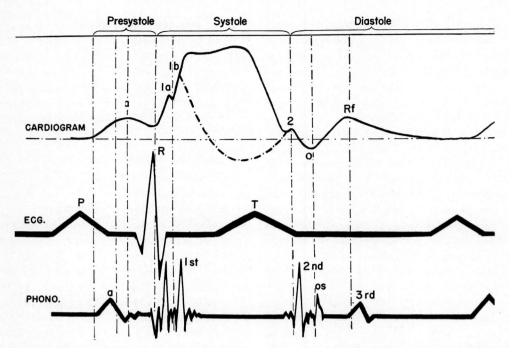

Fig. 54. The cardiogram with its physiological variations compared with the electrocardiogram and phonocardiogram.

two simultaneous tracings can be recorded: one of them is a tracing of the high frequency vibrations of the chest corresponding to a stethoscopic phonocardiogram; the other is a low frequency tracing of the chest, or cardiogram. The funnel records pulsations from about two intercostal spaces in the adult.

The following areas of the precordium can be investigated: *apex, midprecordium, pulmonic area, aortic area,* and *tricuspid area.*

The normal precordial tracing (figs. 54, 55 and 57) is the resultant of several factors:

a) *Movements* of the heart (especially of the apex) together with better contact of the ventricular wall with the chest wall due to rotation of the apex and stiffening of the ventricular mass during the tension period.

b) *Changes in volume* of the heart due to decrease of the ventricular mass during ejection, and its increase during diastole.

c) *Pulsations* of the large arteries, more or less directly transmitted.

The movements of the heart are particularly well recorded over the apex when the subject is either lying on his left side or sitting. The volume changes are recorded better over the mid-precordium in the supine position. The arterial pulsations are recorded best at the base.

A small upright and rounded wave can be observed in the cardiogram during *presystole* (wave 4). This is related to atrial contraction and is caused by *rapid inflow of blood entering the ventricles,* as proven by cases of complete heart block. The curve starts to rise at the *beginning of ventricular systole;* the onset of motion occurs between the Q and R waves of the electrocardiogram and with the first slow wave of the phonocardiogram in cases of atrial fibrillation. This rise, due to *hardening of the ventricular mass during the tension period, reaches a peak which is simultaneous with that part of the first sound indicating the closure of the a-v valves (point 1a).* Following a notch, the curve frequently rises again at the be-

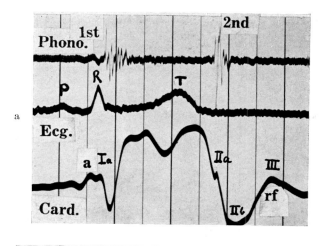

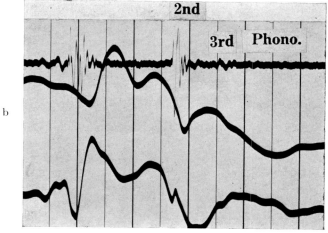

FIG. 55. Cardiograms recorded at the apex in a normal individual in the supine position. a, Cardiogram with positive plateau. ECG and sound tracing. b, Comparison of the cardiogram with carotid and sound tracings.

ginning of ejection, simultaneously with the opening of the semilunar valves (*point 1b*).

Two main types may be seen. In the first, a *systolic plateau* constitutes the main part of the tracing; this indicates predominance of motion phenomena in the tracing. In the second, a *deep, inverted wave occurs during most of systole*, changes of volume having predominance over evidence of motion. In both tracings, the curve has a notch, which is simultaneous with the closure of the semilunar valves (*point 2a*). From this point on, the various cardiograms are similar, whatever direction the waves had during systole.

Since *diastole* is accompanied by two phases of rapid inflow, there are two main diastolic waves in the cardiogram. The first is the *wave of rapid filling during early diastole*. This is usually well-defined and its peak is simultaneous with the third heart sound (*point 3*). A deep depression follows the notch which accompanies the main vibration of the second sound and precedes that simultaneous with the third. Its lowest point occurs at the time of, or slightly before, the *v* wave of the jugular and hepatic tracings (opening of the a-v valves) (*point 2b*). The second phase of rapid filling is caused by *atrial contraction* and takes place just before the following ventricular systole (*point 4*).

REGIONAL VARIATIONS

a) *Pulmonic area.* The waves are usually small but amplification facilitates their study. There is a *relatively high presystolic wave,* and a well-defined *positive wave during early systole.* The former is probably due to contraction of the *left atrium,* indirectly transmitted through intermediate organs. Whenever there is a pulsation during the ejection period, this is caused by the *pulse of the pulmonary artery (wave p).*

b) *Aortic area.* The waves are usually small. There is a well-defined wave *during the tension period* and a *positive wave during early systole.* The former is transmitted from the left ventricle; the latter is an arterial wave caused by the *pulse of the ascending aorta (wave p).* Closure of the aortic valves is marked by a notch.

c) *Tricuspid area.* The cardiogram shows a *high presystolic wave,* small systolic notches, and a well-defined, early-diastolic wave. The first is probably due to the *contraction of the right atrium* because of the proximity of this chamber; the latter is due to *rapid inflow* into the right ventricle.

Cardiography has lost much of its importance for the diagnosis of arrhythmias of the heart, having been replaced by electro-cardiography. It still has a place in the study of valvular and septal defects. Interesting cardiographic data may be found in cases of hypertensive or coronary heart disease, or cor pulmonale. In all of them, cardiography may be used in order to recognize the phase and significance of the sounds recorded by phonocardiography. The value of cardiograms for recognition of diastolic sounds is great, and is superior to that of jugular tracings. Cases of adhesive pericarditis and of aortic aneurysm often require an accurate cardiographic study. Personal studies (201) have shown that the comparison of the apex cardiogram with the epigastric tracing is of value for recognition of right or left ventricular enlargement.

Epigastric Tracing

Epigastric tracings were recorded long ago by students of cardiology (25, 26, 27). The present technique is identical with that of cardiograms (page 95). The bell should be placed as high as possible in the epigastric triangle, even to the extent of including part of the xiphoid process, but more on the left side. The patient may be studied in either the supine or the sitting position. The latter gives rise to larger respiratory oscillations, which, however, can be avoided by using a special filter. A rubber strap keeps the microphone in place without undue pressure. If an epigastric tracing is recorded together with an apex phonocardiogram, two microphones should be used: one should be placed over the apex; the other is used as a support for the bell, over the epigastrium. The bell of the latter should be connected to a linear microphone, and the tracing is recorded by the electrocardiograph.

NORMAL EPIGASTRIC TRACING

The following factors should be considered:

a) Pulsations transmitted through the diaphragm from the heart, mainly the right heart.

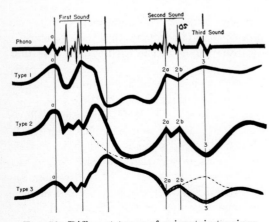

FIG. 56. Different types of epigastric tracings

b) Effect of changes of intrathoracic pressure on the diaphragm.

c) Pulsations of the liver.

d) Pulsations of the abdominal aorta.

Epigastric tracings are by no means identical. Even in different normal individuals, an amazing variety of records can be obtained (fig. 56). Some parts of the tracing are common to all while others vary. Again, a terminology similar to that of the cardiogram is suggested.

A high positive wave is usually present during *presystole* (*wave 4*). During the *period of tension*, the curve either falls below the base line or has two small notches caused by the two valvular events of this phase (*1a* and *1b*). A positive wave may be present in the phase immediately following; however, in most tracings, a deep *negative plateau* takes place during a large part of systole. A positive wave, simultaneous with the arterial pulse, occurs in others (*wave p*). Closure of the semilunar valves is marked on all records by a well-defined notch (*2a*) which may be either upright or inverted. The *opening of the a-v valves* is well-defined in most records (*2b*). *Rapid filling* of the ventricles is also indicated by a deep wave which may be either upright or inverted (*wave 3*).

The presystolic wave is largely due to the mechanical movement of the *right atrium*, transmitted through the diaphragm. The two notches *1a* and *1b*, when present, are caused by the valvular events of early systole and probably more by those of the right heart. The *high systolic wave* represents the beginning of a systolic plateau, abruptly interrupted by the following *systolic collapse*. It is likely that the plateau is due mostly to motion of the right ventricle; the collapse, to its volume changes. The high wave of other tracings, on the contrary, occurs later in systole and is a *transmitted aortic pulsation*.

Different types of tracings can be recognized (fig. 56). *Type 1 tracings reveal the predominant influence of ventricular events*

during systole and early diastole. *Type 2 tracings show mainly the effect of changes of intrathoracic pressure. Type 3 tracings are largely influenced by the aortic pulsations* but still show effect of motion during presystole and early systole; effect of thoracic pressure changes during diastole. *Type 4 tracings are pure hepatic tracings* and occur when the enlarged liver occupies the epigastrium (page 103, figs. 58 and 59b).

If it is true that the right heart has a particular influence on the epigastric tracing, information about dynamics of the right atrium and ventricle will be obtained by the study of this record. Simultaneous (or immediately subsequent) tracings of the apex and the epigastrium complete, therefore, our knowledge of the dynamics of the two halves of the heart. The atrial wave of the tracing is larger in the epigastric tracing than in any other record of cardiac pulsations. In cases where a hepatic tracing is necessary, this should always be compared with the epigastric tracing in order to avoid confusion between liver pulsations and transmitted pulsations. Comparison of the epigastric tracing with the apex cardiogram is of value for recognition of right or left ventricular enlargement (201).

Jugular Vein Tracing (Phlebogram)

Venous pulsations may be very striking and accordingly they were described early and studied in detail (28–31). Increasing progress of electrocardiography lessened the importance of the phlebogram. More recent studies, related in general to phonocardiography and particularly to cases of bundle branch block and mitral stenosis, again made use of venous tracings.

Early studies were made by lightly applying a funnel over the bulb of the right jugular vein. The funnel was connected with a Marey tambour. Necessity of avoiding any, even slight, compression of the vein led to description of many ingenious devices, such as a little sambucus ball moving a delicate lever (32). Progress was later made by substituting a Frank's capsule for the Marey's tambour. Later, a small mirror, reflecting a light beam, was pasted on the skin of the cervical region or the patient was directly interposed between the source of light and the camera (33).

The best system consists of a special applicator and a crystal microphone (21). The *applicator* is a double circular cup. The inner chamber is used for picking up the venous pulsations; the outer chamber, connected with the bulb, develops a suction for fastening the cup to the patient's skin. The venous pulsations set up changes of pressure in the funnel. These are transmitted through a short tube to a linear microphone which converts them into equivalent electric pulsations. The electric waves are recorded

by the camera after amplification and transmission to a galvanometer.

The *suction cup* is applied either over the external jugular vein or over the jugular bulb. The right side of the neck is usually preferred owing to the greater proximity of the great veins to the right atrium. In normal people and in most patients, the venous pulse is recorded in supine position, with the head nearly at the level of the heart. In cardiac patients, a good tracing can sometimes be obtained in a semirecumbent position because of the higher venous pressure. In persons with low venous pressure, a tracing can be obtained either by placing the head slightly lower than the heart or by slightly compressing the vein.

The normal venous tracings show three

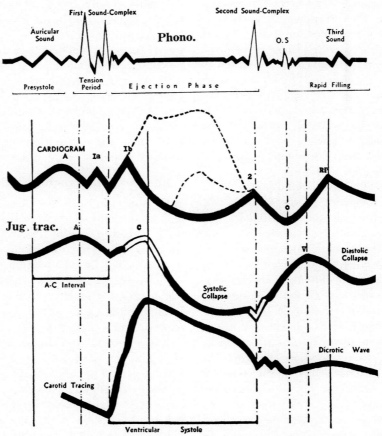

FIG. 57. The jugular tracing (phlebogram) compared with the other tracings. In black, that part of the tracing which has a venous origin. In white, that part of the tracing which has an arterial origin.

positive and three negative waves (30) (figs. 57, 58 and 59a).

The presystolic wave (*a*) is positive and occurs during and after atrial contraction. It is usually a rounded wave followed by a sharp drop during early tension of the ventricles. However, tracings recorded through an amplifier frequently present a tall and peaked presystolic wave.

The systolic wave (*c*) is positive and occurs during early systole, after the opening of the semilunar valves. It is a peaked wave followed by a long and slow *depression* (*x*, or *systolic collapse*) which lasts through most of the ejection period and slightly beyond it. Toward its end, a little notch may mark the closure of the semilunar valves.

The early-diastolic wave (*v*) is also positive. It is a peaked wave which coincides with the opening of the a-v valves and marks, therefore, the beginning of ventricular filling. This is followed by a *depression* (*y*, or *diastolic collapse*). When diastole is long, another small positive wave (*h*) may be found after *v*.

Two types of jugular tracings are most commonly recorded in normal subjects:

a) The *atrial pressure* type. Here the *c* wave is characterized by a sharp decline at the onset of systolic ejection and during the traction on the atrio-ventricular septum, just as in atrial pressure curves.

b) The *modified arterial* type. The *c* wave is high and rapid, due to impact of an adjacent artery. It often resembles the first part of a central arterial pulse.

It has been shown (36) that each wave of the venous tracing is the result of *changes of volume, of pressure, and velocity*. The relation between these three factors (volume, pressure, and velocity) varies from moment to moment. It seems likely, moreover, that in high venous pressure, changes of pressure predominate over changes of volume because the veins are already distended.

The *presystolic* (*a*) *wave* is undoubtedly related to the contraction of the right atrium as shown by the fact that it is absent in

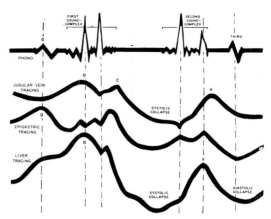

Fig. 58. The jugular tracing compared with the hepatic and epigastric tracings.

cases of atrial fibrillation. Its beginning marks the beginning of atrial contraction; its peak, the end of the same phase. The *a* wave is largely a pressure wave with additional volume and velocity components. Actual regurgitation of blood is minimal in normal subjects but may become more important when venous pressure is high and the superior cava is dilated. The wave occurs about 0.10 second after the corresponding rise of pressure within the right atrium. The wave is much larger when simultaneous contraction of the atria and ventricles leads to important regurgitation of blood into the venous system as in nodal rhythm, nodal premature beats, and a-v block.

The *systolic* (*c*) *wave is a pressure wave*. In many cases it is due to transmission of the strong pulsation of the underlying subclavian or carotid artery and the wave is an unavoidable artefact. In other cases, the wave is venous and is caused by an arterial pulsation, transmitted from the ascending aorta to the superior vena cava. The same is true of the small notch marking the closure of the semilunar valves (fig. 57). It has been shown (39, 40, 41) that *occasionally a double* (*c*) *wave may be seen*, the first component being due to closure of the tricuspid valve; the second, to arterial pulsation.

The *early diastolic wave* (*v*) is connected to the opening of the tricuspid valve. The

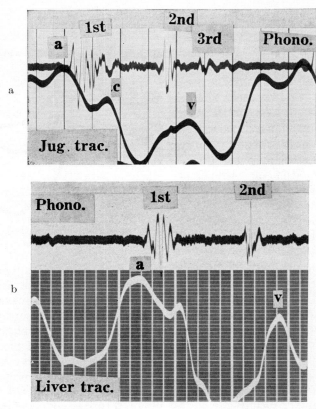

Fig. 59. a, Jugular tracing of a normal young man in the supine position. Phonocardiogram. b, Hepatic tracing of a normal young man. Phonocardiogram.

rise preceding its peak is the expression of the gradual filling of the right atrium. Therefore, the *v wave is chiefly a volume wave.* However, as the fall of the curve is caused by the opening of the tricuspid valve, *the descending limb is almost exclusively due to a drop in pressure.*

A *depression* occurs during early tension of the ventricles. Its depth is greater when the interval between atrial and ventricular contractions is longer. The *depression (x) (systolic collapse)* occurs during the ejection phase of ventricular systole. It is due to suction caused on the venous system by the outflow of blood from the thorax and by the downward movement of the a-v septum. It is, therefore, a wave due to *increased speed* of the blood and *decreased volume* of the vein.

The depression (y) (diastolic collapse) fol-

lows the *v* wave. Slow filling of the right atrium terminates this depression. Sometimes it is followed by a small positive wave which has been attributed to floating of the tricuspid valve.

There is no constant relation between the waves of the phlebogram and those of the electrocardiogram, except for a close time relationship between the intervals *a-c* and *P-Q.*

The waves of the jugular and hepatic tracings practically coincide, except for the *c* wave which is nearly absent in the latter.

The fourth (atrial) sound slightly precedes the peak of the *a* wave of the venous tracing. This concidence is due to the fact that both events *follow* the atrial contraction; the fourth sound is due to the blood hitting the ventricular wall while it takes some time for the transmission of the *a* wave from the right atrium to the vein. The descending limb of the *a* wave is so slow that it ends after the start of the first sound.

The main vibration of the *second sound* precedes the peak of *v* by about 0.10 second, while the *third sound* falls during the descending limb of *v*, e.g. 0.064 to 0.078 second later. However, there may be a much shorter interval between *v* and the third sound, and there may even be coincidence. This fact, due to occasional slower transmission of the *v* wave, reduces the importance of the jugular tracing for identification of an early diastolic sound.

The jugular tracing is of definite value: a) in valvular defects, chiefly tricuspid lesions, b) in heart failure with functional insufficiency of the tricuspid valve, c) in bundle branch block, and d) in cases with low voltage of the *P* wave of the electrocardiogram or where the former is masked by other waves. The jugular tracing gives information concerning mechanical events of the right heart. In this respect it still holds a special place, together with the hepatic and epigastric tracings, among graphic methods.

Record of Pulsations of the Liver (Hepatic Tracing)

The hepatic tracing is recorded without difficulty when the liver is enlarged or lowered; tracings of normal individuals are obtained less readily.

The hepatic tracing was studied many years ago (29, 42). The importance of this record is due to the fact that 1) the liver is influenced by changes of flow and pressure in the inferior vena cava, and 2) there is no underlying arterial vessel (corresponding to the carotid artery under the jugular vein) which may affect the record. Old records were obtained by means of Marey tambours (25, 37, 43, 44). More recent studies of normal hepatic tracings were made by means of a Frank's capsule (45).

Modern procedure is based on the fact that a crystal microphone of a "linear" type transforms pulsations of the air contained in the applicator into electrical waves. These are recorded by the galvanometer of an electrocardiograph and are transcribed photographically or by direct-writing methods. Another sound or mechanical tracing should be simultaneously recorded in order to time accurately the waves. Whenever the waves are small and magnification is necessary, a preamplifier may be introduced between the crystal microphone and the galvanometer. The sensitivity of the linear microphone is such that the round bell normally used for taking low frequency tracings of the chest is sufficient for recording hepatic tracings. A microphone, connected to the cup as a support, is placed over the right upper quadrant of the abdomen and is held by a rubber strap. If respiration is forceful and irregular, the microphone may be held by hand; however, this procedure is not recommended because slight movements of the hand may be recorded by the microphone. In normal individuals, the same procedure may be used on that part of the liver which crosses the epigastrium by firmly applying the cup below the right costal arch. Respiratory movements possess an amplitude far greater than the hepatic waves; therefore it is necessary for the patient to "hold his breath" for a few seconds during the taking of the tracing. If the patient is unable to do so, closing of the nose and mouth by hand for a few seconds may be necessary. Otherwise, a high pass, electric filter may be used. This reduces the amplitude of all slow waves, so that the shape of certain hepatic waves is somewhat changed. Detection of a plateau might be more difficult with the use of the filter.

The hepatic tracing shows a *small, positive wave during presystole (a wave)* (figs. 58 and 59b). It is due to presystolic swelling of the liver when atrial contraction arrests the venous inflow. Regurgitation of blood in presystole is minimal in normal individuals while it may be important in subjects with high venous pressure. The *a* wave of the jugular tracing and that of the hepatic tracing are practically simultaneous. However, the jugular *a* wave may precede the hepatic *a* wave, especially if the former is recorded through an amplifier. The rise of the *a* wave of the hepatic tracing precedes the 1st sound at the apex by about 0.15 sec. Tracings of patients with high venous pressure and distended liver may present an atrial wave which is much higher in the hepatic than in the epigastric tracing, proving the hepatic origin of this wave. In exceptional cases a double presystolic wave may be recorded. The first (*a*) is transmitted through the diaphragm via the epigastrium; the second (*a*¹) is a real hepatic wave.

The beginning of ventricular contraction is revealed by a small, positive wave (*wave 1*), probably transmitted through the diaphragm; following this, there is a deep collapse. In normal individuals, the *systolic collapse* recorded below the right costal arch is far deeper than that recorded below the left costal arch. Therefore, the former is the result of decreased hepatic volume while the latter is due to rise of the diaphragm with decrease of abdominal pressure. Sometimes a small notch can be seen during that part of the 1st sound which coincides with the opening of the semilunar valves and during the wave *1b* of the cardiogram; it is probably transmitted through the diaphragm.

The tracing rises gradually at first, rapidly later, with a peak (*v* or *2b*) at the time of the opening of the tricuspid valve. Following this, the curve falls, forming a *deep and rounded negative wave*, variable in shape and depth because of the effect of respiration on venous return. The lowest point of this wave coincides with the wave of rapid filling of the cardiogram, and should be named *3*. It may also be called *diastolic collapse*.

It should be kept in mind that a right ventricular impact is transcribed as an early systolic wave followed by a deep depression

while the positive hepatic pulse of tricuspid insufficiency consists of a positive systolic plateau (page 270).

In conclusion, the normal hepatic tracing is formed by a *deep negative wave, the systolic collapse*. This is preceded by an *atrial posiive wave* and is followed by a *diastolic collapse* (figs. 58 and 59b). The main causes for these waves are changes of flow in the inferior vena cava. Smaller notches may be transmitted from the heart through the diaphragm.

The hepatic tracing may yield important data in diseases of the tricuspid valve, in heart failure, and in constrictive pericarditis. The absence of an underlying artery, giving a powerful systolic pulsation, may make the hepatic tracing superior to the jugular vein tracing.

Pulsations of the Heart Recorded Through the Esophagus (Esophagocardiogram)

The esophagocardiogram was first recorded by using a Marey tambour (48–56); then, by a Frank's capsule (57, 58). The linear microphone should be preferred and gives accurate tracings. A phonocardiogram can be recorded together with the esophagocardiogram.

The best type of stomach tube is one of 5-mm. internal bore. This may be connected to a rubber cylinder having a metal support or a small balloon slightly distended by air.[29] The tube should be marked in centimeters and should be radio-opaque, so that its penetration may be followed by fluoroscopy. It should be kept in mind that the esophagus curves in its lower section and proceeds from the vicinity of the spine into the anterior mediastinum below the heart. According to the position of the tip, four types of curves can be obtained:

a) At the aortic level, 25 to 30 cm. from the dental arch.

[29] A thin (0.1-mm.) rubber membrane tied around the tip of a stomach tube may be used for the purpose.

b) At a high atrial level, 30 to 35 cm. from the dental arch.

c) At a low atrial level, 35 to 40 cm. from the dental arch.

d) At the ventricular level, 40 to 45 cm. from the dental arch.

Each of the tracings present interest. However, those of positions b and c are the most important.

a) *Tracing at the aortic level.* The characteristics of this are the following. A small, negative wave during presystole, 0.05 to 0.08 after the beginning of *P* in the electrocardiogram (*wave 4*); a small, diphasic wave at the beginning of systole with inscription of the first large vibration of the first sound (*wave 1a*); a deep systolic collapse during the ejection period, interrupted by a small positive wave simultaneous with the *c* wave of the jugular tracing; a rapid rise coinciding with the second sound and the incisura of the carotid pulse (*wave 2a*); a rapid rise with a positive peak at the time of the third sound (*wave 3*).

b) *Tracing at the high atrial level.* Usually, a negative wave is present during presystole (*wave 4*); a positive peak is simultaneous with the first sound (*wave 1*); then there is a small dip and a small peak, synchronous with the *c* wave of the jugular tracing; later, a rounded, negative wave occurs during ejection and culminates with a positive peak at the time of the second sound (*wave 2*); last, a negative peak is present during rapid filling of the ventricles (*wave 3*).

c) *Tracing at the low atrial level (true atrial tracing)* (fig. 60). There is a negative wave during presystole with a peak which follows by 0.03–0.04 that of the P wave of the electrocardiogram (*wave 4*); this wave may be double-peaked. After this, and starting after R, a small positive wave (*wave 1a*) occurs during the first part of the first sound. This is followed by a small drop and another small, positive wave, synchronous with the second part of the first heart sound (*wave 1b*). Then there is a systolic collapse and a positive or negative peak at the time of the

second sound (*wave 2*). Rapid ventricular filling is marked by a deep collapse (*wave 3*).

d) *Tracing at the ventricular level.* The presystolic wave (*4*) is more frequently positive than negative. The systolic collapse is poorly visible. There are large vibrations caused by the valvular events and simultaneous with the heart sounds *1a*, *1b*, *2a*. Rapid filling is marked by a high positive wave called *3*.

Several factors act on the intra-esophageal pressure and give rise to the waves of the esophagocardiogram:

a) *The variations of intrathoracic pressure.* One of the main effects is the deep systolic collapse of the tracing at the aortic level.

b) *The changes in volume of the left atrium.* This chamber is in the near proximity of the esophagus and its presystolic contraction causes a negative wave in the tracing at the low atrial level (sometimes also in that at the high atrial level). Lowering of the atrio-ventricular floor by the left ventricle causes the systolic collapse at the low atrial level.

c) *The pulsation of the descending aorta.* It may be observed in the tracing recorded at the high atrial level as a positive systolic wave.

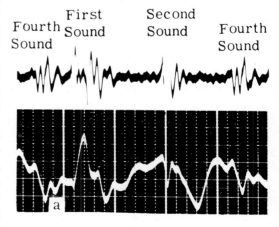

FIG. 60. Sound tracing from the esophagus, and esophagocardiogram at high atrial level in a normal adult.

d) *The impact of the ventricular contraction.* It can be observed in most tracings, chiefly during the tension period.

e) *The vibrations of the heart sounds.* These are inscribed in most of the tracings.

Until a few years ago, the esophagocardiogram had a unique position. This tracing, recorded at the atrial level, presented direct evidence of the movements of the left atrium. Its usefulness was particularly marked in patients with a systolic murmur where a differential diagnosis between rheumatic mitral disease and other cardiac diseases was necessary. At present, electrokymography represents an easier and better tolerated method of study. Still, esophagocardiography presents some interest. In particular, whenever a fluoroscope and an electrokymograph are not available, the esophocardiogram may be the method of choice.

Pulsations of the Heart Recorded Through the Air Passages (Internal Pneumocardiogram)

Physiologic studies of the past (59, 60) showed that the heart beat is accompanied by changes of pressure within the thorax causing a movement of air through the nostrils and mouth. In the presence of disease, this movement may be so great that the observer becomes aware of it (61–63). Older studies were made through the use of either a Marey tambour (64, 65) or a Frank's

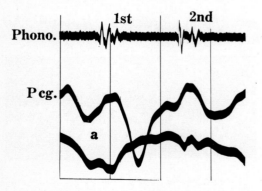

Fig. 61. A normal pneumocardiogram (Pcg.) compared with a sound tracing (Phono.).

capsule (66). The use of the pneumotachograph connected to a Frank's capsule (67) or to a string anemometer (68a) later permitted a more careful study of the different waves. A study of the pneumocardiogram by means of an *intrabronchial catheter* (68) confirmed that the recorded waves are caused mainly by differences between inflow to and outflow from the chest.

Use of the *linear microphone with a filter* and recording of the pneumocardiogram together with a phonocardiogram constitutes the present technique (69). The filter is used for decreasing the intensity of the slow, respiratory, waves without curtailing the rapid pulsations caused by the heart beat.[30] A rubber tube is connected to the microphone. It ends in an "olive" which is inserted in one of the nostrils of the patient. The patient is placed in a comfortable sitting position with complete muscular relaxation. A semi-recumbent position may also be employed. The patient is instructed to breath normally through the nose with his mouth closed.

The normal pneumocardiogram has five negative waves, each having a definite connection with some phase of cardiac action. Only two positive waves are usually present but, as the junction between some of the negative waves may become more positive and reach a point above the base line, they may increase in number (figs. 50 and 61).

A negative wave (*a*) is present *during presystole*. Residual arterial outflow from

[30] The electrical filter does not remove every trace of the low-frequency waves caused by respiration. Thus, some waves may be seen in the pneumocardiogram in one cycle and not in another because of the unlike rhythms of respiration and cardiac action. These respiratory components are more marked in children and excitable adults. Pneumocardiographic waves may be differentiated from respiratory waves because they occur in every succeeding cardiac cycle, although they may be somewhat modified in contour. Difference between different cycles, however, is more than an artefact; it is partly due to changes of venous return by effect of the different respiratory phases.

the thorax plus the cessation of venous return causes a suction of air and therefore a depression in the pneumocardiogram. Later, a small, positive wave is simultaneous with the wave *1a* of the apex beat before the rise of the carotid pulse. The a-v valves are slightly raised at the beginning of the tension period, then are lowered by the contraction of the papillary muscles. This movement creates a slight aspiration of blood into the right atrium with a resulting small outflow of air from the thorax. This notch is called p^1 (*contraction of the papillary muscles*, or *first positive wave*).

During the *first half of systole*, blood leaves the thorax through the branches of the aortic arch and abdominal aorta. Considerable aspiration of air into the thorax exists in this phase with a resulting negative wave in the pneumocardiogram. This wave, which is often the most marked of all, has been called v^1 (*1st ventricular wave*).

After the first part of systole, the aspiration exerted on the veins by the increased negative pressure within the thorax and by the lowering of the atrio-ventricular septum causes a quick inflow into the right atrium (as shown by the jugular and hepatic tracings) which may be greater than the outflow of arterial blood. The pneumocardiogram shows an upright notch which usually does not reach the zero line but may occasionally becomes positive. The pulsations of the pulmonary arteries and of the tracheal and nasopharyngeal vessels also contribute to the formation of this wave (*wave* p^2 = *peripheral pulse or 2nd positive wave*).

Little blood enters the thorax during the *second half of systole* since the right atrium is nearly filled. At the same time, the blood continues to flow into the peripheral vessels, and another negative wave occurs in the pneumocardiogram, evidence of a suction of air into the thorax. This wave (v^2 = *second ventricular wave*) is, at times, larger than v^1.

An upright notch (s = *semilunar valves*) occurs simultaneously with the 2nd sound and with the *incisura* of the carotid pulse. A small downward wave (d^1) or a straight line occurs later.

The opening of the tricuspid valve causes a sudden inrush of blood from the veno-atrial reservoir into the right ventricle. The moment of transition is indicated by an upright notch which may become a decidedly positive wave (t *wave* = *tricuspid valve opening*). It occurs simultaneously with the point o of the cardiogram and with, or before, the peak of the v wave of the jugular tracing. An increased amount of blood leaves the thorax at the time of the *dicrotic wave* in the aorta. Blood flows from the large veins into the right atrium but its amount is less than that which leaves the thorax through the arteries. Therefore, an inflow of air into the thorax occurs, revealed by a deep, negative wave in the pneumocardiogram (d^2 = *second diastolic wave*). The peak of the wave rf of the cardiogram and the *3rd heart sound* occur at the point of maximum depression of d^2.

Normal persons show *larger waves of the pneumocardiogram during inspiration, smaller waves during expiration*. The best tracings are obtained either in a *sitting* or in a *semi-recumbent position* with the patient complete relaxed. Other positions (such as supine, sitting erect, sitting bent forward, or standing) may produce important changes in the pneumocardiogram (68) which can be explained as the result of an altered venous return. In general, the difference between the sitting and semi-recumbent positions is unimportant. Somewhat different results have been obtained by others employing different techniques (68b).

Arterial Pulse Tracings (Sphygmograms)

A *sphygmogram* is a tracing of the changes in volume of an artery, consequent to internal changes in pressure. It can be divided into three types: aortogram, cervical sphygmogram, and peripheral sphygmogram.

The old *sphygmographs* recorded the pulsation of the radial artery by placing over it a button with a tension such that the extra-arterial approximated the intra-arterial diastolic pressure (Marey's principle). First, systems of levers or tambours amplified the excursions of the arterial wall (18, 19, 70–73). Then an improved record was obtained by the use of a pneumatic cuff, inflated to a known pressure, and of a differential capsule (oscillometric capsule of Pachon-Boulitte) (74). Further improvement was obtained by using a Frank's optical capsule and by photographic recording. The optic method was later adapted to the differential capsule as well as to an open cup pressed to the skin over the carotid artery. The latest improvement is the combination of pneumatic cuff, differential capsule, and crystal microphone (154) (p. 161).

The *aortogram* may be recorded readily over three points: the *2nd right interspace*, the *suprasternal notch*, and *the abdomen* (fig. 62). The first record, already described with the cardiogram, shows a typical aortic pulse but still has some waves caused by cardiac action. The second type of aortogram is nearly free from cardiac waves. Whenever the aortic arch is dilated, or blood pressure is increased, excellent tracings are obtained in this area. The abdominal aortogram is recorded about 1 inch above the umbilicus. Poor results are obtained when the abdomen is distended or obese. In lean individuals, on the contrary, it is obtained easily. In aortic lesions, this tracing is of interest.

In all three types of aortogram, a small cup, connected to a linear microphone, is

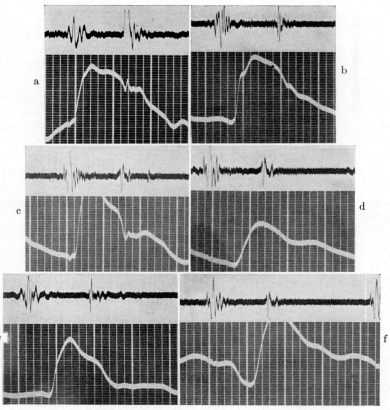

FIG. 62. Pulse in different arteries compared with the sound tracing over the aortic area in normal young people. a, suprasternal notch; b, abdominal aorta; c, subclavian artery; d, radial artery; e, femoral artery; f, tibial artery.

pressed against the skin over the vessel. In the case of the suprasternal notch, the pressure is made by hand; in the other two instances, a rubber band holds the cup. The simplest way is to use the microphone as a support for the cup. Thus, a simultaneous recording of the arterial sounds is possible.

The *cervical pulse* may be obtained over either the carotid or the subclavian artery. The best way to obtain such a tracing is again by the use of an open cup, pressed on the artery either behind the sterno-cleido-mastoideus (carotid), or above the clavicle (subclavian) (fig. 62).

The *peripheral pulse* of the extremities (arm, forearm, wrist, thigh, leg, foot) is recorded easily by an apparatus consisting of a *double chamber pneumatic cuff connected to a linear microphone and an amplifier* (75). It utilizes both the principle of the differential manometer and that of the crystal microphone. It has the advantage that the records are taken from a cuff maintained at a constant pressure, while the pressure is modified at will in another cuff. Furthermore, it gives two simultaneous records: that of the arterial pulse and that of the arterial sounds. Therefore, in addition to sphygmographic purposes, the apparatus may be used also for graphic recording of the blood pressure (page 161).

The pulse of the fingers or toes can be recorded by means of a *photoelectric cell* (transillumination of the part) (173).

AORTIC TRACING

The aortogram is essentially a tracing of *central pulse* (fig. 61 a, b). Tracings recorded in normal subjects at the 2nd right interspace or at the suprasternal notch may present additional waves due to changes of cardiac volume and inscription of vibrations which are simultaneous with the heart sounds.

An atrial wave in presystole (*wave 4*); a small wave during the tension period (*wave 1a*); and a wave of rapid filling in early

diastole (*wave 3*), may be observed. The tracing shows a steep rise at the beginning of ejection and a small depression in the ascending limb of the pulse (*anacrotism*). This is followed by a slower rise, a rounded peak, and a slow decline. The end of ventricular contraction and the onset of ventricular relaxation are marked by a sudden drop of the tracing (*incisura*). After this, one or more coarse vibrations take place indicating the rebound of the blood on the closed aortic valve; then a slow decline of the tracing can be seen.

As soon as the ascending aorta and the aortic arch are dilated, the blood wave moves rapidly into the abdominal aorta and reaches the arteries of the legs. The movement of blood during systole is complicated by the *low natural frequency* of the aortic wall and by *reflected waves* from regions with sudden narrowings and branchings (73). It has been proven that the pulse wave presents gradual changes so that it gradually acquires a higher peak and a simpler contour. This is due to the existence of a "standing wave" created by alternate accelerations and decelerations (203). The arch and the upper part of the descending aorta accommodate more blood during the first part of ejection; the lower aorta and its branches, more blood during the second half. For this reason, the abdominal aortogram has a more pointed peak and shows less well the various details of the tracing.

The aortogram is of interest in:

a) Diffuse enlargement (aortitis) or local dilatations (aneurysms) of the ascending aorta and aortic arch due to luetic heart disease (2nd space and suprasternal notch).

b) Aortic stenosis (2nd space and suprasternal notch).

c) Coarctation of the aorta (abdominal aorta).

d) Arteriosclerotic dilatation of the abdominal aorta (abdominal aorta). Differential diagnosis with tumors or masses with transmitted pulsation.

CENTRAL PULSE

The tracing of a central pulse, as recorded over the *cervical area*, reveals the following details (fig. 62).

a) One or two small waves are present during presystole and during the tension period of the ventricles.

b) There is a rapidly *ascending phase* (the *anacrotic slope*) which frequently presents a change of speed (*anacrotic depression*). The rise of the curve coincides with that large vibration of the 1st sound which is caused by opening of the aortic valves.

c) The *peak* or *summit of the percussion wave* is attained at about the middle of systole and is followed by a slight depression.

d) A second, more rounded, wave (*tidal wave*) occurs during the second part of systole and is followed by the beginning of the *descending phase* (*catacrotic slope*).

e) In coincidence with the main vibration of the 2nd sound (closure of the aortic valve), the curve presents a sudden drop (*incisura*), often followed by one or two small vibrations.

f) The curve rises again forming a slow positive wave, the *dicrotic wave*.

g) Later, the tracing gradually falls to its lowest level which is attained just prior to the rise of the following pulse wave.

Reflected waves from peripheral subdivisions may be superimposed on the curve if this is taken at a high level of the carotid artery (upper carotid pulse); the changes are noticeable during early ejection soon after the time of the incisura. They occur earlier if there is hypertonus or sclerosis of the wall so that the speed of the pulse wave is increased. On the contrary, low tonus of the wall is revealed by a high-peaked tracing.

The *small waves* which precede the rise of the pulse curve are transmitted from the heart. The first is caused by atrial contraction; the second, by bulging of the aortic valve during the tension period. The rapid, ascending phase of the pulse curve is due to the *ejection of blood* into the aorta. The anacrotic change of slope is due to the fact

that at first the inertia prevents a large displacement of blood while later a more rapid flow occurs (76). The tonic-elastic reaction of the aorta may also contribute to it. The formation of a *summit* when about one-half of the blood has left the left ventricle may be attributed to the fact that the volume of blood entering the aorta is then smaller than that leaving the aorta through the various branches. The *tidal wave* seems due to the summation of the still-moving wave with multiple waves reflected from the periphery.

The aorta and the left ventricle are still a single chamber at the beginning of ventricular diastole. Ventricular relaxation causes a sharp drop of pressure in the aorta which is quickly terminated by closure of the semilunar valves; this causes the *incisura*. While pressure eddies complete the closure of the aortic valve, the retraction of the aortic wall forces blood toward the heart as well as toward the periphery. This sets up a negative wave which follows the main wave (*incisura*). After closure of the aortic valve, the blood column rebounds from its surface and sets up a second, positive wave (*dicrotic wave*) which follows the main wave toward the periphery.

The tracing of the central pulse is useful mainly for timing the waves of other tracings. For example, hepatic tracings or electrokymograms are frequently timed by means of a carotid tracing. The tracing of the central pulse gives accurate information about the time of opening of the aortic valve (rise of the pulse) and its closure (incisura of the pulse). Therefore, this tracing presents interest in bundle branch block. Abnormal patterns are found in atherosclerosis of the aorta, coarctation of the aorta, aortic stenosis, and aortic insufficiency. The tracing helps in the differential diagnosis of these conditions.

PERIPHERAL PULSE

The peripheral pulse of *normal subjects* is much simpler than the central pulse. The ascending phase is straight, the incisura is replaced by a *rounded depression*. The *dicrotic wave* is also rounded. After the dicrotic wave, other secondary vibrations may occur (figs. 62, 63).

The reaction of the peripheral arteries deepens the predicrotic notch, transforming it into a valley, and rounds out the dicrotic wave. Therefore, the peripheral pulse shows no evidence of the tidal wave.

The *abnormal sphygmogram* may show marked variations:

a) The *water-hammer type* has a steep, ascending slope and a rapid drop. There is a turbulent condition at the front of the wave which may be revealed by a small *anacrotic notch* and is felt as a *thrill* upon palpation (76). It is typical of aortic regurgitation.

b) The *anacrotic pulse* has a deep notch in the ascending slope. It is found in aortic stenosis, hypertension, and marked bradycardia (pages 252).

c) The *dicrotic pulse* has a high dicrotic wave. It is found in fever, anemia, and hyperthyroidism.

d) *Pulsus alternans* is a regular pulse which has alternatively a large and a small wave. It is found in cases with severe myocardial damage (page 373).

e) *Pulsus paradoxus* is the name for the periodical waxing and waning of the pulse connected with respiration and is typical of constrictive pericarditis (page 454).

A measurement which seems to have a certain clinical value is that of *crest time*. This is measured in seconds between the rise of the pulse and the highest point of the main wave (204). Normal crest time of the radial pulse is between 10 and 16 per cent of the total duration of the pulse cycle, from rise of one pulse to rise of the next.

THE ABSOLUTE SPHYGMOGRAM

The sphygmogram is a pressure tracing of the artery. However, it does not reveal that important element of pressure which is between the foot of the wave and zero. In order to quickly evaluate the different elements, a diagram has been suggested,

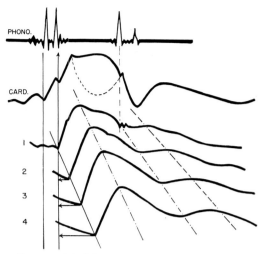

FIG. 63. Modification of the accidents of the pulse tracing from the central to the peripheral arteries. Phono., sound tracing; card., cardiogram; 1, subclavian pulse; 2, brachial pulse; 3, radial pulse; 4, tibial pulse.

which is called the *absolute sphygmogram*. In this diagram, the ordinates represent *pressure*, as measured by clinical evaluation, while the abscissae represent *time* and are modified by the pulse rate.

The sphygmogram can be used for the following studies.

1) *Speed of the pulse wave*. For this purpose the sphygmogram should be recorded together with another tracing. If speed from the heart to a certain artery is studied, a cardiogram may be used. However, the simplest way is to record the heart sounds simultaneously over the aortic area and the arterial pulse. *The distance between the second large vibration of the 1st sound (opening of the semilunar valves) and the rise of the pulse wave gives the speed of the wave if compared with the time lines of the record.* When, on the other hand, one wishes to record the speed of the pulse wave in a certain artery, two simultaneous sphygmograms are recorded over different points of the artery. It is a good precaution to take them at the level of the diastolic pressure in order not to alter the local flow.

2) *Shape of the pulse wave*. Three records should be taken; at diastolic pressure, at mean pressure, and at two-thirds of the way from the diastolic upwards. The latter may show great prominence of all secondary waves including the anacrotic notch.

3) *Study of arterial sounds (phonoarteriogram)*. The sound tracing is automatically recorded together with the sphygmogram by using the above-described apparatus (pages 107 and 161).

4) *Irregularity of the heart*. Simultaneous electrocardiograms and sphygmograms are taken. The former gives information about the type of arrhythmia; the latter shows the peripheral effect of the disorder.

5) *Study of the peripheral circulation*. The study of the arterial pulse may be very important in cases of arteritis, thrombosis, or embolism. The pneumatic cuff is successively applied to different sections of the limb, and the sphygmogram is recorded at the lowest pressure capable of giving a good record. Crest time is measured in both the tracing of the medium-sized arteries and in that of fingers or toes.

6) *Measure of stroke volume*. A method for calculating stroke volume on the basis of the study of the pulse was described (205). As the difference between the values found by this and those found by the Fick method may reach 50 per cent, the method is unreliable.

The Diastolic Waves in the Various Tracings

A. Atrial wave. The interval between right and left atrial contractions is so small in normal individuals that very little difference in the time of appearance of the waves is to be expected. Even so, a marked difference can be found between apex and epigastrium. On the contrary, patients with fibrosis of the atrial myocardium are more apt to give evidence of increased delay between right and left atrial contraction. Studies made on such patients (201) have proven the following data (fig. 64):

a) Tracings recorded over the 2nd right interspace frequently show *left* atrial contraction as a downward wave. Tracings recorded over the 2nd left interspace frequently show it as a high positive wave.

b) Tracings of the apex usually show a positive wave for *left* atrial contraction, sometimes preceded by a negative wave for *right* atrial contraction.

c) Tracings of the epigastrium show mainly the effect of *right* atrial contraction which is revealed by a high positive wave. Sometimes a negative phase follows this at the time of left atrial contraction.

The tracings of the apex and epigastrium seem to show the effect of presystolic filling

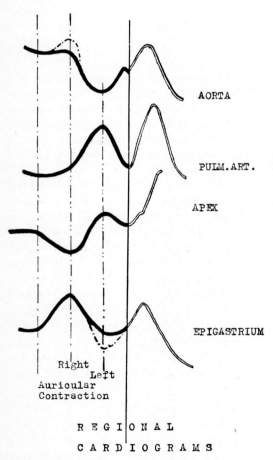

FIG. 64. The atrial wave in the tracings recorded over different areas of the chest.

of the respective ventricle while the waves recorded at the base seem due to indirect transmission of the atrial waves.

The atrial wave (wave 4) presents good development and an unusual height in certain types of patients (201): a large atrial wave in the 2nd and 3rd left interspaces is present in most cases of rheumatic heart disease with mitral lesions or mitral plus aortic defects; a large atrial wave in the epigastric tracing is found in cases of cor pulmonale; in some of them, the atrial wave of the epigastric tracing is much larger than that of the apical tracing.

In cases of a-v block, the atrial waves are high both at the epigastrium and at the apex. In all of them, the atrial waves are far more pronounced in the low frequency tracings than in the phonocardiogram.

B. Wave of rapid filling. The wave of rapid filling (wave 3) may present typical changes. In a large percentage of cases with mitral stenosis this wave is low and poorly defined. This indicates *slow filling of the left ventricle due to mitral obstruction* (page 229).

Mechanical Events During Systole

The simplest way to obtain data concerning systole is by means of the carotid pulse tracing. The rise of the pulse wave occurs within 0.02 second from the opening of the semilunar valves of the aorta; the incisura, within 0.03 second from their closure. However, this time relationship occurs between carotid pulse and *left* ventricular ejection. Exact knowledge about the right ventricle is more difficult. It is true that both the jugular and the hepatic tracings are influenced by right ventricular systole. However, both have many disadvantages. The utilization of the jugular tracing is impaired by delay of the waves over mechanical events of the heart, marked variability of the waves, and the influence of left ventricular systole (c wave, notch 2). That of the liver tracing is impaired by delay of the waves over mechanical events of the heart, influence of transmitted pulsations

through the diaphragm, and influence of changes of thoracic pressure.

Two other tracings should be preferred to the venous tracings. They are the *internal pneumocardiogram* and the *epigastric tracing.* The former records opening and closing of the valves of the right heart through their effect on intrathoracic pressure. The latter records mechanical events of the right heart through transmitted pulsation of the right ventricle.

Record of the Vibrations of the Body Caused by Heart Dynamics (Ballistocardiogram)

A ballistocardiogram is a tracing of the movements of the human body as a result of cardiac action. These may be recorded either in the lying position (longitudinal movements) or in the sitting position

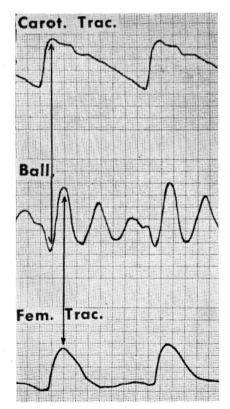

Fig. 65. Ballistocardiogram, carotid tracing, and femoral tracing.

(vertical movements). The original apparatus of *Starr* (78) consisted of a bed suspended from the ceiling and restrained by a spring. Motions of the body were followed by small oscillations of the bed and were magnified by a moving mirror and an optical system. A modification of this (205) consists of the critical damping of all waves. The electromagnetic and the photoelectric (206) types are smaller and simpler. Both use a crosspiece placed over the legs of the patient. The oscillations of the body are picked up by a magnet in the former, by a phototube in the latter. The resulting electrical pulsations are recorded by the galvanometer of an electrocardiograph.

The photoelectric apparatus consists of: a) a *crosspiece* of light wood containing the source of light and placed transversely over the legs of the patient; and b) a *phototube*, contained in a separate unit and so placed that the light beam enters the opening; this is revealed by a prism projecting the light on a frosted glass at the top of the unit. The phototube is connected with the galvanometer of an electrocardiograph. Accurate records are obtained only with a completely immobile table and with a light beam absolutely perpendicular to the phototube. The tracings can be recorded by a direct writing or photographic electrocardiograph at speeds of 10, 25, 50 or 75 mm. per second.

Calibration can be obtained by hitting the foot of the bed (in the case of Starr's method) or the head of the patient (in the case of the magnetic or photoelectric methods) with a known force. However, it is preferable to place a small scale, exerting a known force (600 gm.) against the head of the patient, then release it suddenly. There should be an upward displacement of 20 mm. in the tracing.

The main complex of the ballistocardiogram is the triphasic wave H-I-J-K-L (figs. 65, 66 and 67). The interpretation of this is based on the following principles:

a) Any *acceleration* of the blood in the main arterial trunks is accompanied by a movement of the body in the *opposite* direction; any *deceleration* of the blood is accompanied by a movement of the body in the *same* direction.

b) *Rapid ejection* causes displacement of a large mass of blood and acceleration, first in a headward direction (ascending aorta), then in a footward direction (descending aorta).

c) The *braking effect* of the branchings and smaller vessels, particularly in the lower extremities results in a deceleration.

The ballistocardiogram consists of the rapid succession of positive and negative waves; the time relationship of each peak is easily ascertained; on the other hand, only the first branch of a wave should be considered, the second branch being already the main component of the following wave (fig. 67).

The most useful graphic tracings for the interpretation of the BCG are the phonocardiogram and the arterial tracings, while the other tracings are of help only in special cases.

F wave. The beginning of the cardiac cycle which should be called F (207), occurs from 0.02 to 0.04 second before the first vibration of the first sound.

G wave. The first part of this small, negative (footward) wave is made of a descending branch which is simultaneous with the initial part of the first sound. The peak of G takes place at the time of that large vibration of the first sound which marks the closing of the a-v valves.

H wave. The ascending branch of this small, positive (headward) wave takes place during the central part of the first sound complex. Its peak coincides with that large vibration of the first sound which marks the opening of the semilunar valves and the rise of the carotid pulse.

I wave. The descending branch of this large negative (footward) wave starts at the beginning of ejection, together with that vibration of the first sound which marks the opening of the semilunar valves. Its nega-

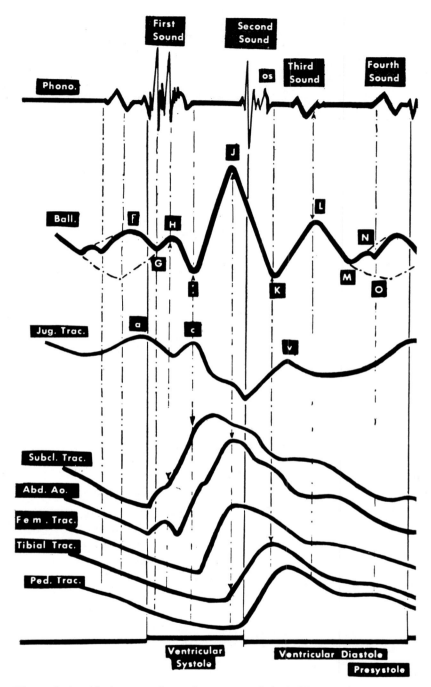

F𝗂G. 66. Time relationship between the various waves of the ballistocardiogram and those of other tracings.

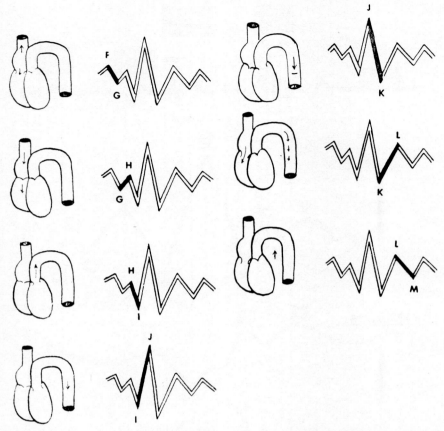

FIG. 67. The waves of the ballistocardiogram and the mechanism of their production

tive peak coincides with the peak of the carotid pulse.

J wave. The ascending branch of this large positive (headward) wave takes place during the first half of ventricular ejection. The peak precedes considerably the second sound. It is simultaneous with the peak of the femoral pulse.

K wave. The descending branch of this deep negative (footward) wave takes place during the end of systole and during the isometric relaxation period. Therefore, it overrides the main vibration of the second sound, at least in normal subjects. It is simultaneous with a small vibration of the second sound complex which marks the opening of the a-v valves. It coincides with the peak of the tibial pulse and slightly precedes that of the pedal pulse.

L wave. The ascending branch of this positive (headward) wave takes place in early diastole, during rapid passive filling of the ventricles. Its positive peak follows the third sound by a short interval (0.04 to 0.06 second). It takes place during the dicrotic wave of the pulse in the aortic arch, as revealed by suprasternal and carotid tracings.

M wave. This negative (footward) wave is variable in shape and is markedly affected by the heart rate. Its descending branch takes place during mid-diastole. Its negative peak may coincide with the dicrotic wave of the abdominal aorta and of the tibial arteries. On the other hand, there may be a single wide negative wave with a peak at the time of the fourth sound.

Respiration modifies considerably the height of the various BCG waves by changing the position of the heart in relation to the long axis of the body and the venous return to either ventricle. It is typical to observe an increased height of the I and J waves in inspiration, a decrease in expiration.

Ballistocardiograms have been studied in an attempt to estimate either *stroke volume*[31] or *cardiac strength*. Should the accuracy of calculations for measuring them be confirmed, ballistocardiography would represent an easy and practical way for determination of these values. Even if absolute values should be inaccurate, variations of the values in the single case would still be of clinical and experimental interest.

The patterns revealed by the tracing are of value in coarctation and in atherosclerosis of the aorta. Abnormal patterns are present in coronary heart disease, peripheral arteriosclerosis, bundle branch block, hypertension, and heart failure. Future experience should prove whether or not these patterns are more typical or more easily detected than with other graphic methods.

[31] The method is based on:

a) Measurement of aortic section (s) by orthodiography.

b) Pulse pressure (PP) measurement by sphygmomanometry.

c) Determination of the speed of the pulse (a) through comparison of carotid and femoral tracings.

d) Determination of length of the pulse wave (l) from peak of the main wave to peak of the dicrotic wave.

Stroke volume (V) is calculated by formula 1:

$$(1) \qquad V = \frac{2PP}{E}$$

E is the coefficient of elasticity of the vascular segment from the aorta to the femoral artery and is calculated by formula 2:

$$(2) \qquad E = \frac{1.06 \times a^2}{S\frac{l}{4}}$$

1.06 is the specific gravity of the blood.

Tracings of Volume (Plethysmograms) and Temperature Changes of Different Parts of the Body

A *plethysmogram* is a tracing of the volume change of some part of the body as affected by changes in its blood content. In order to obtain such a tracing, the body section should be enclosed in a rigid container. The in- and outflow of blood should be unhampered by the membrane which insures closure of the container around the part of the body. The most common plethysmograms are those of the limbs (forearm, leg) or parts of them (fingers, toes). A plethysmogram of the intestines is possible in man. (80, 84).

General rules (80). The container has rigid walls. It is closed around the limb by means of a rubber membrane, carefully applied. Water at body temperature fills the container and transmits volume changes to a recording apparatus which should work with very little change of tension at any level. Air transmission has been also used but is less exact. Every rapid undulation of the tracing is an arterial pulsation. Every slow movement of the curve is caused by change in the blood content, often due to changes of vascular tonus.

Plethysmography of either the *forearm* or the *leg* was used by various authors (18, 81, 82). That of the *ear* did not find many applications. Plethysmogram of *one finger* (83) has also been used with good results in the study of peripheral circulation.

Tracings of volume changes have been employed chiefly in the study of the peripheral circulation, for testing the action of drugs on the vessels, and for evaluating the reactivity of the autonomic nervous system.

Evaluation of the blood flow in different regions may be obtained by *separate skin temperature measurements*. The apparatus consists of a small temperature-sensitive electric unit connected to a recording instrument. Accurate measurements of axillar, skin surface in any area, sublingual or rectal temperature, are indicated on a dial or recorded automatically on a chart. As changes of blood flow and temperature in a certain area are parallel, the simultaneous recording of different temperatures may be substituted for plethysmography.

The plethysmogram of various superficial parts of the body can be obtained also by means of a photoelectric cell, coupled with a galvanometer (173). Extremely interesting results have been obtained by this method. Five types of waves, the faster superimposed on the slower, have been observed:

a) *Pulse waves* caused by the contraction of the heart. They represent the differences between arterial inflow and venous outflow at each cardiac beat. They have a cardiac rhythm, and their amplitude varies considerably following vasomotor changes. They are smaller with vasoconstriction.

b) *Respiratory deflections*. They follow the respiratory rate and are due to respiratory fluctuations of both the arterial and the venous flow.

c) *Alpha waves*. These waves are present in all parts of the body; they are not related to variations of arterial pressure but seem due to local changes of vascular tonus. Their rate is about 10 times per minute.

d) *Beta waves*. These are large, slow, and irregular waves occurring at a rate of about 1 to 2 per minute.

e) *Gamma waves*. These are the slowest of all, including cycles of from 1 to 8 hours. They represent extensive changes in volume.

The study of the pulse of the fingers and toes should be correlated with that of the radial and tibial pulses and their *crest times* should be compared (208). In normal subjects, *digital crest time* is equal to, or not longer than 4 per cent above, radial crest time. The increased amplitude of the pulse after exertion is used as a functional test about the efficiency of the peripheral arteries.

Electrocardiogram

The old observation that electrical phenomena occur during heart action was fol-

lowed by attempts to record them on a tracing by means of a *capillary electrometer*.

At the beginning of the twentieth century, *Schweigger* described the first *string galvanometer* and soon afterwards *Einthoven* applied this instrument to the graphic registrations of cardiac electric currents (85).

The physical principle upon which the string galvanometer is based is the same as that used in electric motors. The moving part of the instrument is a very fine filament, called *the string*, which carries the current to be registered and moves in proportion to its magnitude. The movement is magnified by an optical system and recorded on a photographic film.

With this galvanometer, Einthoven succeeded in laying down the fundamental rules of electrocardiography. However, Einthoven's original apparatus was large, cumbersome, and rather intricate. As time went on, the electrocardiograph was perfected, so that today it is a *portable instrument*, capable of simple operation.

In Germany, not many years after the first string galvanometer was described, a rotating mirror and coil-type instrument was perfected with sufficient sensitivity to register cardiac potentials (*mirror galvanometer*). This did not receive wide recognition, being more sluggish than the string galvanometer.

With the perfection of the thermionic vacuum tube, which took rapid strides in the early 20's, it became possible to register electrocardiograms by means of oscillographic units coupled with electronic amplifiers. *Electronic electrocardiographs* are popular because of their flexibility, high galvanometer speed, and fine photographic detail.

Bedside electrocardiography has been made possible by the fact that modern apparatus is light, compact, and accurate, so that the physician can easily carry it with him. Even simultaneous recording of electrical, mechanical, and sound tracings can be effected at the patient's home.

Prolonged vision of the electrocardiogram

is possible by means of a *cardioscope* or an *oscilloscope*. The cardioscope is based on the property of fluorescent substances of retaining their induced light for some time. The oscilloscope is a cathode-ray apparatus which projects a beam of light on a screen.

The *continuous study* of the electrocardiogram has been made possible by another apparatus which records the electric currents of the heart continuously on a microfilm (87). The study can be continued for 24 hours and even during the patient's sleep without any assistance. The interesting parts of the film can be magnified.

The *direct writing* method avoids the need for photographic processing of the film and is now currently used. The possibility of immediate inspection of the film renders this method preferable whenever delicate multiple tracings are recorded, and for bedside use. The method is based on the color change of a special film, caused by a heated stylus. Ink writing devices are less perfect and can be used only for mass work.

TECHNIQUE

Calibration. Evaluation and comparison of electrocardiograms (ECG's) includes the knowledge that a certain height of deflection corresponds to a certain difference of potential. Therefore, all apparatus are provided with a calibration device. This consists of a button which introduces a current of 1 millivolt into, or excludes a resistance of 1 millivolt from, the circuit. The button is depressed while the film is moving and the sensitivity is adjusted until a positive deflection of 1 centimeter is recorded. The button for calibration (or standardization) is also used in order to check the characteristics of the apparatus. The angles of the rectangle should be square with minimal evidence of rounding. Otherwise, an incorrect picture of the various waves would be obtained.

Electrodes. The normal limb electrodes are 3- x 5-cm. rectangles of German silver. The chest electrodes, made of the same alloy, are round and have a diameter of 3 cm.[32]

Preparation of the patient. A supine or semirecumbent position is preferable because it insures complete muscular relaxation and avoids superimposition of currents of skeletal muscles on those of the heart. A long, wide, and comfortable cot with adjustable back can be used. If the patient has orthopnea, his back should be raised and propped up with pillows. If the tracing is taken in the sitting position, a large chair should be used. The feet of the patient should be raised from the floor and should rest on a nonmetallic, low stool. It may be necessary to shave the chest and limbs of a male patient, if there is excess of hair. In general, however, a generous supply of *electrode jelly*[33] avoids the need for this procedure.

Electrocardiographic leads. Bipolar lead is the name given to any lead using two electrodes placed at the opposite sides of, and at some distance from, the source of electric currents (heart). The record represents the algebraic summation of two potentials of opposite polarity. Examples are the old *standard leads. Semi-unipolar lead* is the name given to any lead using one electrode near the source of the electric currents (heart) while the other is at a greater distance. The record again represents the algebraic summation of two potentials; one of them is of a high value because it is recorded near the source; the other has a smaller value because it is recorded at a greater distance from the source of currents. Examples are the old *lead IV* (anteroposterior), and the various *CF* and *CR leads. Unipolar lead* is the name given to that lead using one electrode near the source of electric currents (heart) while the other is in an area of zero potential (e.g. at an "infinite distance" from the source of currents). The record represents the expression of the

[32] In infants and young children, a chest electrode of ½ cm. in diameter should be used.

[33] This contains sodium chloride or zinc sulfate, pumice powder, and glycerine.

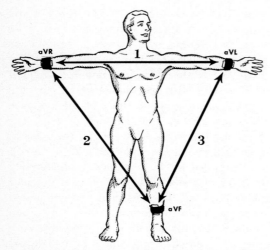

FIG. 68. The classic bipolar limb leads and the unipolar limb leads of the electrocardiogram.

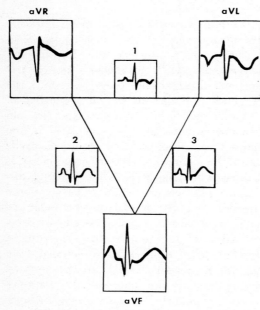

FIG. 69. Electrocardiogram of a normal person. Unipolar and classic bipolar limb leads. The voltage of the latter has been purposely reduced in order to focus the attention on the former.

"absolute" changes of potential in the area lying under the electrode near the source of currents (heart) because it registers the difference in potential between that point and zero. The concept of a "zero potential electrode" is extremely valuable but of difficult

realization. The best solution seems to be the "central terminal" of *Wilson* (see below). In both the semi-unipolar and the unipolar leads, the electrode placed near the heart is called the *exploring electrode* while the other is called *semi-indifferent* or *indifferent*.

A. Standard limb leads. The standard limb leads were the only ones used from 1905 to 1935 and are still currently employed. These *bipolar limb leads* are the following (fig. 68): *lead 1*, connecting the right with the left arm; *lead 2*, connecting the right arm with the left leg; *lead 3*, connecting the left arm with the left leg. Each bipolar limb lead represents the algebraic summation of the potentials of two limbs.

Lead 1 reports the variations of potential of the left lateral cardiac wall minus those of the atrial and ventricular cavities; lead 2, the variations of potential of the diaphragmatic surface of the heart minus those of the atrial and ventricular cavities; lead 3, the variations of potential of the diaphragmatic surface of the heart minus those of the left lateral cardiac wall.

B. The "unipolar" limb leads. Following *Wilson's* suggestion (177), it is possible to study the variations of potential of any point of the body without interference from currents of other points. In order to do this, the three limbs are connected by three wires and three resistances of 5000 ohms or more. To this central point of connection, called the *central terminal*, is attached one of the cables of the electrocardiograph. Based on the principle of Einthoven's triangle, the "central terminal" is supposed to have zero potential and to act as an *indifferent electrode*.[34] The other cable of the electrocardiograph is connected with any point of the body by means of an electrode, called the *exploring electrode*. In the case of the limb leads, the exploring electrode is connected successively with the right arm,

[34] Actually, the *central terminal* has small changes of potential which can be disregarded in clinical tracings.

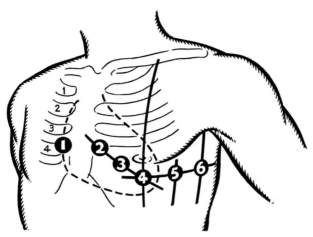

FIG. 70. Various locations of the electrodes for the chest leads. The outline of the heart has been made larger in order to show that point 4 may be within the apex in the case of an enlarged heart.

the left arm, and the left leg. The three tracings are called VR, VL and VF (fig. 68).

It has been suggested (175) to eliminate the electrical resistances of the central terminal and to disconnect the wire of the limb under study in order to increase the amplitude of the waves. These leads are called *augmented unipolar leads* and their symbols are *aVR*, *aVL*, and *aVF*. Successive studies (212) have confirmed that disconnecting the wire of the extremity under study does not change the shape and polarity of the waves while increasing their magnitude. On the other hand, the presence of the resistances is necessary in order to have a central terminal of "zero potential". Therefore, present-day technique embodies the best features of the Wilson terminal but with alternate disconnection of the wire of the terminal from the limb under study. For simplicity's sake, the symbols of the three limb leads with this technique can be called *R*, *L* and *F*. Connection of the three wires with the central terminal and disconnection of the wire of the limb under study is obtained automatically in most modern apparatus.

C. *The chest leads. Semi-unipolar chest leads* have been taken for several years by placing one electrode on the chest while the galvanometer was connected with the

electrode of any of the limbs. The symbols used were: chest-right arm = CR leads; chest-left arm = CL leads; chest-left leg = CF leads.

The *unipolar chest leads* are now generally accepted. They are taken by placing a round *exploring electrode* on the chest while the galvanometer is connected with Wilson's central terminal (*indifferent electrode*). The symbols used are: *CV leads*, or simply *V leads*.

Six chest locations (leads V1 to V6) are now commonly used (fig. 70). To these, several others have been added for use in special cases: a) *three posterior locations* for the study of high posterior potentials of the heart (leads V7, V8, V9); b) one *xiphoid* or *ensiform location* for the study of postero-diaphragmatic potentials (VE); c) *three high antero-lateral locations* for the study of the high antero-lateral potentials (high V4, high V5, high V6); d) *one high right sternal lead* for the study of right atrial potentials (high V1); e) *three* right chest leads for the study of potentials of the right heart in cases with right heart enlargement (V3R, V4R, V5R)[35]; and f) *four esophageal*

[35] *V1* is the topographic equivalent of *V2* on the right chest. *V3R* is the equivalent of *V3* on the right chest. *V4R* is the equivalent of *V4* on the right chest.

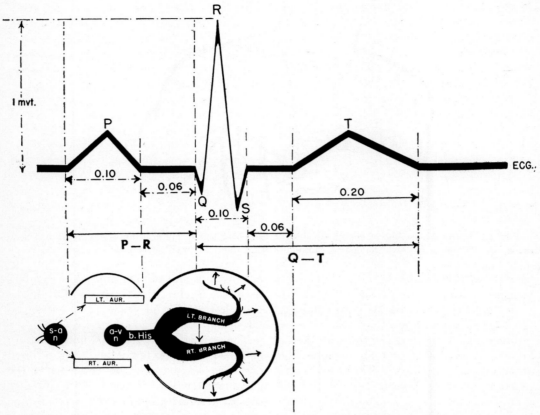

Fig. 71. Duration and height of the waves and intervals of the electrocardiogram. Comparison with a scheme indicating origin and spread of the stimulus.

leads for the study of postero-inferior potentials (left atrial and ventricular).

THE WAVES OF THE ELECTROCARDIOGRAM AND THEIR INTERPRETATION

The Electrocardiogram in General

The *electrocardiogram* (ECG) is a composite curve in which various accidents, or waves, have a definite position. These waves are called P, Q, R, S, and T (fig. 71). The first part of the ECG, composed of the P wave and of minor accidents, is called the *atrial* (or *auricular*) *complex* because it bears a definite relationship to the activity of the atria (auricles). The second part of the ECG, composed of an initial rapid complex QRS and a slow final deflection (T), is called the *ventricular complex* because it is connected with the activity of the ventricles.

Atrial complex. The excitation of the s-a node is not recorded in clinical tracings but can be recorded by means of an intra-atrial electrode. As there is no way of detecting it in routine cases, it is assumed that it precedes the beginning of P by a small fraction of a second (0.05 sec.?). The *P wave* is the resultant of the *activation* (or *depolarization*) *of both atria*. It is a blunt deflection, lasting from 0.08 to 0.10 second in normal individuals. Whenever transmission of the impulse to the left atrium is impaired, or the wall of the left atrium is distended or hypertrophied, the P wave shows a double peak or a diphasic configuration. In such cases, the first, or upward, phase of P is due to the right atrium; the second, or downward, phase of P is due to the left. This is frequently apparent in leads V1, aVF, and 3.

Inactivation (or *repolarization*) of the atria is usually not revealed by the ECG. However, cases with prolonged a-v conduction or a-v block may show a small dip, called the atrial T wave (*Ta wave*), due to repolarization of the atrial myocardium.

Atrioventricular interval. The P wave is normally followed by a period during which the electrocardiogram reveals no deflection. The stimulus starts to spread at the beginning of P and reaches the a-v node *during P*; activation of the a-v node and diffusion along the bundle of His takes place between P and Q. The interval between the initiation of P and that of QRS (called *P-R interval*) measures the sum of: a) sino-nodal and sino-atrial conductions; b) nodal latency; and c) nodo-septal conduction. Normal duration of the P-R interval is between 0.12 and 0.20 second.

The *ventricular complex* is composed of a rapid initial complex, the *QRS complex*, and a slow final wave, the *T wave*. The beginning of the initial complex may be represented by a small Q wave. This is explained by the fact that depolarization starts on the *left* side of the septum and spreads from there toward the *right* side of this structure. While the small Q wave of chest leads V5-V6 is a septal Q, the small R wave of chest leads V1-V2 has been explained as due to depolarization of either the septum or the right ventricle. After this initial stage, the wave of depolarization spreads along the Purkinje fibers into the ventricular walls *from the endocardium toward the epicardium.* This causes the upward deflection R of the tracing. As the left ventricular mass is greater, its potentials are greater than those of the right; the sum of depolarization of the ventricles is revealed as an upward deflection in V5-V6; as a downward deflection in V1-V2. When depolarization has spread to the subepicardial layers, the cavity and surface of the ventricles reach a stage of equilibrium and no changes of potential are recorded. The phase of balancing of the forces is represented by the descending branch of R. For these reasons, *QRS represents the period between beginning and completion of ventricular depolarization.*

The *T wave* reflects the stage of *ventricular repolarization.* It is sometimes followed by a small positive wave, the *U wave*, the mechanism of production of which is still obscure.

The *atrial contraction* takes place during the second half of P and during the first isoelectric period. It can be measured approximately by the distance from the peak of P to that of Q. The *ventricular contraction* starts during QRS and lasts throughout the second isoelectric period and during T. It can be measured approximately by the distance from the peak of Q to the end of T (so called *Q-T interval*). According to an agreed standardization, the earliest upward wave is called R; any downward preceding wave is called Q; any downward following wave is called S. If a second upward wave follows S, it is called R[1] and this may be followed by S[1] (fig. 73-I).

The Three Intervals of the Electrocardiogram

The P-R interval. That part of the tracing which is between the beginning of P and the beginning of QRS is called the P-R interval (it should be called more accurately P-Q) (fig. 71). The importance of this interval is that it measures the time necessary for the atrio-ventricular conduction. When the P-R interval is prolonged, there is a disturbance of conduction either in the atrial myocardium or (more usually) in the tissues of the a-v node and bundle of His. This may occur: a) in congenital heart disease; b) in acute myocarditis; c) in myocardial fibrosis caused by coronary arteriosclerosis or following an acute inflammatory process; d) after digitalis; e) during vagal stimulation. A very common cause of prolongation of P-R is rheumatic carditis. On the contrary, P-R is usually normal in the thyrotoxic heart and in bacterial endocarditis.

The QRS interval. This interval is measured from the beginning of the first rapid wave to the end of the last. The QRS interval measures the time required by the stimulus to spread to and through the ventricular wall. When prolonged, it indicates *impaired spreading of the stimulus*, either in the septum (bundle branch block) or within the ventricular wall (intraventricular block, periinfarction block, focal block). Exceptions are represented by ventricular premature beats, ventricular tachycardia, and the preexcitation syndrome (Wolff-Parkinson-White syndrome).

The Q-T interval. This interval measures the *duration of electrical systole* of the ventricles. Its duration varies with the heart rate, becoming shorter with a more rapid rate and vice versa.[36]

Aspect, Duration, and Nomenclature of the Different Waves

The *P wave* may be modified as far as voltage (tall or low), duration (broad), and configuration (notched, slurred, diphasic, peaked or gothic). It is usually upright in leads 1 and 2, may be occasionally inverted in 3, is frequently small or inverted in some of the chest leads, and is normally inverted in aVR. It is usually blunt and

---

[36] The figures of the *expected Q-T* or *average Q-T* are obtained by means of *Bazett's* formula $Q\text{-}T = K \sqrt{R\text{-}R}$ (K is equivalent to 0.37 second in men and 0.40 in women). The ratio between the actual $Q\text{-}T$ and the expected $Q\text{-}T$ (r = act. $Q\text{-}T$/exp. $Q\text{-}T$) indicates whether or not the duration of electrical systole is prolonged. Any ratio higher than 1 indicates prolongation. Calculation of the ratio can also be made by the use of a nomogram.

Expected Q-T

RATE	AVERAGE	MINIMUM	MAXIMUM
	sec.		
50	0.43	0.39	0.47
60	0.39	0.35	0.43
70	0.36	0.32	0.40
80	0.34	0.30	0.38
90	0.32	0.28	0.36
100	0.30	0.26	0.34
110	0.29	0.25	0.33
120	0.27	0.23	0.31

lasts from 0.06 to 0.11 sec. in the normal subjects (fig. 71).

QRS complex. The initial ventricular complex may be monophasic, diphasic, or polyphasic. Slurring or notching is more common in aVF and in lead 3. Normal amplitude is from 5 to 15 mm. but it may be much larger in chest leads. It lasts from 0.06 to 0.10 sec. in normal subjects. The QRS complex has a different nomenclature according to the direction of the first wave and to the number of subsequent waves. This can be conveyed to the reader by using capitals or small letters according to the height of the waves and by giving to each wave its symbol in sequence (fig. 73-I).

The *T wave* may be modified as far as voltage (tall or low), polarity (positive or negative), and configuration (diphasic, symmetrical or asymmetrical). It is normally upright. However, it is normally inverted in aVR and may be inverted in aVL; it is normally inverted in V1 and V2 (or even V3 and V4) in infants. It lasts from 0.16 to 0.25 second.

The *S-T segment* may be isoelectric (normal), displaced upwards or downwards. The direction and form of the S-T segment may indicate the difference between the *coronary* (or *cove-shaped*) *T wave* and the *digitalis T wave* (fig. 73-II). It normally follows the basal line but may be slightly raised (not more than 1 mm. = $\frac{1}{10}$ mv.). The displacement may reach about 2 mm. in the chest leads.

Special Features of Certain Leads

A. Unipolar right arm lead (VR, aVR, or R). The ECG presents typically inverted waves: the P wave, the main rapid ventricular deflection, and the T wave are directed downwards. The heart has its base directed upwards and toward the right; the thin vascular and atrial walls contribute little to the tracing and leave free passage to the stronger ventricular potentials. The stimulus, after reaching the septum and the endocardial surface of the ventricular walls,

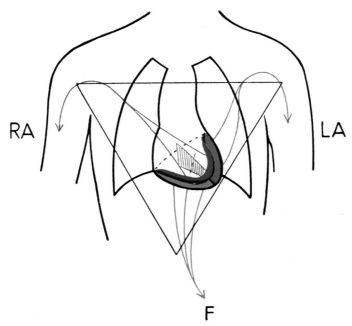

RA LA

F

FIG. 72. The spreading of potentials from the normal heart in average position. In red, endocardial or cavitary potentials. In blue, epicardial potentials from left ventricle. In green, epicardial potentials from right ventricle. (From Holzmann).

spreads outwards toward the epicardium. This causes a vector directed away from the electrode (so called *negative potentials within the cavities*) and explains the inverted QRS and T waves of VR (fig. 72). The QRS complex is similar to that obtained by introducing an electrode within the upper part of the right atrial cavity. The currents of both ventricles are recorded. This lead is only slightly influenced by the position of the heart within the chest.

B. *Unipolar left arm lead (VL, aVL, or L).* This lead has usually positive waves. The picture strongly varies according to changes in position of the heart with subsequent shifting of the electric axis. It reflects the variations of electric potential presented by the *anterior and lateral epicardial surfaces of the heart.*

C. *Unipolar left leg lead (VF, aVF, or F).* This lead has usually positive waves. It is strongly influenced by the position of the heart within the chest and by the resulting shifting of the electric axis of the heart. It

reflects the variations of electric potential presented by the *posterior and diaphragmatic epicardial surfaces of the heart.*

D. *Standard leads (1, 2, and 3).* These present normally positive waves. P may be diphasic in 3. QRS may have a deep S in 1 or an rS in 3 if the electric axis of the heart is unusually shifted to the left. T may be inverted in 3 due to the same cause.

E. *Chest leads.* The anterior surface of the heart, including parts of both ventricles, lies closer to the surface of the body (anterior chest wall and left axilla) than any other part of the heart. Leads from various anterolateral points of the chest (V1 to V6) resemble *direct epicardial leads* more than any other lead from the body surface. Still, it should be kept in mind that they are not identical with them because the tracing is much less influenced by the small fraction of muscle lying in contact with the electrode, and it includes potentials from the surrounding areas. For this reason, an intrinsic

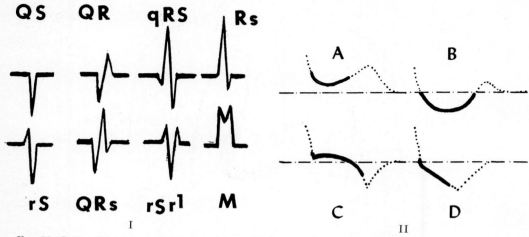

FIG. 73. I. Possible changes of the ventricular complex. II. Possible changes of the S-T tract (black) and T wave (dotted). A, raised S-T; B, depressed S-T; C, cove-shaped ST and inverted T; D, S-T and T changes due to digitalis.

deflection[37] cannot be recognized in a chest electrocardiogram.

V1 and V2 give the best information about right ventricular potentials (fig. 74). VE records the potentials of the diaphragmatic or postero-inferior aspect of both ventricles. The R wave is smallest in V1 and increases gradually in height from V1 to V5 or V6 where it is tallest (fig. 74). The S wave is deepest in V1 or V2 and decreases gradually from right to left until it disappears. Q waves are present over the left side of the precordium but are small. Normal QRS should not last more than 0.10 second. In V1, the intrinsicoid deflection begins 0.006 to 0.02 second after the onset of QRS; in V5 or V6, it starts about 0.035 second after it. The T waves are upright in all leads but may be inverted in V1 (occasionally in V2). It should be noted that, in certain normal subjects, V1 and V2 seem to present an inverted initial deflection (type QS) on account of the extreme smallness of R. The

[37] Intrinsic deflection is the name given to the sharpest and largest downward deflection which represents depolarization of the muscle under an electrode. The similar deflection recorded by the chest leads is called *intrinsicoid deflection* and is supposed to represent depolarization of the heart muscle in the area which is *nearest* to the electrode.

S-T segment may be slightly above the base line; this displacement usually does not exceed 1 mm. but may reach 2 mm.

NORMAL VERSUS ABNORMAL ELECTRO-CARDIOGRAMS

It is impossible to draw a sharp line between normal and abnormal tracings. In reaching a decision, the observer must consider the possible occurrence of a certain variation in the ECG of a normal person. Statistical tables have been made and reference to them may be useful. However, personal experience and additional clinical and laboratory data determine whether or not an abnormality should be considered pathological.

PRACTICAL APPLICATIONS

1) Electrocardiography may be useful for an *exact evaluation of the atrial and ventricular rates and for the location of the pacemaker*. Thus, diagnosis of abnormal rhythms and their focus of origin, is made possible.

2) *The electric axis can be determined; dextrocardia can be diagnosed*. The data are of help in the study of congenital malformations, valvular disease, chronic cor pulmonale, etc.

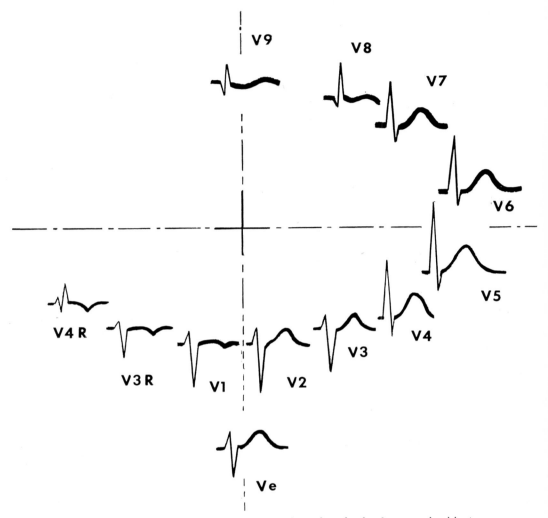

FIG. 74. The electrocardiogram in the various chest leads of a normal subject

3) *Delayed a-v conduction, a-v block, bundle branch block, or intraventricular block,* are recognized.

4) Evidence of *diffuse myocardial damage* or *metabolic unbalance,* is obtained. This includes infectious lesions and digitalis effect.

5) Evidence of *localized myocardial ischemia* or *damage* is secured. This is of great importance for the diagnosis of coronary heart disease and the differential diagnosis with pulmonary infarction, dissecting aneurysm of the aorta, and pericarditis.

It should be emphasized that, in most conditions, *repeated registration of electrocardiograms* is necessary; then interpretation will be far more accurate than after a single tracing.

In requesting an electrocardiogram, the physician should give information about the following points: a) presence of valvular defects; b) level of blood pressure; c) administration of digitalis or allied drugs or other drugs acting on the myocardium (quinidine, emetine, insulin); clinical diagnosis or reason for requesting a tracing.

The time relationships between the electrocardiographic waves and those of other tracings are the following:

a) Initial evidence of right atrial contraction (mechanical cardiogram, electrokymogram, atrial sound by esophageal route) is found 0.04 to 0.06 after the rise of P. The atrial sound recorded at the apex follows the peak of P by a longer interval.

b) The beginning of any evidence of ventricular contraction (mechanical cardiogram, electrokymogram, first sound at apex) is found between Q and R; coinciding with R; or between R and S.

c) The end of the T wave usually coincides with the end of mechanical systole of the ventricles. However, a dissociation between the two phenomena may occur in abnormal conditions.

d) There is no relationship between the U wave and the phase of rapid ventricular filling.

ESOPHAGEAL ELECTROCARDIOGRAM

A thin rubber tube ending with a metal tip and carrying inside it the connecting wire, is introduced through the nose or mouth (better if under fluoroscopic control). The tip is used as an *exploring electrode* while the *indifferent electrode* is represented by Wilson's *central terminal*. Thus the tracings are unipolar esophageal leads and should be marked with the symbols VEs and a notation of the depth of the electrode from the nostrils or the dental arch.

A different method, employed by the author, made use of a rubber tube with two silver rings at 10 mm. from each other and two internal wires. This bipolar esophageal lead presents certain advantages because it gives larger atrial deflections (92). Four *standard esophageal leads* should be studied: 1) VEs 30–35—atrial lead; 2) VEs 35–40—low atrial lead; 3) VEs 40–45—ventricular lead; 4) VEs 45–55—low ventricular lead.

At the atrial level (*position 1*), *the P wave is prominent* and shows an "intrinsic" deflection similar to that usually seen in the ventricular complex. A deep, inverted, initial ventricular deflection and an inverted T wave are normally seen. The nearness with the left atrium explains the high voltage and the diphasic aspect of the atrial complex. The ventricular wave is inverted and indicates "cavity potentials" which spread through the thin atrial wall. In *position 2*, transitional tracings are obtained. In *position 3*, usually a different pattern is observed. It consists of a *positive P*, an initial ventricular complex with a qR or QR pattern, and a diphasic or positive T wave. Considerable differences are noted according to the position of the heart. In *position 4*, the electrode has reached the diaphragmatic surface of the heart and records a tracing similar to VE or aVF: a positive P, variable QRS patterns, usually positive but occasionally inverted T waves.

The differentiation between a Q caused by normal cavity potentials and a Q due to posterior myocardial infarct is based on the fact that, in the first instance, there is a QS pattern and an inverted T wave while, in the case of infarction, there frequently is a qR pattern and T may be upright.

INTRACARDIAC ELECTROCARDIOGRAM

A catheter for cardiac catheterization with a small silver electrode connected to the silver mandril is introduced into the cavities of the right heart following the usual technique of right heart catheterization (page 157). The position of the tip of the catheter is determined by means of fluoroscopy, pressure readings, and oxymetry. The endocardial electrode is connected with the wire commonly used for chest leads and serves as an *exploring electrode*. The *central terminal* completes the circuit.

Intracardiac leads can be considered as *direct* leads from the endocardial surface of the heart. The *atrial electrogram* consists of a series of rapid deflections (S, e, i, o waves) and a final slow wave (Ta). S has been considered as due to the activity of the s-a node and precedes by 0.05 second the onset of P in the limb leads. The *Ta* wave represents the final phase of repolarization of the atria and is visible only in cases of a-v block. The interval from the beginning of P in the limb leads to the end of Ta measures from 0.34 to 0.42 second but may be much longer.

The *right ventricular electrogram*, recorded directly from the ventricle, shows an initial *positive* deflection (*r*) due to depolarization of the septum (and possibly of the right ventricle), a large inverted deflection (*S*), and an inverted *T* wave. The *left ventricular electrogram* shows a QS type of initial ventricular complex; there may be some degree of elevation of S-T, possibly due to pressure of the catheter. The P wave is positive. Above the aortic valve, the electrogram has an "atrial" type and presents negative P and T waves and an initial complex of the qR type.

FUNCTIONAL TESTS

Several functional tests have been suggested in order to evaluate the efficiency of the coronary system. They can be used whenever the history of a patient seems to indicate coronary heart disease while the electrocardiogram is normal. The most used are the anoxemia test and the exercise test.

1) *Anoxemia test* (209). It is performed in the following way. The patient inhales a mixture of 10 per cent oxygen with nitrogen which is insufficient for the normal oxygen supply to the tissues. A tracing is recorded before the test and at 5-minute intervals during the inhalation for 20 minutes. Normal persons have only slight electrocardiographic changes consisting of decreased height of T in all leads and occasionally an inversion of T in leads 2 and 3.

A positive test consists of the following changes:

a) The sum of S-T deviations in leads 1, 2, 3, and V4 should be greater by 3 mm. or more, than in the control tracing.

b) There is a partial or complete reversal of the direction of the T wave in 1, accompanied by S-T deviation of 1 mm. or more in this lead.

c) There is a complete reversal of the direction of the T wave in V4 regardless of any associated S-T deviation in this lead.

A tank of 100 per cent oxygen is incorporated in the circuit so that oxygen can be rapidly administered if needed.

2) *The "two step" exercise test* (210). Since normal persons submitted to excessive exercise may present electrocardiographic changes, the exercise has been standardized for age, weight and sex. The procedure is the following. The weight of the subject and a control electrocardiogram are recorded. Then the patient is invited to walk up one side of a two-step stool[38] and down the other. He makes a trip only when a count is given and the required number is completed in $1\frac{1}{2}$ minutes. The electrocardiogram is then recorded, and at 2 and 6 min. after cessation of the exercise.

Criteria for an abnormal electrocardiographic response are:

a) Depression of S-T of more than 0.5 mm. below the isoelectric level in 1, 2, or V4.

b) Change from an upright T wave to an isoelectric or inverted T wave (or becoming upright of a previously inverted T).

c) Onset of arrhythmias immediately after exercise.

3) *Amyl nitrite test* (211). After a short rest in recumbent position, the ECG is recorded. Then an ampule of amyl nitrite is broken and the patient is instructed to breathe deeply. As soon as flushing of the face occurs, an ECG is again recorded, and the tracing is repeated at 1-minute intervals until normalization.

The sudden drop of blood pressure caused by amyl nitrite determines coronary insufficiency whenever the coronary arteries are sclerotic. Evidence of abnormal response is: displacement of S-T of more than

---

[38] This stool is made of two steps having a height of 22 cm. (or 9 inches). It is easily built by a carpenter.

1 mm. from the base line, flattening or in-version of the T wave in any lead, and premature contractions. This test is harmless because the ischemia is of short duration, and the vasodilating properties of the drug prevent functional disturbances. The result of the test usually coincides with that of the two-step exercise test.

ELECTRICAL AXIS

According to an assumption of Einthoven, the right shoulder, left shoulder, and left hip form the apices of a triangle. If it is assumed that they are equidistant from the center of the triangle, and that the heart is located at this center; if it is further admitted that the conducting media are homogeneous, various important calculations can be made from the tracings recorded in the standard limb leads.

Positive and negative charges (dipoles) appear on the surface of a cell whenever there is a change in the permeability of its membrane. Each charge can be thought of as exerting a force, and its *magnitude* is proportional to the strength of the charge. Each charge exerts its greatest force along a line which connects the charges (from the negative to the positive) and which repre-

sents the *direction* of the force. These two elements, magnitude and direction, as well as *sense*, have been used in order to represent the charges as *vectors*.

The electrical field around the heart is the result of depolarization and repolarization of several fibers; the combined effect can be found by determining the *sum of the vectors* representing the various charges, or *manifest vector*. The force resulting from this vector can be easily determined by drawing perpendicular lines from the origin and end of the vector line to each side of the triangle. These perpendiculars indicate the magnitude and sense of the deflections in leads 1, 2, 3 at any instant. At the beginning of depolarization, the septum is activated from left to right; at the end of this phase, the postero-basal region of the left ventricle is activated from right to left. This causes the various vectors forming the initial QRS complex. The phenomena associated with repolarization and causing the T wave can also be projected onto the three lines, resulting in another vector (fig. 75).

The concept of the equilateral triangle (a rough approximation) was used by Einthoven in order to calculate the magnitude of electromotive forces of the heart as projected

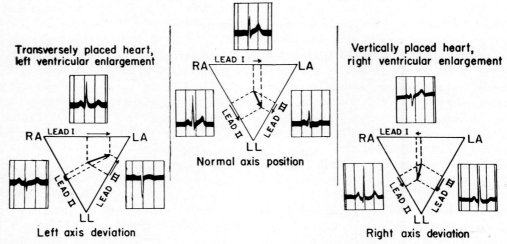

FIG. 75. Determination of axis deviation. Conventional geometrical construction to determine degree and direction of the electrical axis. (From H. Hecht. Courtesy of the author and Charles C Thomas, Publisher.)

on the *frontal plane* of the body. Determination of the *electrical axis* and measure of the *axis deviation* on the basis of the above method have been made in clinical cases for several decades. This procedure is the following (fig. 75).

a) The magnitudes of either P, QRS, or T in leads 1 and 3 (mmV) are traced upon two sides of an equilateral triangle inscribed within a circle marked in degrees, in order to determine the mean axes of P, QRS, or T. That of QRS is the most commonly studied.

b) Perpendicular lines are drawn from the points obtained.

c) A line is drawn from the center of the triangle to the point of intersection of the perpendiculars. This line represents the direction and magnitude of the electrical forces projected upon the frontal plane of the body.

d) The line drawn in step c is prolonged to intersect the circle, and the *degree of inclination* of the axis is read directly on the circle.

In general, the term "electric axis" is used as applied to the axis of QRS. Degrees from 0 to +90 represent *normal axis*. Degrees from 0 to −90 represent *left axis deviation*, degrees from +90 to +180 represent *right axis deviation*. A right axis deviation indicates that the potentials of the left arm are lower than those of the right. A left axis deviation indicates that they are higher. Determination of the axis by plotting the direction and height of the waves is a practical but only approximate procedure; a correct procedure should be based on plotting *both the direction and the surface of the waves*.

A *system of six axes*, by which determination of the electrical axis by the use of either the standard or the unipolar limb leads is possible, has also been described.

VECTORCARDIOGRAM (221)

The line indicating the axis has direction, magnitude, and sense. Therefore, it can be called a *vector*. Such a vector can be constructed for each of the points and for each of the waves of an electrocardiogram. All vectors have their origin at zero and vary in direction and size according to the changes of the electrical field of the heart recorded in the electrocardiogram. Each of these vectors is called an *instantaneous electrical axis*. The end points of the various vectors can be connected by a line which describes a *loop* for each electrocardiographic wave (loop of P, loop of ARS, loop of T). The largest diameter of each loop is identical with the *modal electrical axis* of a given deflection. The loop connecting the end points of all possible instantaneous axes, called *frontal vectorcardiogram*, has an irregular shape and can be constructed graphically. However, a simpler way is that of connecting the electrocardiographic wires with an *oscilloscope*. Then the light beam of a cathode ray tube traces automatically the outline of the loop on the fluorescent screen. A photograph of this loop may be used to reproduce the vectorcardiogram.

Various geometric arrangements have been suggested for placing the electrodes necessary to record the various vectors, not only in the frontal plane but also in the antero-posterior plane.

The vector method represents a different point of view in comparison with other methods of interpretation of the electrocardiogram even when the same electrode positions are used and the same deflections are studied. The vector method has the following advantages over empirical methods basing their interpretation on the "pattern" of the various leads:

a) It simplifies clinical interpretation by eliminating the need to memorize patterns.

b) It is more accurate and objective because the deflections are reduced to a few simple measurements of the electrical field.

c) It is easier to separate normal tracings

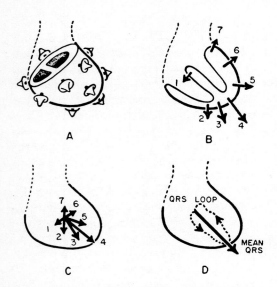

FIG. 76. The QRS vectors of the heart. A, Each QRS vector is directed perpendicularly to the surface of the region where it is generated. The T vectors have a similar direction in the normal subject. B, Frontal plane cross-section of the heart, illustrating the magnitude, direction, and effective source of resultant QRS vectors from instant to instant during a single QRS cycle. C, The instantaneous vectors from the previous figure are drawn as if they all originated at the same point, the relative zero point of the electrical field in the frontal plane. D, The pathway of the terminus of the QRS vector from instant to instant in a single QRS cycle (QRS loop), and the mean of the instantaneous vectors (mean QRS vector) as projected in the frontal plane of the body. (From Grant and Estes, courtesy of the authors and the Blakiston Co.)

and positional changes from tracings caused by myocardial abnormalities.

However, vectorcardiography can only supplement, and should not supplant, conventional methods of pattern interpretation (fig. 76).

VENTRICULAR GRADIENT

The term *gradient* (G) is used to indicate the rapidity of a variation (like those of pressure, temperature, or electricity). As this variation is characterized by three values, e.g. sense, direction and magnitude, it complies with the definition of a vector. When a muscular fiber is stimulated, the currents generated by the stimulus can be theoretically considered as the resultant of two monophasic waves of opposite polarity. Comparison of the *surfaces* or *areas* (A) of these waves shows that they are identical. Being of opposite polarity, their algebraic sum is zero and there is no gradient. If the waves have a different duration, then the algebraic sum of the areas of the two waves is not equal to zero and represents a *gradient* of value x.

In the mammalian heart, several conditions (high pressure, low blood supply) contribute to slow down the process of depolarization in the subendocardial layers. Therefore, the subendocardial layers which were depolarized first are repolarized last. For this reason, the areas of QRS (A QRS) and T (A T), which represent the resultant of the various vectors of depolarization and repolarization in the subendocardial and subepicardial layers, have surfaces of different values. The difference between the two surfaces is the *ventricular gradient*. A similar comparison can be repeated for the atrial potentials in order to study whether or not there is an *atrial gradient*.

A change of the area of T (AT) may be the result of changes of the area of QRS (A QRS) because variation of the order of depolarization of the various bundles is necessarily followed by a corresponding change in their order of repolarization. In other words, *a change of the area of T may be the result of an abnormality of QRS*, as in ventricular hypertrophy, bundle branch block, ventricular extrasystoles, or the preexcitation syndrome: there is *a secondary change of T* and *the gradient is normal*. On the contrary, a change of the area of T may be due to abnormal metabolism of certain areas of the myocardium which does not affect QRS: there is *a primary change of T* and this is revealed by *a modification of the ventricular gradient*.

A wave or deflection of the electrocardiogram may be defined by its *duration* in seconds and by its *height* in microvolts (or tenths of a millivolt). These two factors determine the *area* included in one wave. The same geometrical construction which is used for determination of the electrical axis may be employed in order to obtain the area of a certain wave from the areas found in two standard limb leads. The area of QRS (called A QRS) is the *mean electrical axis of QRS*, is two-dimensional, and is identical with the frontal vectorcardiogram for QRS. The area of T (AT) is the mean electrical axis of T and has the same respective properties.

THE ELECTROCARDIOGRAM IN THE VARIOUS POSITIONS OF THE HEART

The electrocardiograms of normal subjects were recorded for many years only by means of the standard limb leads. It soon became apparent that the patterns of certain normal subjects were similar to those of patients with abnormal hearts. In particular, the ECG of the vertical heart sometimes was confused with that of right ventricular hypertrophy; that of the horizontal heart, with the tracing of left ventricular hypertrophy. A new era was opened with the study of unipolar chest leads and unipolar limb leads.

The heart of a normal subject may be in different positions within the chest. Accordingly, a greater or lesser part of either ventricle may "face" one or the other shoulder, or the left leg. Tracings recorded by means of the unipolar limb leads explain the cause of several physiologic variants which are necessarily followed by variants of the tracings in the standard limb leads.

Several types of "rotations" of the heart have been recognized. Those around the *anteroposterior axis* cause the vertical, semivertical, intermediate, semihorizontal, and horizontal rotation. Those around the *longitudinal axis* cause the clockwise and counterclockwise rotation. Those around the *transverse axis* cause the forward and backward rotation of the apex. Certain displacements around one of these axes are usually accompanied by displacement around another, thereby limiting the number of possibilities. Judgment on whether the heart is "vertical" or "horizontal" can be drawn by comparing aVL with aVF, or leads 1 with 3. The low esophageal leads give a pattern which is similar to that of aVF. Thus, in the *vertical heart*, they present a left ventricular pattern; in the *horizontal heart*, a right ventricular pattern. It should be emphasized that correlation between anatomical shifts and rotations and electrocardiographic rotations is only approximate and sometimes nonexistent.

The *average vertical heart* has nearly always some degree of clockwise rotation around its longitudinal axis. Therefore, the right ventricle becomes more anterior; V3, and occasionally V4, may show a right ventricular pattern rS. The unipolar lead of the right shoulder may present a QS complex and an inverted T wave because it "faces" the cavity of the left ventricle (fig. 77). If a *severe clockwise rotation* is present, the vertical heart presents a right ventricular pattern, not only in V3 and V4, but also in V5, and even in V6. In all types of vertical heart, the main direction of QRS in aVL is directed downwards; in AVF, upward. Mnemonically, they look like two hands directed toward each other (the same is true for leads 1 and 3) (fig. 79).

The *average horizontal heart* is usually accompanied by some degree of counterclockwise rotation around the longitudinal axis. Therefore, leads V4 to V6 "face" the epicardial surface of the left ventricle and have a qR pattern (fig. 78). Even though seldom found in normal subjects, an horizontal heart may have a marked counterclockwise rotation around the longitudinal axis. Then all chest leads V1 to V6 have a qR pattern because they "face" the epicardial surface of the left ventricle, and the unipolar lead of the left shoulder has an inverted T. An important differential point between this type of physiologically horizontal heart and one with left ventricular hypertrophy

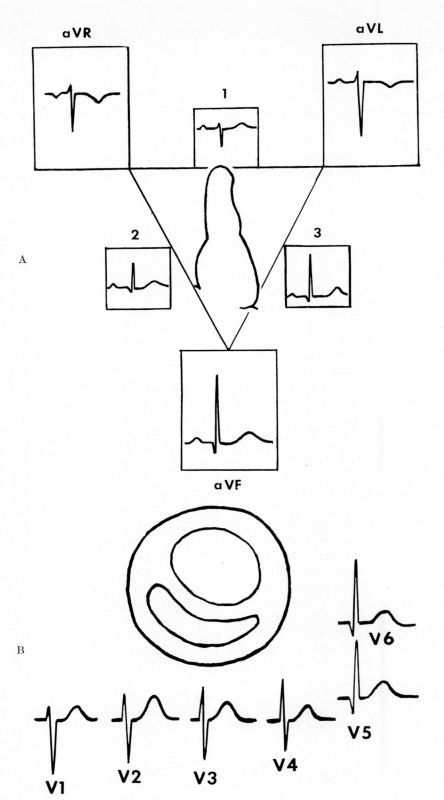

A

B

aVR   aVL

1

2   3

aVF

V6

V5

V1   V2   V3   V4

Fig. 77. A, Electrocardiograms in the *classic bipolar* and in the *unipolar limb leads* of a person with "vertical" heart. Scheme. B, Electrocardiograms in the *chest leads* of a person with "vertical" heart. Scheme.

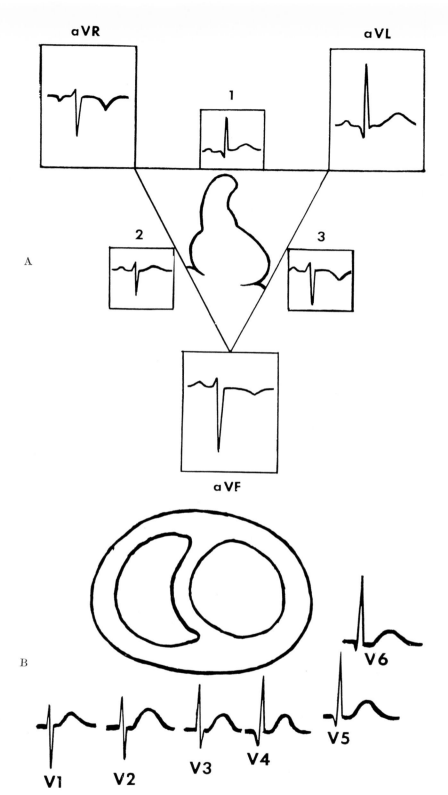

Fig. 78. A, Electrocardiograms in the *classic bipolar* and in the *unipolar limb leads* of a person with "horizontal" heart. Scheme. B, Electrocardiograms in the *chest leads* of a person with "horizontal" heart. Scheme.

is that, in the latter, the downward T in aVL is associated with depressed S-T, wide QRS, and inverted T in the chest leads.

Forward rotation of the apex is rare in a normal subject. If present, V1 and V2 have a right ventricular pattern; aVL has an upright T (it may have an inverted T if there is counterclockwise rotation).

Marked clockwise rotation around the longitudinal axis causes the right ventricle to become anterior. Then all chest leads may show a right ventricular pattern rS.

In all types of *horizontal heart*, the main deflection of QRS in aVL is directed up-

wards; in aVF, downwards; and the same is true for leads 1 and 3; mnemonically, they look like two hands directed away from each other (fig. 79).

Fetal electrocardiogram. It may be recorded by means of an electroencephalograph or with an electrocardiograph having an increased sensitivity (2–3 cm. per millivolt). The best leads are those on the maternal abdomen; most authors have employed a vertical lead from the epigastrium or umbilical region to the suprapubic region. Transverse or diagonal leads have been used also.

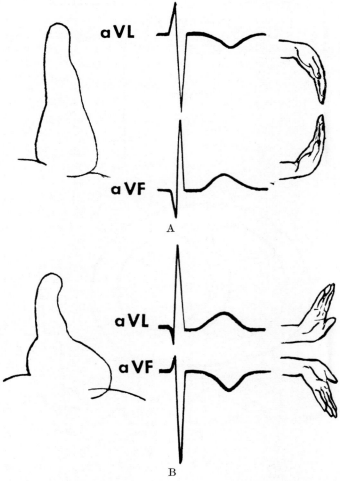

FIG. 79. *Right* (A) and *left* (B) *axis deviation* in the various positions of the heart and mnemonic key based on comparison of leads aVL and aVF.

ELECTROCARDIOGRAM OF THE CHILD

At birth, the standard leads reveal *right axis deviations*; the unipolar limb leads indicate a *vertical heart*; the chest leads reveal a *predominance of the R over the S waves*. The T waves are inverted, diphasic, or isoelectric from V1 to V4, V5, and even V6. As the child grows older, a tendency to diphasism of the complex with actual presence of S, is noted. At the age of 10, usually an adult type of electrocardiogram is recorded and the T wave is usually upright in V4.

Roentgenology (Radiology)

Application of the x-ray apparatus to the examination of the heart and large vessels supplies important data about the size, shape, position, and movements of these organs.

Roentgenology includes fluoroscopy, orthodiagraphy, and teleradiography, which can be accomplished by most radiologists. It further includes roentgenkymography, roentgencinematography, electrokymography, and angiocardiography.

FLUOROSCOPY

Fluoroscopy is the procedure which should be carried out as a first step befor any further x-ray study. Proper adaptation of the pupils to the dark is necessary. This can be obtained either by long waiting in a dark room or by wearing red goggles for some time prior to the examination. X-ray intensity should not exceed 5 milliampères. Gloves and apron protection, and reduction of the aperture by the shutters, are customary protections for the observer.

Skeletal details, costophrenic angles, motion and position of the diaphragm, mediastinum, and lungs, will be observed as a preliminary procedure. Then the heart is observed in the three classic positions:

a) *Postero-anterior* (PA) = chest toward the observer.

b) *Left anterior oblique* (LAO) = left shoulder toward the observer, rotation of 45 degrees (fig. 80).

c) *Right anterior oblique* (RAO) = right shoulder toward the observer, rotation of 45 degrees (fig. 80).

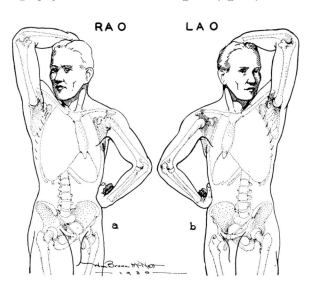

RAO   LAO

FIG. 80. Positions for anterior oblique views. Degree of rotation to be determined for each individual by means of fluoroscopy. a, right anterior oblique view; b, left anterior oblique view. (From *Clinical Roentgenology of the Cardiovascular System*, 2nd Ed. Courtesy of Dr. H. Roesler and Charles C Thomas, Publisher)

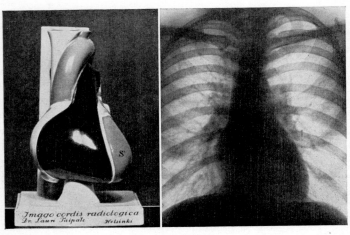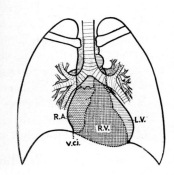

FIG. 81. The heart in posteroanterior position (P-A). Left, model. Center, actual x-ray film. Right, isolation of the different elements. R. A., right atrium; R. V., right ventricle; L. V., left ventricle; V.C.i., vena cava inferior.

In most cases it will be also useful to study:

d) *Right or left lateral* view.

e) *Dorsal position* (AP) = the patient's back is toward the observer.

Correlation of the different parts of the heart with x-ray models and x-ray findings is shown in figures 81 to 84.

Postero-anterior (fig. 81). *The right border of the heart* (to the left of the observer) is formed, from above downwards, by: superior vena cava, ascending aorta, right atrium, and, in certain cases (on deep inspiration), the right ventricle. The *left*

border of the heart (to the right of the observer) is formed, from above downwards, by: aortic arch (aortic knob), pulmonary artery with its left branch (pulmonary knob), left atrial appendage, and left ventricle.

Left anterior oblique (fig. 82). The *anterior border* (to the left of the observer) is formed by the ascending aorta and the right ventricle. The *posterior border* is formed by the left atrium and the left ventricle.

Right anterior oblique (fig. 83). The *anterior border* (to the right of the observer) is formed, from above downwards, by:

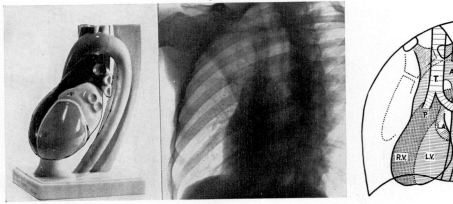

FIG. 82. The heart in left anterior oblique (LAO). T, trachea; A, aorta; P, pulmonary artery; L.A., left atrium; R.V., right ventricle; L.V., left ventricle.

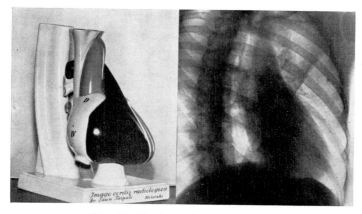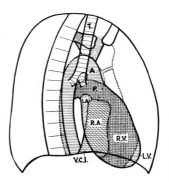

FIG. 83. The heart in right anterior oblique (RAO) (see figure 81)

the aortic arch, the pulmonary artery, the infundibulum of the right ventricle, and a thin anterior portion of the left ventricle. The *posterior border* (to the left of the observer) is formed by the aorta and the left atrium.

The right anterior oblique gives the earliest view of left atrial enlargement and of enlargement of the pulmonary artery. The left anterior oblique confirms the left atrial enlargement and clearly shows an early dilatation of the ascending aorta.

Slight enlargement of the left atrium is present when the left atrial shadow cannot be dissociated from that of the vertebral column at a 45° angle, but only at a 65° angle. A great enlargement exists if the two shadows cannot be dissociated even in the lateral positions.

Lateral views. The lateral positions show that a clear space exists both before and behind the cardiac shadow (fig. 84). Both may become obscure in mediastinal and pericardial processes, and in cardiac enlargement. Enlargement of the descending aorta may obscure the posterior space. *Enlargement of the right ventricle increases the anterior contact between cardiac shadow and sternum, thus decreasing the anterior clear space.*

The fluoroscopic examination consists not only of appreciating changes of size and shape of the different parts of the heart, but also of evaluating cardiac dynamics. The observer can easily follow the systolic contraction of the ventricles and the systolic expansion of the large arteries. The atrial contraction is better observed when

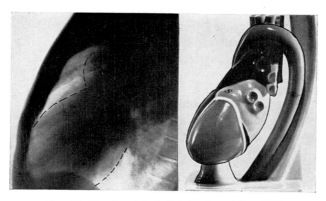

FIG. 84. The heart in left lateral position (LL)

NORMAL TRANSVERSE HEART

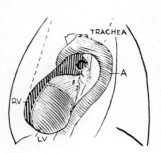
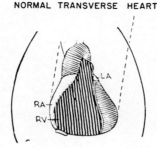
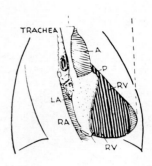

NORMAL VERTICAL HEART

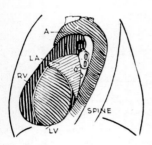
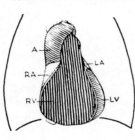
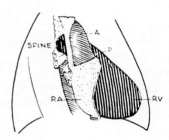

Fig. 85. The normal transverse heart compared to the normal vertical heart. (Courtesy of Dr. Herrmann and the C. V. Mosby Co.)

the heart rate is slow. In addition to the pulsation of the pulmonary artery, it is possible to observe, in certain conditions, a rapid systolic expansion of the hilar vessels. This was called the *hilar dance* (104) and is caused by increased pulse pressure in the pulmonary arterial vessels, as typically seen in pulmonary regurgitation.

Abnormal systolic traction of the heart on the left diaphragm (adhesions); the presence of *a large pulsating shadow* (aneurysm); *intracardiac calcifications* (calcification of the heart valves); and *extracardiac calcifications* (pericardial calcification), should be looked for and interpreted.

Administration of a *barium meal* to the patient permits the study of the esophagus and its relationship with the descending aorta and the left atrium. When enlarged, these parts make a definite and sharp defect in the esophageal shadow.

Administration of any *gas-producing drink* permits a better view of the lower heart border because the gas, accumulating in the stomach, facilitates visualization (105).

The *Valsalva* and the *Mueller tests* cause opposite changes in the size of the heart, which are of interest (106) (page 85).

The *"cardiac apex"* is actually a rounded nose, just above or below the diaphragm or bisected by it. In cases where the diaphragm is high, localization of the position of the apex may be difficult. It is necessary then to ask the patient to breathe slowly and deeply, and the extreme inspiratory position frequently reveals the apex.

A scheme of fluoroscopic observations follows.

POSTEROANTERIOR

1) Lungs

a) Vascularity
   normal
   decreased
   increased
b) Hilar shadows
   normal (with or without expansive pulsations)

decreased
increased (with or without expansive pulsations)

2) Basal Peduncle

a) Normal
b) Enlarged
c) Aortic arch
   normal
   enlarged
   small
   absent
d) Pulmonary arch
   normal
   straight
   enlarged
   absent
e) Vena cava superior
   normal
   enlarged
   pulsating
f) Thymus

3) Cardiac Contour

a) Heart enlarged
   to the left
   to the right
   totally
b) Rhythmic pulsations of the right atrium

LEFT ANTERIOR OBLIQUE

a) Amount of rotation necessary to clear the spinal column (check with a barium swallow) for evaluating the size of left atrium

b) Relationship between right ventricle and anterior chest wall
c) Relationship between right ventricle and ascending aorta
d) Pulmonary window

RIGHT ANTERIOR OBLIQUE

a) Size of the right ventricle
b) Size of the pulmonary conus
c) Size and development of the aortic arch
d) Size and configuration of the left atrium (check with a barium swallow)

ORTHODIAGRAPHY

Orthodiagraphy is the most accurate method for measurements of the size of the heart. The method used in fluoroscopy does not eliminate the distortion and the enlargements of the cardiac shadow caused by the divergent course of the x-ray beams. In order to avoid this cause of error, an immobile glass screen is placed in front of the fluoroscope. Then the x-ray tube and the fluoroscopic screen are moved to different points, taking care that at each station only the central part of the beam (revealed by a lead mark) coincides with the profile of the heart. The observer successively records the most important landmarks of the heart (apex, left border, right border, etc.), marking with a pencil the different

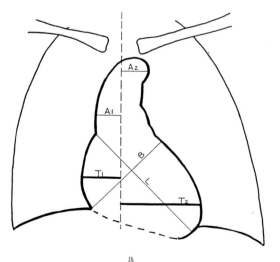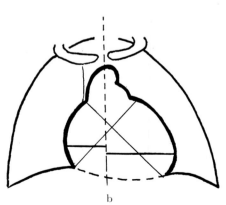

FIG. 86. The different diameters of the heart and aorta: a, in the adult; b, in the infant. A1 + A2, aorta; T1 + T2, transverse diameter; B, broad diameter; L, long diameter.

stations either on the glass or on a special paper. Later, the profile of the heart is drawn by connecting the different points (*orthodiagram*). As the orthodiagram represents an actual-size reproduction of the heart, measurements can be made with a fair degree of accuracy on the tracing.

The following diameters can be drawn on the frontal orthodiagram (fig. 86):

Long diameter, which extends from the junction of the cardiac shadow with the vascular pedicle on the right to the apex on the left (actually, to the junction of the left ventricle with the diaphragm).

Broad diameter, which is the greatest diameter of the cardiac shadow, perpendicular to the long diameter. In order to draw a single line, it may be necessary to artificially extend the lower right heart border, following the natural curve.

Transverse diameter, which is the sum of the longest transverse lines to the right and left heart borders from the midline.

Evaluation of cardiac enlargement can be made only by knowing the normal size of the heart at any height, weight, and age of the patient. A complex table of the transverse diameter in comparison with all these variables has been made for the orthodia-

gram (107) and a simpler one for the teleroentgenogram (108). As simplicity is the basis for any clinical study and no exact formula can take care of *all* variables, so that a certain margin of approximation should be always considered, a simplified table is shown here, both for the orthodiagram and the teleroentgenogram. The table of the transverse diameter of the heart is made from data of *Ungerleider* (108).

A more complete appreciation of the cardiac diameters is possible, however, if both the long and broad diameters are measured. The accompanying tables have been made from data of *Moritz, Dietlen* and *Groedel* (107b). They represent average figures which may vary by about 10 per cent in both directions in different individuals. The fact that the figures of the German authors for the transverse diameter are higher than those of *Ungerleider* can be partly explained

TABLE 11

HEIGHT	WEIGHT	TRANSVERSE DIAMETER	
		Orthodiagram	Teleroent-genogram
in.	*lbs.*	*mm.*	*mm.*
60–64	83– 92	95	100
60–68	92–104	100	105
60–72	101–121	104	110
60–76	110–140	109	115
60–76	120–152	114	120
60–76	130–165	119	125
60–76	141–178	123	130
60–76	152–192	128	135
60–76	163–207	133	140
60–76	175–222	138	145
60–76	187–237	142.5	150
60–76	200–253	147	155
70–76	250–270	152	160
74–76	276–284	156	164

TABLE 12. *Average heart measurements for orthodiagrams based on age*

PATIENT AGE	HEART	
	Transverse diameter	Long diameter
yrs.	*mm.*	*mm.*
19–29	125	135
30–39	130	140
40–45	130	136

TABLE 13. *Average heart measurements for orthodiagrams based on height, weight, and sex*

	PATIENT		THORAX	HEART		
	Height	Weight	Transverse section	Transverse diameter	Long diameter	Broad diameter
	in.	*lbs.*	*mm.*			
Males	60–64	88–110	250	110	120	90
	64–72	110–165	270	125	130	100
	72	165	290	130	140	100
Females	58–62	88–110	210	105	115	90
	62–65	100–130	230	115	120	90
	66	130	250	120	130	90

by the fact that their orthodiagrams were taken in the supine position.

The *diameter of the aortic arch* can be measured by making the sum of the two lines from the midline to the maximum extensions to right and left borders of the vascular pedicle. This diameter may not be accurate because the shadow of the superior vena cava or other mediastinal structures may interfere. Another procedure is that of completing the natural curve of the aortic knob.

TELEROENTGENOGRAPHY

A photographic record of the heart is taken on a film by using a distant source of x-ray. The tube is placed at 2 meters (6.5 feet) so that its rays are practically parallel. The magnification of the cardiac shadow over the actual size is about 5 per cent, a fact which should be considered in taking cardiac measurements. When making the exposure, the subject is properly centered and respiration should be suspended in inspiration. The exposure should be taken in the erect position, if possible.

The size of the cardiac shadow may vary considerably from systole to diastole, and since diastole is usually longer, the picture is more often taken in diastole, showing a somewhat larger heart.

In measuring the diameters, attention should be paid to the fact that an *extrapericardial fat pad* may obscure the apex; that deformity of the thorax may render the accurate determination of the heart size difficult; and that a high diaphragm also may considerably displace the heart and change the profile.

Measurements of cardiac and aortic sizes can be made on teleroentgenograms by the same method as that used on orthodiagrams. Comparison of the transverse diameter with height and weight has been given already (see table).

Determination of the heart volume has been tried either on the basis of the frontal area or by considering the three dimensions in both frontal and lateral pictures (109). This is still in the experimental stage and needs further study.

A set of diameters has also been proposed for studying the enlargement of the individual heart chambers (110). In spite of all speculations, these diameters add little to our knowledge.

ROENTGENKYMOGRAPHY

This is a special technique for recording the movements of the heart on a film. In order to record the pulsations of numerous points along the cardiac borders simultaneously, *a grid with multiple slits* is used. One type employs many horizontal slits (111a); another, on the contrary, many adjustable slits which are placed perpendicularly to the different sections of the cardiac shadow (111b). During suspended respiration, the film is moved about 12 mm. in 1 to 2 seconds, so that 1 to 3 complete cardiac cycles are recorded. As the film moves downward, the beginning of exposure is at the lower margin.

When the lead diaphragm of the fluoroscope is narrowed to a thin slit, single points of the cardiac border can be seen to pulsate inward and outward with cardiac systole and diastole. If an x-ray film is substituted for the fluoroscopic screen and either the film or the grid is made to move at constant speed, the pulsation of a point of the border is recorded as a section of a curve.

Atrial, ventricular, and vascular waves can be observed. To interpret them, one should turn the film 90° counterclockwise (and look into a mirror) for the study of the *left* cardiac border; 90° clockwise, for the study of the *right* cardiac border. Each trough is the result of an *inward* movement (systole, contraction, depression); each crest is caused by an *outward* movement (diastole, expansion, pulsation) (fig. 87).

A complete description of the waves will be given later (page 147) on account of the

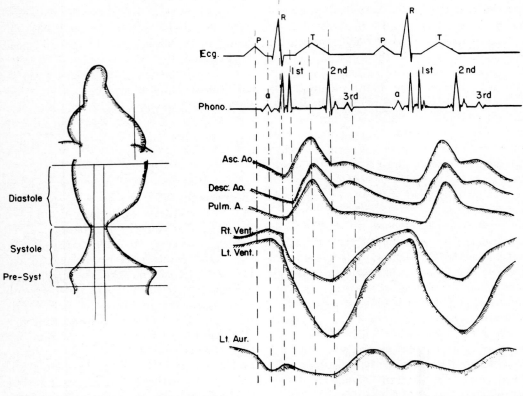

FIG. 87. Roentgenkymographic tracings compared with the electrocardiogram and phonocardiogram. To obtain the tracings, special rotations and magnification of the film are necessary. At left, actual motions of the two margins at ventricular level (magnified and placed near each other).

similarity of the electrokymographic and roentgenkymographic waves.

The *technical limitations* in the use of roentgenkymography are: 1) Difficulty of applying the apparatus in a position perpendicular to the contour to be plotted because of the rigidity of the slits. 2) Short duration of the records obtained (only three or four cycles in Stumpf's multiple-slit kymograph). 3) Insufficient speed of the tracings. 4) Poor distinction and small amplitude of the waves. 5) Inability to record simultaneously other tracings, such as an electrocardiogram, a phonocardiogram, or a sphygmogram. Attempts to overcome these weaknesses by faster recording over a longer period of time, or densometric transcription did not result in a great improvement.

ELECTROKYMOGRAPHY[39]

Following unsuccessful attempts by several authors (112a), Henny and Boone (112b) developed the first practical apparatus in 1945 and called it *electrokymograph*. They applied it to the study of border motions of the right atrium, the aortic and pulmonary knobs, and the left ventricle. A year later, Marchal (112c) built, independently, a similar device for the study of density changes of the lungs. In 1947 the author, working with *Fleischner* and *Rappaport* (113), described an instrument which operated on the same principle as that of *Henny* and *Boone* but combined several modifications. With this, a

[39] Alternate terms suggested: fluorocardiography (113); kinedensigraphy (112c).

systematic study of the border motions and density changes of the heart, great vessels, and lungs was made in several positions of the subjects.

The setup for electrokymography consists of: 1) fluoroscope; 2) pick-up fastened to the fluoroscopic screen (photo-multiplier tube, slitted diaphragm, and small fluorescent strip); 3) electrical arrangement to transform a.c. into d.c., and device for rapid changes of amplification; 4) electric filter suppressing the flicker of the x-ray tube; 5) galvanometer transcribing the tracing on a moving film; 6) microphone to be connected with a sound recorder; and 7) device for electrical tracing of the carotid pulse.

Any upright fluoroscopic stand can be used for the seated patient; for children or sick patients, a horizontal table is used. A commercial tilt-table can be employed for both purposes.

The main part of the apparatus is an electron multiplier *phototube*. A strip of *fluorescent screen* is cemented to the glass cover of the phototube in front of the cathode. When the x-rays strike this screen, the light generated by the screen is picked up by the cathode, transformed into equivalent electrons, amplified, and fed into the electrocardiographic channel. Thus the electrical output varies in proportion to the amount of x-rays which reach the fluorescent screen. A good analysis of the waves can be done only if the film moves at speeds of between 50 and 100 mm. per second. If, on the other hand, one is interested in the magnitude of the waves, film speeds of between 2.5 and 10 mm. per second should be used.

The polarity of the apparatus is so arranged that an increase of light causes a downward movement of the tracing. Therefore, a drop of the curve indicates either an *inward motion* of the cardiac border (border tracing) or a *decrease in the thickness* of the structure (densogram). The former may be due to either contraction or displacement.

Any wave occurring before the first large vibration of the first sound is *presystolic*; any wave occurring after the last vibration of the second sound is *diastolic*: any wave taking place between the beginning of the first sound and the end of the second is *systolic*.

In general, the tracings should be recorded during voluntary apnea in an intermediate phase because it has been shown that the pulsations of the lung (and, to a lesser extent, those of the hilar shadows and pulmonary artery) are greater in inspiration than in expiration. It is difficult, however, to obtain reliable tracings in children, patients in failure, and patients with chronic lung diseases, who are unable to control their respiration because of dyspnea. A high-pass filter, made of several condensers, is then interposed between the electrokymograph and the galvanometer; this filter modifies the time constant, so that the tracing does not wander off the paper. A slight error, proportional to the amount of reduction and consisting of a slight change of phase and configuration of the waves is the result. Therefore, such filter should not be used in cases where plateau-like waves are suspected because these are basically altered by the device.

Several *standard positions for the slit* can be used with the patient in either the sitting or the recumbent position (fig. 89). As a routine, with the patient in the posteroanterior position, one starts *on the left side*, plotting the *apex* of the heart, the *upper part of the left ventricle*, the *appendage of the left atrium* (often better visualized by a 10° to 15° rotation toward one of the oblique positions), the *pulmonary knob*, and the *aortic knob*.

On the *right side*, one traces the *right atrium*, the *ascending aorta* (10° left oblique), the *superior cava* (seldom satisfactory), and the *inferior cava* (deep inspiration); one can also plot the *right hilar shadow* and the *peripheral pulmonary pulsations* (these are densograms).

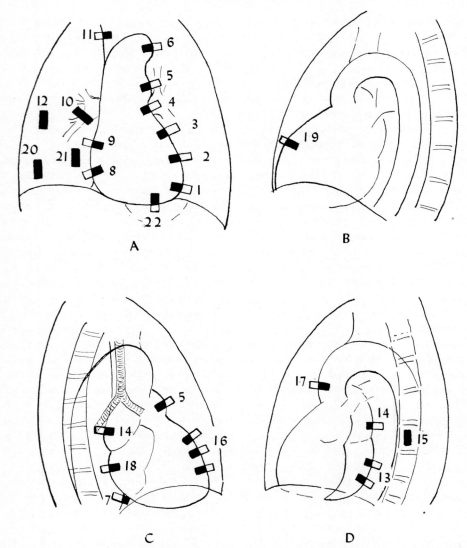

Fig. 88. Standard positions of the slit for recording electrokymograms. Positions for border tracings are marked with black and white rectangles; positions for densograms are marked with black rectangles. *A, Posteroanterior projection:* 1, apex; 2, 3, higher positions on left ventricle; 4, left auricular appendage; 5, pulmonary arch, 6, aortic arch; 8, 9, right atrium; 10, right hilum; 11, superior cava; 12 and 20, right lung; 21, pulmonary veins; 22, left ventricle (inferior aspect). *B, Left lateral:* 19, right ventricle. *C, Right anterior oblique:* 5, pulmonary arch; 7, inferior cava; 14, left atrium; 16, left ventricle (anterior aspect); 18, right atrium. *D, Left anterior oblique:* 13, left ventricle (posterior aspect); 14, left atrium; 15, descending aorta; 17, ascending aorta.

The *left oblique* is used for the study of the *left atrium,* the *descending aorta,* and the *posterior aspect of the left ventricle.* The *right oblique* is used for the study of the *left atrium* and the *anterior aspect of the left ventricle.*

The pulsation of the *right ventricle* is best picked up in the straight lateral view just above the point where it separates from the anterior chest wall (the best tracings are obtained with the subject in the recumbent position). The *pulmonary veins* can be studied with the slit placed vertically between convexity of the right atrium and right hilum in the posteroanterior position.

In the study of the various cardiovascular structures, the following data should be considered:

a) *Amplitude of pulsation.* It can be evaluated by comparing the amplitude of pulsation of one structure with that of another, if they are recorded with the same degree of amplification.

a) *Shape and time of various waves.* They can be evaluated by the use of optimum amplification and by timing the waves of the EKY with those of other records.

c) *Abnormal movements.* Transmitted and inherent pulsations can be differentiated by comparing a border tracing with a densogram of the same organ.

d) *Dissociation between various chambers* (dissociation between the atria; bundle branch block; A-V block). This study is best accomplished by simultaneously recording the pulsations of two chambers (two electrokymographs).

The Waves of the Normal Tracing and Their Interpretation

It should be kept in mind that the electrokymogram (EKY) is used for the study of entirely different structures; atrial, ventricular, arterial, and venous (figs. 89 and 93). According to the structure and its function, the tracing should be compared with a physiological or clinical tracing of atrial or ventricular contraction, or of arterial or venous pulsation.

The EKY tracings represent the summation of: volume changes of a chamber or vessel, motions due to rotation or total shift of the heart, and tractions from other structures. In particular, each atrium shows the effect of traction by its respective ventricle.

Left ventricle (fig. 90). *Apex.* A *small positive wave* can be recorded immediately before or during the first group of vibrations of the first sound. This is due to left atrial

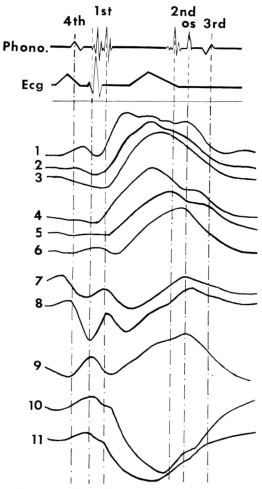

FIG. 89. Comparison of various schematic electrokymograms with the phonocardiogram (phono.) and the electrocardiogram (Ecg.) Electrokymograms: 1, ascending aorta; 2, aortic arch; 3, descending aorta; 4, pulmonary artery; 5, hilum; 6, lung; 7, right atrium; 8, left atrium; 9, pulmonary veins; 10, left ventricle; 11, right ventricle.

contraction which pushes a certain amount of blood into the left ventricle. The tension period is accompanied by *a small depression,* probably due to torsion of the heart. The main ventricular wave consists of a *large downward deflection* which starts at the time of that large vibration of the first sound which is due to opening of the aortic valve. The descending branch of this wave reaches *its lowest point* at a time which varies in different subjects and with various positions on account of variable influence of rotation and displacement of the apex. In most cases, this point slightly precedes that large vibration of the second sound which is due to closure of the aortic valve. The brief interval corresponds to the protodiastole. Early diastole is marked by a *small rebound* and a *rapidly ascending slope* which ends at the time of the third heart sound (phase of rapid filling); then by a *more gradual slope* or a horizontal line, which continues until the beginning of the following cycle. The *isometric relaxation period* lies between the

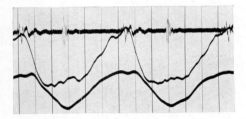

Fig. 90. Simultaneous electrokymograms of the left ventricle. Upper tracing, phonocardiogram. Middle tracing, EKY of the apex. Lower tracing, EKY of the left ventricular margin at medium level. There seems to be precession of the apex due to its rotation during the tension period.

lowest point of the ventricular wave and the beginning of the rebound in early diastole.

Convexity of the left ventricle. The waves reproduce volume changes of the ventricle more faithfully and denote to a lesser degree the effect of motion.

Other points on the ventricular surface. The left ventricle can be studied in various projections, such as the left anterior oblique (posterior aspect) and the right anterior oblique (anterolateral aspect). Tracings recorded in the oblique positions present the same type of waves as the left margin in the P. A. position, except that they are smaller; the lowest part of the main wave is frequently made of a shallow curve.

Right ventricle. Indirect evidence of right

ventricular activity may be found in tracings of the right atrium in the P. A. view; however, the data cannot be considered accurate because of influence from venous return. The best tracings are recorded in the lateral views with the slit placed where the cardiac shadow separates from that of the anterior chest wall, or just below this spot.

Left atrium (figs. 89 and 93). The typical tracing shows a *rapid downward wave in presystole* starting about 0.14 second before the first sound. If the heart rate is rapid, there may be only one slow wave in diastole with a negative peak at the end of left atrial contraction. This peak usually coincides with the first vibration of the first sound but may take place slightly before. If a fourth (atrial) sound is present, it occurs during the first (downward) branch of the atrial wave. The presystolic wave is deeper in patients with left atrial hypertrophy and disappears in patients with atrial fibrillation. After this wave, the tracing rises sharply to a *small positive notch* during the first part of the first sound. After this, two negative waves are present, one in systole and the other in diastole. The *systolic collapse* of the left atrium is related to the dynamics of the left ventricle. The left ventricular contraction lowers the a-v septum and creates a suction within the atrial cavity which is slowly compensated by increased flow of blood. Therefore, an inward movement of the free atrial wall takes place. The highest level of the tracing is reached slightly after the end of systole, when the mitral valve opens. After this positive notch, there is a *diastolic collapse* which is probably due to passive flow of blood into the left ventricle after the opening of the mitral valve.

Right atrium. The tracing recorded over the margin of the right atrium is similar to that of the left (fig. 89). Contraction of the atrium during presystole is manifested by a *small and rounded downward wave.* After this, the tracing either reaches the baseline or rises above it, but drops again during ventricular systole. The latter is manifested by a sharp downward wave (*systolic collapse*) which is usually deeper than the atrial wave. The subsequent course of the atrial tracing varies with the position of the subject. In the sitting position, the tracing rises slowly and attains its maximum height at the time of tricuspid opening; in the recumbent position, the rise is quicker and there may be a convex line which brings the tracing above the baseline. Another drop, however, takes place after the opening of the tricuspid valve (*diastolic collapse*). In summary, there is a presystolic collapse, a systolic collapse, and, frequently, an early-diastolic collapse.

Ascending aorta (fig. 91). The tracing of the ascending aorta presents a typical pattern. It has an early systolic drop; a rapid rise; an early peak; a slight descent (or none at all) during the second half of systole; a small incisura; a high and occasionally prolonged wave after the incisura. The lowering of the aortic root by ventricular systole and the medial displacement of the ascending aorta by rotation of the heart in the same phase apparently reduce the height of the aortic wave. Opposite movements, taking place in diastole, add their effect to that of the dicrotic wave and create a high positive wave. The proximity of the ascending aorta to the left ventricle may contribute to the fact that, in some subjects, the profile of the aortic pulse during systole greatly resembles a tracing of intraventricular pressure.

Aortic arch (fig. 91). The tracing of the aortic arch presents: a) a small positive wave during the first part of the first sound, probably due to a rise of the aortic valve during isometric contraction; b) a sharp rise, after the second large vibration of the first sound (opening of the aortic valve); c) an anacrotic depression in the first part of systole; d) a peak during the last part of systole but well before the second sound; e) a predicrotic notch, which may coincide with, or last slightly beyond, the second sound; f) a dicrotic wave, which is usually small and rounded; and g) a few small aftervibrations.

Descending aorta (fig. 91). Since the descending aorta does not present a sharp contour on fluoroscopy, only a *densogram* is possible in normal subjects. The tracing is similar to that of the aortic arch, but shows a slight delay in the rise of the pulse in comparison with that in the arch.

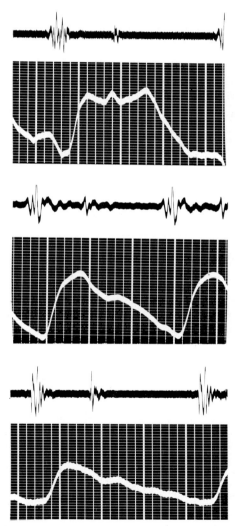

FIG. 91. Electrokymograms of the aorta. a, ascending aorta (slight rotation toward LAO); b, aortic arch (PA); c, descending aorta (LAO).

Pulmonary artery (fig. 92). The tracing of the pulmonary arch is usually easily obtained. However, a large left hilar shadow or a dilated descending aorta may modify the tracing. The pulmonic pulsation starts with the opening of the pulmonic valve (second part of the first sound) and rises sharply, occasionally with an anacrotic depression. The peak is reached at about two-thirds of ventricular systole. The predicrotic notch is deep and occurs 0.06 and

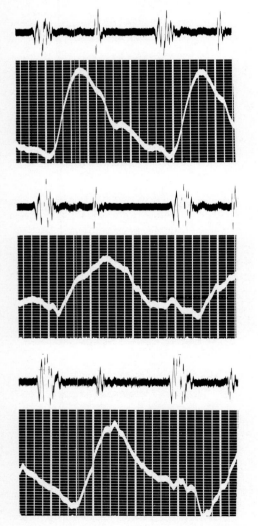

FIG. 92. Electrokymograms of the pulmonary arterial wave. a, pulmonary knob; b, right hilum; c, visible base of the right lung.

0.08 second after the main vibration of the second sound. The dicrotic wave is well-defined and has a peak from 0.10 to 0.12 second after the main vibration of the second sound. Another positive wave may be seen in late diastole.

Hilar shadows (fig. 92). The tracings of the hilar shadows are *densograms* and represent the variations of opacity of the hilar regions caused by changes in the blood content. The amplitude of the normal hilar pulsation is between one-half and two-thirds of that of the pulmonary arch. Following a small drop, the tracing presents *a large positive wave* about 0.04 second after the pulse of the pulmonary artery and 0.12 second after the beginning of the first sound. The peak of the pulse wave is reached at or about the time of the main vibration of the second sound. It may be followed by a small notch and by a small dicrotic wave. The positive wave of the hilar pulse indicates the arrival of the arterial pulse into the branches of the pulmonary artery. However, the pulsations of the pulmonary veins also influence the tracing and the early systolic depression may be due to acceleration of the venous flow.

Pulmonary veins. The typical tracing shows a *presystolic positive wave* (increased volume), synchronous with the negative wave (contraction = decreased volume) of the left atrial tracing. Later on, a *systolic collapse*, a *positive peak* at the time of mitral valve opening, and a *diastolic collapse*, are present. In other words, the tracing is a typical "venous" tracing.

Lungs (fig. 92). The *densogram* of the lung is a tracing which resembles that of the hilum. However, there are some differences: there is a greater delay in the rise of the pulse wave (this takes place about 0.04 second after the rise of the hilar pulse; there may be a greater delay of the peak (this occurs from 0.08 to 0.10 second after the main vibration of the second sound); the curve is more rounded and exhibits no evidence of a dicrotic wave.

Superior cava. Occasionally, it is possible to obtain a record similar to the jugular tracing and which shows the three typical, positive waves *a*, *c*, and *v*. Smaller vibrations are frequently superimposed.

Inferior cava. There is a small, presystolic, positive wave, due to slower flow of blood at the time of atrial contraction ("*a*" wave). This is followed by a deep negative wave (*systolic collapse*). Then follows a slow rise culminating in a single or double wave about 0.10 second after the second sound ("*v*" wave). This is due to slow engorgement of the vein until the tricuspid valve opens. The subsequent drop reaches its maximum after the middle of diastole (*diastolic collapse*). No "*c*" wave is present.

The tracing of the inferior vena cava is similar to the hepatic tracings of normal subjects and is the result of the same physiologic phenomena.

The method is simple to handle, accurate, and satisfactory for the study of cardiac and vascular structures. It may be applied to the study of:

a) Physiology and pharmacology of the heart and vessels. b) Rheumatic and luetic heart disease. c) Congenital heart disease. d) Coronary heart disease. e) Pericarditis and adhesive pericarditis. f) Aneurysms and mediastinal tumors.

ANGIOCARDIOGRAPHY

Angiocardiography was first described for the study of the pulmonary vessels (114a) and then applied to the visualization of the cardiac chambers in children (114b). Later, it was modified, so that visualization of the cardiac chambers in the adult was made possible (115, 116).

Present technique consists of the rapid intravenous injection of 30 to 50 cc. of 70 per cent *diodrast* (2 seconds or less) in the adult (1 cc. per Kilo in children). The arrival of undiluted contrast medium into the heart takes place about 2 seconds later when a series of roentgenograms is started. When circulation is slower, the correct exposure

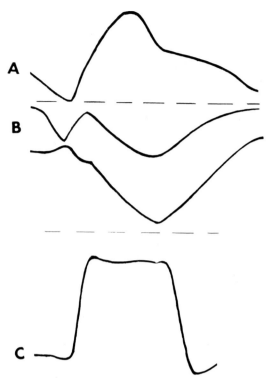

Fig. 93. The various electrokymographic patterns. A, Pattern of expansion (aortic arch, pulmonary arch, hila, lungs). B, Pattern of contraction (atria, ventricles). C, Pattern of intraventricular pressure (ascending aorta, normal; left atrium, mitral regurgitation; left ventricle, infarct).

time is found by means of circulation time tests (page 156).

In order to obtain complete vision of the various chambers, it is often necessary to obtain several films at extremely short intervals. This can be obtained by various devices. Most of them, including the "roll-film magazine" driven by a motor unit, take films at half-second intervals.

According to the timing of the exposure, two main pictures can be obtained: that revealing the chambers of the right heart (*right angiocardiography*) and that revealing the chambers of the left heart (*left angiocardiography*) (figs. 94 to 97).

The *left anterior oblique* gives the best picture of the heart. The different cardiac

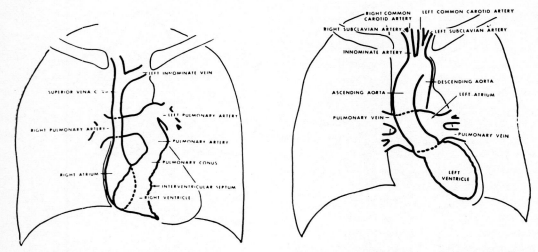

Fig. 94. Idealized angiocardiographic outlines in posteroanterior projection. A, right heart. B, left heart. (From Dotter and Sternberg's *Angiocardiography*. Courtesy of the authors and of Paul B. Hoeber, Inc.)

chambers are then visualized one after the other so that important informations about the shape and size of the *chambers*, the size of the *valvular openings*, and the condition of the *septa*, can be secured.

Among the disadvantages of this procedure are: a) nearly constant thrombosis of the vein; b) unpleasant general sensations during the injection; c) need for general anesthesia in infants and children; d) occasional febrile reaction; and e) some mortality (about 0.5 per cent).

Angiocardiography is particularly useful in the complex congenital malformation of the heart and large vessels.

COMPLEMENTAL PROCEDURES

Whenever difficulties in the interpretation of x-rays of the heart are found, complemental maneuvers may be used.

They are:

a) *Distention of the stomach by gas* (gas-producing mixture in water).

b) *Distention of the transverse colon by air* (injection of air via the rectum).

c) *Diagnostic pneumothorax* (customary technique of pneumothorax; injection of air under negative pressure with manometric control).

d) *Diagnostic pneumoperitoneum*. This is done by injecting from 1 to 2 liters of air in the peritoneal cavity by means of a blunt needle. The procedure is used in order to visualize the lower border of the heart and the upper border of both the liver and spleen. It is used almost exclusively in cases with ascites (page 457).

e) *Diagnostic pneumopericardium*. This procedure is adopted only in cases with pericardial effusion. The injection of air is preceded by evacuation of fluid (page 448).

f) *Diagnostic pneumomediastinum* (117, 118). This procedure gives visualization of the anterior mediastinum whenever the obscuration is caused by enlargement of the heart. Anterior adhesions are often visualized. Mediastinal tumors and extensive adhesions persist as dense shadows. Injection of 40 to 60 cc. of air is made in the anterior mediastinum by means of a curved needle sliding along the posterior surface of the sternum (fig. 98). The procedure seems devoid of danger.

g) *Administration of a barium meal* for the study of the esophagus and its relationship to the heart and aorta.

In conclusion, *roentgenology of the heart* supplements the information obtained by

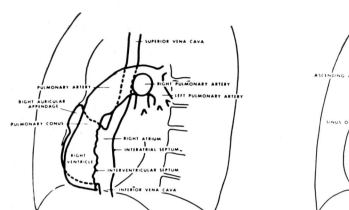
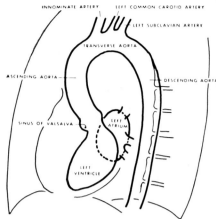

FIG. 95. Idealized angiocardiographic outlines in the left anterior oblique projection. A, right heart; B, left heart. (From Dotter and Sternberg's *Angiocardiography*, courtesy of the authors and of Paul B. Hoeber, Inc.)

other methods and gives exact data about the size, shape, and position of the heart and large vessels.

Tracings of the Atomic Discharges of Radioactive Materials Within the Heart (Radiocardiography)

The passage of radioactive substances through the cardiac chambers can be graphically recorded with the aid of a Geiger-Mueller tube. The carefully shielded Geiger-Mueller tube is placed in front of the precordium and is connected with a count-rate meter and either an ink-writing device (217) or a direct-writing electrocardiograph, as used by the author (218). The curve records the concentration of a radioisotope in the structures underlying the tube as represented by the number of disintegrations of the radioactive element per unit of time.

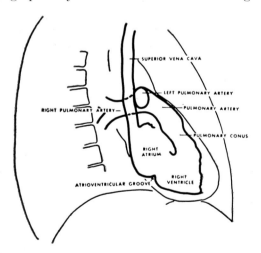
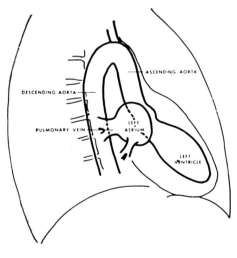

FIG. 96. Idealized angiocardiographic outlines in the right anterior oblique projection. A, right heart; B, left heart. (From Dotter and Sternberg's *Angiocardiography*, courtesy of the authors and of Paul B. Hoeber, Inc.)

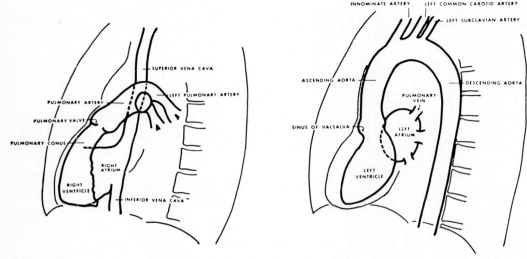

FIG. 97. Idealized angiocardiographic outlines in the left lateral projection. A, right heart; B, left heart. (From Dotter and Sternberg's *Angiocardiography*, courtesy of the authors and of Paul B. Hoeber, Inc.)

In the original description, the curve was corrected for the random bursts by taking the mean of the counts over a half-second period. In the suggested modification, the characteristics of the counter and the electrocardiograph are so adjusted that a slower curve, representing the mean of counts, is automatically recorded.

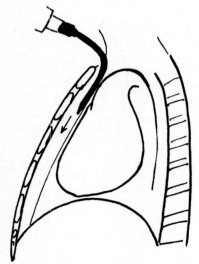

FIG. 98. Technique of introduction of air in the performance of anterior pneumomediastinum.

Either radiosodium (Na^{24}) in a dose of 100 to 200 microcurie (217) or di-iodofluoresceine (I^{131}) in a dose of 20 to 50 microcurie (218) can be injected into an antecubital vein. The latter has a half-life of 7 days and is eliminated in extremely minute daily amounts so that no special precautions in the handling of urine and feces are necessary.

The tracing consists of *two main waves* sometimes connected by a plateau-like transitional zone. The first wave is sharp; it starts from 0.25 to 2 seconds after the injection and lasts from 3 to 4 seconds. It is due to penetration of the drug into the *right heart* and therefore it is called *R wave*. The second wave is more rounded and may be lower; it starts 5 to 7 seconds after the injection and lasts 5 to 7 seconds. It is due to penetration of the drug into the *left heart* and therefore it is called *L wave*. Return of the tracing to norm indicates that all the blood containing the isotope has left the heart.

The method may be used for the determination of residual blood within the heart. It may give interesting data in heart failure, chronic cor pulmonale, coronary heart disease, congenital shunts, adhesive pericarditis, and obstructions to the venae cavae. Slower passage of blood to or through one of the ventricles is revealed. Controversial problems concerning right and left heart failure may be solved by the use of this technique.

Determination of Cardiac Output and of the Blood Gases

CARDIAC OUTPUT

Knowledge of the *oxygen consumption* per minute and of the *rate* of oxygen yielded by a definite amount of blood to the tissues can be used for calculating the amount of blood which is necessary in order to deliver this oxygen (121). The first is determined by measuring the amount of oxygen taken from the air in 1 minute; the second, by the difference between the volumes per cent of oxygen in the mixed venous blood and in the arterial blood. Mixed venous blood can be withdrawn in man from the pulmonary artery during right heart catheterization (page 157) while arterial blood can be obtained by puncture of the brachial or femoral artery. Thus it is possible to use this *direct method* in man.

Numerous *indirect methods* have also been developed for determination of oxygen content of the arterial and venous bloods (122). They are based upon the rate of absorption of a foreign gas through the lungs.

A technique for calculating cardiac output is based on a simple equation (125).[40] The most common procedure, however, is that of rebreathing a mixture of 15 per cent

---

[40] *Cardiac output* =

$$\frac{\text{O}_2 \text{ consumption (normal)} - \text{O}_2 \text{ consumption (rebreathing)}}{\text{Arterial O}_2 \text{ content (normal)} - \text{Arterial O}_2 \text{ content (rebreathing)}}$$

The procedure involves the determination of oxygen consumption and two analyses while breathing deeply from a bag of *nitrogen* for 20 to 30 seconds.

---

acetylene in air from a 3-liter bag until a homogeneous mixture is obtained in the lungs-bag system (122). Samples of this gas are analyzed for oxygen and nitrogen, or acetylene, at the beginning, after 5, and after 23 seconds, from the beginning of rebreathing. These methods are valuable but have certain limitations; their accuracy should not be overestimated. Other methods are based upon the intravenous injection of *a nondiffusible dye* (213), *radioactive material*, or *tagged red cells* (214), and the determination of their mean concentration in the blood of a peripheral artery.

The *cardiac output per minute* of an average normal individual under basal conditions (page 44) has been found to be 5.6 liters (124) with variations caused by the difference in size and weight of different individuals. Division of the figure of cardiac output by that of the heart rate per minute gives the figure of *systolic discharge*, which averages 84 cc. (page 43).

BLOOD GASES

Determination of the oxygen and carbon dioxide content of the arterial and venous blood may have different purposes in addition to that of evaluating cardiac output. Among them are:

a) *Determination of oxygen intake by the blood in the lungs.* It is reduced in pulmonary diseases and in heart failure.

b) *Evaluation of oxygen transportation to the tissues.* Slow circulation due to heart failure deprives the tissues of oxygen to a greater extent. This is known as "stagnation anoxemia."

c) *Recognition of blood mixture, caused by congenital shunts.* If blood passes from the lesser to the greater circulation, the arterial blood contains a lower percentage of oxygen (incomplete saturation).

Venous (right atrial) blood is aspirated through a thin catheter after its introduction through an arm vein into the right atrium (page 157). *Arterial blood* is obtained directly through puncture of one of the femoral arteries at the groin. Precautions should be taken that the blood sample does not come in contact with the air. One of them is the presence of paraffin oil in the syringe. The sample is transferred to a blood-gas apparatus (*Van Slyke or Scholander*). Then all oxygen is freed from the hemoglobin by the addition of potassium ferricyanide, or carbon dioxide is freed from combination by the addition of acid.

The oxygen capacity is evaluated by exposing the blood to air and determining the amount which it contains after saturation. The ratio of oxygen content to oxygen capacity per 100 cc. gives *the percentage saturation of the blood with oxygen*. If the oxygen capacity is 20 cc. and the arterial blood contains only 19 cc., there is a saturation of 95 per cent. If the venous blood contains 15 cc. of oxygen, its saturation is 75 per cent. In certain cases of congenital heart disease, the oxygen saturation has been found as low as 58 per cent (127, 128).

The following figures may be considered normal for the blood:

Oxygen capacity............ 19–22 vol. %
Arterial content............. 18–21 vol. (94–96%)
Venous content............. 10–16 vol. (60–85%)
pH (serum)................. 7.35–7.45

Blood Quantity and Circulation Time

BLOOD QUANTITY

Evaluation of the blood quantity can be determined in patients but the figure must be considered as actually referring to the *amount of circulating blood*. Present technique is far from accurate but, as the range of clinical variations is far wider than the margin of error, interesting results can be obtained. The methods are based on the intravenous injection of a colloidal dye which promptly diffuses into the plasma but is not absorbed by the tissues (120). If determination of the dye is then made in the venous blood at regular intervals, knowledge of the amount of circulating blood will be obtained. One of the most frequently used dyes is Evans blue.

The following technique is used (216).

a) A sample of blood is obtained and the plasma–corpuscles ratio is obtained by using the hematocrit.

b) Ten cc. of physiologic salt solution containing 25 mg. of Evans blue is injected into an antecubital vein.

c) At regular intervals, samples of blood are removed from the vein by means of another syringe. Sodium oxalate is mixed with these samples, then they are centrifuged. Comparison of the samples with known standards is made by means of a colorimeter. In normal individuals, mixing of the dye with the blood is complete in 9 minutes after the injection. In congestive failure, the mixing time may be prolonged to 15 minutes or more.

Normal individuals have an average of 77.5 grams of blood per kilogram. Accumulation of blood in the blood reservoirs and slow circulation of blood in capillary districts may change the amount of circulating blood in a remarkable way. Whenever the amount of the circulating blood is increased, the term *plethora* is used.

CIRCULATION TIME

Circulation time is studied by means of the intravenous injection of a chemical substance and by the study of its effect after it has passed through a certain part of the circulatory apparatus.

Three types of circulation time tests are used: a) arm-to-periphery, b) arm-to-lung, and c) lung-to-periphery.

Arm-to-periphery. Circulation of these chemicals includes part of the venous circulation, the heart, the pulmonary circulation, and part of the arterial circulation. The drugs used are studied through the effects they have on the carotid body or the respiratory center (sodium cyanide (129), papaverine (130a), aminophyllin (131)); on the color of the face (histamine (132)); on the taste (saccharine (133), decholin (134)); on the color of the pupil or oral mucosa with ultraviolet radiation (fluorescein (135)). In the author's opinion, the easiest test is the decholin test.

Arm-to-tongue time with Na dehydrocholate (decholin). The injection is made in a superficial vein of the forearm. Three cc. of a 20 per cent solution of decholin (134) are injected within 3 seconds. The arrival of the drug at the tongue is felt by the patient as a bitter taste. *The arm-to-tongue time* averages 15 seconds from the end of the injection.

Arm-to-lips time with fluorescein. This is to be preferred in infants and children. About 0.7 cc. per 5 kg. of body weight of a 5 per cent sodium fluorescein in 5 per cent sodium bicarbonate is rapidly injected into an antecubital vein. The room is darkened, and an ultraviolet lamp, concentrated on the lips, reveals greenish fluorescence as soon as the drug reaches the oral mucosa. Circulation time varies from 5 to 8.5 seconds (average 6.5) from birth to 2 years; from 5 to 12.5 seconds (average 8.5) from 2 to 13 years.

Arm-to-lung (136). This test is made by rapidly injecting one-third cc. of ether plus one-half cc. of physiologic saline solution. The arrival is marked by the subjective (patient) and objective (observer) perception of ether vapor in the breath of the patient. Arm-to-lung time is short, averaging from 4 to 8 seconds.

Lung-to-ear (215). The patient is made to inhale nitrogen. The decreased oxygen saturation of the arterial blood is revealed by an electrical oximeter applied to the ear-lobe. Average lung-to-ear time in the adult is 5.12 seconds.

The arm-to-periphery tests show a *shorter time* whenever there is a shunt between lesser and greater circulations with blood passing from the former to the latter; they show a *prolonged time* in congestive failure and may demonstrate either a slower pulmonary circulation (arm-to-lung) or a slower peripheral circulation (lung-to-ear).

Catheterization of the Heart

I. *Catheterization of the right heart.* The method is based on the introduction of a thin catheter into one of the superficial veins of the forearm; the catheter is carefully pushed through the venous system until it reaches the heart (123, 124, 183). A single lumen catheter (size 9 French) of woven silk and radio-opaque, with the orifice at the tip, is employed. It is 100 to 125 cm. in length, flexible but stiff enough to permit rotation without buckling. The patient lies on a fluoroscopic table with a spot-film device. Observations are intermittent and exposure of each part of the body is as brief as possible.

An incision is made through the skin over the median basilic vein of either side under local anaesthesia and in aseptic conditions. The catheter is threaded into the vein and advanced under fluoroscopic control until it reaches the various chambers of the heart.

The catheter is passed into the axillary vein, the superior cava and the right atrium; hence into the right ventricle, the main trunk of the pulmonary artery and either of its branches.

Clotting of blood in the catheter is prevented by a continuous perfusion of normal saline solution from a reservoir.

This method can be used for several studies which include pressure determinations, gas studies, and intracardiac electrocardiography.

A. Pressure measurements (cardiomanometry). Pressure of the cardiac chambers or vessels should be taken by means of graphic records. These are obtained through the use of a manometer (an electromanometer is preferable) and supply information also about phasic changes of pressure.

As venous spasm may prevent introduction of the catheter, it is advisable to push this as far as possible and to proceed to the various pressure and oxygen determinations during withdrawal. The following records can be taken: a) pulmonary capillary pressure, b) pulmonary artery pressure, c) right ventricular pressure, d) right atrial pressure, and e) superior caval pressure.

Pulmonary capillary tracing. This is essentially a venous tracing, the waves being due to changes of pressure transmitted from the pulmonary veins through the capillaries of the lungs. The tracing shows: a positive atrial wave, an early-systolic dip followed by a systolic collapse and an early-diastolic rise, and a mid-diastolic collapse. Differences between this tracing and that of the right atrium are: a higher mean pressure, a delay of the waves of about 0.08 seconds, and a deeper diastolic collapse. Mean pressure is about +3 mm. Hg.

Pulmonary artery tracing. It is a typical arterial tracing (page 108). The *anacrotic notch* is usually well visible. The *peak* is rounded (except if artefacts mar the record with superimposed vibrations). The *incisura* is deep. The *dicrotic wave* is well visible and followed by a few aftervibrations. Pressures vary between +20 to +25 (systolic) and +5 to +8 (diastolic).

Right ventricular tracing. The tracing presents the plateau-like configuration which is typical of intraventricular pressure tracings. A small positive wave indicates completion of filling by the atrial contraction. A rapid rise of the curve takes place during the tension period and terminates with a small notch which marks the *closure of the tricuspid valve.* After further rise, a second notch marks the *opening of the pulmonic valve.* During ejection, a steady line is typical (plateau-like curve) but a rounded contour may be observed. A sudden drop indicates the end of ejection. This is followed by two vibrations; the first marks the *closure of the pulmonic valve;* the second, the *opening of the tricuspid valve. Rapid filling* is usually not accompanied by rise in pressure proving that the right ventricle dilates gradually with the incoming blood. Pressures vary between +20 to +25 (systolic) and 0 (diastolic).

Right atrial tracing. The tracing presents a small positive wave in presystole due to atrial contraction. This is followed by a depression (systolic collapse) during ventricular contraction. The pressure rises during the last part of systole and reaches a peak

at the time of tricuspid valve opening. Following this, there is a slow fall of pressure until the following atrial contraction. The pressure varies between 0 and 3 mm. Hg with marked respiratory oscillations.

Various calculations can be made upon data supplied by cardiomanometry. The most important are: a) determination of mitral area, b) determination of mitral regurgitant area, and c) determination of regurgitant flow. These determinations involve complex mathematical formulas and their accuracy has not been established as yet. If confirmed, they would have a special importance in mitral valve lesions.

Two interesting refinements of technique are *catheterization of the renal veins* (188) or *the coronary sinus* (189).

B. Oximetry. Oximetry is done by evaluating chemically or photoelectrically the oxygen content and saturation of samples of blood drawn through the catheter. It is likely that, within a few years, oximetry will be done graphically and automatically from the tip of the catheter.

Evaluation of oxygen saturation supplies essential data for calculation of both the systemic and the pulmonary blood flow. The existence and size of a shunt can also be determined.

The *estimated systemic blood flow* (Qs) is equal to oxygen consumption in the tissues (i.e. oxygen intake in the lungs) divided by the difference between oxygen concentration in the aorta or peripheral artery[41] (Cao) and in the right atrium (Cra):

$$Qs = \frac{O_2}{Cao - Cra}.$$

The *estimated pulmonary flow* (Qpa) is equal to oxygen consumption divided by the difference between oxygen concentration of the blood of the left atrium (Cla)[42] and that

[41] The blood sample is usually drawn from the brachial, radial, or femoral artery.

[42] This is of course identical with that of a peripheral artery if there are no shunts between the ventricles or the large arteries.

of the blood in the pulmonary artery (Cpa):

$$Qpa = \frac{O_2}{Cla - Cpa}.$$

When the oxyhemoglobin concentration of the arterial blood is decreased far below the normal figure of 96 per cent, either right-to-left shunt or pulmonary pathology will be suspected.

In the study of persons without congenital heart disease, it has been found that, when multiple samples of blood are obtained from different chambers, the greatest normal variation in oxygen content between *superior vena cava* and *right atrium* is 2.3 volumes per cent; between right atrium and *right ventricle*, 1.8 volumes per cent; and between *right ventricle* and *pulmonary artery*, 0.5 volumes per cent. Therefore, in any given case, a rise of more than this amount indicates the entry of oxygenated blood into the chamber through a shunt. The existence of a moderate shunt, however, is compatible with a difference which is still within the above mentioned variations.

II. *Catheterization of the left heart or aorta. Catheterization of the human aorta* has been used for the study of aortic pressure pulses. The procedure seems to be no more hazardous than catheterization of the right heart. The contour of the pulse closely resembles that of the aortic pulse in the dog. Catheterization of the *left atrium* has been done in cases of atrial septal defect by passing the catheter through the defect. *Catheterization of the left ventricle* has been attempted in man, first in cases with aortic regurgitation, then in normal subjects. The technique is based on: isolation of the left brachial artery; introduction of the catheter into the artery; penetration of the catheter into the aortic arch, then, through the aortic valve, into the left ventricle. The *procedure is to be advised against on account of the dangers which it entails* (rupture of the aorta, occlusion of a coronary artery, rupture of an aortic leaflet, attacks of ventricular tachycardia or flutter). The tracing of pressure of the left ventricle is similar to that of the right ventricle in regard to the various details. The systolic pressure is similar to that of the aorta; the diastolic pressure is 0 in normal subjects.

Together with determination of oxygen content, measurement of pressure within the chambers of the right heart and the pulmonary vessels is of great importance in the diagnosis of congenital heart diseases. Low-speed tracings are used in order to obtain objective determinations of pressure. High-speed tracings are useful for the study of the various details of the curves and for solving problems of cardiac physiology in the normal and diseased heart. Important observations have been made in congestive failure, chronic cor pulmonale, tricuspid valve defects, and constrictive pericarditis. The shape of the tracing may have a diagnostic value in the last two types of disease.

Arterial Pressure (Blood Pressure)

DIRECT REGISTRATION

Direct registration of pressure in man is possible through puncture of either the brachial or the femoral artery and use of a manometer (139–143). Although this method is invaluable and may be used in particularly important cases, the procedure of inserting a cannula into the artery of a patient is a decided limitation from a clinical standpoint. Moreover, possible errors exist owing to spastic contraction of the artery, psychic factors, difficulty at times in ascertaining the exact zero level, and occasional errors in the transmission of pressure.

The *pressure of the pulmonary artery* can be recorded directly through a catheter passed along the arm veins into the heart (page 157). It can be recorded directly by means of a needle introduced through the anterior chest wall under x-ray control (187).

INDIRECT REGISTRATION

Indirect registration of pressure is the common clinical procedure and is based on either the oscillatory or the auscultatory method.

Oscillatory Method

The first practical oscillometer was the *Pachon* apparatus (144), still in common use, though somewhat modified. It is composed of an aneroid manometer which indicates the cuff pressure and of a constantly balanced, manometric capsule which indicates the magnitude of the arterial oscillations. The procedure is repeated step by step every 5 mm. Hg, as the cuff pressure is brought down from above systolic to below diastolic pressure.

As the cuff pressure is gradually lowered, the following phases occur (fig. 99).

a) Oscillations of small amplitude caused by the ram action of the pulsating stump of the occluded artery. These are called *supramaximal oscillations* and start far above systolic pressure.

b) An abrupt increase in amplitude of the oscillations marking the level of the *systolic pressure*.

c) A progressive increase in the amplitude of the oscillations until a maximum is reached, then a gradual decrease. This is called *the phase of maximal oscillations.*

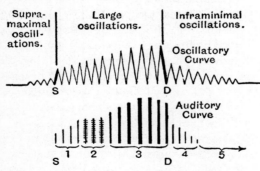

FIG. 99. Comparison of curves obtained by the use of the oscillatory and auditory methods for estimating arterial pressure. Curves to be read from left to right, showing vertical correspondences between the levels of S (systolic pressure) and D (diastolic pressure). The figures below the auditory curve refer to the five phases of sound: 1, clicks; 2, loud sounds with murmurs; 3, thuds; 4, muffled sounds; 5, no sound.

d) *An abrupt decrease* of the amplitude of the oscillations, marking *the diastolic pressure.*

e) Some small, terminal oscillations, progressively decreasing, called *the inframinimal oscillations.*

The level of diastolic pressure, first thought to coincide with the maximal oscillation, was later placed much lower, where a marked change in amplitude occurs (145–147).

A double-pouch cuff was later applied to the oscillometer (148), thereby suppressing the supramaximal oscillations and easing the reading of systolic pressure.

The data which can be secured by the use of the oscillometer are: the *systolic pressure*, the so-called *mean pressure*,[43] the diastolic pressure, and the oscillometric index.[44]

These data can be obtained over any limb, or section of a limb, and are very helpful in the study of the peripheral circulation. Cases with vascular disease, coarctation of the aorta, auscultatory gap (page 252), or low intensity of the arterial sounds, especially indicate the use of the oscillometer.

Auscultatory Method

This is based on the original apparatus of *Riva-Rocci* and on the *Korotkow method* (152). A pneumatic cuff is applied around the arm and a stethoscope is placed over the brachial artery below the cuff. Auscultation of the artery is then made during the decompression of the cuff from a high level (higher

[43] It was thought that *the level of the maximal oscillation would indicate the clinical mean pressure,* e. g. that continuous pressure which would be equivalent to the clinical rhythmic pulsation. In spite of many studies (149, 150), proof that this is obtained is still lacking. In most cases, a *conventional mean pressure,* placed midway between systolic and diastolic, is sufficient.

[44] *Oscillometric index* is the amplitude of the largest oscillation at any pressure level. The figures of the index are the conventional figures of the oscillometer's quadrant.

than the systolic pressure). Five distinct phases may be successively heard (fig. 99).

a) Faint, dull sounds.

b) Louder sounds, each followed by a hissing murmur.

c) Very loud and booming sounds, no longer followed by murmurs.

d) Muffled sounds or thuds.

d) Complete silence.

It was soon recognized that the *systolic pressure is marked by the first sound which appears*. On the contrary, differences of opinion have been expressed as to location of the diastolic pressure. Contradictory official statements are made (153, 217). The author's belief is that *the true level of diastolic pressure is where the arterial sounds become muffled*.

Auscultatory blood pressure can be evaluated also at the lower part of the leg by placing the stethoscope over the arteria dorsalis pedis. Still, the most common and the only comparatively accurate reading is obtained on the arm.

Among the possible causes of error which may lead to wrong readings, *the auscultatory gap* should be mentioned. This is caused by soundless arterial pulsations between the levels of systolic and diastolic pressures. This phenomenon, which is even more misleading when the gap is either at the upper or at the lower border (gap-open-upwards or gap-open-downwards), has been found in heart failure, hypertension, aortic stenosis, and, by the author, in severe bradycardia. *The auscultatory gap has been connected with the presence of a change of speed in the front of the pulse wave (anacrotism)* (149).

GRAPHIC REGISTRATION

Graphic registration of blood pressure can be accomplished routinely by means of a device which simultaneously registers both the pulse and the sounds of an artery (154). This graphic device eliminates the human element in the appreciation of the physiologic signs and gives an objective and permanent document.

The apparatus consists of:

a) A double-chambered pneumatic cuff (upper part = pressure chamber; lower part = registration chamber).

b) A manometer with valve and pump.

c) A differential crystal microphone.

d) The recording apparatus (electrophonocardiograph).

The lower chamber is inflated far below diastolic pressure (20 mm.); the upper chamber, on the other hand, is inflated above systolic, then gradually deflated. During deflation, a continuous tracing of both the arterial sounds and the arterial pulsations is recorded.

In the *pulse tracing*, the systolic pressure is revealed by the first sharp oscillation; the diastolic pressure is revealed by the *first wave which is undistorted during its negative phase*.

In the *sound tracing*, systolic pressure is revealed by the *first distinct sound* which occurs at the time of the first oscillation of the pulse tracing. The diastolic pressure is revealed by the *first muffled and small sound vibration* and corresponds to the above-mentioned change in the pulse tracing.

Graphic tracings can be obtained on any section of the limbs. They are especially valuable in cases with difficult evaluation of blood pressure and in vascular diseases.

The graphic method requires a few seconds for the registration. A continuous tracing of the blood pressure is still not obtainable in patients, despite many attempts in this direction.

SPECIAL TESTS

Among the different tests which have been described for the study of vascular reactivity, either in patients with abnormal blood pressures, or in those with peripheral vascular disease, the following two deserve special mention.

Cold Pressor Test (156)

After a rest of 20 to 60 minutes in a supine position and several determinations of blood pressure in one arm, the patient's hand on the opposite side is immersed in iced water. Further readings are made at the end of 30 and 60 seconds. Then the hand is removed from the water and more readings are made.

Normal people experience an average increase of about 12 mm. of systolic and 11 mm. of diastolic pressure with a maximum variation of 22 mm. Hg.

Hyperreactive people have a much greater increase, with an average of about 30 mm. systolic and 25 diastolic.

Patients with essential hypertension have an even greater reaction (page 501).

Static Blood Pressure Test (157)

After a preliminary period of rest in the supine position, the cuff of an oscillometer is applied to the forearm of the patient. A *first reading* is made with the forearm at the level of the right atrium (hand on a pillow). A *second reading* is made with the hand passively held as high as possible above the body (*raising test*). A *third reading* is made

with the hand passively hanging out of the bed, as far below the level of the body as possible (*lowering test*).

Normal people experience a decrease of about 25 mm. systolic and 25 mm. diastolic in the raising test and an increase of the same proportion in the lowering test. *Hypotensive patients* at times show a curious reaction consisting of marked increase of the pulse pressure in the raising test and marked reduction of the pulse pressure in the lowering test (page 521).

BLOOD PRESSURE IN VARIOUS DISTRICTS

Blood pressure is slightly lower at the forearm than at the arm; it is slightly higher at the leg than at the arm (fig. 100). This relationship varies in valvular defects, hypertension, hypotension, or aortic lesions.

Venous Pressure

Before the determination of venous pressure, the patient should rest in the recumbent position for 15 to 20 minutes. The vein which is used for the determination (usually one of

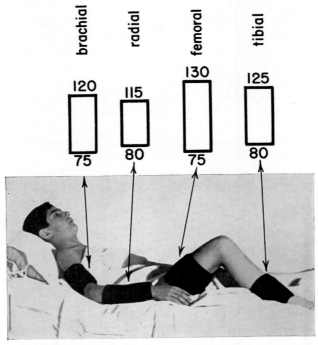

FIG. 100. Normal blood pressure in different arteries

the superficial veins of the forearm) should be on a level with the right atrium. Two methods can be used.

DIRECT METHOD

The apparatus consists of an 18-gauge needle connected by means of rubber tubing to a manometer and to a container of normal saline or citrate solution (158).

Both the zero point of the manometer and the arm vein are placed 10 cm. above the level of the bed. The needle is inserted into the vein after compressing its proximal end, and saline solution is permitted to enter the vessels. The point at which the fluid stops flowing represents the venous pressure level.

A quicker method measures the column of blood directly in an L-shaped glass manometer (159). Another modification is represented by the use of an aneroid manometer (160). In all these methods, readings are made in centimeters of water (actually saline or citrate solution).

INDIRECT METHOD

This method makes use of a small, metal air chamber, covered by a glass disc, which is fastened over a vein of the forearm or hand. The chamber is connected with a water manometer and a pump. Air is pumped in until the vein collapses and the pressure at that moment represents the venous pressure (163).

Normal venous pressure varies between 4 and 11 cm. of water by all methods, and shows different physiological and pathological variations (164).

Venous pressure is decreased in all veins in *shock* (page 520) and is increased in all veins in *congestive failure* (page 571), as well as in *constrictive pericarditis* (page 450). Normal pressure in the veins of the arms with elevated pressure in the veins of the legs is found in *ascitis, pregnancy, various surgical conditions of the abdomen,* the *inferior caval syndrome* (page 464), and certain cases of *constrictive pericarditis* (pages 454 and 458). Normal pressure in the veins of the legs with

elevated pressure in the veins of the arms is found in the *superior caval syndrome* (page 463), in certain *aneurysms of the aorta* (page 480), and in some cases of *constrictive pericarditis* (pages 454 and 458).

FUNCTIONAL TESTS

A test which can be employed to evaluate *the efficiency of the right heart,* is based on *the compression of the right upper quadrant of the abdomen.* In normal individuals, the temporary increase of venous return to the heart does not affect the venous pressure of the arm. In initial heart failure, a rise of 1 to 5 cm. of water may occur after 1 minute of compression (16).

The venous filling test. This functional test consists of the occlusion of the proximal section of the vein by means of the blood pressure cuff. The latter is inflated up to the level of diastolic pressure after introducing the needle into the vein. The duration of venous pressure increase and the level reached by the latter, are recorded (162). As any connection with the right heart is blocked, *the level* of venous pressure is dependent upon the work of the left ventricle. *The time* necessary for reaching it is dependent upon the freedom of flow through the small peripheral vessels. The normal time is from 90 to 115 seconds with a maximum of 3 minutes in elderly people (163). The level of venous pressure reached at the end of this time is between 6 and 7 cm. of water (163b).

The oscillations of venous pressure may be studied by means of *continuous graphic tracings* (186). These reveal rapid changes due to transmitted arterial pulsations; slower changes connected with respiration; and very slow undulations of the tracing caused by variations of venous tonus.

CAPILLARY PRESSURE AND RESISTANCE

Measurement of the capillary pressure can be made either by a direct or by an indirect method.

Direct Measurement

A micropipette controlled by a micro-manipulator is introduced into a capillary under microscopic observation. The pipette is filled with saline solution, flowing from a container, and is connected to a manometer. Pressure is applied until only a few red cells remain at the tip of the pipette. Normal readings are 32 mm. Hg in the arterial limb, 20 in the loop, and 12 in the venous limb (165a).

Indirect Measurement

Indirect measurement of the capillary pressure is obtained by compressing the capillary loops of the nail bed under microscopic observation. The pressure necessary for stopping the flow of blood in one of the capillaries is *the capillary pressure of that single loop*. The procedure consists of observing the nail bed under oblique light, after having applied cedar oil over the skin. An enlargement of 100 diameters is sufficient. The compression is obtained in different ways by various apparatus.

The *Kylin device* consists of a glass disc compressing the skin (166). The pressure of a chamber partly made of extensible rubber pushes the disc downwards on the nailbed. Visualization of the loops is obtained through the disc. Many technical objections have been raised against this device which gives inaccurate results (167).

Another apparatus has been described by the writer (167). It consists of a round metal chamber covered by a flat glass top. The finger is introduced into the chamber and a special device avoids air escape around its root. The compression is exerted by the air surrounding the finger, thereby avoiding any faulty transmission. A manometer, pump, and microscope complete the apparatus. The capillary pressure, as recorded by the indirect methods, varies between 15 and 25 mm. Hg.

CAPILLARY RESISTANCE

The original method for testing capillary resistance (168) has been slightly modified (169). A pneumatic cuff is applied to the arm and is successively inflated at 35, 50 and 65 mm. Hg. Each test is prolonged for 15 minutes. A circle, 6 cm. in diameter, is marked on the anterior surface of the elbow before the pressure is applied, and *petechial hemorrhages* are counted later in this area. Normal subjects show no hemorrhages with any of the three pressures. Occurrence of petechiae is an expression of reduced capillary resistance (increased capillary fragility), a condition which is frequently encountered in subacute bacterial endocarditis as well as in other diseases outside of the realm of cardiology.

Other Laboratory Methods

EXAMINATION OF THE BLOOD

Routine blood examination is important in many cases of heart disease.

Anemia may be the cause of many cardiovascular signs and symptoms. *Polycythemia* may be the cause of cyanosis and of different symptoms. The presence of *abnormal endothelial cells* has been described in subacute bacterial endocarditis. An *increased*

TABLE 14. *Hematologic values (172)*

DETERMINATION	MINIMUM QUANTITY REQUIRED	NORMAL VALUE
	cc.	
Bleeding time..........	—	Below 4½ min
Clotting time..........	10	5–8 min.
Sedimentation rate (two methods)...... {	4	Less than 0.40 mm./min.
	4	Less than 15 mm./hr.
Hematocrit (percentage volume of packed red cells)............	2	Male, 40–54%; female, 37–47%
Hemoglobin............	0.05	14–16 gm./10 cc.
Mean corpuscular volume..............	—	80–94 cu. μ
Mean corpuscular hemoglobin............	—	27–32 μg.
Mean corpuscular hemoglobin concentration.................	—	33–38%

number of white blood cells may be due to myocardial infarction; a reduced number contraindicates treatment with sulfa drugs. Further data will be given in the following chapters.

SEDIMENTATION RATE, SEROLOGY, BLOOD CULTURE, PROTHROMBIN LEVEL

The rate of settling of red blood cells in blood containing an anticoagulant gives a very valuable index of inflammation and often of infection.

No standard method for determining the erythrocyte sedimentation rate (ESR) has been adopted. In common use are the procedures of Westergren, Cutler, Rourke and Ernstene, and Wintrobe and Landsberg. Numerous others have been described, including several micromethods utilizing capil-

lary blood, and more elaborate systems using apparatus with photographic records of sedimentation rate. The Westergren value represents mm. of fall in 1 hour while the Rourke-Ernstene reading is expressed in mm. settled during the fastest minute.

Rourke-Ernstene method (190). Special tubes are used, having a capacity of 1.2 to 1.25 cc. and graduated in 2-mm. divisions. Three cc. of blood are drawn without venous stasis into a dry syringe and transferred immediately to a tube containing 2 mg. of heparin. The blood is allowed to stand for at least 15 minutes but not for more than 3 hours. When the test is ready to be started, the blood is again mixed by inverting the tube back and forth for 2 to 3 minutes; the sedimentation tube is filled to the zero mark and placed in the vertical position. The de-

TABLE 15. *Blood, plasma or serum values (172/191)*

DETERMINATION	MATERIAL ANALYZED	MINIMUM QUANTITY REQUIRED	NORMAL VALUE
		cc.	
Amino acids (CO$_2$ of carboxyl carbon)	Plasma	2	5–8 mg./100 cc.
Bilirubin (van den Bergh test)	Serum	2	Direct, 0.4 mg./100 cc.
Calcium	Serum	2	9–11 mg./100 cc.
Carbon dioxide (content)	Serum	0.5	26–28 mEq./liter
Chloride	Serum	0.5	560–630 mg./100 cc.
Cholesterol esters	Serum	0.5	65% of total cholesterol
Glucose	Blood	0.1	80–120 mg./100 cc. (fasting)
Magnesium	Serum	2	1.5–3 mEq./liter
Nonprotein nitrogen	Serum	0.5	25–35 mg./100 cc.
Urea nitrogen	Serum	1	10–15 mg./100 cc.
Uric acid	Serum	1	2–4 mg./100 cc.
Oxygen:			
Capacity	Blood	3	19–22 vol. %
Arterial content	Blood	3	18–21 vol. %
Arterial percentage saturation	—		94–96%
Venous content	Blood	3	10–16 vol. %
Venous percentage saturation	—		60–85%
pH (reaction)	Serum	0.2	7.35–7.45
Phosphorus, inorganic	Serum	0.2	2.5–4.5 mg./100 cc.
Potassium	Serum	3–4	4.1–5.7 mEq./liter
Protein:			
Total	Serum	0.5 (macro) 0.05 (micro)	6–8 gm./100 cc.
Albumin	Serum	0.5	3.5–5.5 gm./100 cc.
Globulin	Serum	0.5	1.5–3.0 gm./100 cc.
Sodium	Serum	0.5	136–145 mEq./liter

gree of settling is recorded on a graph at frequent intervals until two readings indicate a decreased rate of settling because of packing of the red cells. The sedimentation tube is then transferred to a centrifuge and spun at 3000 rpm for 30 minutes to obtain the hematocrit reading. The slope of the period of constant fall is calculated from the graph and is plotted against the hematocrit value on a reference chart prepared by the author. The final reading, corrected for abnormality in cell volume, is expressed in mm. settled in the fastest minute. *Normal range is from 0.05 to 0.40 mm.*; a slight increase is from 0.4 to 0.6; a moderate increase is from 0.6 to 1.0; a severe increase is from 2 to 2.5 mm.

A high sedimentation rate is constant in *rheumatic disease*. A high sedimentation rate is present after *myocardial infarction* (170) and it has been stated that the patients should not be allowed to arise until the sedimentation rate has returned to normal.

Serologic examinations for syphilis should be made in every case.

Blood cultures should be done repeatedly in patients with evidence of valvular defects and fever because bacterial endocarditis may be the cause of the increased temperature (page 206).

PROTHROMBIN DETERMINATION

Prothrombin time is an empiric interval representing the minimal time required for oxalated or citrated plasma to clot when provided with optimal amounts of thromboplastin and calcium. It is between 12 and 14 seconds in normal subjects.

Prothrombin concentration is the actual level of prothrombin in the plasma and is expressed in percentage (prothrombin per cent) of the value found in normal subjects. In the two-stage technique, this value is expressed in units, and averages 300 units per cc. in the normal plasma.

Prothrombin activity, also expressed in percentage of normal, is calculated by interpolation of the observed prothrombin time on a standardization curve.

Prothrombin determination is very important in any form of occlusive disease including coronary thrombosis and pulmonary infarction, and in the peripheral arterial and venous diseases. It is a basic requirement for correct use of anticoagulant therapy.

URINE

The urine should be collected and the total volume of the 24-hour period measured. This allows measurement of *total intake and output*. A rise of the output in cases of congestive failure under action of certain drugs is frequently noted.

The main data of urinalysis in a cardiac patient are: *specific gravity, albumin, sugar,* and *sediment.*

The specific gravity will be further studied after functional tests. Among them, the

TABLE 16. *Urine* (172)

DETERMINATION	MINIMUM QUANTITY REQUIRED	NORMAL VALUE
	cc.	
Albumine (quantitative)	10	0
Creatine	24-hr. sample	Less than 100 mg./24 hr.
Creatinine	24-hr. sample	15–25 mg./kg.
Diastase	2	Dilution of 1:4 to 1:16
Sugar, total (quantitative)	5	0
fermentable	1	0
fructose	1	0
lactose	6	0
Urobilinogen	10	Dilution of 1:4 to 1:30

TABLE 16a. *Renal-function tests* (172)

DETERMINATION	AMOUNT ADMINISTERED (I.V.)	MATERIAL ANALYZED	MINIMUM QUANTITY REQUIRED	NORMAL VALUE
	cc.		cc.	
Phenolsulfonphthalein	1	Urine	Total output	25% or more in the first 15 min.; 40% or more in 30 min.; 55% or more in 2 hr.
Urea clearance	0	Blood and urine	Blood, 1 cc.	75 to 125% of normal
			Urine, two 1-hr. samples	

concentration test and the *dilution test* are simple and useful (171).

The *concentration test* is done by putting the patient on a diet containing a minimum of fluid and excluding all fluids for 12 hours. The urine is collected every 2 hours; its amount and specific gravity are recorded.

The *dilution test* is made by giving the patient from 1200 to 1500 cc. of water early in the morning. The urine is collected every 2 hours and the same data recorded.

The specific gravity of the urine rises up to 1030–1035 in a normal person after the concentration test. It drops to 1003–1005 after the dilution test. The entire amount of fluid will be eliminated within 4 hours in a normal person.

In hypertensive patients, the routine urine examination will be supplemented by the separate analysis of the urine of each kidney, by an intravenous pyelogram, and by special functional tests.

SPUTUM

Examination of the sputum may be of interest in chronic pulmonary conditions which may cause *chronic cor pulmonale*.

BASAL METABOLISM

Determination of the basal metabolism is important: a) when the possibility of a "thyroid heart" is considered, b) in cases of thyroid insufficiency, c) in angina pectoris, d) in congestive failure, and e) in hypertension.

Thyroidectomy or radioactive iodine therapy have been advocated in the last three conditions, and a preliminary study of the BMR is imperative.

VITAL CAPACITY

The measurement of vital capacity in cardiac patients may be of interest. The test is done by using a common spirometer and its practicability has been enhanced by the appearance of small, portable apparatus.

The patient is instructed to take the fullest possible inspiration, to close his lips around the mouthpiece of the instrument, and to effect a forceful, complete expiration. The number of cubic centimeters of the expired air represents the vital capacity which varies from 2 to 5 liters. Special tables give the average expected figure on the basis of sex, height, and weight.

Reduction of vital capacity may be due to lack of training, weakness, or pulmonary conditions. When these factors are excluded, the reduction may be attributed to pulmonary congestion. Repeated tests are of greater value than a single test, as they help to follow the progress of cardiovascular insufficiency. When a sharp drop in vital capacity is recorded, it may be attributed to either pulmonary congestion or poor function of the diaphragm, on account of liver enlargement. However, only a marked enlargement of the liver inhibits the free movement of the diaphragm. Therefore, if no increase of the size of the liver is detected by palpation, and there are no apparent bronchial conditions, a sharp drop in vital capacity may be accepted as evidence of engorgement of the vessels of the lungs.

BIBLIOGRAPHY

1. EINTHOVEN, W. Arch. Néerl. Sciences Exactes et Natur., 1907, **12,** 401.
2. FRANK, O. Zeit. Biol., 1908, **50,** 281; and 1914, **64,** 125.
3. GERHARTZ, H. *Die Registrierung des Herzschalles.* Berlin, 1911.
4. OHM, R. *Venenpuls und Herzschallregistrierung.* Berlin, Hirschwald, 1914.
5. WIGGERS, C. J., AND DEAN, A. L. Am. J. Physiol., 1917, **42,** 476.
6. TRENDELENBURG, F. *Klaenge und Geraeusche. Methoden und Ergebnisse der Klangforschung.* Berlin, Springer, 1935.
7. RAPPAPORT, M. S., AND SPRAGUE, H. B. Am. Heart J., 1941, **21,** 257; and 1942, **23,** 591.
8. HOUSSAY, B. A. Presse Méd., 1936, **2** (1), 353.
9. ORIAS, O., AND BRAUN-MENÉNDEZ, E. *The Heart Sounds in Normal and Pathological Conditions.* New York, Oxford Univ. Press, 1939.
10. WOLFERTH, C. C. Heart Sounds. In *Cyclo-*

pedia of Medicine. Philadelphia, Davis, 1943, vol. 3.

Also: WOLFERTH, C. C., AND MARGOLIES, A. Heart Sounds: In Stroud's *Diagnosis and Treatment of Cardiovascular Disease.* Philadelphia, Davis, 1945, vol. 1.

11. TAQUINI, A. C., AND BRAUN-MENÉNDEZ, E. Rev. Soc. Arg. Biol., 1935, **11,** 410.

12. BRAUN-MENÉNDEZ, E., AND SOLARI, L. A. Rev. Soc. Arg. Biol., 1936, **12,** 112.

13. CAEIRO, A., AND ORIAS, O. Rev. Arg. Card., 1937, **4,** 71.

14. LUISADA, A. A. Arch. Ped., 1943, **60,** 498; and Bull. New England, Med. Center, 1945, **7,** 183.

15. LUISADA, A. A., AND MAUTNER, H. Exper. Med. & Surg., 1943, **1,** 282.

16. MELIK-GUELNASARIAN, E. A. Zeit. ges. exper. Med., 1932, **81,** 390.

17. ROUTIER, D., AND VAN BOGAERT, A. Arch. Mal. Coeur, 1934, **27,** 588.

18. MAREY, E. J. *Physiologie Médicale de la Circulation du Sang.* Paris, Delahaye, 1863. Also *La Méthode Graphique dans les Sciences Expérimentales.* Paris, Mason, 1885.

19. JAQUET: Muench. med. Woch., 1902; also Verh. Congr. inn. Med., 1901, **19,** 579.

20. FRANK, O., AND HESS, O. Verh. 25 Kongr. inn. Med., Vienna, April, 1908 (Wiesbaden, Bergmann, 1908).

21. MILLER, A., AND WHITE, P. D. Am. Heart. J., 1944, **21,** 504.

22. WEITZ, W. Deut. Arch. klin. Med., 1917, **124,** 134.

23. WEBER, A. Zeit. exper. Path. Ther., 1920, **21,** 252.

24. COSSIO, P. Rev. Arg. Cardiol., 1943, **10,** 145.

25. MACKENZIE, J. *The Study of the Pulse, Arterial Venous and Hepatic, and of the Movements of the Heart.* New York, Macmillan, 1902.

26. DRESSLER, W. *Die Brustwandpulsationen.* Vienna, Maudrich, 1933. Also Arch. Int. Med., 1937, **60,** 225, 437, 441, 654 and 663.

27. FUKUI, N. Wien. Arch. inn. Med., 1928, **15,** 349.

28. FRIEDREICH, N. Deut. Arch. klin. Med., 1865, **1,** 241.

29. POTAIN, P. C. E. Mem. Soc. Méd. Hôp., Paris, 1867, **4,** 3.

30. MACKENZIE, J. Am. J. M. Sci., 1907, **134,** 12.

31. WENCKEBACH, K. F. Zeit. klin. Med., 1899, **36,** 181.

32. OHM, R. Zeit. exp. Path. Ther., 1912, **11,** 531.

33. PARKINSON, J. Heart, 1915, **6,** 57.

34. GIBSON, A. G. Lancet, 1907, **2,** 1380.

35. HIRSCHFELDER, A. D. Am. J. M. Sci., 1906, **132,** 378.

36. CAEIRO, A. *El Pulso Venoso Normal.* Buenos Aires, S. de Amorrortu, 1942.

37. LEWIS, T. *The Mechanism and Graphic Registration of the Heart Beat.* London, Shaw and Sons, 1925.

38. WENCKEBACH, K. F., AND WINTERBERG, H. *Die Unregelmaessige Herztaetigkeit.* Leipzig, Engelmann, 1927.

39. RIHL, J. Zeit. exp. Path. Ther., 1909, **6,** 619.

40. EDENS, E. *Die Krankheiten des Herzens und der Gefaesse.* Berlin, Springer, 1929.

41. LUISADA, A. A. Rev. Arg. Cardiol., 1942, **9,** 169.

42. MACKENZIE, J. Am. J. M. Sci., 1907, **134,** 12.

43. VAQUEZ, H. *Maladies du Coeur.* Paris, Baillière, 1928.

44. HAY, J. *Graphic Methods in Heart Disease.* London, Oxford Univ. Press, 1921.

45. KAPFF, W. Deut. Arch. klin. Med., 1914, **113,** 459.

46. HITZENBERGER, K. Wien. Arch. inn. Med., 1923, **5,** 451; and 1924, **9,** 205.

47. DRESSLER, W. *Clinical Cardiology.* New York, Hoeber, 1942.

48. LUCIANI, L. *Fisiologia dell'Uomo.* Milan, S. E. L., 1923.

49. KRONECKER, H., AND MELTZER, S. J. Arch. f. ges. Phys., 1883, Suppl. Festgabe, 338.

50. JOACHIM, G. Berl. klin. Woch., 1907, **42,** 215.

51. FREDÉRICQ, L. Arch. de Biol., 1887, **7,** 230.

52. PACE, D. Rif. Med. (Naples), 1909, **25,** 533, 567 and 594.

53. VAQUEZ, H., CLERC, A., AND ESMEIN, C. Bull. Soc. Med. Hôp., 1909, **28,** 802.

54. LIAN, C. Arch. Mal. Coeur, 1909, **2,** 391.

55. WEBER, A. Muench. Med. Woch., 1913, **60** (II), 553.

56. WEITZ, W., AND SCHALL, L. Deut. Arch. klin. Med., 1919, **129,** 309.

57. BOECKELMAN, A. J. Erg. inn. Med., 1929, **36,** 91.

58. TAQUINI, A. C., *Exploración del Corazon por Via Esofágica.* Buenos Aires, El Ateneo, 1936.

59. LANDOIS. Physiologie des Menschen. Wien, 1880.

60. MOSSO, A. Arch. di Bizzozero, 1878, **2,** 4.

61. LUCIANI, L. Arch. di Bizzozero, 1877, **2,** 2.

62. GALVAGNI, E. Clin. Med. Ital., 1904, **43,** 436.

63. CHEESMANN. New York Herald, March 3, 1888.

64. FISCHER, G. Muench. med. Woch., 1903, **50,** 821.

65. LANG, G. Deut. Arch. klin. Med., 1912, **108,** 35.

66. KLEWITZ, F. Deut. Arch. klin. Med., 1918, **124,** 460.

67. Luisada, A. A. Min. Med. (Turin), 1928, **8**, 1139.
68. a) Holzloehner, E. Zeit. Biol., 1932, **92**, 293.
    b) Groedel, F. M. Exper. Med. & Surg., 1945, **3**, 361.
    c) Bence, A. E., Segura, R. G., and Lanari, A. An. Cáted. Pat., Clin. Tuberc. (Buenos Aires), 1945, **7**, 1.
69. Luisada, A. A. Am. Heart J., 1942, **23**, 676.
70. v. Frey, M., and Krehl, L. Arch. Anat., Phys. (Phys. sect.), 1890, 31.
    Also v. Frey, M. *Die Untersuchung des Pulses.* Berlin, 1891.
71. Schliep. Berl. klin. Woch., quoted by H. Straub: *Abderhalden Handb. biol. Arbeitsmeth.*, 1922, **5** (4), 367.
72. Frank, O., and Petter, J. Zeit. Biol., 1907, **49**, 70.
73. Wiggers, C. J. *Pressure Pulses in the Cardiovascular System.* New York, Longmans, Green and Co., 1928.
74. Pachon, V. Presse Méd., 1913, **21**, 229. Also Gallavardin, L. Presse Méd., 1922, **30**, 776.
75. Rappaport, M. B., and Luisada, A. A. J. Lab. & Clin. Med., 1944, **29**, 638.
76. Bramwell, C. In *The Principles and Practice of Cardiology* by Bramwell and King. London, Oxford Univ. Press, 1942.
77. Bramwell, C., Downing, A. C., and Hill, A. V. Heart, 1923, **10**, 289.
78. Starr, I., and co-workers. Am. J. Physiol., 1939, **127**, 1 and 1941, **134**, 403; also J. Clin. Investigation, 1940, **19**, 437; also Am. Heart J., 1943, **25**, 81.
79. Wiggers, C. J. *Physiology in Health and Disease.* 4th Ed. Philadelphia, Lea and Febiger, 1944.
80. Straub, H. Plethysmographie. In Abderhalden's *Handb. der Arbeitsmeth.*, 1922, **5** (4), 447.
81. Mosso, A. Arch. Ital. Biol., 1884, **5**, 130.
82. Mueller, O. Arch. Anat. Phys. (Phys. Section), 1904, Suppl., 203.
83. Soldati de, L., Cabanne, E. A., and Introzzi, A. S. Rev. Arg. Cardiol., 1941, **8**, 383.
84. Weber, E. Arch. Anat., Phys. (Phys. section), 1907, 293.
85. Einthoven, W. Arch. ges. Phys., 1895, **60**, 101; also Ann. Physik., 1903, **12**, 1059; and 1904, **14**, 182.
86. Asher, G., and Hoecker, F. Am. Heart. J., 1938, **16**, 51.
87. Likoff, W. B., Rappaport, M. B., and Levine, S. A. Am. Heart J., 1944, **28**, 98.
88. Macleod, A. G., Wilson, F. N., and Barker, P. S. Proc. Soc. Exper. Biol. & Med., 1930, **27**, 586.
89. Wilson, F. N. Am. Heart J., 1930, **5**, 599.
90. Wood and Woolferth. J. Clin. Investigation, 1932, **11**, 815.
91. Groedel, F. M. Deut. Ges. Kreislauff., 1933; also Cardiol. (Basel), 1940, **4**, 1.
92. Luisada, A. A. Cuore e Circ. (Rome), 1935, **19**, 77.
93. a) Lieberson, A., and Liberson, F. Proc. Exper. Biol. & Med., 1934, **31**, 441.
    b) Brown, W. H. Am. Heart J., 1936, **12**, 1.
94. Am. Heart Assoc. and Cardiac Soc. of Great Britain and Ireland. Am. Heart J., 1938, **15**, 107; and 1943, **25**, 535.
95. Wilson, F. N., Johnston, F. D., Macleod, A. G., and Barker, P. D. Am. Heart J., 1934, **9**, 447.
96. White, P. D. New England J. Med., 1944, **231**, 863.
97. Einthoven, W. Arch. ges. Phys., 1908, **122**, 517.
98. Einthoven, W., and co-workers: Arch. ges. Phys., 1913, **150**, 275.
99. American Heart Assoc. Am. Heart J., 1943, **25**, 528.
100. Katz, L. N. *Electrocardiography.* Philadelphia, Lea and Febiger, 1941.
101. Calabresi, M. *Elettrocardiografia Clinica.* Bologna, Cappelli, 1935.
102. Kreutzer, R. Rev. Arg. Card., 1944, **11**, 240.
103. a) Goldberger, E. Am. Heart J., 1945, **30**, 341.
    b) Wilson, F. N. Form of the Electrocardiogram. In Stroud's *Diagnosis and Treatment of Cardiovascular Disease.* Philadelphia, Davis Co., 1945, vol. I.
104. Pezzi, C. Cuore e Circ. (Rome), 1927, **11**, 381.
105. Assmann, H. *Die klinische Roentgendiagnostik der inneren Erkrankungen.* Leipzig, Vogel, 1934.
106. Crowden, G. P., and Harris, H. I. Brit. M. J., 1929, **1**, 439.
107. a) Hodges, F. J., and Eyster, J. A. E. Arch. Int. Med., 1926, **37**, 707.
    b) Ungerleider, H. E., and Gubner, R. Am. Heart J., 1942, **24**, 494. Also Ungerleider, H. E. In Stroud's *Cardiovascular Disease.* Philadelphia, Davis, 1945.
108. a) Groedel, F. M. *Die Roentgendiagnostik der Herz- und Gefaessezkrankungen.* Berlin, Meusser, 1912. Also *Die Roentgenuntersuchung des Herzens.* Muenchen, Lehmann, 1924.
    b) Moritz. Quoted by Assmann (105).

c) DIETLEN. *Herz und Gefaesse im Roent-genbild.* Leipzig, Barth, 1923.

109. COMEAU, W. J., AND WHITE, P. D. Am. J. Roentgenol. 1939, **17**, 158.

110. VAQUEZ, H., AND BORDET, E. *Le Coeur et l'Aorte.* Paris, Baillière, 1928.

111. a) STUMPF, P., WEBER, H. H., AND WELTZ, G. A. *Roentgenkymographische Bewe-gungslehre innerer Organe.* Leipzig, Thieme, 1936.

b) CIGNOLINI, P. *Roentgenchimografia Car-diaca e Regmografia.* Bologna, Cappelli, 1934.

112. a) HECKMANN, K. Erg. inn. Med., 1937, **52**, 569.

b) HENNY, G. C., AND BOONE, B. R. Am. J. Roentgen., 1945, **54**, 217. Also HENNY, G. C., BOONE, B. R., AND CHAMBERLAIN, W. E. Am. J. Roentgenol., 1947, **57**, 409.

c) MARCHAL, M. Ctr. Acad. Sciences, 1946, **222**, 973, and Arch. Mal. Coeur, 1946, **39**, 345.

d) LIAN C., AND MINOT, G. Arch. Mal. Coeur, 1946, **39**, 339.

113. a) LUISADA, A. A., FLEISCHNER, F. G., AND RAPPAPORT, M. B. Meet. Am. Heart Assoc., June 1947.

b) LUISADA, A. A., FLEISCHNER, F. G., AND RAPPAPORT, M. B. Am. Heart J., 1948, **35**, 336 and 348.

c) LUISADA, A. A., AND FLEISCHNER, F. G. Proc. Soc. Exper. Biol. & Med., 1948, **66**, 436.

d) FLEISCHNER, F. G., ROMANO, F. J., AND LUISADA, A. A. Proc. Soc. Exper. Biol. & Med., 1948, **67**, 535.

114. a) EGAS MONIS, LOPO DE CARVALHO, AND ALMEIDA LIMA. Presse Méd., 1931, **39**, 996.

b) CASTELLANOS A., PEREIRA, R., AND GARCIA, A. Presse Méd., 1938, **46**, 1474.

115. ROBB, G. P., AND STEINBERG, I. Ann. Int. Med., 1939, **13**, 12.

116. GRISHMAN, A., STEINBERG, M. F., AND SUSS-MAN, M. L. Am. Heart. J., 1941, **41**, 365.

117. CONDORELLI, L. Min. Med. (Turin), 1936, **27**, (1), 81.

118. CONDORELLI, L. Cardiol. (Basel), 1937, **1**, 26.

119. ROESLER, H. *Clinical Roentgenology of the Cardiovascular System.* Baltimore, Thomas, 1943.

120. KEITH, N. M., ROWNTREE, L. G., AND GERAGHTY, J. T., Arch. Int. Med., 1915, **16**, 547.

121. FICK. Sitzungsber. phys.-med. Ges. zu Wuerz-burg, 1870, 16.

122. GROLLMAN, A. *The Cardiac Output of Man in Health and Disease.* Baltimore, Thomas, 1932.

123. FORSMANN, W. Muench. med. Woch., 1931, **78**, 489.

124. a) COURNAND A., AND CO-WORKERS. Proc. Soc. Exper. Biol. & Med. 1941, **46**, 462; also J. Clin. Investigation, 1945, **24**, 106.

b) BURWELL, C. S., AND DEXTER, L. Mo. Conc. Cardiov. Dis., 1947, **16**, N. 4.

125. DONAL, J. A., JR. J. Clin. Investigation, 1937, **16**, 879.

126. BOCK, A. V., AND CO-WORKERS. J. Physiol., 1929, **68**, 277.

127. WHITE, P. D. *Heart Disease.* New York, Macmillan, 1944.

128. TALBOTT, J. H., AND CO-WORKERS. Am. Heart J., 1941, **22**, 754.

129. ROBB, G. F., AND WEISS, S. Am. Heart J., 1934, **9**, 2.

130. a) ELEK, S. R., AND SOLARZ, S. D. Am. Heart J., 1942, **24**, 821.

b) BERK, L., AND SAPEIKA, N. Am. Heart J., 1945, **30**, 365.

131. KOSTER, H., AND SARNOFF, S. J. J. Lab. Clin. Med., 1943, **28**, 812.

132. a) WEISS, S., ROBB, G. F., AND BLUMGART, H. L. Am. Heart J., 1929, **4**, 1.

b) BLUMGART, H. L., AND WEISS, S. J. Clin. Investigation, 1927, **4**, 15, 149, 173, 199, 399 and 555; and 1928, **5**, 343 and 379; and 1928, **6**, 103.

133. HITZIG, W. M., KING, J. T., AND FISHBERG, A. M. Arch. Int. Med., 1935, **55**, 112.

134. a) WINTERNITZ, M., DEUTSCH, J. AND BRULL, Z. Med. klin., 1931, **27**, 986.

b) GARGILL, S. C. New England J. Med., 1933, **209**, 1089.

135. LIAN, C., AND BARRAS, E. Bull. Mem. Soc. Hôp. Paris, 1930, **54**, 175 and 179.

136. HITZIG, W. M. Am. Heart J., 1935, **10**, 1080.

137. GROSS, D. Am. Heart J., 1945, **30**, 19.

138. BRUMLIK, J. Klinica Vrozenych poruch Srdce a cev (Prague) 1937, **5**, 109.

139. GALATÀ, G. Cuore e Circ. (Rome), 1925, **9**, 441.

140. POILLET, P., DODEL, P., AND BOUCOMONT, R. Bull. Acad. Med., 1932, **107**, N. 27.

141. VAN BOGAERT, A., BEERENS, J., LEQUIME, J., AND SAMAIN, L. Presse Med., 1934, **42**, 791.

142. GIROUX, R. Presse Méd., 1934, **42**, 1388.

143. DAMESHEK, W., AND LOMAN, J. Am. J. Physiol., 1932, **101**, 140.

144. PACHON, V. Presse Méd., 1913, **21**, 229.

145. MACWILLIAM, J. A., AND MELVIN, G. S. Heart, 1913–14, **5**, 153.

146. GALLAVARDIN, L. Presse méd., 1922, **30**, 776.

147. PACHON, V., AND FABRE, R. Bull. Mem. Soc. Biol., 1921, **84**, 871; and 1923, **89**, 951.

148. GALLAVARDIN, L. *La Tension Artérielle en Clinique.* Paris, Masson, 1923.

149. FABRE, P. *La Mécanique des Phenomènes Sphygmomanométriques*. Paris, Doin, 1925.

150. GLEY, P., AND GOMEZ, D. M. Presse Méd., 1931, **39**, 284; also J. Phys. Path. Gen., 1931, **29**, 38.

151. RIVA-ROCCI, S. Gazz. Med. di Torino (Turin), 1896, **47**, 981.

152. KOROTKOW, N. S. Mitt. klin. med. Akad. (St. Petersburg), 1905, **11**, 365; and Arch. Int. Med., 1910.

153. Am. Heart Assoc. and Cardiac Soc. Great Britain and Ireland: Am. Heart J., 1939, **18**, 95.

154. RAPPAPORT, M. B., AND LUISADA, A. A. J. Lab. & Clin. Med., 1944, **29**, 638.

155. a) VON RECKLINGHAUSEN, H. Zeit. klin. Med., 1930, **113**, 1, 91, 157, 433 and 663.
    b) BAZETT, H. C., AND LAPLACE, L. B. Am. J. Physiol., 1933, **103**, 321; and 1935, **112**, 182.

156. HINES, E. A., AND BROWN, G. E. Proc. Staff Meet. Mayo Clin., 1932, **7**, 332; and Am. Heart J., 1936, **11**, 1.

157. LUISADA, A. A. Cuore e Circ. (Rome), 1924, **8**, 291.

158. MORITZ, F., AND V. TABORA, D. Deut. Arch. klin. Med., 1910, **98**, 475.

159. TAYLOR, F. A., AND CO-WORKERS. Proc. Soc. Exper. Biol. & Med., 1930, **27**, 867.

160. CLAUDE, H., AND CO-WORKERS. Rev. Méd., 1914, **34**, 393.

161. OPPENHEIMER, B. S., AND HITZIG, W. M. Am. Heart J., 1936, **12**, 257.

162. GOVAERTS, A. Presse Méd., 1924, **32**, 161.

163. a) VILLARET, M., ST. GIRONS, F., AND JUSTIN-BESANÇON, L. *La Pression Veineuse Péripherique*. Paris, Masson, 1930.
    b) CASTELLOTTI, F. Cuore e Circ. (Rome), 1925, **9**, 112.

164. SCHLEITER, H. G. Venous Pressure. In STROUD's *Cardiovascular Disease*, Philadelphia, Davis, 1945, vol. II.

165. a) LANDIS, E. M. Heart, 1930, **15**, 209; and Physiol. Rev., 1934, **14**, 404.
    b) DE GRAFF, A. C., AND KOSSMANN, C. E. Capillary Circulation. In STROUD's *Cardiovascular Disease*. Philadelphia, Davis, 1945, vol. II.

166. KYLIN, E. Zentralbl. inn. Med., 1921, **42**, 785.

167. LUISADA, A. A. Cuore e Circ. (Rome), 1926, **10**, 55.

168. LEEDE, C. Muench. Med. Woch., 1911, **58**, 1673.

169. GOETHLIN, G. F. Skand. Arch. Phys., 1931, **61**, 225.

170. RABINOWITZ, M. A., AND CO-WORKERS. Am. Heart J., 1931, **7**, 52.

171. VOLHARD, F., AND FAHR, T. *Die Brightsche Nierenkrankheit*. Berlin, Springer, 1914.

172. Data reported from New England J. Med., 1946, **234**, 224. The source of the original data is quoted in the article.

173. a) MATTHES, K. Arch. exper. Path., Pharm., 1935, **179**, 698.
    b) HERTZMAN, A. B. Proc. Soc. Exper. Biol. & Med. 1937, **37**, 290; also Am. J. Physiol., 1938, **124**, 328.
    c) DILLON, J. B., AND HERTZMAN, A. B. Am. Heart J., 1941, **21**, 172.

174. a) LUISADA, A. A., RUBINO, A., AND CANELLA, C. Cardiol. (Basel), 1937, **1**, 280.
    b) LENÈGRE, J., AND MAURICE, P. Arch. Mal. Coeur, 1945, **38**, 298.
    c) HECHT, H. Am. Heart J., 1946, **32**, 39.

175. GOLDBERGER, E. *Unipolar Lead Electrocardiography*. Philadelphia, Lea and Febiger, 1947.

176. BURCH, G., AND WINSOR, T. *A Primer of Electrocardiography*. Philadelphia, Lea and Febiger, 1945.

177. a) WILSON, F. N., AND CO-WORKERS. Am. Heart J., 1934, **9**, 447; and 1944, **27**, 19. Also Trans. Assoc. Am. Phys., 1941, **61**, 258.
    b) KOSSMANN, C. E., AND JOHNSTON, F. D. Am. Heart J., 1935, **10**, 925.

178. MEYERS, G. B., AND KLEIN, H. A. Am. Heart J., 1948, **35**, 727.

179. HOLZMANN, M. *Klinische Elektrokardiographie*. Zuerich, Fretz and Wasmuth, 1945.

180. SODI PALLARES, D. *Nuevas Bases de Electrocardiografia*. 2nd Ed. Ed. del Inst. Nac. de Cardiol., 1949.

181. a) SPRAGUE, H. B., AND WHITE, P. D. J. Clin. Investigation, 1925, **1**, 389.
    b) BATTRO, A., AND BIDOGGIA, H. Am. Heart J., 1947, **33**, 604.

182. a) BERNSTEIN, P., AND MANN, H. Am. J. Obst. & Gynec., 1942, **43**, 21.
    b) BLONDHEIM, S. H. Am. Heart J., 1947, **34**, 35.

183. SOSMAN, M. C. Radiology, 1947, **48**, 441.

184. LUISADA, A. A., MENDOZA, F., AND ALIMURUNG, M. M. Brit. Heart J., 1949, **11**, 41.

185. LUISADA, A. A., ROMANO, F. J., AND TORRE, J. M. Proc. Soc. Exper. Biol. & Med., 1948, **3**, 308.

186. JANDOLO, C., AND DE RYSKY, C. Cuore e Circ. (Rome), 1945, **29**, 97.

187. VACAREZZA, R. F., LANARI, A., AND ALBERTI, V. A. J. Rev. Arg. Cardiol., 1946, **13**, 205.

188. DEXTER, L. Radiology, 1947, **48**, 451.

189. BING, R. J., AND CO-WORKERS. Proc. Soc. Exper. Biol. & Med., 1947, **66**, 239.

190. ROURKE, M. D., AND ERNSTENE, A. C. J. Clin. Investigation, 1930, **8**, 545.

191. GOTTLIEB, J., AND CHAPIN, M. J. Maine M. A., 1942, **33**, 10.

192. LUISADA, A. A., HANTMAN, H., AND WEISZ, L. Cardiol. (Basel), 1944, **8**, 63.

193. DUKES, H. H. *The Physiology of Domestic Animals*. 6th Ed. Ithaca, Comstock Publ. Co., 1947.

194. LUISADA, A. A., ALIMURUNG, M. R., AND LEWIS, L. Am. J. Physiol., 1952, **168**, 226.

195. COUNIHAN, T., MESSER, A. L., RAPPAPORT, M. B., AND SPRAGUE, H. B. Circ., 1951, **3**, 730.

196. CALO, A. Tunisie Méd., 1950, N. 4.

197. LUISADA, A. A. Acta Med. Scand., 1952, **142** (Suppl. 266), 685.

198. WELLS, B. G., RAPPAPORT, M. B., AND SPRAGUE, H. B. Am. Heart J., 1949, **37**, 586.

199. LUISADA, A. A., AND MONTES, P. Ann. Int. Med., 1950, **33**, 56.

200. LUISADA, A. A. *The Heart Beat. The Graphic Methods in the Diagnosis of Cardiovascular Diseases*. New York, P. Hoeber, 1953.

201. LUISADA, A. A., AND MAGRI, G. Am. Heart J., 1952, **44**, 545.

202. JOHNSTON, F. D., AND OVERY, D. C., Circ., 1951, **3**, 579.

203. HAMILTON, W. F., AND DOW, P. Am. J. Physiol., 1939, **125**, 48 & 60.

204. HERTZMAN, A. B., AND DILLON, J. B. Am. Heart J., 1940, **20**, 750; and Am. J. Physiol., 1947, **150**, 122.

205. NICKERSON, J. L. Federation Proc., 1945, **4**, 201.

206. DOCK, W. AND TAUBMAN, F. Am. J. Med., 1949, **7**, 751.

207. LUISADA, A. A., AND CONTRO, S. Acta Card., 1951, **6**, 847.

208. DILLON, J. B., AND HERTZMAN, A. B. Am. Heart J., 1941, **21**, 172.

209. LEVY, R. L., WILLIAMS, N. E., BRUEN, H. G., AND CARR, H. A. Am. Heart J., 1941, **21**, 634.

210. MASTER, A. M., Ann. Int. Med., 1950, **32**, 842.

211. CONTRO, S., HARING, O. M., AND GOLDSTEIN, W. Circ., 1952, **6**, 250.

212. RAPPAPORT, M. B., WILLIAMS, C. AND WHITE, P. D. Am. Heart J., 1949, **37**, 892.

213. HAMILTON, W. F., AND CO-WORKERS. Am. J. Physiol., 1931/1932, **99**, 534; and 1948, **153**, 309.

214. NYLIN, G. Am. Heart J., 1949, **37**, 543.

215. CALLEBAUT, J., LEQUIME, J., AND DENOLIN, H. Acta Card. (Brussels), 1950, **5**, 137.

216. GREGERSEN, M. J. Lab. & Clin. Med., 1944, **29**, 1266.

217. Recommendations of Am. Heart Assoc. J.A.M.A., 1951, **147**, 632.

218. a) PRINZMETAL, M. AND CO-WORKERS. Science, 1948, **108**, 340.
    b) PRINZMETAL, M. AND CO-WORKERS. J.A.M.A., 1949, **139**, 617.

219. LUISADA, A. A., GOLDFARB, A. R., MAGRI, G., AND SAFFIAN, R. Science, 1953, **117**, 299.

220. DOTTER, CH. T., AND STEINBERG, I. *Angiocardiography*. New York, Hoeber, 1951.

221. GRANT, R. P., AND ESTES, E. H. *Spatial Vector Cardiography*. New York, Blakiston, 1951.

CHAPTER 6

Causes of Cardiovascular Diseases—Modes of Origin of Cardiovascular Disturbances

Causes of Cardiovascular Diseases

The etiology of diseases of the cardiovascular system is such an important subject that it deserves an exhaustive description. However, only a summary will be given in the following pages while each chapter will contain a paragraph devoted to discussion of specific etiology.

Abnormal circulation may result from the following possibilities:

1) It may be caused by a purely functional disorder, such as a sudden attack of rapid heart beat or a regurgitation due to dilatation of the mitral ring.

2) It may be caused by a functional disorder which is related to a structural lesion as the shortness of breath of a patient with a lesion of the aortic valve or the swelling of the legs of a patient with pericardial effusion.

There is also another possibility, namely:

3) The occurrence of a structural lesion which does not cause any sign or symptom.

This means that the physician should always bear in mind the double sequence of events and recognize both the abnormality in structure and the functional disorder.

Any cause of structural lesion or any cause of disturbed function may be at the basis of heart disease.

A structural lesion may be due to either an *abnormal development* during fetal life (congenital lesion) or soon after birth, or to an *acquired process* (acquired lesion). It may be caused by an acute, subacute, or chronic *inflammation*, or it may be due to a process of *atherosclerosis*.

Even though many possible causes of heart disease are known, the gradual disappearance of certain infections has reduced the main causes of heart disease to two: *rheumatic disease* and *arteriosclerosis*. The former originates myocardial, pericardial, and valvular lesions; the latter causes the great majority of the coronary lesions and of the cerebrovascular accidents, and possibly the majority of cases of hypertensive heart disease. For this reason, even though no etiological agent escapes accurate study, rheumatic and arteriosclerotic heart diseases are the object of concerted efforts for prevention and therapy.

According to official data, the cause of death in the United States in 1950 was as follows: cardiovascular disease 51.4 per cent; other causes 48.6 per cent. Cardiovascular disease included arteriosclerosis (47.5 per cent); myocardial degeneration (coronary heart disease) (9.4 per cent); vascular lesions affecting the central nervous system (20.9 per cent); hypertension (13.0 per cent); rheumatic heart disease (3.0 per cent); and various others (6.2 per cent).

At the same date, 9 million were estimated having cardiovascular-renal disease; 5 million, heart disease; and 4,600,000, hypertension.

A. RHEUMATIC DISEASE (RHEUMATIC FEVER) (page 189)

According to a widespread belief, rheumatic fever is a *collagen disease*. The concept of "collagen disease" is a departure from conventional thinking because it introduces the concept of "tissue disease" in contrast to that of "organ disease." This concept signifies that, in certain diseases, *the structural changes lie in the connective tissue and*

in the vascular walls of the entire body.
These diseases include rheumatic fever,
rheumatoid arthritis, lupus erythematosus,
scleroderma, Buerger's disease, polyarteritis
nodosa, and dermatomyositis. The structural changes of the connective tissue
include necrosis followed by proliferation
and fibrosis, and a variable degree of
vascular involvement. It is admitted that
"collagen diseases" represent a general
reaction of the mesenchymal tissues with
changes of the ground substance of the
connective tissue as a response to allergic,
toxic, or bacterial influence. If the various
stimuli set in motion definite correlated
processes, the final effect on the connective
tissue may be identical. It has been said
that the "alarm reaction" and the "adaptation syndrome" represent similar processes.
This is conceivable because all three groups
of steroid hormones of the adrenal cortex
exert a deep influence upon the ground
substance of the connective tissue, through
changes of membrane permeability or by a
direct action.

It should be kept in mind that, in the
causation of rheumatic fever, two major
factors are involved: a) *predisposition* to the
disease, which seems to be transmitted as a
recessive mendelian factor, and b) the
result of *an infection* with the hemolytic
streptococcus. The connection between
streptococcus and disease seems represented
by an allergic reaction; the predisposition
seems to consist of an inherited abnormal
sensitivity to a specific antigen, possibly
favored by hormonal unbalance (page 189).

Rheumatic disease is the most frequent
cause of lesions of the endocardium with
resulting deformity of the cardiac valves. It
also causes myocardial, pericardial, and
vascular lesions and, occasionally, serosal,
pulmonary, renal, and cerebral lesions
(page 190).

B. MICROBES AND OTHER ORGANISMS

Different bacteria may cause cardiac
lesions. If the heart is not previously
weakened by some process, only extremely
virulent germs are able to produce primary
heart disease. Among them, the *Streptococcus
hemolyticus* is the most frequent, followed by
the *Pneumococcus*, the *Meningococcus*, the
Gonococcus, different *Staphylococci*, and the
Typhoid bacillus. These germs may cause an
acute bacterial endocarditis or an *acute
myocardial* or *pericardial process*, resulting at
times in the formation of pus.

When, on the contrary, the bacteria are
less virulent, they may localize on the
cardiac structures only if they have been
previously damaged by another process. In
such cases, they cause a slow, progressive
syndrome, called *subacute bacterial endocarditis*. Localization on the myocardium or
pericardium is seen less frequently in such
cases of endocarditis. The most frequent
invader among the milder germs is the
Streptococcus viridans but a wide variety of
organisms may act in the same way, even
including *amebae*, *spirilli*, and *fungi* (page
206).

In many cases, the germs originate in
focal infections, traveling through the blood
stream to reach the heart. However, routine
interventions on the tonsils, the teeth, and
the appendix, have caused little change in
the frequency of both rheumatic heart
disease and bacterial infections. This should
advise caution concerning too radical ex-
tirpations as a preventive measure.

Syphilis was a common cause of cardiovascular lesions but its importance is
decreasing. The most frequent localization
of the *Treponema* is the ascending aorta,
with common extension to the aortic valves.
Aortitis, aortic aneurysm, aortic insufficiency, and lesions at the mouths of the
coronary arteries, are frequent (page 201).

Direct localization of the *tubercle bacillus*
on the heart and vessels is rare but possible.
Chronic pericarditis or polyserositis is, on
the other hand, relatively frequent. Repercussions on the heart of mediastino-peri-
cardial lesions and of chronic lesions of the
lungs due to tuberculosis, cause typical
clinical entities.

Among the *parasitic diseases*, those caused

by malaria, amebiasis, and the South American trypanosomiasis, should be mentioned.

C. ARTERIOSCLEROSIS

Arteriosclerosis is a common cause of heart disease. The most frequent localization is on the coronary arteries, resulting in different clinical pictures. However, lesions of the aorta and of the peripheral arteries may cause various cardiovascular pictures, and lesions of the renal arteries are believed to be an important factor in the so-called *essential hypertension*. Thus probably arteriosclerosis is the most common cause of cardiovascular disease.

For a long time, arteriosclerosis was considered as the disease of the aged. However, studies on the frequency of coronary heart disease have shown how frequently it is present in relatively young people. The part played by the metabolism of cholesterol is still incompletely known but is definitely preponderant (page 525).

D. HYPERTENSION

Hypertension is a cause of heart disease because its lasting effects may result in heart strain and finally in heart lesions. On the other hand, there may be a clinical syndrome causing important symptoms without the existence of hypertensive heart disease. Therefore, hypertension will be considered as a disease in itself and described as such (page 491).

The connections between heart and kidneys and the fact that high blood pressure, when prolonged, creates abnormal cardiac work and coronary flow, should be emphasized.

A counterpart of hypertension of the greater circulation is represented by hypertension of the lesser circulation which causes strain of the right ventricle (*cor pulmonale*) (page 507).

E. CONGENITAL HEART DISEASE

The great majority of congenital abnormalities of the heart and large vessels is due to a disturbance of development taking place in an early stage of intra-uterine life (14). The development of the cardiac septa and the torsion of the primitive cardiac tube take place between the 5th and the 8th week of development. Any interference with these processes alters the relationship between the different parts, so that serious deformities result. Some of the more common abnormalities are caused by *incomplete torsion*, preventing obliteration of the right aortic arch with closure of the left, or fusion of the right with the left (15).[45]

Heredity is important in some cases, as shown by the association of congenital heart disease with abnormality of various organs. However, the most common cause of congenital heart disease lies in the conditions surrounding the embryo (14); abnormal conditions may be caused by disease or by toxic or otherwise depressing conditions, acting on the mother during early pregnancy. Among them, *lues* may play a role (14) but *rubella* (German measles), acting between the 5th and 8th week of pregnancy, seems to have the greatest importance (26).

The possibility that viruses other than rubella may injure the fetus without killing it, is being considered. However, there is no proof of this fact, so far.

It should not be forgotten that some of the common congenital lesions are due to the fact that one or more changes, which normally occur at or after birth, do not take place (closure of the foramen ovale and of the ductus arteriosus).

F. DISORDERS OF NUTRITION—BLOOD DISEASES—ENDOCRINE DISORDERS

Nutritional deficiencies sometimes may cause heart disease. The most common is *vitamin B deficiency*, because this vitamin has an important part in the metabolism of the cardiac muscle.

Anemia may cause dilatation of the heart,

---

[45] This leads to conditions which more or less reproduce those existing in reptiles, where the persistence of the right aorta is normal.

relative insufficiency of the valves, coronary insufficiency, and even congestive failure.

Polycythemia is a frequent cause of vascular complications including coronary and cerebral thrombosis.

Among the endocrine disorders, the chief cause of heart disease is represented by *thyroid disturbances* (page 407). The importance of *hyperthyroidism* (*thyrotoxicosis*) is such that its possibility should be always kept in mind, whether or not other cardiac diseases are present.

Deficiency of the thyroid may also be a cause of heart disease, as shown by the enormous size of the heart in some cases of myxedema (page 408). As this tremendous enlargement is caused by improper muscle metabolism, a similarity between beriberi heart and myxedema heart has been advocated.

Diabetes is frequently associated with early arteriosclerosis, including coronary arteriosclerosis. The arterial lesion seems to be favored by the metabolic disorder, and is not specific. Repercussions of diabetes on cardiac metabolism are less known. Over 50 per cent of all diabetics die as a result of cardiovascular lesions (16).

Abnormal secretion of *epinephrine* is a possible cause of vascular disorders both when the secretion is increased (*adrenal tumors*) and when it is deficient (*Addison's disease*). In the latter case, a simultaneous cortical deficiency usually adds its effects to the deficiency of the adrenal medulla.

G. LESS FREQUENT CAUSES OF HEART DISEASE

These are represented by *tumors* of the heart, *parasites* of the heart, *trauma* to the heart, and *deformity of the thorax*.

H. LESIONS OF UNKNOWN ETIOLOGY

These may be at the basis of cardiac and vascular disorders. Among them, *von Gierke's disease*, affecting the myocardium, *endocardial fibrosis*, and *Buerger's disease*, affecting the peripheral vessels, are well known examples.

I. FUNCTIONAL DISTURBANCES

Cardiovascular diseases become apparent largely through functional disorders of the circulation.

In some cardiac patients, *the entire syndrome is purely functional.* Many cases having *premature beats* or *paroxysmal tachycardia* and most of those with *neurocirculatory asthenia* or *hypotension* have no recognizable cardiovascular lesions.

A second category of patients suffers from functional disorders, but these are connected with a lesion which at times may be only suspected, while, at other times it is obvious. Many patients, suffering from essential hypertension, angina pectoris, or dyspnea are in this group. The complaint is definitely connected with the anatomical lesion but the part played by the functional elements varies from case to case and may lead to quite different disorders, even if the lesions are equivalent.

It is appropriate to note that *an exact evaluation of the anatomical lesion is often impossible.* The data supplied by the x-ray are largely influenced by functional elements. Those supplied by the electrocardiograph are partly modified by functional elements and may be misleading. Those obtained by the pathologist are usually collected at a later date, when a progressive process has increased the severity of the lesion or even complicated the case. Any attempt to overestimate the anatomical lesions may be refuted by mentioning similar cases where an equivalent lesion was well tolerated and was recognized only at autopsy.

J. STRAIN AND STRESS

The part played by mental and physical strain and by severe effort cannot be discussed in general. In each clinical entity and in each case, these factors should be properly evaluated. Even if there is a tendency on the part of many patients to overemphasize the importance of strain in the causation of some disturbance, this possibility should not be dismissed too lightly. Numerous publications debate the importance of this element which has many legal and insurance aspects.

The value of the "stress syndrome" as a cause of cardiovascular disturbances has been repeatedly emphasized (29). Changes of the pituitary and cortico-adrenal functions are now recognized as important in several syndromes, from rheumatic fever (and in general the "collagen" diseases) to the syndrome of shock.

Mode of Origin of Some Cardio-Vascular Disturbances

HEART MURMURS

A heart murmur may be due either to lesion of one of the valves or to abnormalities in the size of the cardiac chambers, in the function of the myocardium, or in the composition of the blood (page 409). Each valve may present one of the two following abnormalities:

a) An imperfect closure of the leaflets (insufficiency, incompetence, regurgitation).

b) A narrowing (stenosis).

Both a-v valves and both semilunar valves may be considered together, as far as murmurs are concerned, because they open and close at the same time.

Insufficiency of the A-V Valves

These valves *close* at the beginning of systole and *open* after the end of this phase. If the leaflets do not close properly during systole, a backflow from the ventricle into the respective atrium takes place, and a murmur arises during this phase (*systolic murmur*). It is usually a *soft* murmur which starts soon after the 1st sound complex and gradually decreases in intensity (fig. 101) (*murmur in decrescendo*).

Insufficiency of the Aortic and Pulmonic Valves

These valves *close* at the end of systole and *open* again only at the beginning of the ejection period of the following cycle. If they do not close properly, regurgitation of blood from the artery into the ventricle occurs *during diastole*. The murmur produced is loud at the beginning of this phase and then gradually decreases. Therefore, there is a *soft, blowing, diastolic murmur*, having its

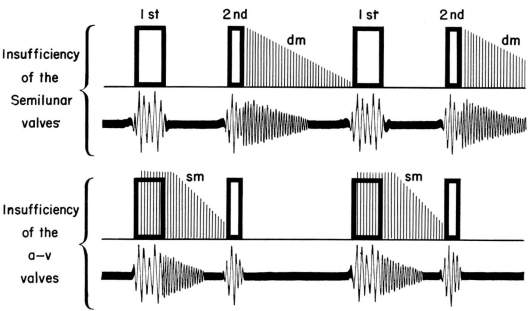

FIG. 101. Murmurs caused by valvular insufficiency. Above, the auditory impression. Below, the vibrations of the sound tracing. 1st, first sound; 2nd, second sound; dm, diastolic murmur; sm, systolic murmur.

maximum intensity immediately after the main vibration of the 2nd sound complex (fig. 101) (*murmur in decrescendo*).

Stenosis of the A-V Valves

The blood passes through the a-v valves during diastole (ventricular filling). Narrowing of one of these valvular openings causes a *diastolic murmur*. This murmur is rough and harsh as are all murmurs caused by stenosis. It is loud during the two phases of rapid filling of the ventricles (page 40), namely early-diastole and presystole (fig. 102). The latter will be even more apparent to the ear because it is more high-pitched and is prolonged by the first sound (*murmur in crescendo*).

Stenosis of the Aortic and Pulmonic Valves

The blood passes through these valves during the ejection period of ventricular systole. Therefore, if one of these openings is narrow, there is a *systolic murmur*. This is usually *harsh* and *rough* and reaches a maximum at the time of the peak of the pulse wave (fig. 102) (*diamond-shaped murmur* in the tracings).

The cause of the murmurs due to organic lesions has been debated, some authors advocating the role of whirlpools and others that of vibrations of solid structures. Studies of *Bondi* have given an experimental basis to the theory that the murmurs are due to turbulence of the blood. However, the possibility of vibrations of the solid structures cannot be absolutely excluded, especially in the case of severe valvular narrowing with a loud murmur.

A systolic murmur of one of the a-v valves may be caused by the following functional elements (fig. 103-I).

a) Abnormal modality of contraction of the ventricles. This may be caused by myocarditis or myocardial weakness.

b) Failure of valvular closure because of enlargement of the opening. This is present with severe dilatation of the ventricles (*relative insufficiency*).

c) Increased blood flow or rapid cardiac action. Turbulence of the blood and myocardial elements may both play a role.

d) Low viscosity of the blood, as in severe anemia.

A diastolic murmur of one of the a-v

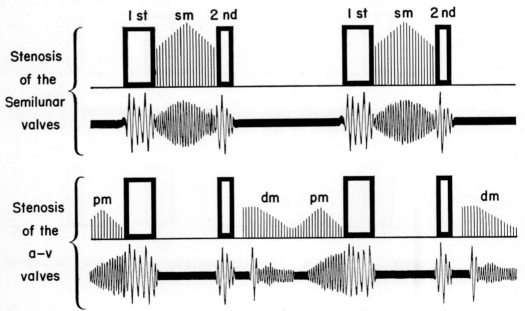

Fig. 102. Murmurs caused by valvular stenosis. Above, the auditory impression. Below, the vibrations of the sound tracing. pm, presystolic murmur; other symbols same as those in figure 101.

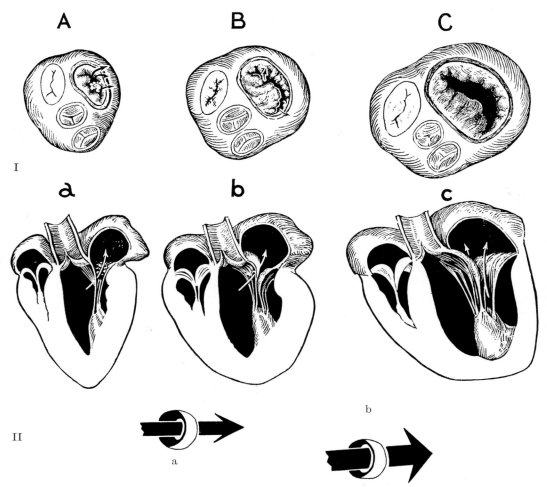

Fig. 103. I. Murmurs caused by structural and relative insufficiency of the mitral valve. A, organic insufficiency; B, relative insufficiency due to stretching of the papillary muscles; C, relative insufficiency due to dilatation of the ring. (From Hirschfelder's *Diseases of the Heart and Aorta*. Courtesy of The J. B. Lippincott Co.) II. Diagram to illustrate relation between size of valvular orifice (ring) and velocity or volume of blood flow (arrow) in creating cardiac murmurs. a, normal; b, increased flow. (From Bramwell and King.)

valves may be caused by the following functional elements:

a) Dilatation of one ventricle without proportional dilatation of the a-v opening (*relative stenosis*) (16) (fig. 104).

b) Presence of extra-sounds during diastole, simulating a diastolic rumble (page 237) (*pseudo-stenosis*).

A systolic murmur of one of the semilunar valves may be due to the following functional elements:

a) Dilatation of the vessel, not ac-companied by dilatation of either the opening or the ventricle (*relative stenosis*).

b) Stretching of the ring, causing a triangular opening (*functional stenosis, trigonoidation*) (17).

c) *Increased flow*, which is equivalent to a relative stenosis (fig. 103-II).

A diastolic murmur of either the aortic or the pulmonic valves may be due to the following functional causes:

a) Extreme dilatation of one of the ventricles.

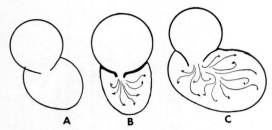

FIG. 104. A, normal mitral orifice; B, organic mitral stenosis—large left atrium, narrow mitral valve; C, "relative" or "functional" mitral stenosis—normal mitral valve, large left ventricle.

b) Lack of support due to incomplete rupture of the vessel (only in the aorta) (18).

c) High pressure in the artery.

CYANOSIS

Cyanosis is an abnormal blue color of the skin and mucous membranes. Often it is more marked over the lips, nose, earlobes, and nailbeds, or it may be present only in the extremities (*acrocyanosis*). *Cyanosis is due to an abnormally high amount of reduced hemoglobin in the capillary blood.*

It is necessary that the amount of reduced hemoglobin be increased at least 30 per cent above the normal level in order to have a visible cyanosis (*threshold of cyanosis*). Thus, a patient with a severe anemia (e.g. under 50 per cent hemoglobin), even though severely anoxemic has not enough reduced hemoglobin in the capillary beds to show cyanosis.[46]

Two mechanisms of cyanosis are possible, the central and the peripheral (19).

Central Cyanosis

This is caused by the fact that the arterial blood is poor in oxygen on account of insufficient oxygen intake in the lungs (fig. 105). It may be caused by:

a) *Pulmonary lesions of an obstructive type* (atelectasis, pneumonia, bronchial obstructions, emphysema, fibrosis).

[46] It has been said that four factors are involved in cyanosis: the *L* factor (lungs = oxygenation); the *D* factor (periphery = deoxygenation); the alpha factor (venoarterial shunt); and the *T* factor (total Hb content of blood).

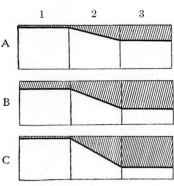

FIG. 105. Diagram of the percentage of reduced hemoglobin (shaded) and oxyhemoglobin in the blood in cases of cyanosis. 1, arteries; 2, capillaries; 3, veins; A, normal; B, central cyanosis with decreased oxygen content in the arterial blood; C, peripheral cyanosis with normal oxygen content in the arterial blood and greater loss in the capillaries. (From Cossio.)

b) *Low oxygen tension in the air* (high altitude flying, high mountains).

c) *Existence of a shunt* with passage of blood from the lesser to the greater circulation (congenital defects) or from a pulmonary artery to a pulmonary vein (congenital a-v fistula). At least 30 per cent of the blood must flow from the shunt into the arterial system in order to cause visible cyanosis in the absence of anemia.

d) *Small volume of the blood reaching the lungs* (pulmonic stenosis).

Peripheral Cyanosis

This is caused by slow circulation in the peripheral capillaries with the result that more oxygen is ceded by the blood to the tissues (fig. 105).

This may be due to: a) heart failure; b) venous obstruction (local cyanosis); c) improper function of the peripheral vessels (*acrocyanosis*); d) abnormal structure of the capillaries, often found in congenital heart disease; or e) abnormal composition of the blood, as in *polycythemia*.

Central cyanosis is a diffuse, universal color. If it is due to disturbed oxygen intake as in chronic cor pulmonale, oxygen administration may decrease the blue color.

If central cyanosis is due to a shunt, any increase of intrathoracic pressure, like that caused by crying, *increases* the amount of blood passing through the shunt and, therefore, the cyanosis.

In all these cases, the difference in the oxygen saturation of the arterial and venous blood (*arterio-venous difference*) is *normal*.

Peripheral cyanosis may be diffuse or localized. It is *diffuse* when due to heart failure, intra- or extracardiac obstruction, or abnormal development of the capillary network. It is *localized* when caused by venous obstruction (thrombophlebitis, venous compression) or by local disturbance of the peripheral circulation (cyanosis of the extremities or acrocyanosis). In peripheral cyanosis, the *hot bath test* and *elevation of the limb* relieve the cyanosis. In all these cases, the difference in the oxygen saturation of the arterial and venous blood (*arterio-venous difference*) is *increased*.

Mixed Cyanosis

Mixed cyanosis, caused by both central and peripheral elements, is not unusual. Patients with heart failure often have both a peripheral and a pulmonary slowing of the circulation. Thus, a central factor is added to the main peripheral factor. Patients with congenital malformations of the heart may also have malformations of the capillaries. Thus a peripheral factor is added to the main factors, which are central (shunt, often also pulmonic ischemia). If heart failure occurs in these patients, another factor is added (20).

EDEMA OF TISSUES AND EFFUSION OF SEROSAL CAVITIES

Edema in general is a serous infiltration of the interstitial tissue. When present in the subcutaneous tissue, it is called *subcutaneous edema*; when diffuse over the whole body, it is called *anasarca*.

Typical *cardiac edema* is present mainly in the *lower parts of the body* (*dependent edema*); in the legs, when the patient stands or sits; and over the sacrum and the back, when he lies down. The name *gravitational edema* is due to the apparent action of gravity in causing this type of edema. On the contrary, edema resulting from other causes, such as renal dysfunction, is less influenced by gravity and starts typically on the dorsal aspect of the hands and on the eyelids.

A renal patient, sooner or later, may have cardiac insufficiency; a cardiac patient, sooner or later, has renal and hepatic dysfunctions. For this reason, each category of patients has a definite type of edema at the beginning but often develops a mixed type later.

Initial cardiac edema is revealed by the fact that the finger, compressing the skin against a solid, bony plane (malleolus, shin) leaves a well defined depression (*pitting edema*). When the edema is recent, the skin is smooth and shiny; when the edema persists, the skin becomes dry and peels off. If it lasts a long time, the skin becomes thick and brown.

As previously stated (page 61), the passage of fluid through the capillary wall is influenced by both hydrostatic and osmotic pressures (fig. 105). Hydrostatic pressure favors filtration of fluid and is influenced by both arterial and venous pressure. Osmotic pressure is particularly dependent upon the content of blood proteins. As the hydrostatic pressure is higher at the arterial than at the venous end of the capillary and the osmotic pressure normally is constant, a double movement of water takes place under normal conditions. *Water leaves the capillary wall at the arterial end and reenters at the venous end* (fig. 105).

In *cardiac edema*, the venous pressure is higher than normal; the effect of gravity adds to it in the dependent parts, and the filtration pressure will be higher than the osmotic pressure, enhancing fluid escape through the capillary wall (fig. 106). In *renal edema*, the osmotic pressure becomes too low because of loss of albumin. There-

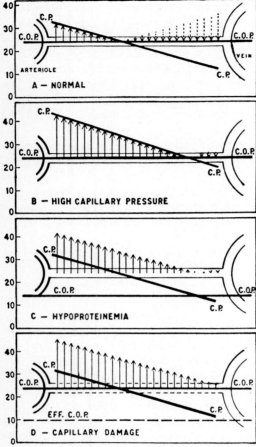

FIG. 106. Diagram illustrating filtration and absorption through the capillary wall in relation to capillary blood pressure (C.P.) and colloid osmotic pressure of the plasma proteins (C.O.P.). (The figures at the left are pressures in mm. Hg). a, Normal. In the anteriolar end of the capillary, where capillary pressure exceeds colloid osmotic pressure, fluid leaves the vessel (upward arrows). At the venous end, where the opposite conditions exist, fluid is drawn into the capillary (downward arrows). b, Increased filtration due to high capillary blood pressure. c, Increased filtration due to lowered colloid osmotic pressure. d, Increased filtration due to capillary damage. Loss of protein through the capillary wall then reduces the *effective* colloid osmotic pressure of the blood. (Courtesy of Dr. E. M. Landis.)

fore, fluid escapes through the capillary walls into the tissues (fig. 106).

The following list indicates the various factors leading to *edema* in cardiac patients (27) (fig. 106).

Elevated capillary pressure. Increased venous pressure. Increased blood volume. Increased intrapleural (intrathoracic) pressure.

Lowered colloid osmotic pressure. Loss of albumin (urine, ascites, etc.). Inadequate protein intake. Dietary restriction and impaired absorption. Impaired synthesis of plasma proteins. Anemia and hepatic damage (chronic cases). Increased blood volume.

Damage to capillary wall. Anoxemia from cyanosis or anemia.

Lymphatic obstruction. Increased venous pressure effects. Decreased physical activity and poor muscular tonus.

Capillary dilatation. Increased filtering surface.

Low tissue pressure. Predilection of certain tissues for early edema. Loss of weight and poor muscular tonus.

High salt (NaCl) intake. Increases edema if water is available.

High fluid intake. Increases edema if salt (sodium ion) is available.

Warm environment. Increases all types of edema.

Disturbed innervation. Increases edema of paralyzed extremities.

Miscellaneous. Vitamin deficiency? Hormonal abnormalities? Unknown factors.

Other diseases. Edema of mixed etiology in cardiac disease associated with liver disease, nephritis, or anemia.

CLUBFINGERS

Clubbing of the fingers, toes, and, occasionally, tip of the nose, is caused by swelling without any other apparent abnormality, and is often unnoticed by the patient. Clubbing of the fingers and toes is typical of *congenital heart disease* with cyanosis. However, it may be present in *chronic conditions of the lungs* (pulmonary abscess, bronchiectasis). Clubbing of the fingers is common also in *subacute bacterial endocarditis* and has been observed in chronic infections, not associated with heart disease or cyanosis. Congenital heart

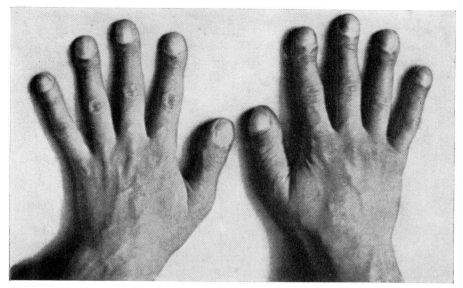

Fig. 107. Clubfingers in congenital heart disease

diseases and pulmonary lesions have one important factor in common: the type of cyanosis (central cyanosis). The other conditions, on the other hand, have the factor of chronic infection in common. Therefore, two different causes seem to be at the basis of this condition which is still somewhat mysterious.

Clubfingers are accompanied by no lesion of the bony structures, as shown by the x-ray; only the soft parts are enlarged while the nails are curved (*watch-glass nails*) (fig. 107).

The capillaries (possibly only the a-v anastomoses) of the soft parts are dilated, and a rapid circulation seems to be present in them (21). Abnormality of the lymphatic circulation is also probably present.

It should be emphasized that patients with acquired valvular defects having cyanosis do not present clubbing of the fingers.

DYSPNEA

The name *dyspnea* is applied to any form of augmented and labored breathing associated with unpleasant sensations. There is usually an increased respiratory rate and an abnormal ratio of inspiration to expiration.

Three main types of dyspnea exist

a) *Exertional dyspnea (effort dyspnea)* in which shortness of breath is caused by physical exercise.

b) *Continuous dyspnea*, which is present all the time.

c) *Paroxysmal dyspnea* in which a sudden attack of shortness of breath has no apparent connection with effort.

In the last two types, the shortness of breath is increased by the recumbent position and decreased by sitting or standing; therefore, the name *orthopnea*. On the contrary, dyspnea decreased by supine position occurs in cases with ball-valve thrombus or intracardiac pedunculated tumor, and may be observed in certain patients with deformity of the chest.

A particular type of exertional dyspnea may be observed in congenital heart diseases. Children with certain malformations of the heart (pulmonic or tricuspid stenosis, tetralogy of Fallot) crouch after effort in a *squatting position*, and breathe heavily (28). It is likely that such a position increases venous return and forces more blood through the lungs by compressing the abdominal viscera.

In some cardiac patients, a *periodic type of breathing* may occur (*Cheyne-Stokes' respiration*).

The following factors should be considered: a) engorgement of the pulmonary capillaries with decreased alveolar space and slower circulation, b) accumulation of carbon dioxide and lactic acid in the blood, c) increased venous pressure in the cerebral circulation, and d) reflexes.

Chemical determinations fail to detect any changes in the blood returning from the brain to the heart (22). Therefore a greater emphasis is given to reflex elements, due to stimuli arising in the lungs, as well as in the various cardiac and vascular receptors (24, 25).

These factors are analyzed in detail in chapters XXIX and XXX.

ENLARGEMENT OF THE HEART

Cardiac enlargement is a common and important sign of heart disease. However, heart disease may be present with little or no enlargement.

Whenever an increase in the work of the heart is required, *the heart dilates*. This physiological dilatation is demonstrated in a striking way by heart-lung preparations (page 30). If the increased work persists for a long time, the myofibrils undergo *hypertrophy* and a greater thickness of walls is present. A further increase in work may call for further dilatation.

However, dilatation of the heart may also occur without a greater demand of work, if lesions of the cardiac walls lead to reduced efficiency. Therefore two causes of dilatation are present: a) a greater demand on the heart, and b) a reduced efficiency.

The latter is typical of cardiac failure and was the only cause known to older physicians. *Coronary heart disease* and *myocarditis* are the two most common causes of reduced efficiency. It should be further noted that any extreme degree of hypertrophy gradually leads to reduced efficiency of the coronary vessels and, therefore, to coronary insufficiency. Prolonged coronary insufficiency frequently causes an increase of connective tissue (*myocardial fibrosis*) which contributes to the increase of thickness of the ventricular wall.

Not only dilatation, but also hypertrophy, may be *reversible*, if the cause of the change disappears.

When the greater demand is limited to only one chamber, dilatation and hypertrophy may be so limited. They may extend later to the other chambers but only to a lesser extent. A typical example of this occurs in certain valvular defects and in hypertension. Hypertension of the greater circulation places a greater demand on the left ventricle; hypertension of the lesser circulation, on the right.

A *sectional enlargement* may lead to predominant localization of coronary sclerosis and myocardial fibrosis in the wall of the affected chamber. It may cause changes of the electric axis and auscultatory signs (triple rhythm), limited to one part of the heart.

The classic division of hypertrophy into *concentric* and *eccentric* should be abandoned, since it has no real meaning. The greater or lesser dilatation found in the postmortem examination, largely depending on whether the heart stopped in systole or diastole, had much to do with the original division.

Decreased cardiac work may lead to *cardiac atrophy* if it is prolonged for years. This atrophy, which consists of decreased thickness of the ventricular walls and is accompanied by alterations of the myofibrils, has been described in constrictive pericarditis (chapter 20), chronic neoplasms, and chronic infections (29).

BIBLIOGRAPHY

1. McEwen, C. Rheumatic Heart Disease. In *Cyclopedia of Medicine*. Philadelphia, Davis, 1943. Also in *Stroud's Cardiovascular Disease*. Philadelphia, Davis, 1945.
2. Coburn, A. F. *The Factor of Infection in the*

Rheumatic State. Baltimore, The Williams & Wilkins Co., 1931.

3. a) Swift, H. F., and co-workers. J. A. M. A., 1928, **90,** 906.

   b) Swift, H. F. *Rheumatic Fever. Nelson Loose-Leaf Medicine.* New York, Nelson, 1941, vol. 1.

4. Schwentker, F. F., and Comploier, F. C. J. Exper. Med., 1939, **70,** 223.

5. Schweinburg and Warren. Personal communication. Unpublished studies.

6. Schlesinger, B., and co-workers. Lancet, 1935, **1,** 1145.

7. Eagles, G. H., and co-workers. Lancet, 1937, **2,** 421.

8. a) Birkhaug, K. E. J. Infectious Dis., 1928, **43,** 280.

   b) Copeman, W. S. C. Ann. Rheum. Dis., 1944, **4,** 37.

9. Ravenna, P. Ann. Rheum. Dis., 1939, **1,** 167; and 1940, **2,** 1: also Min. Med. (Turin), 1936 (I), 202.

10. Dionisi, A. *Anatomia Patologica della Malaria.* Rome, Ferri, 1927.

11. Gallenga. Quoted by Dionisi (10).

12. Zieman. Quoted by Dionisi (10).

13. Kern, F. Arch. Int. Med., 1945, **76,** 88.

14. Abbott, M. E., and Dawson, W. T. Internat. Clin., 1924, **4,** 155. Also *Nelson Loose-Leaf Medicine.* New York, Nelson, 1941, vol. iv.

15. Spitzer, A. *Ueber die Ursachen und den Mechanismus der Zweiteilung des Wirbeltierherzens.* Berlin, Springer, 1910.

16. White, P. D. *Heart Disease.* New York, Macmillan, 1944.

17. Chisholm, D. R. Am. Heart J., 1937, **13,** 362.

18. Perry, Th. M. Arch. Int. Med., 1942, **70,** 689.

19. Cossio, P. *Aparato Circulatorio.* Buenos Aires, El Ateneo, 1945.

20. Cossio, P., and Berconsky, G. Arch. Mal. Coeur, 1935, **28,** 19.

21. a) Mendlowitz, M. J. Clin. Investigation, 1941, **20,** 113.

   b) Mauer, E. F. Am. Heart J., 1947, **34,** 852.

22. Means, Davies and Meakins. Quoted by Wiggers (23).

23. Wiggers, C. J. *Physiology in Health and Disease.* Philadelphia, Lea and Febiger, 1944.

24. Harrison, W. G. *Failure of the Circulation.* Baltimore, The Williams & Wilkins Co., 1939.

25. Luisada, A. A. Medicine, 1941, **20,** 229.

26. a) Swan, C., and coworkers. Med. J. Australia, 1943, **2,** 201; 1944, **1,** 409; and 1946, **1,** 645. Also J. Obst. & Gynec. Brit. Emp., 1949, **56,** 591.

   b) Abel, S., and Van Dellen, T. R. J. A. M. A., 1949, **140,** 1210.

27. Stroud, W. D., and Vander Veer, J. B. Pennsylvania M. J., 1940, May.

28. Taussig, H. *Congenital Malformations of the Heart.* New York. The Commonwealth Fund, 1947.

29. Hellerstein, H. K., and Santiago-Stevenson, D. Circ., 1950, **1,** 93.

Chapter 7

Classification—Diagnosis

Classification

The classification of diseases is always difficult. As already pointed out, the so-called cardiovascular diseases are mere clinical entities, i.e. collections of signs and symptoms having a variable connection with cause, lesion, and functional disturbance.

Until the beginning of the century, classifications were based upon *structural lesions* (1). Then greater emphasis was placed on the *functional state* of the heart and vessels (2) and the importance of the lesions was underestimated.

A third phase developed when Cabot (3) properly emphasized the value and meaning of *cause* in the diagnosis and classification of heart diseases. The latter is most important because different lesions, frequently associated, may be placed together under a single heading (rheumatic heart disease, syphilitic heart disease, arteriosclerotic heart disease, hypertensive heart disease). The first etiological classification (3) was undoubtedly incomplete, but it was later supplemented by the addition of many other clinical pictures (4, 5).

It is now recognized that none of the three fundamental elements of diagnosis, *causation* (etiology), *lesion* (anatomical pathology), and *functional disorder* (physiopathology) can be omitted. Therefore, three separate classifications have been proposed (6, 7).

Since these classifications are well known, they are presented in an abridged form in order to ease reference:

I. ETIOLOGICAL CLASSIFICATION

1. *Congenital defects*
2. *Rheumatic disease*
3. *Bacterial infection*
   Acute
   Subacute
4. *Syphilitic disease*
5. *Parasitic disease*
6. *Thyroid disease*
   Hyperthyroidism (thyrotoxicosis)
   Hypothyroidism (myxedema)
7. *Hypertensive disease*
   Systemic (and hypertensive heart disease)
   Pulmonary (and cor pulmonale)
8. *Atherosclerotic disease*
   Coronary
   Valvular
   Vascular
9. *Toxic disease*
   Minerals
   Bacterial toxins
   Other organic toxins
10. *Neoplastic disease*
11. *Traumatic disease*
12. *Functional disease*
    Neurocirculatory asthenia and neurosis
    Arrhythmias

II. STRUCTURAL CLASSIFICATION

1. Displacement of the heart
   Congenital
   Acquired
2. Change in size
   Atrophy
   Hypertrophy
   Dilatation
3. Myocardial disease
   Congenital
   Inflammatory
   Fibrotic
   Infarction
4. Cardiac aneurysm
5. Cardiac rupture
6. Congenital anomalies of cardiac chambers or septa
7. Endocardial disease
   Congenital defects
   Inflammation
   Sclerosis
   Valvular deformities
8. Pericardial disease
   Congenital

Inflammation
Effusion
Adhesion
Calcification
Pneumopericardium, hemopericardium
Neoplasms
9. Vascular disease
Coronary
Aorta
Pulmonary artery
Peripheral arteries

III. FUNCTIONAL CLASSIFICATION

1. Disturbances of the heart rhythm and rate
   A. Changes of vago-sympathetic origin
      S-a tachycardia
      S-a bradycardia
      Sinus arrhythmia
      S-a standstill
      Wandering pacemaker
      Ventricular escape
      A-v nodal rhythm
   B. Disturbances of the pacemaking function
      Premature beats
      Paroxysmal tachycardia
      Atrial flutter
      Atrial fibrillation
      Obscure ectopic rhythms
      Ventricular fibrillation
   C. Disturbances of conduction
      Short P-R interval
      A-v block
      Idioventricular rhythm
      Intra-atrial block
      Intra-ventricular block
      Abnormal axis deviation
2. Faulty cardiac efficiency
   Congestive failure
   Pulsus alternans
   Neuro-circulatory asthenia
   Valvular incompetence
   Angina pectoris
   Adams-Stokes syndrome
3. Faulty vascular efficiency
   Hypertension
   Hypotension
   Vascular spasm
   Vascular dilatation

Discussion of the common cardiac and vascular diseases can be made on the basis of only one of the criteria of classification (cause, lesion, disturbance). However, this is impossible, because it would overlook many important aspects and many possible occurrences. Therefore, two possible courses are open:

1) To describe the cardiovascular diseases on an *etiological basis*, and then to consider them on a *structural basis*. This has been done in a well-known book of cardiology (*P. D. White* (4)).

2) To describe the cardiovascular diseases in a purely *clinical order*; cause, nature of the lesions, and disturbed function are listed in each case. This has been done in another well-known clinical book (*S. A. Levine* (8)).

A *clinical-anatomical line* will be followed in the present book. Practical considerations have led to the grouping of minor lesions, disturbances of function, or even signs in the same chapters where the most important syndromes have their place.

Further classifications may be useful for dividing the patients on the basis of their functional capacity and the restriction of their physical activity. The following was prepared by the New York Heart Association.

FUNCTIONAL CAPACITY OF CARDIAC PATIENTS

Class I. Patients with *no limitation of physical activity.*

Class II. Patients with *slight limitation of physical activity.* (On ordinary physical exertion, fatigue, palpitation, dyspnea or anginal pain, are experienced.)

Class III. Patients with *marked limitation of physical activity.* (The above symptoms are caused by less than ordinary activity.)

Class IV. Patients who are *unable to carry on any physical activity without discomfort.* (Symptoms of cardiac insufficiency, or cardiac pain are present at rest.)

THERAPEUTIC CLASSIFICATION OF CARDIAC PATIENTS

Class A. Patients whose physical activity need *not* be restricted.

Class B. Patients who should be advised against severe or competitive efforts.

Class C. Patients whose ordinary physical activity should be *moderately restricted,* and whose more strenuous habitual efforts should be discontinued.

Class D. Patients whose ordinary physical activity should be *markedly restricted*.
Class E. Patients with cardiac disease who should
be *at complete rest* (bed or chair).

POTENTIAL HEART DISEASE

Patients in whom no cardiac disease is
discovered, but whose course should be
followed by periodic examinations because
of the presence or history of an etiological
factor which might cause heart disease.

POSSIBLE HEART DISEASE

Patients with symptoms or signs referable
to the heart but in whom a diagnosis of
cardiac disease is uncertain.

Diagnosis

Diagnosis should include the following:

a) Recognition and evaluation of the
functional disturbance (functional diagnosis).

b) Recognition of the *structural lesion*, if
any (anatomical diagnosis).

c) Recognition of the *cause* of the
disturbance and of the lesion (etiological
diagnosis).

The order in which the three types of
diagnoses should be made is that outlined
above. It is self evident that knowledge of
the previous or present existence of a
disease does not imply cardiac damage and
that physical or technical data demonstrating such damage are required before
admitting it.

When the previous occurrence or the
existence of such a disease is unknown to the
patient, and clinical data (serology, hema-
tology, apparent lesions of other organs, or
exposure to infection) are lacking, etiological
diagnosis will be admitted only as a probability. On the other hand, in many cases,
only the functional disturbance is apparent.
Knowledge that this is not based on
structural lesions or impossibility to determine the latter may induce the physician
to leave the structural diagnosis in the
realm of possibility or probability.

BIBLIOGRAPHY

1. VAQUEZ, H. *Les Maladies du Coeur*. Paris, Baillière, 1924.
2. MacKENZIE. Quoted by WHITE (5).
3. CABOT, R. C. J. A. M. A., 1914, **63**, 1461.
4. WHITE, P. D., AND MYERS, M. M. J. A. M. A., 1921, **77**, 1414.
5. WHITE, P. D. *Heart Disease*. New York, Macmillan, 1944.
6. N. Y. Heart Assoc. *Nomenclature and Criteria for Diagnosis of Diseases of the Heart*. New York, Little and Ives, 1953.
7. SPRAGUE, H. B., AND WHITE, P. D. *Classification of Cardiovascular Diagnosis. In Modern Cyclopedia of Medicine*. Philadelphia, Davis, 1943.
8. LEVINE, S. A. *Clinical Heart Disease*. Philadelphia, Saunders, 1945.
9. VAQUEZ, H., AND DONZELOT, E. *Les Troubles du Rythme Cardiaque*. Paris, Baillière, 1926.
10. GALLAVARDIN, L. J. Med. Lyon, 1937, **18**, 489.

CHAPTER 8

Rheumatic Disease

Rheumatic Fever, Acute Rheumatism, Rheumatic Polyarthritis

Rheumatic disease is a chronic condition, characterized by active, often febrile, stages and quiescent or silent stages.

Cause

Rheumatic disease is the result of a complex process which takes place in certain predisposed individuals as a reaction to bacterial invasion. Thus, a complete understanding of its mechanism includes a double problem, that of the agent and that of the host.

Agent. It is now admitted that the only agent of rheumatic disease is the *Streptococcus hemolyticus beta, group A* (2). This agent is the common cause of the streptococcic sore throat, with or without scarlatiniform rash, and of erysipelas. It is frequently present in the throats of patients with upper respiratory infections or diphtheria.

The action of a specific *filterable virus*, possibly carried by the streptococcus, has been advocated (6–9) but no convincing evidence has been brought forward in its favor.

The host. While there is no proof that only certain individuals may become "rheumatic," evidence has been collected demonstrating the importance of *hereditary factors* (10). Predisposition to rheumatic disease seems to be transmitted as a recessive gene. Therefore, it is particularly important in the offspring of two "rheumatic" patients. The inherited tendency to rheumatic disease may be a hormonal defect that prevents metabolization of surplus globulin (48).

The reaction. During a streptococcal infection, antibody globulin forms in excessive amounts; circulating plasma volume increases, and large amounts of the globulin penetrate the tissues. Increase of serum globulin, fall of serum albumin, and instability of fibrinogen, seem to be the result of an *allergic reaction*, possibly of the hyperergic type (3–5). Among the various theories, one advocates development of auto-antibodies, as a result of denaturation of certain tissues caused by the toxins of the streptococcus. The allergic theory explains the usually observed *latent period* of 12–20 days between upper respiratory infection and onset of rheumatic disease.

Epidemiology. Rheumatic disease is one of the most widespread illnesses. It is difficult to evaluate its real extent on account of frequently silent onset, poor symptomatology (especially in children), and variability of symptoms in different countries.

Rheumatic disease is said to be more frequent in the cold and temperate regions than in the tropical. However, statistics based on the occurrence of rheumatic heart disease show that the difference is far less marked than expected. Therefore, it is possible that a large part of the difference is due to greater frequency of arthritis in the northern regions.

Atmospheric conditions, leading to sudden chilling, seem to favor the onset of the disease. Not only cold and humid weather but also variability of the temperature may be important as concurrent elements.

Rheumatic disease is more frequent in the crowded sections of large cities than in the country. Poorer families, living in damp houses, are more subject to it. This is probably due to the concurrence of various factors including increased possibility of transmission of the agent and modified resistance of the body (poor nourishment).

The importance of a *stress reaction* has been advocated (49). This was suggested by the frequency of rheumatic disease in children of school age, in young recruits of the Army, and under the stress of emergencies. It should be noted, however, that all these conditions increase the possible transmission of streptococcal infections. However, the importance of pituitary-adrenal elements in combating inflammation and allergy has been demonstrated. Therefore, exhaustion of these glands following repeated stress may contribute to the particular type of reaction that causes rheumatic disease.

Rheumatic disease is most common in adolescents and young adults. However, it may occur in young children and even in infants. It should be kept in mind that the younger the patient, the more difficult is the diagnosis, so that, apart from a few well-documented cases, knowledge of rheumatic fever in the first years of life is gained only through occasional autopsies or, indirectly, by finding well-established rheumatic heart disease in children between 3 and 5.

Rheumatic disease may initiate in mature or old individuals (50). This occurrence, even though not common, should not be considered as exceptional.

The influence of *focal infections*, such as tonsillitis, gingivitis and chronic sinusitis or otitis media, has been emphasized. There is no doubt that removal of the foci is sometimes followed by improvement in the signs of the disease. On the other hand, preventive removal of the tonsils, teeth, and appendix, has failed to change the frequency of rheumatic disease.

Lesions

Myocardium. The essential lesions, present in the interstitial tissue, are the *Aschoff bodies.* They are rounded, fusiform, or spindle-shaped nodules in close relation to the arterioles. They range in size from 0.1 to 0.8 mm. and are seldom visible to the unaided eye. They consist of: a) a central necrotic zone, containing fibrin; b) typical giant cells with one or more nuclei arranged in the center (not in a circle as in Langhans' cells); and c) a marginal ring of lymphocytes, plasma cells, and polymorphonuclear leucocytes (fig. 108).

Endocardium. Inflammation of the endocardium is almost always present. It is more frequent, but by no means exclusive, of the valves of the left heart. The typical lesion is represented by minute, cauliflower-like *vegetations*, 1 to 2 mm. in diameter, situated in a row along the line of closure of the valves. These vegetations, or *verrucae*, may cover the entire line of closure of the mitral valve (fig. 111) while the aortic and tricuspid valves are more often affected only in part (13). The vegetations begin very early and lead to formation of scar tissue. Lesions of the same type may be found in the parietal endocardium and on the chordae.

Gross, coarse lesions occur frequently *in the endocardium of the left atrium,* accompanied by Aschoff bodies (14, 15). The area of involvement may be small, or it may affect the entire surface of the atrium. After healing, the lesion becomes scarred and may become calcified.

Pericardium. Serofibrinous pericarditis is common, either in localized areas or diffuse. *Aschoff bodies* are frequently found in the pericardium. Formation of an *abundant effusion* is not unusual. *Adhesions* frequently develop during the healing stage.

Blood vessels. Specific lesions have been described in the *aorta* (16), *coronary arteries* (14), and *pulmonary artery* (17), as well as in the *peripheral arterioles.*[47] *Venous thrombosis* is rare.

Aschoff bodies often develop in the adventitia of the coronary arterioles. They probably last for weeks or even months

[47] Among the vascular lesions, those of the renal blood vessels, various other viscera (18), nose, and throat (19) deserve mention.

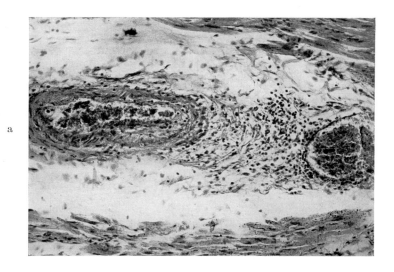

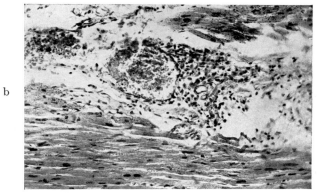

FIG. 108. *Aschoff's nodules* in a case of acute rheumatic myocarditis. a, Nodule in the initial phase near a vessel; perivascular edema; abundant cellular reaction. b, Nodule in a more advanced stage; giant cells.

and then are replaced by scar tissue. Cases where the bodies are located *in the specific tissue of the s-a node* or *in the conducting system* are not uncommon.

Pleurisy is frequent; *pneumonia* may occur. The *kidneys* present acute nephritis only in exceptional cases.

A *meningoencephalitis* with arteritis is present in some cases and explains the occurrence of *chorea*. A *peritonitis* with local predominance (*perihepatitis* or *perisplenitis*) is not rare (1a).

The *synovial membranes* of the affected joints are swollen, congested, and occasionally ecchymotic. There is periarticular edema. The fluid of the articular cavity is usually of moderate amount and turbid but not purulent. It contains a high percentage of albumin and a few fibrin flakes (11). Two types of response have been demonstrated: one is *exudative* and the other *proliferative* (1b). The latter results in the formation of *Aschoff bodies* in the periarticular structures.

Symptoms and Signs

The disease often starts with an upper respiratory infection, usually a tonsillitis. Children frequently have a history of repeated *nosebleeds*, *sore throats*, recurrent *sinusitis*, or earaches; more rarely, gastrointestinal disturbances (diarrhea, abdominal pain, nausea, vomiting). In some cases, a long history of *loss of weight, gastrointestinal symptoms*, and *malaise*, reveals that the disease had really started long before the apparent beginning.

It has to be emphasized that *rheumatic disease is a chronic condition whose symptoms are often mild or latent*. Acute and severe attacks may be superimposed upon this condition but statistical evidence shows that acute episodes may be absent.

Fever. The degree of fever is an index of the intensity and persistence of the disease. The *temperature* usually ranges between 102 and 104°F. (38.5 to 39.5°C.). High temperature is observed in some cases (105 to 108°F. or 40 to 42°C.), with delirium, stupor and convulsions, rapid pulse, and cyanosis. After the acute stage, the temperature may have an irregular, subfebrile course, sometimes of a long duration.

Pulse. The pulse rate is usually proportional to the fever. However, extreme pain raises the pulse rate and cardiac involvement is frequently accompanied by an abnormally high pulse rate or arrhythmia. A *rapid pulse* is evidence of a cardiac lesion, especially if the patient is in the subacute or chronic stage. While *tachycardia* is the most common occurrence, *bradycardia* or *severe respiratory arrhythmia*, may occur.

Sweating. Severe and profuse sweating is typical of rheumatic disease and is frequently followed by a diffuse rash (*sudamina*).

Arthritis. This is a frequent but not necessary manifestation. In children, joint involvement may be so mild or transitory as to be represented by the so-called *"growing pains"* and is frequently absent. The successive involvement of *many joints*, both large and small, is typical. Arthritis is usually accompanied by redness, swelling, tenderness, and increase in local temperature. Any slight movement and even the slightest touch then may cause intense pain.

Nodules. Subcutaneous nodules are characteristic of the disease. They vary from 1 mm. to 2 cm., are not tender, and are mainly localized in the surroundings of the joints.

Erythema. Various types of skin manifestations have been described but the most constant is *erythema marginatum*. This consists of a series of reddish macules, usually appearing on the trunk and more rarely on the limbs. The macules are from 5 to 10 mm. in diameter, then increase rapidly in size while their center becomes normal again. The evolution of a single area may take place within a few hours. These manifestations may appear months before or after an acute rheumatic attack. They indicate the existence of the rheumatic condition in its chronic form.

Petechiae have been described in some cases.

Kidneys. Albuminuria is rather frequent during the acute stages. Red cells and casts may be observed for 4 to 10 weeks after the onset of an acute attack, indicating congestion and cloudy swelling of the renal parenchyma.

HEART

Rheumatic carditis is the most common result of rheumatic disease. Diagnosis often centers upon recognition of carditis, especially in children.

The most important data are the following:

a) Evidence of cardiac enlargement (x-ray).

b) Auscultatory changes consisting of murmurs, triple rhythm, friction rubs (auscultation, phonocardiography).

c) Changes of rate and rhythm (pulse, ECG).

d) Evidence of involvement of the conducting bundles, irritability of the myocardium, and abnormal duration of ventricular systole (ECG).

e) Clinical data (precordial pain, congestive failure).

Evidence of cardiac enlargement is supplied by serial chest films. The oblique positions should be always taken in order to detect changes in the size of the left atrium.

The *auscultatory changes* are important; however, they may be misleading, especially in ambulatory cases, on the one hand suggesting an already established valvular damage, on the other hand frequently being accepted as *innocent* manifestations.

A *triple rhythm* is common. It is evidence of strain of either ventricle, more often the left, and is favored by tachycardia and by delayed a-v conduction. It may be of either the *ventricular* or the *summation* type (page 370).

The most common murmurs are *systolic* and found over the pulmonic area and the apex (51). The *pulmonic murmur* is usually a grade 2 or 3 systolic murmur which may be soft or harsh and even musical. The statement that a musical murmur is usually "innocent" (52) cannot be accepted by the author who observed that a musical murmur may appear and disappear in the course of rheumatic disease. This murmur may be explained with "relative stenosis" of the pulmonic valve on account of dilatation of the pulmonary artery (page 267). The latter may be connected with *arteritis* or may be due to increased pressure of the pulmonary circulation (left ventricular strain, mitral incompetence). The *apical murmur* is a grade 1 or 2 systolic murmur which is usually soft but may be musical (seagull cry). It is a "myocardial murmur" in the first few weeks or months of the disease and is due to the carditis which causes *insufficiency of the mitral valve* through dilatation of the mitral ring or edema of the papillary muscles.[48] The latter might explain the possible musical quality of the murmur. In later stages, a valvular lesion is established and a "valvular murmur" is present.

A *diastolic rumble* is not unusual. It may be misleading because it simulates the murmur of organic mitral stenosis. It is probably due to "relative stenosis" of the mitral valve because of left ventricular dilatation (page 237).

A *systolic* or *early-diastolic aortic murmur* may be heard. This is usually of late appearance being due to organic lesion of the aortic valve. It should be stated, however, that a *soft, early-diastolic, aortic murmur* may be heard during the acute stage and then may sharply decrease or even disappear. The mechanism of production of this murmur is still obscure.

Changes of the heart rate and rhythm. The most common feature is an increased heart rate due to *sinus tachycardia* (page 329). *Sinus bradycardia* (page 330) with a rate of 50 to 60, and *sinus arrhythmia* (page 332), may be observed in certain cases. *Premature beats* are not unusual and may reveal either a focal or a more diffuse myocardial lesion (page 346).

A lesion of the conducting bundles may lead to periodic irregularities (incomplete a-v block) or slow rate of the ventricles (complete a-v block) (page 355). *Atrial fibrillation* and *paroxysmal attacks of tachycardia* may occur, frequently in conjunction with congestive failure.

Pericarditis is not unusual. It starts with the auscultatory finding of *friction rubs* over the precordial area. This phase is frequently followed by a phase of *effusion* (page 444).

Congestive failure is due to active carditis. It implies a severe prognosis because the *myocardium* of these patients responds less readily to digitalis than that of chronic cardiac patients. However, children with severe failure and enlarged heart, whose outlook seems very poor, frequently present an amazing recovery. This is due to healing of the myocardial lesions and to the fact that the valvular lesions are usually slight, unless previous attacks have occurred.

BLOOD

A *leucocytosis* is the rule during the acute stages, with figures between 12,000 and

---

[48] The term *functional insufficiency* should be avoided because this is frequently considered as a harmless or "innocent" phenomenon.

20,000 per cmm. and occasionally higher figures (1a). Polymorphonuclears predominate. The count may range between 10,000 and 15,000 in the chronic stages, indicating the existence of a persistent infection.

A "secondary" anemia is typical of the rheumatic disease. The most frequent is *hypochromic anemia* with reduction of hemoglobin far outranging the decrease in the number of red cells.

The *rate of sedimentation* of the red blood cells is a valuable index of infection, even if not specific. From the normal figures of 7 (males) to 11 (females), *values of 50 to 80 may be reached*. The rate drops as soon as improvement occurs but it often remains between 20 and 40 for a long time.

The *mucin-clot prevention test* for measurement of streptococcal *hyaluronidase* in the blood serum shows high figures in rheumatic disease during the active stage. The mean titer was found 580 as compared to 30 to 36 in normal subjects (52). The *antistreptolysin titer* is also elevated: from a base line of 250 it may rise to above 500. However, children below 5 have a much lower base line. As this titer indicates streptococcal infection, it is of value only in cases with questionable diagnosis of rheumatic disease. Cardiac surgery has revealed the possibility of active carditis in cases with normal sedimentation rate and normal antistreptolysin titer.

ELECTROCARDIOGRAM

The *electrocardiogram* reveals the various changes of rate and rhythm. It may show a broadening of QRS and changes of S-T and T due to pericarditis. The most typical changes are:

a) A *prolongation of the P-R interval* (grade 1 a-v block) which is observed in about one-fifth of the cases. It should not be considered specific because it may take place in any type of myocarditis (22). It is due not only to anatomical lesions (edema or Aschoff bodies in the bundle of His) but also to *vagal stimulation* (23, 24). If the latter is not due to irritation of the vagus

center in the medulla (23) but to a reflex, it is likely to be the result of a diffuse myocardial involvement. Thus, the meaning of the prolonged P-R interval may change from that of a local to that of a diffuse lesion.

b) A *prolongation of the Q-T interval* which measures the duration of ventricular systole (page 124) (43). This is an extremely common occurrence having important diagnostic and prognostic meanings.

c) Various changes of the P and T waves may be observed in one or more leads through a serial study of the electrocardiograms. A change of the electric axis may be due to ventricular dilatation.

PHONOCARDIOGRAM

The sound tracing of patients with rheumatic disease supplies data which are of help for confirmation or clarification of the auscultatory findings and also often for establishing a correct diagnosis (51).

The most common findings are (fig. 109):

1) A *prolonged first sound* or a *systolic murmur* at the apex and midprecordium. This may be a murmur "in decrescendo" or may consist of a few regular vibrations of high pitch and small amplitude during the central phase of systole ("sea gull cry" type of murmur).

2) A *systolic pulmonic murmur* which is normally "diamond-shaped" and lower pitched than the apical murmur.

3) A *split second sound* over the pulmonic area.

4) Increased loudness of the *third sound* at the apex creating a triple rhythm (older terminology—"gallop rhythm") (p. 370).

5) A loud and low-pitched *diastolic rumble* over the midprecordium (only in severe carditis with cardiac enlargement).

APEX CARDIOGRAM (LOW FREQUENCY TRACING)

The cardiogram may be useful in order to ascertain the phase of the additional diastolic sounds and in the differentiation between loud third sound (ventricular gallop) and opening snap of the mitral valve. The latter has a more serious meaning because it indicates a well-established lesion of the mitral valve and probably an initial mitral stenosis.

ELECTROKYMOGRAM

Electrokymographic tracings of the left atrium present great interest (51). Some cases of rheumatic disease with a systolic murmur present a normal tracing; others present evidence of increased pressure and initial regurgitation; most of them, however, present a new plateau-like pattern indicating mitral regurgitation (p. 219). Thus, the EKY of the left atrium permits to evaluate the nature of the systolic murmur and the severity of mitral regurgitation.

Course

Rheumatic disease presents an *inactive stage* and *stages of activity*. The former is revealed only by the scars left by the inflammatory process, chiefly those causing valvular defects. Active rheumatic disease occurs either in the form of *repeated acute attacks* or as a *latent*, persistent activity of inflammation.

The classic description of the clinical picture is unsatisfactory because it applies only to the most apparent phases of the disease. Rheumatic disease has been divided into four stages (55): a) preparatory, b) pre-rheumatic, c) obvious rheumatic (classical or allergic), and d) quiescent.

The *preparatory phase* may start early in infancy and is revealed by irritability, fatigability, poor appetite, labile cardiac rate with rapid sleeping pulse, and a short systolic blowing murmur. Diagnosis is difficult and only a suspicion of rheumatic tendency can be advanced.

The *initial rheumatic phase* is characterized by more marked fatigability, occasional joint and muscle pains, emotional instability, nosebleeds, acute abdominal pain and recurrent upper respiratory infections. Low grade fever, tachycardia,

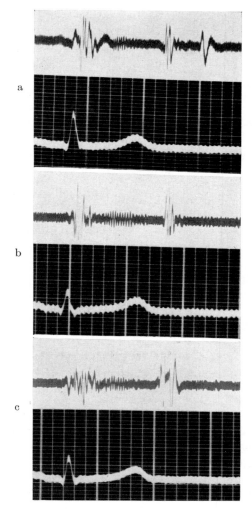

Fig. 109. Phonocardiograms in a boy of 8 with rheumatic disease. a, Apex: short systolic murmur, ventricular type of triple rhythm. b, Musical systolic murmur over third left interspace. c, Prolonged first sound, systolic murmur, and split second sound over pulmonic area.

slight changes of P-R, fullness of the pulmonary conus, cardiac murmurs, and high sedimentation rate are present. In some cases, this represents the only obvious stage, so that the subsequent evolution of the carditis, leading to typical valvular defects, may take place without more striking symptoms.

The *obvious rheumatic phase*, with the

classical symptomatology including poly-arthritis, chorea, and severe carditis, occurs only in a minority of cases. This stage is connected with exudative, allergic phenom-ena and has been considered as a "stress reaction". It has been stated that these obvious cases are becoming less frequent and that prophylaxis is able to prevent only this stage and not the evolutionary cardiac lesion. However, this pessimistic view is not justified.

Following the obvious phase, the patient continues with mild carditis or passes into a *quiescent stage.* If carditis continues, prognosis is less good, bacterial endocarditis is more frequent and less readily treated by antibiotics, and survival seldom lasts beyond 35 to 40 years of age. On the con-trary, if the quiescent stage is reached, prognosis is good and the lifespan is normal unless recurrences cause new damage and a new cycle.

Several clinical types have been recog-nized:

a) A *fulminating type,* which is rare and occurs almost exclusively in children (21). The disease is accompanied by high tem-perature, leucocytosis, and heart failure; death may occur after a few days of sick-ness.

b) *Chronic active type.* The evidence of activity decreases slowly without entirely disappearing. A subacute or chronic state exists for many months or even years. During this time, anemia, malaise, fatiga-bility, low-grade fever, and high sedimenta-tion rate, persist. Once the patient has recovered, a remarkable reduction in size of the heart takes place (fig. 110).

c) *Recurring type.* This is a rather fre-quent clinical form. The periods of activity occur every few years, separated by long periods of inactivity during which cardiac efficiency is good.

d) *Persistently inactive type.* One single attack starts the disease which, after a few months, becomes inactive. No further attacks occur. This type is rather rare.

e) *Latent type.* The acute attack is so mild that it is not recognized. Differential diag-nosis may be difficult but the subsequent course usually reveals the true nature of the disease. This type is frequent.

Sudden death may occur in a small per-centage of cases. The cause of the fatalities seems to be *acute allergic coronaritis* super-imposed upon a low-grade rheumatic car-ditis (41).

Diagnosis

The diagnosis is easy when the complete picture, with evidence of carditis and joint manifestations, is present. In some cases, there is knowledge of an old attack of rheumatic disease and it is known that rheumatic heart disease is present with typical valvular lesions. The diagnostic problem is then limited to ascertaining whether or not a new episode represents a *new attack* of the disease. In such cases, attention should be paid to: fever, increased sedimentation rate, changes of the electro-cardiogram, changes in the type of cardiac murmurs, antistreptolysin titer, and evi-dence of cardiac enlargement or apparent congestive failure. When present, they indicate activity of the disease and may be useful for diagnosis in doubtful cases.

All these data will also have great im-portance in cases with multiple acute joint lesions, where suspicion of *tubercular poly-arthritis type Poncet* is justified by other tubercular lesions.

The P-R interval has been repeatedly in-vestigated owing to its importance in the diagnosis of rheumatic heart disease. Inter-vals of 0.18″ to 0.24″ are not normal for children but have, on rare occasions, been recorded without any pathology (25). Therefore, a variation of the P-R interval in successive tracings is even more signifi-cant than one single finding. However, it should be known that spontaneous varia-tions in the length of P-R are occasionally seen in healthy children (25).

The increase in the duration of the Q-T

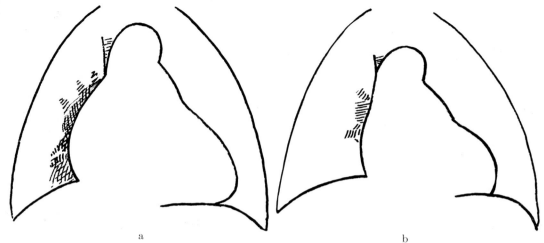

Fig. 110. Dilatation of the heart (a) and its subsequent reduction in size (b) during and after acute rheumatic disease. No pericarditis; murmurs present in a. (Inspired by originals of Paul D. White.)

interval, on the contrary, has a definite diagnostic importance.

The phonocardiogram and the electrokymogram of the left atrium have proven of help in the evaluation of cardiac murmurs (51).

The differential diagnosis between *rheumatic heart disease* and *bacterial endocarditis* is frequently necessary. It will be discussed later (page 000).

Hyperthyroidism, with its accompanying tachycardia, cardiac murmurs, and even low-grade fever, may simulate rheumatic heart disease. The lack of joint or skin manifestations, the absence of increased sedimentation rate and leucocytosis, and the electro- and phonocardiographic data are of help in excluding rheumatic disease.

Sickle-cell anemia, *leukemia*, and *undulant fever* sometimes lead to the erroneous diagnosis of rheumatic disease. Careful blood and serologic studies and the electro- and phonocardiographic data usually lead to the correct diagnosis.

Prognosis

The mortality of acute attacks of rheumatic disease in patients having undamaged hearts prior to the onset has been evaluated as between 1 and 4 per cent. About 20 to 30 per cent of rheumatic children either do not develop evidence of cardiac disease or develop signs which later disappear. Their prognosis is undoubtedly good.

Once rheumatic heart disease is apparent, the prognosis is definitely worse. However, it is impossible to say what the course will be after the first attack. The real entity of the lesions is usually apparent only after some years, when valvular defects are established.

It should be kept in mind that a certain percentage of rheumatic patients become *cardiac cripples* and may be obliged to lead a sedentary life.

Before accepting the existence of murmurs as evidence of already established valvular damage, it should be considered that they may be due to active carditis causing dilatation of the heart. Moreover, undeniable evidence of valvular defects may later disappear (30). This probably occurs with slight valvular lesions which are compensated by the heart muscle.

When valvular defects are established, their accurate evaluation is important. Valvular insufficiency is less important than valvular stenosis; tight stenosis has a more serious prognosis than slight stenosis; onset of stenosis at an early age is more serious than when it develops later; lesions of many valves have a worse prognosis than the lesion of one valve.

After establishment of a chronic condition of rheumatic inactive heart disease, the prognosis will be influenced by: a) *Heart size.* b) *Evidence of heart failure.* c) Age, activity, sex, and possibility of avoiding strenuous exertion. d) Possibility of new attacks of rheumatic disease or bacterial endocarditis. (e) Possible influence of prophylaxis.

Treatment

I. *Prophylaxis.* Prevention of attacks should be attempted: a) in children of rheumatic parents or having rheumatic siblings; b) in patients with an acute streptococcic sore throat; and c) in patients who have recovered from an acute attack of rheumatic disease.

Prophylaxis can be done with *sulfadiazine* (17)* (0.5 gm. twice a day) or *oral penicillin* (18) (200,000–300,000 units twice a day). It has given good results (31–34) causing a remarkable decrease of rheumatic disease or rheumatic recurrences. In patients with an acute streptococcic infection, large doses of penicillin by injection (or sulfa by mouth) should be used in order to terminate quickly the infection. Oral prophylaxis should be continued for 2 to 4 years, or until the adolescent is out of school.

II. *Therapy.* Three drugs have shown definite utility but their relative merits are still discussed. They are *ACTH, cortisone,*

and *salicylates.* All three of them decrease rheumatic activity. ACTH and cortisone were started following the studies of *Hench* and co-workers (54). Their effects may not be statistically different from those of aspirin. Still, individual cases benefit from one of the drugs and not from the others. Therefore, subsequent individual trials are sometimes necessary. ACTH and cortisone seem slightly more rapid in their initial action; salicylates have greater effect on joint manifestations. Therefore, ACTH (74) or cortisone (75) seem to be more appropriate in cases with acute congestive failure or heart block while salicylates (14, 16) are more indicated in poliarthritis and in milder cases. It should be kept in mind:

a) That both ACTH and cortisone require supportive therapy with mercurials, potassium administration, and salt restriction, because they favor water and salt retention.

b) That they may cause secondary disturbances (Cushing's syndrome, hirsutism, amenorrhea).

c) That all three drugs depress the inflammatory and exudative processes without abolishing them; therefore, they should be given *for a long time*, until the "natural" course of the disease is approaching its end.

d) That all three drugs should be given in gradually decreasing doses in order to avoid the flare-up which may follow a sudden withdrawal.

The duration of treatment should last at least 6 weeks and probably 8 weeks or more. A hormonal treatment may be prolonged or integrated by salicylate therapy.

Doses of the three drugs are shown in table 17.

Patients using cortisone or ACTH experience a sharp curtailing of water and salt elimination. Therefore, patients using these drugs should be treated with mercurial diuretics, restriction of sodium in the diet, and administration of potassium by mouth, in order to avoid onset of congestive failure.

Acetylsalicylic acid (aspirin) by mouth

TABLE 17. *Six-week treatment of rheumatic disease —daily dose*

PERIOD	ACTH	CORTISONE	ASPIRIN
	mg.	*mg.*	*gm./kg.*
1st–4th day	120–150	250–300	0.10
5th–7th day	100–120	150–250	0.08
2nd week	80–100	100–150	0.07
3rd week	60–80	75–100	0.06
4th week	40–60	50–75	0.05
5th and 6th week	20	30–50	0.03

(14) can be used instead of the classic treatment with sodium salicylate and alkali. An adequate salicylate blood level is between 30 and 40 mg. per cent (27). This blood level should be evaluated at regular intervals. Administration of *ascorbic acid* (67) prevents possible dangers of prolonged salicylate therapy.

Aminopyrine (15) in dose of 0.3 gm. four or five times a day occasionally gives striking results. The possibility of idiosyncrasy resulting in granulocytopenia must be kept in mind and administration of the drug will be promptly discontinued if the white blood count is below 6000.

Bedrest is very important. In certain cases, it should be prolonged for several months because it avoids the strain placed by exertion on the damaged heart and, therefore, limits the extent and severity of cardiac lesions. The difficulty of such treatment in children is overcome, and its possible side effects are prevented, if treatment is effected in specialized institutions where the young patient's minds are kept occupied.

Acute carditis seems to be favorably influenced by *oxygen therapy* and may also improve by the intravenous administration of *glucose* and *insulin* (46). *Digitalis* is used if there is evidence of failure or the heart rate is above 140. Toxic symptoms, revealed by nausea and vomiting, premature beats, or persistent tachycardia, should be avoided. The fact that the myocardium of these patients is more excitable than the average indicates the need for caution in the dosage of digitalis. Among the various glycosides, *gitalin* (7) has the best results on account of its wide margin between therapeutic and toxic dose.

Climate. Even if the change of climate does not fulfill all the wonders which have been described, it may have an important part in preventing recurrence of attacks. Dry, warm locations are the best. If the patient is unable to move to a completely new climate, at least care should be taken that

he does not live in a crowded section and in a damp and poorly heated house. He should not go out on humid and windy days and should avoid strenuous exercise and competitive sports for some years.

Tonsillectomy. In spite of the limited statistical results, tonsillectomy in children having large or infected tonsils is a good precaution.

Rheumatoid Arthritis

It is usually stated that the hearts of patients with rheumatoid arthritis are normal. However, in contrast with the usually negative clinical findings, postmortem studies reveal rheumatic heart lesions in about one-half of the cases (35, 39). This indicates either late onset or mild rheumatic lesions of the heart. It also suggests the possibility of a closer relationship between the two diseases.

BIBLIOGRAPHY

1. SWIFT, H. F. a) *Rheumatic Fever.* In *Nelson's Loose Leaf Medicine.* New York, Nelson, 1941.
   Also b) J. Exper. Med., 1924, **39**, 497.
   Also c) J. A. M. A., 1928, **90**, 906.
2. a) COBURN, A. F., AND PAULI, R. H. J. Clin. Investigation, 1939, **18**, 141.
   b) COBURN, A. F. *The Factor of Infection in the Rheumatic State.* Baltimore, The Williams & Wilkins Co., 1931.
   c) COBURN, A. F. AND YOUNG, D. C. *The Epidemiology of Hemolytic Streptococcus During World War II in the U. S. Navy.* Baltimore, The Williams & Wilkins Co., 1949.
3. a) WEINTRAUD, W. Berl. klin. Woch., 1913, **50**, 1381.
   b) KLINGE, F. Virch. Arch. path. Anat., 1930, **278**, 438.
   c) FREEMAN, J. *Report on Chronic Rheumatic Diseases.* London, Lewis, 1935.
4. SCHWENTKER, F. F., AND COMPLOIER, F. C. J. Exper. Med., 1939, **70**, 223.
5. SCHWEINBURG AND WARREN. Personal communication. Unpublished studies.
6. SCHLESINGER, B., AND CO-WORKERS. Lancet, 1935, **1**, 1145.
7. EAGLES, G. H., AND CO-WORKERS. Lancet, 1937, **2**, 421.

8. a) BIRKHAUG, K. E. J. Infectious Dis., 1928, **43**, 280.
   b) COPEMAN, W. S. C. Ann. Rheum. Dis., 1944, **4**, 37.
9. RAVENNA, P. a) Ann. Rheum. Dis., 1939, **1**, 167 and 1940, **2**, 1.
   b) Arch. Ital. Anat., Istol. Pat., 1934, **5**, 423.
   c) Min. Med. (Turin), 1936, (I), 202.
10. a) WILSON, M. G. *Rheumatic Fever*. New York, Commonwealth Fund, 1940.
   b) PAUL, J. R. *The Epidemiology of Rheumatic Fever*. 2nd Ed. New York, Metropolitan Life Insurance Co., 1943.
   c) READ, F., CIOCCO, A., AND TAUSSIG, H. B. Am. J. Hyg., 1938, **27**, 719.
11. SACKS, B. Am. Heart J., 1926, **1**, 2.
12. LUISADA, A. A., AND ANTONIAZZI, E. Cuore e Circ., (Rome) 1931, **15**, 89.
13. LIBMAN, E. J. A. M. A., 1923, **80**, 813.
14. MACCALLUM, W. G. a) Bull. Johns Hopkins Hosp., 1924, **35**, 329 and J. A. M. A., 1925, **84**, 1545.
15. VON GLAHN, W. C. Am. J. Path., 1926, **2**, 1.
16. PAPPENHEIMER AND VON GLAHN. Am. J. Path., 1926, **2**, 15.
17. KUGEL, M. A., AND EPSTEIN, E. F. Arch. Path., 1928, **6**, 247.
18. GRAY AND AITKEN. Quoted by SWIFT (1a).
19. HOLSTI, O. Arb. a. d. Path. Inst. d. Univers. Helsingfors, 1927, **5**, 110; and 1928, **5**, 401.
20. URRUTIA, D. M., AND VAISMAN, S. B. *La Enfermedad Reumatica*. Santiago, La Sud-America, 1941.
21. MCEWEN, C. *Rheumatic Heart Disease in Stroud's Cardiovascular Disease*. Philadelphia, Davis, 1945.
22. CANDEL, S., AND WHEELOCK, M. C. Ann. Med., 1945, **23**, 309.
23. BRUENN, H. G. Am. Heart J., 1937, **13**, 413.
24. KEITH, J. D. Quart. J. Med., 1938, **7**, 29.
25. BEYERSBACH, G. Mo. Conc. Cardiov. Dis., 1941, **10**, n. 5.
26. SMULL, K., WÉGRIA, R., AND LELAND, J. J. A. M. A., 1944, **125**, 1173.
27. COBURN, A. F. Bull. Johns Hopkins Hosp., 1943, **73**, 435.
28. MEYER, D. D., AND BERYL, H. Proc. Soc. Exper. Biol. & Med., 1943, **53**, 234.
29. WATSON, R. F., ROTHBARD, S., AND SWIFT, H. F. J. A. M. A., 1944, **126**, 274.
30. BLAND, E. F., DUCKETT JONES, T., AND WHITE, P. D. J. A. M. A., 1936, **107**, 569.
31. COBURN, A. F., AND MOORE, L. V. J. Clin. Investigation, 1939, **18**, 147.
32. THOMAS, C. B., AND CO-WORKERS. J. A. M. A., 1941, **116**, 551.
33. CHANDLER, C. A., AND TAUSSIG, H. B. Bull. Johns Hopkins Hosp., 1943, **72**, 42.
34. THOMAS, C. B. J. A. M. A., 1944, **126**, 490.
35. YOUNG, D., AND SCHWEDEL, J. B. Am. Heart J., 1944, **28**, 1.
36. BOYER, N. H. New England J. Med., 1943, **228**, 509.
37. a) COBURN, A. F. *Mass Chemoprophylaxis*. Publ. 284, Govt. Print. Office, Washington, D. C., 1944.
   b) WESSELHOEFT, C., AND WEINSTEIN, L. New England J. Med., 1945, **232**, 531.
38. a) RICH, A. R., AND GREGORY, J. E. Bull. Johns Hopkins Hosp., 1943, **73**, 239.
   b) CAVELTI, P. A. Arch. Path., 1947, **44**, 119.
39. a) ROBLES, G. J. Arch. Card. Mexico, 1948, **18**, 774.
   b) ROSENBERG, E. F., BISHOP, L. F., WEINTRAUB, H. J., AND HENCH, P. S. Arch. Int. Med., 1950, **85**, 751.
40. MILZER, A., KOHN, K. H., AND MACLEAN, H. J. A. M. A., 1948, **136**, 536.
41. GRIFFITH, G. C., AND HUNTINGTON, R. W. Ann. Int. Med., 1946, **25**, 283.
42. MAGALHÃES GOMES, E. *Diagnóstico das Formas Anátomo-Clínicas da Cardite Reumatica*. Jornal do Commercio, Rio de Janeiro, 1947.
43. TARAN, L. M., AND SZILAGYI, N. Am. Heart J., 1947, **33**, 26.
44. SAMPSON, J. J., AND KAPLAN, P. C. Am. J. M. Sci., 1946, **212**, 321.
45. CAHALL, L. Med. Clin. North America, Nov. 1946, 1332.
46. TARAN, L. M. Med. Clin. North America, May 1947, 557.
47. COCCHI, C. Riv. Clin. Ped. (Florence), 1947, **45**, 31.
48. BRADLEY, W. H. Proc. Roy. Soc. Med., 1950, **43**, 979.
49. SELYE, H. J. Clin. Endocrinol., 1946, **6**, 117.
50. KAUFMAN, P., AND POLIAKOFF, H. Ann. Int. Med., 1950, **32**, 889.
51. LUISADA, A. A., AND MAGRI, G. Am. Heart J., 1952, **44**, 545.
52. ASH, R. Am. Heart J., 1948, **36**, 89.
53. a) HARRIS, T. N. Am. J. M. Sci., 1949, **217**, 174.
   b) HARRIS, T. N., FRIEDMAN, S., AND HAUB, C. F. Pediatrics, 1949, **3**, 845.
54. HENCH, P. S., SLOCUMB, C. H., POLLAY, H. F., AND KENDALL, E. C. J. A. M. A., 1950, **144**, 1327; and Arch. Int. Med., 1950, **85**, 545.
55. TARAN, L. M. Bull. St. Francis Sanat., 1953, **10**, 9.

CHAPTER 9

Cardiovascular Syphilis

The agent of lues, *Treponema pallidum*, is the cause of several clinicopathological pictures. While both congenital and acquired lues may cause cardiovascular lesions, these are most usually found in the acquired type. Patients with luetic heart disease may be of any age, from birth to old age; the largest group, however, is between 30 and 55 years old.

Evidence of cardiac and vascular lesions usually becomes apparent from 10 to 30 years after the initial infection.

The most common processes are the following: a) *aortitis* (page 475), b) *aortic aneurysm* (page 478), and c) *aortic insufficiency* (page 238). Less frequent lesions include: d) *luetic arteritis of peripheral vessels* (page 530), e) *luetic coronaritis* (page 414), and f) *luetic myocarditis* (page 385).

Early syphilis may give changes of the electrocardiogram due to myocardial lesions which are as yet not clinically evident (1).

Treatment

Treatment aims at improving the functional conditions of the heart and arresting the luetic process without causing harm to the patient. An adequate therapy of syphilis in the early stages prevents cardiovascular lues.

When cardiovascular lues is present, treatment should be started cautiously in order to avoid sudden reactions.[49] If severe lesions are present, the patient should be kept in bed during the early phase of treatment.

If there is congestive failure, this will be treated before undertaking any important antiluetic therapy. However, moderate doses of *potassium iodide* may be given without harm. Then the following scheme will be used:

a) A 2-week intensive course of treatment with *iodides*; potassium iodide, 1 to 3 gm. daily by mouth.

b) A 2-week course of treatment with *mercury*; daily inunctions with strong mercurial ointment (4 gm.). KI is continued.

c) A 6-week course of treatment with *bismuth*; 10 per cent bismuth subsalicylate in peanut oil may be used; one weekly intramuscular injection. KI is continued.

d) A 12-week course of treatment with *arsenicals*; gradually increasing doses of *mapharsen* by weekly intravenous injections (10 to 30 mg.). During this course, KI is discontinued. Instead of arsenicals, *penicillin* can be used. A five million unit course of *procaine G penicillin* in aqueous solution (**19**) is given in 10 days (1 daily injection of 500,000 units) (2). Following this, either a course of bismuth (see b) or a second course of penicillin may be necessary. It is possible that the entire treatment may be reduced to 8 weeks (2 weeks iodide, 4 weeks bismuth, 2 weeks penicillin) but definite conclusions are still not available.

During this treatment, digitalis, diuretics, vasodilators, diet, and other useful procedures, may be used if necessary, as in other cardiac patients.

[49] The two most fearful reactions are *shock* and the *Herxheimer flare-up* of the disease. In patients with latent heart failure, irreversible failure may result.

BIBLIOGRAPHY

1. STEIGER, H. P., CHARLOTTE, N. C., AND EDEIKEN, J. Am. Heart J., 1947, **34,** 674.
2. STOKES, J. H., WOLFERTH, C. C., EDEIKEN, J., FALK, M. S., AND FORD, W. T. J. A. M. A., 1951, **147,** 943.

Chapter 10

Diseases of the Endocardium

Endocarditis

Endocarditis is an acute, subacute, or chronic disease due to an inflammatory lesion of the endocardium. It usually results in a permanent deformity of the cardiac valves.

Cases of endocarditis have been classified in different ways.

a) According to the *cause*, they are divided into toxic, rheumatic, and bacterial.

b) According to the *lesion*, they are divided into verrucose, polypoid, ulcerative, and sclerotic.

c) According to the *severity*, they are divided into benign and malignant.

d) According to the *course*, they may be acute, subacute, or chronic.

The belief that the terms *benign, rheumatic,* and *verrucose* on the one hand and *malignant, bacterial,* and *ulcerative* on the other may be interchangeable is common. In most of the cases this is correct, but it is by no means always so.

Benign Endocarditis

A benign endocarditis is one which usually has a favorable course.

CAUSE

Benign endocarditis may occur during the course of different acute diseases such as *diphtheria, scarlet fever, pneumonia, gonorrhea, typhoid fever,* and *grippe.* An even milder form may be present during *tuberculosis* or *chronic pyogenic infections.* Lastly, *syphilis* should be mentioned because an extension of the luetic process from the aorta to the aortic valves is common. In some of these cases, there is a *direct localiza-*

tion of the main agent of the disease; in others, of *associated germs.*

The endocardial lesion also may be caused by *toxins.* Experimental studies have shown the possibility of causing valvular lesions by injecting *bacterial toxins* or *foreign proteins* and even through *starvation* and *avitaminosis.* This may explain the accidental finding of slight valvular lesions without any apparent cause. *However, all these possible causes are of secondary importance in comparison with the most frequent of all: rheumatic disease.*

As already pointed out (page 190), a rheumatic endocarditis is admitted in cases where a definite and complete clinical picture of rheumatic disease is present in the history. It is also known that the same lesion occurs in many cases with the history of chorea, scarlet fever, erysipelas, streptococcic sore throat, and even diphtheria. In most of these cases, the endocarditis is not caused by the Streptococcus or the diphtheria bacillus but is due to either the more complex relationship between Streptococcus and rheumatic disease (page 189) or an associated lesion. Cases of rheumatic endocarditis without any history of acute disease are frequently encountered.

LESIONS

The most frequent localization of the lesion in the valves of the left heart led to the belief that the mechanical element plays an important rôle as these valves are submitted to a much more severe strain than those of the right heart. In general, the first attack of rheumatic disease causes a lesion of the mitral valve, with or without a similar lesion of the aortic valves. On the

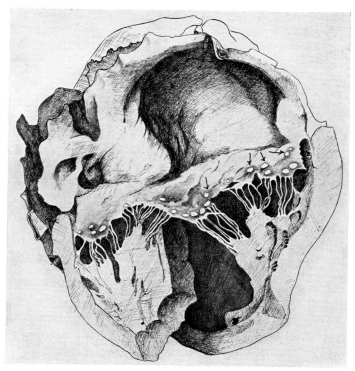

FIG. 111. The verrucae in rheumatic endocarditis.

contrary, benign endocarditis due to the Pneumococcus, Gonococcus, or Staphylococcus has a greater tendency to cause a lesion of the aortic valve first.

Whenever a greater strain is applied to the valves of the right heart, they become the preferred seat of endocarditis. This applies primarily to patients who already have mitral valve lesions with a higher than normal pressure in the pulmonary circulation, as well as to newborn babies and patients with congenital malformations of the heart. The latter may not only present inflammation of the cardiac valves but also of the communicating orifices or of the ductus arteriosus. In general, the tricuspid is a more common site of localization than the pulmonic valve.

Rheumatic endocarditis is typically accompanied by the production of *verrucae*. These are usually present along the *free margin of the leaflets* but they may invade the entire valvular surface (Fig. 111), as well

as the parietal, septal, and papillary endocardium.

The first stage is represented by redness and swelling of the valves; the second, by the production of minute granulations, the *verrucae*, which gradually become firmer and more resistant; and the third stage by the formation of scar tissue which deforms and retracts the valves and may cause narrowing of the valvular openings.

The *verruca* is formed over an *initial necrosis of the endothelium* by exudation of coagulable fluid and the development of a mass which forms like a minute *thrombus* (1). However, a *proliferation* of inflammatory cells in the subendocardial tissue seems to precede the superficial changes. *Aschoff bodies* have been found in the valves (page 108).

Subendothelial fibrous plaques and endocardial fibrosis of the left atrium are considered signs of previous rheumatic endocarditis (2).

Nonrheumatic endocarditis may have the verrucose type. However, it may cause a mild inflammation with swelling and redness of the endocardium without any formation of verrucae. When the acute stage is over, *fibrosis of the valves and of the septal endocardium* remains. If thickening and shortening of the cusps result, it may be difficult to distinguish the process from that caused by rheumatic disease. Fibrosis of the parietal and chordal endocardium may be followed by shortening of one or more chordae tendineae, causing valvular insufficiency.

Tuberculous endocarditis (rare) may produce miliary tubercles, with or without ulceration. Simple fibrosis of the endocardium, caused by tubercular toxins, is frequent.

Syphilitic endocarditis often causes an adhesion of the cusp ends of the aortic valve against the aortic wall, resulting in valvular insufficiency. The fibrosis which follows the acute process may extend to the medial cusp of the mitral causing insufficiency of that valve.

The process of *scarring* of all types of benign endocarditis results in the *fibrosis* of the tissues previously involved. This is a frequent cause of valvular defects. Fibrosis is usually accompanied by the production of minute vessels in the valves which may further favor lesions caused by bacteria. Fibrosis may be followed by *calcification*.

SYMPTOMATOLOGY

There are no definite signs of the endocardial lesion in its early stage, most of those previously described being signs of *carditis* in general. It is possible that a certain *dulness of the 1st sound* and a *soft systolic murmur* are due to edema and inflammation of the mitral valve; however, myocarditis and ventricular dilatation may produce the same result.

In cases of rheumatic disease, these signs of carditis will be sufficient for admitting the existence of endocarditis as a prob-ability. In other cases, on the contrary, it will be necessary to follow the case further before accepting the evidence. A *prolonged and loud systolic murmur*, persisting after the acute stage of the disease, is the proof that there has been an endocarditis.

TREATMENT

Treatment of benign endocarditis is the same as that of the basic disease. That of rheumatic disease has been discussed previously (page 198).

Bacterial Endocarditis (Malignant Endocarditis)

Malignant endocarditis is almost always caused by bacteria. Therefore, malignant and bacterial endocarditis have become synonymous, even if the identification is not always exact.

Acute Bacterial Endocarditis

CAUSE

A variety of bacteria may be the cause of this type of disease. The most common is *Streptococcus hemolyticus* but different other strains of Streptococci (occasionally including *S. viridans*) have been found. The Pneumococcus, Meningococcus, Staphylococcus, are possible agents; other bacteria may cause this disease.

Malignant endocarditis is often due to an association of bacteria. Among them, the possibility of an acute streptococcic endocarditis in patients with rheumatic disease should always be considered.

Acute malignant endocarditis may follow puerperal sepsis, carbuncle, pulmonary abscess, osteomyelitis, purulent cholangitis, meningitis, or pneumonia. It may occur during acute miliary tuberculosis. In a few cases due to various bacteria and in most of those due to nonhemolytic streptococci, no febrile illness precedes the endocarditis which seems to appear suddenly.

LESIONS

The typical lesion of acute malignant endocarditis consists of rapidly formed

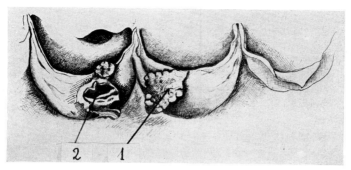

FIG. 112. Acute bacterial endocarditis. 1, polypose formation on a valve; 2, ulceration of a valve.

valvular ulcerations. The initial stage of congestion and edema may last only a few hours and is immediately followed by a process of necrosis and ulceration. There may be formation of *soft vegetations* (fig. 112) which soon soften and slough off, forming numerous small *emboli*. The necrosis first causes a depression and later a *valvular aneurysm*. When this breaks, perforation of the valve takes place. Sudden *breaking of chordae tendineae* may be due to the same process; *perforation of the ventricular septum* may occur as the result of acute purulent myocarditis.

SIGNS AND SYMPTOMS

The patients present the signs of a severe *sepsis*. They also complain of *palpitation, dyspnea, precordial pain*, and a *smothering feeling*. The *pulse is weak* and may be *irregular* as the result of myocardial lesions. The heart is dilated. Auscultation reveals rapid changes in the findings. *The heart sounds become dull and weak and murmurs appear.*

The appearance of both *mitral and tricuspid systolic murmurs* is very frequent. *Aortic or pulmonic diastolic murmurs* also occur often. These murmurs may change from hour to hour: now soft, then harsh, later musical; now brief, then prolonged. A murmur due to stenosis of one valve may appear, then disappear again, owing to the softening and splitting of a mass which obstructed a valvular opening. Breaking of a valve or rupture of a chorda may be a

further cause of valvular defects revealed by auscultation.

Small hemorrhagic petechiae may appear, having a greater frequency on the palms of the hands and on the soles of the feet.

Janeway lesions. These are small, erythematous, and partially hemorrhagic areas which occur mostly on the palms, the soles, and the tips of the fingers and toes. They have no gray center and are not tender. They are from 1 to 4 mm. in diameter, and blanch on pressure.

CLINICAL TYPES

Two types have been described.

Pseudo-typhoid type. The initial stage may simulate typhoid fever. Meteorism, vomiting, diarrhea, and abdominal pain are among the first symptoms. The *fever* presents wide oscillations and there is *chill*. The pulse is rapid, irregular, and unstable. There is severe *dyspnea. The liver and spleen are enlarged.* There may be erythema. There is severe anemia (often hemolytic anemia) and high grade leukocytosis.

Pyohemic type. This type starts suddenly. The fever is typical of the purulent infections. The patient is delirious or confused. There may be signs of meningeal involvement. There is acute glomerulonephritis. The heart is enlarged; the liver and spleen are very large. *Multiple metastatic abscesses* are formed because of purulent emboli which originate from the cardiac valves. *Arteritis* and *phlebitis* are common. *Skin embolisms* are frequent: *hemorrhagic pete-chiae* are formed with a gray center, the embolus. They are usually *tender*.

Several other varieties exist having greater or lesser severity of the above-described signs. Among the possible complications, *perforation of the cardiac septa* is worthy of mention.

An important type is that occurring *in the aged* where the course is often *fulminating* and the diagnosis is often obscure because of the patient's prostration (5).

DIAGNOSIS

The general diagnosis of sepsis is easy and is confirmed by *positive blood culture*. The recognition of *loud variable cardiac murmurs* (among them a diastolic aortic murmur frequently appears) and the occurrence of *embolic phenomena* are fundamental in the diagnosis of acute malignant endocarditis. This diagnosis should not be made without a positive blood culture and the typical cardiac findings.

PROGNOSIS

The prognosis was constantly unfavorable until the development of chemotherapy led to the cure of some cases. It is still serious.

TREATMENT

The only effective methods of treatment are with the *sulfonamides*, or with *penicillin* and other antibiotics. They may *prevent* the occurrence of endocarditis if given during pneumonia, meningitis, or erysipelas. If they are given *during* endocarditis, they may cure the patients, if the treatment is initiated early and continued without interruption until the results are attained. The dose of penicillin varies from 300,000 to 1 or 2 million units every 24 hours.

Cases of bacterial endocarditis, caused by organisms which are not affected by penicillin, should be treated by means of *streptomycin* or other antibiotics.

Blood transfusions may be helpful.

The *diet* should be bland as with any acute infectious disease (Diet I).

Subacute Bacterial Endocarditis (Endocarditis Lenta—Disease of Osler-Libman, 6, 7)

The division of bacterial endocarditis into acute and subacute has been criticized (8) on the basis that the same germs may cause both types. It is the author's view that a clinical separation is still justified.

CAUSE

The great majority of cases is caused by nonhemolytic Streptococci of either the *alpha* (*S. viridans*) or the *gamma* (*S. anhemolyticus*) variety. Some cases are due to the Hemophilus influenzae, Gonococcus, Meningococcus, germs of the Brucella group, and others. The Enterococcus is not exceptional; the others are very rare. Last, infection by higher organisms (Monilia, Leptothryx, Actinomyces, Histoplasma) must be mentioned. Their reported incidence is increasing (10).

MODE OF ORIGIN

This type of endocarditis almost always occurs in patients already having valvular lesions or congenital abnormalities. The most frequent occurrence is in patients with *rheumatic heart disease* and mitral or aortic lesions. *Congenital defects* are frequently involved with localization on the valves, on the rim of a septal opening, or in the patent ductus.[50] *Syphilitic lesions* of the aortic valves may predispose to subacute bacterial endocarditis. *Arteriosclerotic valves* may occasionally become the seat of the endocarditis (11, 15).

[50] In this latter case the name of *subacute bacterial arteritis* is justified, as well as in the cases where the germs are localized in an arteriovenous aneurysm.

The incidence of subacute bacterial endocarditis in congenital lesions is the following (12):

	per cent
Ventricular septal defect	42
Patent ductus arteriosus	28.6
Pulmonary stenosis	19
Bicuspid aortic valve	17.4
Syndrome of Fallot	12.5

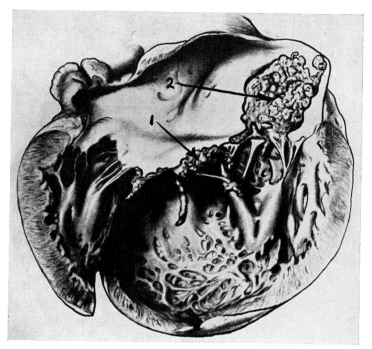

Fig. 113. Subacute bacterial endocarditis. Active lesions over the mitral valve (1) and in the posterior wall of the left atrium (2). (Courtesy of Dr. E. Libman.)

The germs may be present in some *focus* (tonsils, teeth, etc.) and may enter the blood stream after a surgical intervention (frequently after removal of a diseased tooth). *No localization on the endocardium occurs, however, without a previous lesion.* Simultaneous occurrence of new rheumatic lesions in the course of subacute bacterial endocarditis may occur (3, 8).

The old endocardial lesions seem to predispose the tissues to bacterial implantation. on the one hand by providing suitable means for reaching the deep structures of the valves (newly formed vessels, toxic and degenerative processes) and, on the other hand, by increasing the strain and stress on the valves (9).

LESIONS

The most important lesion is constituted by *soft polypoid vegetations* on the valves, the parietal endocardium, and occasionally the large arteries (congenital defects). They are greenish or grayish, friable at first, firmer later. They are larger than rheumatic vegetations and occasionally may determine *ulceration*, *perforation*, or *rupture* of either the valves or the chordae (fig. 113).

The vegetations are composed of fibrin, blood elements, platelets, and bacteria. The latter frequently are adherent to the surface of the vegetations. Early in the course of the disease, embolic fragmentation of the valves occurs.

Infarcts are encountered frequently in visceral organs (spleen, kidneys, brain) and are seen more rarely in the lungs (except with congenital defects, where they are more common). Minute and multiple *emboli* frequently are transported to the brain, kidneys, spleen, retina, and skin, frequently occurring in shower-like episodes. *Arteritis* and *capillaritis* are frequent. The former leads to the formation of aneurysms and is often due to penetration of the germs into the *vasa vasorum*.

The healing process occurs first in the deeper portions of the lesion and causes a characteristic spongy aspect (9).

Myocardial lesions are far more frequent and extensive than previously thought (13, 14, 42, 43). Miliary infarcts and interstitial and perivascular infiltrates or scars are the most common findings.

The most constant renal lesion is *focal glomerulonephritis*, described by *Loehlein* (16). This is due to endothelial lesions followed by thrombosis of minute vessels. Diffuse glomerulonephritis and larger infarctions are not uncommon.

In conclusion, the pathologic changes of subacute bacterial endocarditis consist of:

1) Development of soft vegetations on previously damaged valves or congenital defects.

2) Dissemination of minute bacterial emboli into both the lesser and the greater circulations.

3) Occasional transportation of massive emboli with gross infarctions.

4) Various inflammatory changes depending upon the particular response of the organ or tissue involved.

SYMPTOMS AND SIGNS

The *onset* of the disease is usually *slow and insidious*. The patient is known, as a rule, to be a "cardiac" and the first manifestations, consisting of *weakness*, *fatigue*, and *vague pains* may not be observed. However, if they are noticed and the temperature is taken, *fever* is discovered. Occasionally, a *sudden onset* with sharp increase in temperature and, possibly, *chill* is observed. Headache, abdominal pain, vertigo, urinary symptoms, dyspnea, palpitation, or precordial pain may be present at the beginning.

Once the disease is established, the most frequent symptoms and signs may be grouped under: general, embolic and cardiac (7b).

1) *General symptoms*. They are due to toxemia. *Fever* is a constant feature. It may be irregularly remittent or intermittent. It is usually low at first, higher later. It may present slow undulations, disappearing at times for one or two weeks, then becoming higher. It may simulate malaria or brucellosis. *Chills* are not constant but may occur. *Profuse sweating* is constant when the temperature has sharp oscillations. *Progressive anemia* is also constant. It is usually an hypochromic anemia, due both to hemolysis and poor regeneration. There is a moderate *leucocytosis* (occasionally leucopenia) with *monocytosis*. *Weakness*, *breathlessness*, and *exhaustion* are caused by anemia, toxemia, and fever. *Nausea* and *vomiting* may occur; *loss of appetite* is practically constant. *Diffuse pains*, *tenderness of the sternum*, and *joint pains* are common.

2) *Multiple symptoms caused by either embolism or local inflammation*. These symptoms are extremely variable, owing to the variety of vessels and organs which may be affected. There may be blocking of either large or small arteries. The capillaries may be affected by embolism or by local inflammation. Embolism may cause weakness or paralysis of an extremity, hemiplegia, visual disturbances, and pulmonary, myocardial, splenic, or renal infarctions. *Albuminuria* and microscopic or gross *hematuria* may be seen.

3) *Cardiac signs and symptoms*. These are due to the underlying valvular defects or congenital abnormalities and to the superimposed vegetations. *Cardiac enlargement* is frequent. *Cardiac murmurs* are present since the onset because of the already present valvular lesions. The murmurs will be modified:

a) By addition of *myocardial murmurs*, due to the anemia with secondary cardiac dilatation.

b) By addition of *new valvular murmurs*, due to the vegetations and perforations of the valves (both regurgitation and stenosis of a valve may gradually appear).

Atrial fibrillation is rare but less so than previously thought (34). *Heart block* is rare and occurs only when a concomitant myocarditis with involvement of the septum is present.

Some of the clinical signs deserve further mention.

Pallor of the skin and mucous membranes is constant. It is less apparent when the patient is cyanotic.

Clubbing of the fingers and toes is frequent but not constant. It is very significant if it appears during the course of the disease, but has no meaning when present before the onset (possible congenital cardiac defects). Clubbing may recede if the patient recovers or enters the bacteria-free stage (7b).

Petechiae, with or without a pale yellowish center, are commonly seen. They may be present in the conjunctivae, on the fundus, or on the palate. They may be isolated or occur in showers. They are easily caused by artificially raising the venous and capillary pressure.

Osler nodes. These nodes occur in about one-half of the cases; they are small, raised, red lesions, often of the size of a pea, which are observed mostly on the fingertips, under the nails, or on the soles of the feet. They are always tender and disappear after 4 to 5 days, usually without suppuration (*false whitlows*). The latter, however, may occur if there is bacterial association (7b). These nodes, which have been attributed to embolization may be also the result of inflammation, possibly toxic or allergic (17).

Janeway lesions. These are small erythematous and partially hemorrhagic lesions, of 1 to 4 mm. in size, which may be macular or papular in character. They occur mostly on the palms, the soles, and the tips of the fingers and toes. They are present occasionally over the extremities and trunk. *These lesions are never tender or painful.*

Enlargement of the liver and spleen is constant; that of the latter more so than that of the former.

LABORATORY FINDINGS
Electrocardiogram

There usually is *sinus rhythm.* A *prolongation of the P-R interval*, reaching from 0.21″ to 0.36″, has been described in about 15 per cent of the cases (7b). It is possible, however, that this may have been caused by a concomitant rheumatic carditis (8). *Premature beats are present at times.*

Phonocardiogram

This gives the tracings of the different murmurs. It may be useful for obtaining objective evidence of the changes occurring from day to day.

X-ray

The x-ray reveals the changes in size of the heart and, in general, the results of both the underlying original lesions and the new valvular defects.

Blood

Red cell counts are often between 3 and 3.5 million; *hemoglobin*, between 50 and 70 per cent. *White cell counts* are variable. They show a moderate leucocytosis at times but leucopenia has been encountered. The highest white cells counts are present with visceral infarction. A high polymorphonuclear count is present in cases with leucocytosis; a high lymphocyte count, in those with leucopenia. Sometimes the blood contains large histiocytes or endothelial cells and their number is increased by rubbing the ear before taking the blood.

The *sedimentation rate* is usually accelerated in the active stage of the disease.

Blood culture. Blood cultures, repeatedly made, are usually positive in the *active stage* and negative in the *bacteria-free stage*. They reveal *S. viridans* in about 90 per cent of the cases, other germs in the others. Attention should be paid to the possibility of *fungi* which are likely to be interpreted as due to faulty technique.

The *Wassermann test* has been found positive in some cases of subacute bacterial endocarditis without syphilis.

COURSE AND COMPLICATIONS

The disease may pass spontaneously into a *quiescent stage* in which the blood does not contain bacteria (*bacteria-free stage* of *Libman*) and the cardiac lesions are healing. The patients then may show evidence of great improvement but they may still suffer from cardiac and renal insufficiency, progressive anemia, embolic accidents, or vascular aneurysms. If no effective treatment has been undertaken and the patient survives, the disease may return to an *active stage* and follow its course to the fatal end.

Spontaneous recovery is rare but possible.

The chief complications are due to *embolism* and *infarction* of different organs. Myocardial and pulmonary infarction are not common; splenic infarction, on the other hand, is very frequent. *Heart failure* is frequent.

Active rheumatic disease is a possible complication (8). Bacterial endocarditis may reactivate the rheumatic process or may occur during active rheumatic disease. Tender and swollen joints, epistaxis, atrial fibrillation or prolonged P-R interval, may be evidence of active rheumatic disease when present during subacute bacterial endocarditis.

The *anemia* may become a complication in itself if severe and untreated. *Pneumonia* is favored by the weakness of the patient. *Ball-valve thrombus* of the left atrium has been described (page 214).

VARIETIES

Among the various clinical pictures, one is caused by subacute bacterial endocarditis confined to the right side of the heart or the pulmonary artery (44). Petechiae and systemic embolism are rare in such cases while pulmonary embolism is a common occurrence.

DIAGNOSIS

As the early symptoms of the disease are extremely varied in type, subacute bacterial endocarditis may simulate many other diseases, such as grippe, pulmonary tuberculosis, rheumatic disease, typhoid fever, malaria, heart failure, subphrenic abscess, gastric carcinoma, acute appendicitis, meningitis, undulant fever, or leukemia. The diagnosis will be particularly difficult in the aged and in those patients with cardiac symptoms and signs which are either mild or of difficult interpretation.

Differential diagnosis between subacute bacterial endocarditis and other types of endocarditis is always necessary. *Rheumatic endocarditis* is only one manifestation of a widespread disease; myocardial and joint signs are often present; blood culture is negative. In *acute bacterial endocarditis*, an extensive primary lesion, like osteomyelitis, erysipelas, or pneumonia, is often present.

In *subacute bacterial endocarditis* the symptoms are due to the endocardial involvement or its complications while the primary focus is usually insignificant or obscure. The diagnosis in difficult cases is aided by the result of blood cultures in the *active stages*.

The diagnosis in the *bacteria-free stages* is suggested whenever a patient with valvular defects presents one of the following features: renal insufficiency, severe progressive anemia, multiple emboli, severe splenomegaly, or clubbing of the fingers.

PROGNOSIS

Owing to the small percentage of recovery, the prognosis has been invariably unfavorable until the progress of chemotherapy permitted a definite modification of the course. It should be kept in mind that often these patients die through renal or cardiac failure, even after subsidence of the infection.

TREATMENT

The difficulty in the treatment of this disease is demonstrated by the great number of drugs and biologicals (tried with varying degrees of success) since its first description.

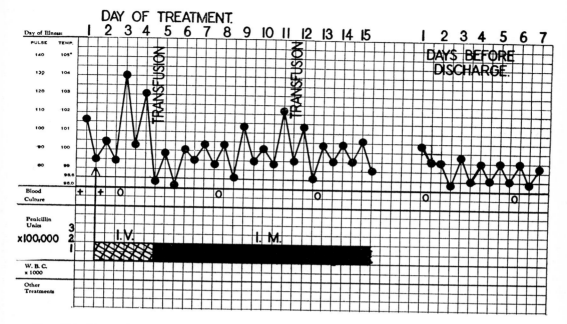

Fig. 114. Chart of a case of subacute bacterial endocarditis treated with penicillin. (From Bloomfield and co-workers (33); courtesy of the authors and of J. Clin. Investigation.)

A definite step was made with the *heparin-sulfonamide treatment* which increased the number of recoveries to about 6 per cent (18, 19).

The next step was the *penicillin treatment* which is of great utility (21–23). Penicillin should be given in adequate dosage (from 1 to 20 million units daily), the larger doses being reserved for the most resistant cases. Treatment will be continued for about 1 month, then repeated with a higher dosage if blood sterility is not obtained (fig. 114).

Experience has shown that *penicillin* is almost always bactericidal. *Streptomycin* seems to reinforce its action. Therefore, penicillin-streptomycin treatment succeeds in many penicillin-resistant cases. *Aureomycin, Chloromycetin,* and *Terramycin* are bacteriostatic in the average doses, while they become bactericidal if used in massive doses (seldom tolerated) or in combination with *streptomycin.* Enterococcal endocarditis is usually cured by *Aureomycin plus Terramycin.* In the other types, treatment with bacteriostatic agents should be followed by *penicillin-streptomycin* therapy. Penicillin-streptomycin combined therapy seems to be effective even in a 2-week period of treatment whenever the agent is sensitive to penicillin.

If the active agent of the disease is unaffected by penicillin, aureomycin, or streptomycin, *emetin* or *neo-arsphenamine* (higher organisms) should be tried.

The possibility of a combined rheumatic and bacterial endocarditis should be kept in mind; in such cases, penicillin treatment should be followed by *cortisone* or *aspirin* (page 198). Cortisone should *not* precede penicillin.

Demonstration that surgical or dental interventions in cardiac patients may lead to occurrence of subacute bacterial endocarditis (page 207) advises *the systematic use of either sulfonamides or penicillin before, during, and after such procedures.* This will prevent a large percentage of infections, even if some of them still seem beyond prophylaxis.

It is probable that a large majority of the patients can be saved; the inevitable percentage of fatalities is due to cardiac or renal failure and to irreversible cerebral lesions. However, early treatment may decrease the number of these complications. If cardiac failure occurs, the patient should be treated as any other patient in failure.

Administration of large doses of *vitamin C* (67) may be of great help in view of the importance of this vitamin in healing wounds and its frequent deficiency in prolonged infections. *Blood transfusions* may be necessary in many cases. *Iron therapy* will be of use in cases with severe anemia.

A *high caloric* and *high vitamin diet* will be given (Diet II) in order to increase the resistance of the patient.

Libman-Sacks' Disease

This disease, once confused with bacterial endocarditis, is actually the result of a "systemic lupus erythematosus" and is considered a "collagen disease" (37–40).

LESIONS

Diffuse or focal fibrinous *pericarditis* occurs frequently. It may result in fibrous pericardial and pleuropericardial adhesions. The endocardium is the site of a *nonbacterial verrucous endocarditis* which may attack *all four valves*. The verrucae are frequently found all over the surface of the leaflets, as well as over the chordae, valve rings, valve pockets, and the parietal endocardium. The valvulitis is characterized by severe fibrinoid degeneration of the collagen fibers, accompanied by necrosis and severe exudation. This leads to formation of granular basophilic masses, the so-called *hematoxylin bodies*. No bacteria can be found in the valves. A similar, milder type of degeneration can be found in the myocardium. A peculiar type of periarterial fibrosis can be found in the spleen. The kidneys are the site of severe lesions, with endothelial proliferation in the glomerular capillaries and the so-called *wire-loop le-*

sions. Pulmonary and neurological lesions may be observed. Skin lesions may be present including the typical *butterfly pattern* on the face.

CLINICAL PICTURE

The clinical picture is similar to that of subacute bacterial endocarditis but no bacteria can be demonstrated in the blood. The blood count reveals leucopenia, thrombopenia, and hypochromic anemia.

TREATMENT

Treatment with *cortisone* or *ACTH* has brought temporary remissions in several cases, and occasional cure. Treatment with sulfadiazine may prevent secondary infections. Exposure to strong light and to sun should be prevented.

Chronic Endocarditis—Endocardial and Valvular Sclerosis—Valvular Calcification

Endocarditis of the benign type may be so mild and so slow in its course as to be completely unobserved. This applies not only to *rheumatic endocarditis* but also to that caused by *bacteria* of low virulence and to that caused by *syphilis*. The latter may be localized on either the parietal or the valvular endocardium without previous aortic localization (24, 25). Mild inflammation of the valves has been encountered during *chronic sepsis* or *chronic nephritis*. It is likely that the valvular lesion is often due to the action of bacterial toxins and metabolites and not to direct localization of germs.

Endocardial sclerosis is found in one of the most commonly fatal diseases of infancy. The cause of this sclerosis is unknown and it is likely that the endocardial lesion, which involves also one or more valves, is only a part of the picture. There is good evidence proving that the endocardial sclerosis is the result of *extensive subendocardial sclerosis* due to coronary insufficiency (page 415). Cardiac enlargement, cyanosis, dyspnea, tachycardia, cough and vomitus

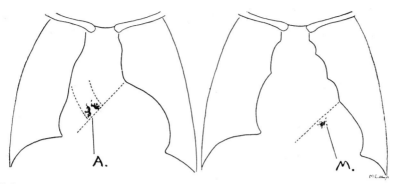

FIG. 115. Calcification of the aortic (A.) and mitral (M.) valves in two different cases (frontal view) (from Menendez de Oliveira).

are common. Cardiac murmurs are atypical and inconsistent and there is no diagnostic electrocardiographic pattern. The patients die with evidence of circulatory failure.

Chronic endocardial fibrosis seems to be rather common in Central Africa. People presenting this lesion usually die in late maturity or early senility. As myocardial and coronary lesions are also found, it might be that the entire picture is due to *coronary heart disease.*

Valvular sclerosis is the process by which the cardiac valves are thickened by fibrous connective tissue without too serious deformity. This may be caused by a mild endocarditis as described above, by tubercular toxins, or by a degenerative process without any preceding active inflammation. *Atherosclerosis* is a very common cause of valvular sclerosis in the aged. The typical manifestations of this process are (page 526) degenerative processes, atheromata, calcification, and even secondary thrombosis. The most common localization is on the aortic and mitral valves. More or less serious valvular defects may result.

Calcification of the cardiac valves is not a rare occurrence and may be due to either previous endocarditis or atherosclerosis. Its most frequent localization is in the mitral and aortic valves. The calcifications appear at the points of greater functional strain, such as the lines of insertion of the valves, and then spread to the surrounding struc-

tures. The seat of predilection is the posterior part of the mitral ring (26). Diagnosis of the calcifications during life may be made by means of x-ray (fig. 115). The differentiation between calcification of the posterior semilunar valve or posterior part of the *aortic* ring and calcification of the ring or anterior valve of the *mitral* may be difficult. However, in the left anterior oblique, the anterior mitral valve is a little under and behind the aortic valve (26). Purely atherosclerotic lesions rarely cause valvular disturbances of the mitral valve; still they cause occasional mitral insufficiency and possibly slight mitral stenosis. They may cause severe aortic stenosis (*calcific aortic stenosis*—page 250).

Anomalies of the Endocardium

Many congenital *anomalies of the cardiac valves* will be described in the following two chapters, devoted to valvular diseases.

Anomalous chordae have been described, in many instances forming a system of fine tendinous threads attached to the lower border of the atrial septum, to the tricuspid valve, and to the right wall of the right atrium. They constitute *Chiari's network* and may cause loud murmurs and, occasionally, favor intracardiac thrombosis. They are probably due to remnants of the right venous valve of the fetus (27–29).

Endocardial pockets (pseudo-valves) have been found in cases with valvular defects, in the upper part of the left ventricle, near the apex, or in the left atrium (27, 28). They resemble folds of endocardium and are favored by the abnormally regurgitating blood caused by valvular insufficiency. Their presence may decrease the severity of regurgitation.

Rupture of Mitral Chordae Tendineae

This lesion may be caused by bacterial endocarditis, rheumatic heart disease, myocardial infarction, or severe trauma on the chest. Its cause is obscure in some cases (30).

Rupture of the chordae is suggested by the *sudden appearance of a loud systolic murmur*, maximal at the apex and in the 3rd left interspace, and accompanied by a *thrill*. The complete picture of mitral regurgitation develops within a short time. Congestive failure may develop only after several months or years or may be abrupt and severe.

Differential diagnosis includes the rupture of a valvular cusp, rupture of a papillary muscle, and perforation of the interventricular septum. The last occurrence produces *a murmur directed toward the right* (page 284) *and no enlargement of the left atrium*. Rupture of a papillary muscle has the most serious effects.

Cardiac Thrombosis

Cardiac thrombosis is the formation of firm blood clots adhering to the wall of one of the cardiac chambers.

ATRIAL THROMBOSIS

The most typical thrombi occur in the atria. *Thrombosis of the left atrium* is common in mitral stenosis and insufficiency, especially when there is aneurysm of the atrium, atrial fibrillation, or heart failure.

The *atrial thrombus* is a globular body, either adherent to the cardiac wall or pedunculated and freely moving (*ball thrombus*). It may vary from the size of a walnut to that of an egg. A gradual *fibrous trans-*

formation with penetration of vessels and connective tissue proliferation usually takes place in the adherent thrombi. Fibromyxosarcomatas of the endocardium are probably due to transformation of thrombi. Pedunculated thrombi have also been called *cardiac polyps*.

A lesion of the endocardium is usually the ultimate cause of blood clotting in the atria but this is favored by slow circulation, by the extreme dilation of one of the cardiac chambers (aneurysm), and by the weak or absent contraction of their walls (atrial fibrillation).

Thrombosis of the left atrium may be so extensive as to cause obstruction of a large part of the chamber. Sometimes a large clot leaves the wall and *nearly occludes the mitral orifice*. Terrific dyspnea, precordial pain, extreme pallor, and violent and irregular pulsation of the heart with impalpable pulse, are the typical signs of this picture which is usually fatal.

A *ball thrombus* may cause repeated and transitory occlusions of the mitral orifice (more rarely of the tricuspid) without being able to pass through owing to its size (fig. 116). Apart from being the cause of multiple emboli, a ball thrombus may cause a typical picture: dyspnea, pallor and cyanosis, precordial pain, and impalpable pulse. *The supine position sometimes determines disocclusion of the mitral orifice and sudden improvement.*

Not only calcified thrombi, but also soft mural thrombi, can be recognized under certain conditions by means of x-ray. Undue prominence of the left atrial appendage is frequently due to thrombosis of its wall (41).

Nonembolic peripheral vascular phenomena may occur. They consist of symmetrical ischemia of the legs, of all four extremities, the tip of the nose, and the ears. They seem to be caused by severe arteriolar constriction and may lead to gangrene (32, 36).

A *thin, pedunculated thrombus* may hang through the mitral valve and cause both valvular insufficiency and regurgitation.

The *murmurs* resulting from this occurrence may be so loud as to keep the patient awake and even to disturb people sleeping in the same room.

VENTRICULAR THROMBOSIS

Mural thrombosis of the ventricular cavity is a frequent complication of myocardial infarction (page 427). Thrombi are usually large and are easily dislodged by the vigorous ventricular contractions. As a result, peripheral embolism is a possible complication.

Tumors of the Endocardium

LESIONS

Endocardial tumors may be *primary* or *secondary*. The most common primary tumor is the *fibromyxosarcoma* (31). This is more frequently observed in the left heart and the most common localization is in the *fossa ovalis* of the left atrium. These tumors may be the result of a previous thrombosis; they may be pedunculated or ball-like; they may cause valvular occlusion or compression of the coronary arteries. They usually cause paroxysmal attacks, often resulting in death.

SIGNS AND SYMPTOMS

The patients usually have the clinical picture of congestive failure and they suddenly present one of the following paroxysmal attacks:

a) Fainting.

b) Paroxysmal dyspnea with wheezing and noisy respiration simulating bronchial asthma or mediastinal tumors.

c) Pulmonary edema.

d) Anginal pain.

e) Acute atrial fibrillation or acute a-v block.

f) Acute suffocation, relieved by the supine position.

Examination of the heart reveals a large precordial dulness. Auscultation reveals *soft systolic murmurs* due to functional insufficiency of the mitral and tricuspid valves, or *bizarre murmurs* as in no other heart disease.

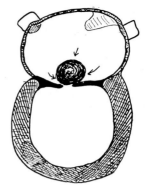

Fig. 116. Scheme of a ball thrombus occluding the mitral orifice.

Blood pressure may be normal and even high, but drops suddenly to the lowest levels compatible with life during the attacks.

The *electrocardiogram* is often normal, but it may present persistent deviation of the S-T segment because of pericarditis or compression of the coronary arteries. Acute atrial fibrillation or acute heart block may be present.

Peripheral embolism, due to minute parts of the tumor, is not uncommon.

COURSE

The course is inevitably progressive, as sooner or later, the fatality is determined by occlusion of one of the valves by the tumor. One-third of the patients die suddenly (31). Others have a slower course with *ice cold extremities* (occasionally associated with gangrene), *extreme cyanosis*, and *small or impalpable pulse* (32).

DIAGNOSIS

Diagnosis is possible when a patient, having no recognizable valvular, coronary, or myocardial lesion, presents a typical picture as described above. At times, the knowledge of a primary tumor in another organ may lead to the correct diagnosis.

Histological study of a peripheral embolus may be of help (35).

The paroxysmal attacks which are alleviated by the supine position are absolutely typical and in contrast to the frequent orthopnea of the cardiac patients. Still, they may be caused by a pedunculated tumor, a pedunculated thrombus, or a ball thrombus. Cardiac thrombosis usually occurs in patients with a long cardiac history while cardiac tumors are found more usually in patients without cardiac precedents. On the other hand, a fibromyxosarcoma may be due to transformation of an old thrombus.

TREATMENT

Surgical removal of endocardial tumors has been suggested but seldom attempted (35).

BIBLIOGRAPHY

1. SACKS, B. Am. Heart J., 1926, 1, 750.
2. MACCALLUM, W. G. J. A. M. A., 1925, 84, 1545. Also KOLETSKY, S. Am. Heart J., 1945, 29, 739.
3. WHITE, P. D. Heart Disease. New York, Macmillan, 1944.
4. a) KEEFER, C. S., AND CO-WORKERS. J. A. M. A., 1943, 122, 1217.
   b) CATALDO, R. J. Ann. Int. Med., 1946, 24, 479.
5. ZEMAN, F. D., AND SHEPPARD, S. Am. Heart J., 1945, 29, 597.
6. OSLER, W. Brit. M. J., 1885, 1, 467, 522, 577 and 607; also Quart. J. Med., 1908–09, 2, 219.
7. a) LIBMAN, E. Bull. Johns Hopkins Hosp., 1906, 17, 218.
   b) LIBMAN, E., AND FRIEDBERG, C. K. Subacute Bacterial Endocarditis. New York, Oxford Univ. Press, 1941.
8. KELSON, S. R., AND WHITE, P. D. Ann. Int. Med., 1945, 22, 40.
9. GROSS, L., AND CO-WORKERS. Arch. Int. Med., 1936, 58, 620. Also Am. J. Pathol., 1937, 13, 769.
10. BEAMER, R., REINHARD, E. H., AND GOODOF, I. I. Am. Heart J., 1945, 29, 99.
11. WILLIUS, F. A. Proc. Staff Meet., Mayo Clin., 1940, 15, 270; and 1944, 19, 497.
12. GELFMAN, B., AND LEVINE, S. A. Am. J. M. Sci., 1942, 204, 324.
13. CLAWSON, B. J. Arch. Int. Med., 1924, 33, 157.
14. BUCHBINDER, W. C., AND SAPHIR, O. Arch. Int. Med., 1939, 64, 336.
15. ZEMAN, F. D. Am. Heart J., 1945, 29, 661.
16. LOEHLEIN, M. Med. Klin., 1910, 6, 375.
17. MERKLEN, P., AND WOLF, M. Presse Méd., 1928, 36, 97.
18. KELSON, S., AND WHITE, P. D. J. A. M. A., 1939, 113, 1700.
19. LEACH, C. E., AND CO-WORKERS. J. A. M. A., 1941, 117, 1345.
20. KELFER, C. S., AND CO-WORKERS. J. A. M. A., 1943, 122, 1217.
21. LOEWE, L. Bull. New York Acad. Med., 1945, 21, 59.
22. DAWSON, M. H., AND HUNTER, T. H. J. A. M. A., 1945, 127, 129.
23. BLOOMFIELD, A. L. J. Clin. Investigation, 1945, 24, 251.
24. BRIN, L., AND GIROUX, L. La Syphilis du Coeur et de l'Aorte. Paris, Doin, 1924.
25. GALLAVARDIN, L. AND CHARVET: Quoted by BRIN AND GIROUX.
26. a) MENENDEZ DE OLIVEIRA, R. Escleroses Valvulares Calcificadas. Rio de Janeiro. Tip. do Patronato, 1943.
   b) FERTMAN, M. H., AND WOLFF, L. Am. Heart J., 1946, 31, 580.
27. COSTA, A. Clin. Med. Ital., 1930, 56, 572.
28. YATER, W. M. Arch. Path., 1929, 7, 418.
29. a) ABBOTT, M. E. Congenital Heart Disease. In Nelson's Loose Leaf Medicine. 4th Ed. New York, Nelson, 1944.
   b) ABBOTT, M. A. Atlas of Congenital Cardiac Disease. Am. Heart Assoc., New York, 1936.
30. BAILEY, O. T., AND HICKAM, J. B. Am. Heart J., 1944, 28, 578.
31. DAVID, J. M., AND SACHS, J. Am. Heart J., 1943, 26, 385.
32. FISHBERG, A. M. Heart Failure. Philadelphia, Lea and Febiger, 1940.
33. BLOOMFIELD, A. L., ARMSTRONG, C. D., AND KIRBY, W. M. M. J. Clin. Investigation, 1945, 24, 251.
34. McDONALD, R. K. Am. Heart J., 1946, 31, 308.
35. MAHAIM, I. Les Tumeurs et les Polypes du Coeur. Paris, Masson, 1945.
36. a) EVANS, M. E. Brit. Heart J., 1948, 10, 34.
   b) EVANS, M. E., AND BENSON, R. Brit. Heart J., 1948, 10, 39.
37. LIBMAN, E., AND SACKS, B. Arch. Int. Med., 1924, 33, 701.
38. KLEMPERER, P., POLLACK, A. D., AND BAEHR, G. Arch. Path., 1941, 32, 569.
39. GROSS, L. Vol. in honor of Dr. E. Libman, New York, Internat. Press, 1932.
40. BAGGENSTOSS, A. H. Proc. Staff Meet., Mayo Clinic, 1952, 27, 412.
41. ARENDT, J., AND CARDON, L. Radiology, 1949, 53, 371.
42. SAPHIR, O., KATZ, L. N., AND GORE, I. Circ., 1950, 1, 1155.
43. PERRY, E. L., FLEMING, R. G., AND EDWARDS, J. E. Ann. Int. Med., 1952, 36, 126.
44. BARKER, P. S. Meet. Am. Heart Assoc., 1948.

Chapter 11

The Valvular Defects of the Left Heart

Mitral Insufficiency

Mitral insufficiency occurs when the left atrioventricular valve is incompetent and does not prevent regurgitation of blood during ventricular contraction. This causes adaptations and changes both in the heart and in other organs, especially the lungs.

CAUSE

Different causes may lead to mitral insufficiency.

a) *Rheumatic endocarditis.* This is the most common cause of mitral insufficiency.

b) *Bacterial endocarditis.* A mild lesion due to the toxins of different germs and occasionally to their localization on the mitral valve may be the cause of mitral insufficiency. Among them, different Strepto- and Staphylococci, Pneumococci, Gonococci, and *E. typhi* have been described. A malignant bacterial endocarditis may also cause insufficiency, at times by perforation of a leaflet or rupture of a chorda.

c) *Syphilitic endocarditis.* This is usually due to the spreading of inflammation from the aortic to the mitral valve.

d) *Atherosclerosis.* This is a process of fibrosis which may be localized primarily on the mitral or spread from the aortic valve.

e) *Coronary heart disease.* Myocardial infarction may be followed by rupture of a chorda tendinea or even of a papillary muscle, causing mitral regurgitation of sudden appearance.

LESIONS

Mitral insufficiency is a common valvular lesion, alone or in combination with others.

Different types of lesions may cause regurgitation. The most common is a *retraction of the leaflets* which causes an imperfect adaptation of their margins (rheumatic endocarditis). There may be *ulceration* or *fragmentation* of the leaflets (malignant bacterial endocarditis). There may be *calcification* and even *ossification* of the valve (both in endocarditic and atherosclerotic types). There may be *shortening of one or more chordae* without lesion of the leaflets (septal and chordal endocarditis), and there may be *rupture* of one of them (bacterial endocarditis, myocardial infarction, old rheumatic lesions).

Both the left atrium and the left ventricle are dilated and their walls are hypertrophied. The right ventricle usually is not affected until late in the disease. The vessels of the pulmonary circulation are distended and have thickened walls.

SIGNS AND SYMPTOMS

Mitral insufficiency can be tolerated for a long time without any symptoms. However, prolonged effort may be followed by symptoms which are evidence of pulmonary congestion and left heart strain: *dyspnea, cough, precordial oppression, palpitation. Dysphagia* may be caused by left atrial enlargement. Physical exercise is followed by dyspnea and a rapid pulse. *The pulse is often of small amplitude.* Other symptoms, if present, are evidence of initial heart failure: pain in the upper right abdominal quadrant, dependent edema, obstinate cough, attacks of nocturnal dyspnea; the patient may present a slight *cyanosis.*

Local Signs

The jugular veins may be slightly distended and often present active pulsations.

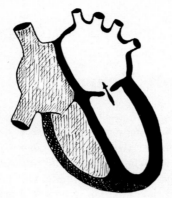

Fig. 117. Changes of the heart in mitral insufficiency.

There may be a *precordial bulge* (mainly in children).

The *apical thrust*, easily visible and sudden, is in the 5th or 6th left interspace. At times, when exceptional hypertrophy of the left ventricle is present, a massive movement of the precordium toward the left may be observed (1). Multiple pulsations in different interspaces are often present, especially in children. Among them, pulsation in the 2nd left interspace is the most common. A systolic pulsation of the right side of the chest has been observed in cases complicated by aneurysmal dilatation of the left atrium (1b).

Percussion reveals a practically normal heart in the initial stages. Later, an *elongated heart* is found (fig. 118).

Auscultation. In initial or slight mitral insufficiency, the *first sound* becomes prolonged, blowing, and impure at the apex. If regurgitation is more severe, a *blowing, soft, systolic murmur* is heard. This starts after the first sound, has its maximum intensity at the apex, and is heard clearly at the left axilla. The murmur may be *musical, harsh,* or resemble *the cry of a sea-gull*. The latter is more common when there is either calcification of the mitral valve or a vibrating broken chorda. When the murmur is very loud, it can be heard all over the precordium and the back.

A *systolic murmur may be present at the*

pulmonic area. This murmur is encountered most easily in the initial stages of the disease. It should be considered as a "functional" murmur, caused by the distention of the pulmonary artery.

BLOOD PRESSURE

It is common to observe a slightly low systolic and normal (or slightly high) diastolic pressure. Normal (or even slightly high) systolic pressure is present in some cases.

The pressure in the *tibial artery* is usually equal to or lower than that in the brachial

GRAPHIC RECORDS

Electrocardiogram

Increased voltage of the ventricular complex in the limb and chest leads is not unusual. *Left axis deviation* may be noted whenever the left ventricle is enlarged; thus QRS has waves mainly directed upwards in aVL and in 1; downwards in aVF and 3; a qR complex is noted in the chest leads V4 to V6. If the left ventricle is markedly hypertrophied (as in advanced cases), some degree of broadening of the complex is present. Left ventricular "strain", revealed by inverted T in aVL, 1, and the chest leads V5–V6, may occur. The P wave is frequently tall, notched, or diphasic, as a result of left atrial enlargement. The P-R interval may be slightly prolonged, reaching from 0.20 to 0.24 second as a result of an old rheumatic lesion of the conducting system. Atrial fibrillation is frequent, especially if the patient is in failure, or has been digitalized for several years.

Phonocardiogram

In initial or slight insufficiency, a simple *prolongation of the central phase of the first sound* is present; later, the vibrations of the first sound continue during the first half of systole with decreasing intensity. When mitral insufficiency is established, three types of murmurs can be recorded (fig. 119).

1) A *systolic murmur* with gradually de-

creasing vibrations, both high- and low-pitched. This systolic murmur *"in decre-scendo"* is the most common finding.

2) A systolic murmur which continues throughout all systole with the same intensity; the vibrations are mostly high-pitched (soft murmur). This *"all systolic"* *murmur* is less common and is found mostly in children.

3) A *late systolic murmur* with increasing intensity before the second sound. This systolic murmur *"in crescendo"* is rare.

The first high vibration of the first sound-complex may be high (*closing snap of the mitral valve*). The second high vibration of the second sound-complex may become more visible and high-pitched (*opening snap of the mitral valve*). This phenomenon, however, is already evidence of a more severe damage to the valve and possibly of initial stenosis.

One of the diastolic sounds (third sound; fourth sound) or both, may become high. When only one of them is loud, auscultation reveals a *triple rhythm* (fig. 119a). When both are loud, a *diastolic rumble* may be heard (fig. 120b). An incorrect diagnosis of mitral stenosis may be made in such cases upon clinical auscultation. This is more common in children but also is frequently observed in adults.

Tracings recorded over the pulmonary artery may show a distinct *systolic murmur* and a *loud* or *split second sound*.

Apex Cardiogram

The low frequency tracing of the apex often shows the following changes: quick rise followed by sudden drop before the end of the first sound-complex; low level of the point 2b; at times, high waves during diastole (both the waves 3 and 4 are high) (fig. 120b).

Low frequency tracings recorded outside the apex (regional cardiograms) show: 1) high atrial wave *4* over the midprecordium (strong left atrial contraction), and 2) high vascular wave *p* at the 2nd left interspace (high pulmonic pulsation).

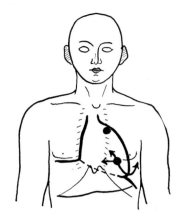

Fig. 118. Cardiac dulness and transmission of the murmur in mitral insufficiency.

Electrokymogram

This tracing is of primary importance for diagnosis. The electrokymogram should be recorded as a *border tracing of the left atrial appendage* and of *the posterior border of the left atrium* in both oblique positions (p. 148) and in one of the lateral positions. A densogram of the left atrium can also be recorded in certain cases.

The normal tracings of the left atrium consist of a sharp negative wave in presystole (inward motion caused by atrial contraction) and a more rounded negative wave in systole (inward motion caused by lowering of the a-v septum, only partly compensated by venous flow into the atrium). In cases of mitral insufficiency, a new pattern is visible:

1) The presystolic negative wave is deeper and broader (unless there is atrial fibrillation) on account of stronger atrial contraction.

2) The systolic negative wave has disappeared and is substituted by *a positive plateau*. There is a rapid rise in early systole; a sharp angle; a straight or concave line in systole; another sharp angle; then a rapid drop after the opening of the mitral valve (fig. 121).

The systolic plateau is the graphic expression of a "systolic swelling" of the left atrium during ventricular systole, caused by the

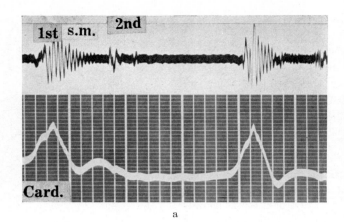

a

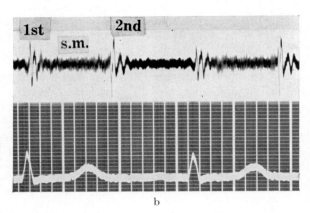

b

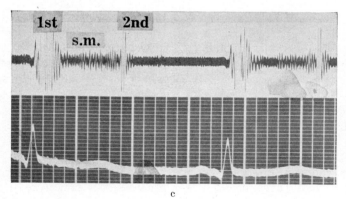

c

FIG. 119. Systolic murmur in three cases of mitral valve disease with predominant regurgitation (phonocardiograms). a, systolic murmur in decrescendo; b, soft continuous systolic murmur; c, systolic murmur in crescendo.

blood which regurgitates from the left ventricle. It is similar to a tracing of intraventricular pressure and quite different from the normal pattern (fig. 122).

The various stages of insufficiency, from the slightest degree to the severe regurgitation, are revealed by successive substitution of the plateau for the normal systolic trough

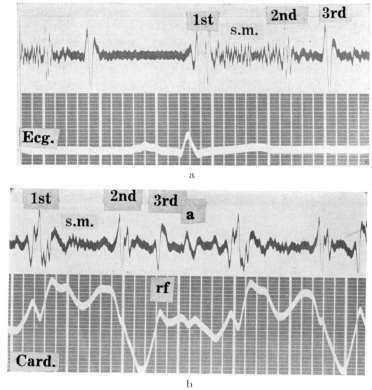

FIG. 120. a, Phonocardiogram of mitral regurgitation. Long and loud systolic murmur. Ventricular type of triple rhythm. b, Phonocardiogram (above) and low frequency tracing (below) at the apex in a case of mitral regurgitation. Faint systolic murmur (s.m.); loud diastolic sounds (*3rd, a*) creating a quadruple rhythm.

(fig. 123). It is likely, though not proven, that this indicates a moderate regurgitation. The existence of this diagnostic pattern, which had been previously detected by roentgenkymography, was demonstrated by the author with Fleischner (70) and confirmed by various other researchers.

Esophagocardiogram

This tracing, recorded at the level of the left atrium, shows a typical pattern. This consists of a high, positive plateau which replaces the normal negative wave present during ventricular systole. This pattern is particularly typical if the tracing is recorded by an electromanometer esophagopiezogram (80). The importance of this tracing is decreased by the ease of recording an elec-trokymogram, and the typical pattern revealed by that method. However, an esophagocardiogram can be studied if one lacks an electrokymograph.

X-RAY

Increased size of the left ventricle is apparent in the frontal view (fig. 124). The oblique positions show *an increase in size of the left atrial shadow* which tends to be confused with the shadow of the spine. There is a displacement of the esophagus toward the right. *The left atrium expands in systole.*

In some cases, the left atrium is so dilated as to be visible on the right side of the right atrium in the frontal position (*aneurysm of the left atrium*, page 394). The right ventricle and the pulmonary artery may be dilated,

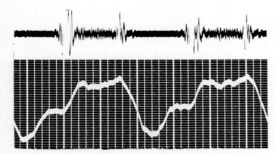

FIG. 121. Electrokymogram of left atrium (border tracing) in a case of mitral regurgitation. Left oblique position.

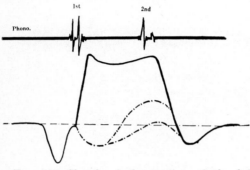

FIG. 122. Sketch of the tracing of the left atrium in a case of mitral lesion with sinus rhythm. The thin dotted line represents the arbitrary baseline; the heavy dotted line indicates normal tracings during ventricular systole. (From Luisada and Fleischner, Am. J. Med.)

but less than the left sections of the heart. The hilar shadows are thicker than usual but present normal pulsations. The dilated left atrium may cause transmitted systolic pulsations of the right hilum (6) and the right bronchus (7).

MODE OF ORIGIN OF THE SIGNS

Mitral insufficiency has a notable importance; it may be isolated or associated to mitral stenosis. As revealed by electrokymographic tracings of the left atrium and by animal experimentation, it causes backflow of an important mass of blood into the left atrium during ventricular systole.

In experiments with models of the circulation, insufficiency of the mitral valve causes both *a rise of the mean pressure of the left atrium and a drop of the mean arterial pressure.* An artificial increase of the ventricular stroke reestablishes normal conditions (9a).

In animal experimentation, insufficiency of the mitral valve causes little change in arterial pressure, rise of left atrial pressure, and no increase in the pressure of the pulmonary artery (9a). The left ventricle compensates later by restoring the systolic discharge to normal.

Mechanical tracings in animals (9a) and electrokymograms recorded over the left atrial border in man indicate that the regurgitation of blood is slight during the tension period and occurs mainly during systolic ejection. The amount of backflow is limited by the rapid development of pressure. If the myocardium is impaired, the rise in pressure occurs more slowly and the effects are more serious. The backflow, taking place during ventricular systole, first causes dilatation of the left atrium, then hypertrophy of its wall. Both of these factors increase the power of the atrium which sends a greater amount of blood to the ventricle in presystole. This will cause dilatation of the left ventricle and hypertrophy of its wall. The backflow causes increased pressure in the left atrium and in the pulmonary veins.

The *systolic murmur* is caused by the stream of blood regurgitating into the atrium. Whether the murmur is due to the whirlpools of the stream or to the vibrations of the wall is still a moot question. While the murmur is a common occurrence, regurgitation may occur even without a systolic murmur, as revealed by electrokymography (70).

Increased pressure and distention of the pulmonary artery taking place in the early stages cause the pulmonic systolic murmur (relative stenosis or trigonoidation—page 179) and the loud or split 2nd sound over the pulmonic area. These findings usually disappear later.

The increased atrial pressure and the stronger atrial contraction cause the loud diastolic sounds frequently recorded.

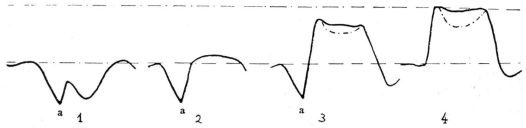

FIG. 123. Schematic tracings of the left atrium in mitral lesions: 1, normal; 2, initial neutralization of systolic collapse; 3, sinus rhythm, positive systolic plateau, no trace of atrial activity. (From Luisada and Fleischner, Am. J. Med.)

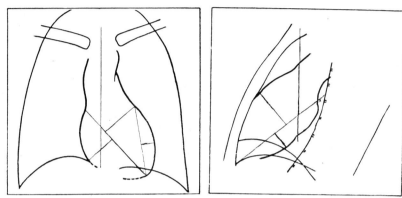

FIG. 124. X-ray configuration of the heart in mitral insufficiency. Frontal and left anterior oblique positions. (From Benedetti and Bollini.)

The dilatation of the pulmonary veins and the anastomoses between pulmonic and bronchial circulation explain the frequent *bronchial catarrh*. When the pulmonary circulation is engorged, some degree of cyanosis may occur.

COURSE AND COMPLICATIONS

Mitral insufficiency, rheumatic in origin, is frequently followed by mitral stenosis. It is, therefore, the first stage of a progressive disease which is liable to become more severe. If, however, many years have passed since the beginning of the valvular defect and no stenosis can be ascertained, this is less likely to occur unless a new attack of rheumatic disease takes place.

Mitral insufficiency of nonrheumatic nature is seldom accompanied by stenosis and bears no danger of increased severity through recurrence of endocarditis.

Chronic distention of the left atrium causes *fibrosis* of its wall. This, on the one hand, favors *atrial fibrillation* or *flutter* and, on the other, a further distention, with possible formation of an aneurysm of the left atrium (65). These complications favor *thrombosis of the left atrium* and possible formation of a ball thrombus (page 214).

Distention of the left atrium may cause *compression of the left recurrent nerve* and of branches of the azygos vein. If the membrane occluding the foramen ovale is not firm, the increased pressure in the left atrium may cause its *rupture* with a clinical picture similar to Lutembacher's syndrome (page 304).

Bacterial endocarditis may be favored by the valvular lesion.

Heart failure is a possible occurrence and presents a typical picture (page 563).

Cases where the insufficiency is caused by

rupture of one of the chordae present sudden onset of the signs and symptoms. Heart failure may be insidious or abrupt in its onset and progressive or remittent in its course. Months and even years may elapse between rupture and the onset of frank heart failure (10).

DIAGNOSIS

The two fundamental signs on which the diagnosis should be based are: 1) *The apical systolic murmur*, and 2) *the systolic expansion of the left atrium*, both caused by the regurgitation of blood. The first can be investigated by auscultation and phonocardiography; the second, by fluoroscopy, esophagocardiography, and electrokymography.

If the data supplied by the latter methods are not available or are not clear, the murmur becomes even more important. The typical area of auscultation, the radiation of the murmur, and the increased intensity of the 2nd pulmonic sound are evidence of an actual regurgitation of blood and not of an inconspicuous or unimportant murmur. A history of rheumatic attacks is also important.

I.v. septal defect. The murmur of an interventricular septal defect is harsh, is accompanied by a thrill, is loudest in the 3rd left interspace, and is well transmitted toward the right but not too well toward the apex. There is no enlargement and no systolic expansion of the left atrium (roentgenkymogram, electrokymogram) (page 284).

Aortic stenosis. The heart is more elongated in aortic stenosis than in mitral insufficiency. The murmur is of maximum intensity over the 2nd right interspace and is transmitted to the suprasternal notch (12) and along the carotid arteries. The pulse is typical. The murmur has a different appearance on phonocardiograms (page 250).

Mitral stenosis. The exclusion of a pure mitral stenosis is easy as the latter has no systolic murmur. The exclusion of a double mitral defect is sometimes more difficult. The x-ray, auscultation, phonocardiography,

and electrocardiography are of help in the diagnosis (page 235).

VARIETIES

The picture given by *rupture of one of the chordae* consists of the sudden appearance of a loud systolic murmur and thrill, maximal at the apex and at the left sternal border (10) (page 214). Bacterial endocarditis, myocardial infarction, and rheumatic heart disease are possible causes. Differential diagnosis includes perforation of the interventricular septum (page 284) and rupture of either a cusp or a papillary muscle.

The *rupture of a papillary muscle* is rare and is usually followed by immediate death. Occasional longer survival may permit diagnosis. This is based on the sudden occurrence of a loud, rough, harsh systolic murmur over the apex and mid-precordium, associated with the clinical picture of myocardial infarction (page 419).

TREATMENT

If mitral insufficiency is due to old rheumatic disease and is well compensated, no treatment is necessary. Avoidance of physical strain and moderation in the quantity of food and drink are good precautions. If the patient complains of palpitation or presents premature beats, *bromides* (32), *quinidine* (24), or *phenobarbital* (29), are indicated.

If rheumatic disease is recent, the patient should be kept under observation for possible prevention and treatment of new episodes (page 190) and also because mitral stenosis may still develop. Congestive failure and atrial fibrillation are possible complications and should receive the necessary treatment (pages 563 and 343).

Surgical repair of severe mitral insufficiency has been tried (76). The earlier attempts were based on the creation of *a new valve* of the *sling* or *hammock* type made of pericardium, vein, or tendon. Better results were obtained by the creation of a pedicle tube graft of pericardium with intact blood supply. Further experiments were based on the passing of a loop of thread around the chordae in an attempt to reduce the size of the valvular opening or on implantation of a plastic valve. So far, surgical therapy of mitral insufficiency is unsatisfactory.

Relative Mitral Insufficiency

The closure of the mitral opening is perfect only if both the ventricle and the atrium are capable of an effective contraction and if the atrial contraction precedes the ventricular. Therefore, mitral insufficiency may be present: a) In myocarditis and myocardial infarction. b) In heart failure, vitamin B deficiency, hypertensive heart, and anemia. c) In toxic conditions (icterus). d) In heart block and in different types of premature beats.

Thyrocardiacs or patients with acute anemia may have an *apical systolic murmur*. This murmur may be due to a muscular weakness, as described above, or may be caused by a different mechanism which does not include blood regurgitation (pages 83 and 178).

In general, the murmur of relative mitral insufficiency is *soft* and not very long; it is clearly heard at the apex and is transmitted toward the axilla only to a limited extent; there are no signs of increased pressure in the pulmonic circulation. It is customary to say that this murmur disappears after physical exercise but this is seldom true.

In general, the electrocardiogram is normal or reflects changes caused by coronary or hypertensive heart disease or by lesions of other valves.

The phonocardiogram presents a series of high-pitched vibrations of poor amplitude during systole. There may be no real systolic murmur while the first sound is prolonged. There may be accentuation of those low-pitched vibrations, caused by vascular distention, which are frequently found in normal subjects and represent the last phase of the first sound (page 91).

The electrokymogram of the left atrium may be entirely normal. However, if the functional disorder causes an actual and important regurgitation of blood, the typical pattern of regurgitation (plateau) may be present.

Mitral Stenosis[51]

Mitral stenosis is a narrowing of the left ventricular orifice. This causes compensations and adaptations in different parts of the cardiovascular apparatus and in extracardiac organs.

CAUSE

a) The most usual cause of mitral stenosis is *rheumatic endocarditis*. Mitral stenosis, caused by *benign nonrheumatic endocarditis* is theoretically possible but not proven.

b) *Bacterial endocarditis* may cause mitral stenosis. The cases were rare in the past but are increasing in number.

c) *Congenital mitral stenosis* is possible but rare. Many cases once labelled as congenital are due to fetal or infantile endocarditis. However, this is often a mild inflammatory process which, while causing slight deformity of the leaflets, prevents a normal development of the valvular opening. Therefore, some aspects may be similar to those of a congenital lesion.

d) *Sudden obstruction* of the mitral valve may be due to a thrombus, polyp, or myxoma of the left atrium (page 214).

e) In elderly patients, *fibrosis* or *calcification* of the mitral annulus may cause mitral stenosis. This process, which is due to atherosclerosis, is independent of aortic calcification of the Moenckeberg type (81). It may be associated to a-v block (66). It may be part of a general process of *calcification of the heart* including the pericardium (67).

LESIONS

Mitral stenosis is a common valvular defect, following in frequency mitral and aortic regurgitation. It is seen somewhat more often in females.

[51] This disease was described by *Duroziez* who attributed it to a congenital lesion.

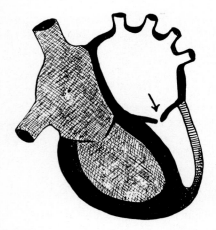

FIG. 125. Changes of the heart in mitral stenosis.

The problem of whether "pure" mitral stenosis exists has been discussed repeatedly. There is no doubt that, in some hearts, the opening is narrowed, while the valves are completely competent. However, this is not the rule. The most typical cases present a small opening at the end of a funnel which is caused by the fusion of the two leaflets and projects into the left ventricle (fig. 126). The opening may be round or oval and is far smaller than normal. Sometimes the entire atrioventricular orifice is smaller than average.

In typical cases, the *left ventricle* is either normal or small. The cardiac apex is then formed by the right ventricle which pushes the left backwards. Both the *left atrium* and the *right ventricle* are severely dilated and have thick walls. The left atrium may occasionally reach the size of a fetus' head. *Mural thrombi* are often present in the left atrial cavity, occasionally also in the right.

A fibrotic process is often seen in the posterior aspect of the left atrium (*body of MacCallum*). This process may occasionally become calcified.

The *pulmonary artery* is dilated and has a thickened wall. It may present atherosclerosis. The branches of the pulmonary artery and the pulmonary veins are distended and have thick, sometimes sclerotic, walls.

Pulmonary, splenic, and renal infarctions are frequent.

Most organs present the customary appearance of chronic stasis. Among them, chronic pulmonary congestion and chronic pulmonary edema are usually observed.

Large varicosities are frequently observed in the bronchial veins (fig. 127).

SIGNS AND SYMPTOMS

Mitral stenosis is often well tolerated for a long time and may be discovered by chance or because circulatory embarrassment arises during pregnancy or after strenuous exercise.

Mitral stenosis is a disease of the young. Nevertheless, greater numbers are discovered in the aged. While many of them acquired the disease in the second half of their life, some patients over 70 had mitral stenosis since adolescence.

Infantilism or dwarfism (mitral dwarfism) may be seen in cases of congenital nature or early onset.

The first revealing symptoms usually follow emotion, exercise, pregnancy, or acute infections. They are dyspnea, palpitation, weakness, and precordial pain. The *pain* is occasionally located in the back at the left of the spine, but is localized more often in the precordium. It may be described as a smothering feeling, or a sticking pain.

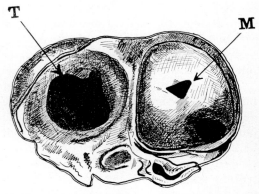

FIG. 126. Section of the heart in mitral stenosis. Narrowing of the mitral valve (M) and dilatation of the tricuspid valve (T). (Inspired by originals of P. D. White.)

The patients often complain of *obstinate dry cough* or bronchial catarrh. *Hemorrhagic sputum* and even *abundant hemoptysis* are not unusual. *Difficulty in swallowing* and *changes of the voice* may occur.

At some stage, *nocturnal dyspnea* and *orthopnea* occur, *pitting edema* is present, and pain is felt in the right upper quadrant of the abdomen. *Weakness* and *oliguria* then complete the picture of heart failure.

These patients are moderately *cyanotic*. The cyanosis is present typically on the lips, nosetip, and earlobes (*facies mitralica*). It may be accentuated at the extremities (*acrocyanosis*) and associated with low skin temperature. Some patients, however, are *pale* and give the impression of being anemic.

The radial pulse is *small* and is frequently irregular. The *jugular veins* are slightly distended and show visible pulsations.

There may be *dysphonia* due to paralysis of the left recurrent nerve (*Ortner sign*). This disturbance, which is due to compression of the nerve by the large left atrium, is sometimes reversible.

Local Signs

If the disease has been acquired in early childhood, a typical *precordial bulge* is present. There may be small venous dilatations over the precordium.

The *apical thrust* may be displaced to the left; it may be replaced by a diffuse pulsation, multiple pulsations, or an *inward thrust of the apex* (1). There may be a *forward thrust of the lower part of the sternum or of the epigastrium.*

On palpation, a snap at the end of systole may be distinguished over the second left interspace. In *the most typical finding the apical thrust is followed by a snap (Cossio's sign).* This is due to the fact that the closure of the mitral valve is delayed and is not simultaneous with the thrust, as in normal people (2).

A *diastolic thrill* may be felt over the 4th interspace and at the apex.

Percussion shows that the cardiac apex

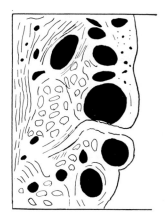

FIG. 127. Varicosities of the bronchial veins (black circles) in severe mitral stenosis. (Inspired by originals of Ferguson.)

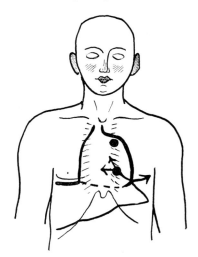

FIG. 128. Cardiac dulness and transmission of murmurs in mitral stenosis.

is often in the normal seat. There is a typical *dulness in the 3rd left interspace.* Cardiac dulness starts far more to the right than with the normal heart. A median heart with a large transverse diameter and a broad base is frequently observed (*coeur en sabot*) (fig. 128).

Auscultation may reveal a *diastolic rumble*, a *presystolic murmur* "in crescendo" ending with a loud first sound, or both. It is possible to hear a *loud snapping sound after the 2nd sound* and no murmurs.

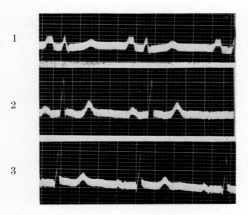

FIG. 129. Electrocardiogram in mitral stenosis. Long P-R, notched P, right axis shift.

A presystolic murmur alone is heard when the diastolic rumble is absent or low-pitched (and, therefore, inaudible). A diastolic rumble alone is the rule whenever atrial fibrillation prevents the possibility of a coordinated contraction of the atria.

The loud snapping diastolic sound is the *opening snap of the mitral valve* described by *Potain* (13). It is audible all over the precordium and is well separated from the 2nd sound. It is due to a creaking noise made by the mitral valve at the time of its opening.

The *2nd pulmonic sound* is usually *loud* and may be *split*. There may be a *systolic* pulmonic murmur of functional nature. A *soft diastolic murmur* of functional nature may be occasionally heard at the pulmonic area (*Graham Steell murmur* (14)).

A systolic murmur at the apex indicates mitral insufficiency.

BLOOD PRESSURE

Blood pressure may be normal, high, or low.

High blood pressure is found more often in middle-aged or elderly people because of association with renal or vascular lesions. However, hypertension may be temporary, resulting from latent heart failure (anoxemia, stimulation of the vasomotor center).

Low blood pressure is common when mitral stenosis is acquired in infancy. Severe mitral stenosis may cause low blood pressure with low pulse pressure.

There is a *relative hypotension in the legs*.

GRAPHIC TRACINGS

Electrocardiogram

Several changes may be observed (fig. 129):

1) High, diphasic, or notched P wave in the limb leads. Diphasic P in V1 and V2.

2) A prolonged P-R interval (0.21–0.24 second).

3) Right axis deviation, revealed by comparing aVL with aVF, or lead 1 with lead 3.

4) A shift of the transitional zone in the chest leads revealing that the right ventricle forms all of the anterior portion of the heart and even the apex (rS complex in V1 to V5).

5) Possible right bundle branch block or intraventricular block.

6) Possible disturbances of the rhythm consisting of atrial premature contractions, atrial flutter or fibrillation, paroxysmal atrial tachycardia, or ventricular tachycardia.

Phonocardiogram

The findings vary with different auscultatory signs and over different areas.

1) There may be a *presystolic murmur "in crescendo" at the apex*. This reveals itself by a series of oscillations in late diastole which then increase in intensity and fuse with the 1st sound (fig. 130b and c). If the conduction time is long, the presystolic murmur may be separated from the first sound and loses its "crescendo" type. In extreme prolongation of conduction, this murmur may even fall in early diastole. This murmur disappears if there is atrial fibrillation.

2) There may be a *rumbling diastolic murmur, also at the apex*. This is revealed by a series of irregular and low-pitched vibrations (fig. 130a, b, d). They start some time after the main oscillation of the second

sound-complex with a small but rapid vibration (the opening snap of the mitral valve); they continue until middiastole or late diastole with decreasing intensity, and then disappear. There may be a pause between this murmur and the presystolic murmur, if diastole is long. If, on the contrary, diastole is short, the diastolic murmur continues and fuses with the presystolic murmur. A loud sound equivalent to a *gallop sound* may be recognized within the murmur if the stenosis is not severe.

3) The *opening snap of the mitral valve* (fig. 130d) is a typical vibration which, alone, is sufficient to diagnose a lesion of the mitral valve, and probably mitral stenosis. It is a rapid vibration which is separated from the main vibration of the second sound-complex by an interval of from 0.08 to 0.12 second. The interval is of variable length from cycle to cycle if there is atrial fibrillation (74). The snap is frequently followed by diastolic vibrations but it may be isolated. It is recorded best at the midprecordium. It should be distinguished both from the physiologic opening sound of the mitral valve and from the third sound (or gallop sound) (fig. 131). It coincides with the point 2b of the cardiogram and with the v wave of the jugular tracing (if the latter is not delayed). It may be recorded over a large area of the chest, at times even outside the precordium.

4) It is common to observe the vibrations of *a systolic murmur over the pulmonic area*. There frequently is a *split second sound* (fig. 131). The distance between the two phases of this split sound varies from 0.04 to 0.08 second. Very seldom is the splitting audible when the interval is below 0.06.

5) There may be an early-diastolic murmur in decrescendo at the pulmonic area, due to pulmonic insufficiency (*Graham Steell murmur*). This murmur is usually of short duration, appearing only during congestive failure. A persistent murmur indicates sclerotic or endocarditic pulmonic insufficiency. An aortic diastolic murmur re-

corded in this region is, of course, extremely common.

When atrial fibrillation is present, the interval between QRS of the electrocardiogram and the main vibration of the 1st sound-complex may vary, becoming longer when the preceding diastole is short on account of delayed mitral valve closure. Thus the interval between QRS and the first high vibration of the first sound may become variable (15, 16, 74).

When no audible murmur exists, either there is no murmur (rare) or there are low-pitched, inaudible, vibrations during diastole (*subsonic murmur*). In both cases, the murmur may appear or become audible after exercise.

Cardiogram

The low frequency tracing of the apex (*apex cardiogram*) may reveal the following phenomena:

1) Slow rise of the tracing during the tension period with a delay of the peak 1a (delayed closure of the mitral valve).

2) Slow descent of the tracing after the point 2a (delayed opening of the mitral valve) and a slow rise afterwards (slow filling in early diastole). (fig. 130b.)

3) Small or absent atrial wave (difficult filling of the left ventricle).

The low frequency tracing of the second left interspace (*regional cardiogram*) often reveals a high systolic wave (large pulsation of the pulmonary artery). That recorded over the third left interspace may present a high atrial wave (large pulsation of the left atrium).

Epigastric Tracing

The epigastric tracing frequently shows a high atrial wave (large pulsation of the right atrium) and a high systolic pulsation (strong contraction of the right ventricle).

Electrokymogram

The electrokymogram of the left atrium frequently reveals the typical pattern of

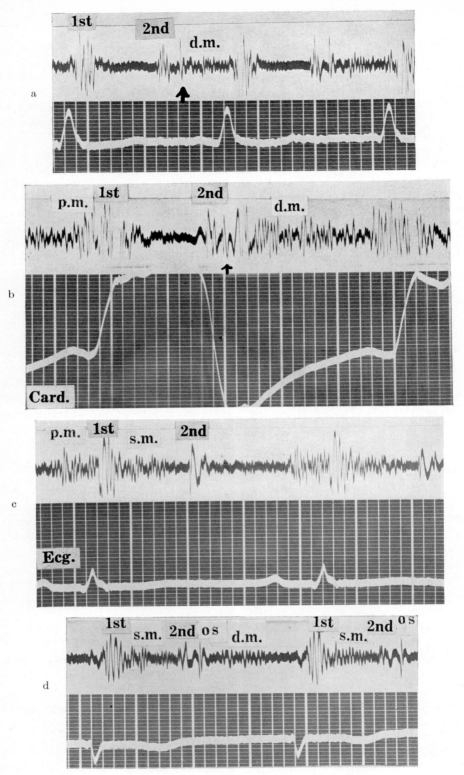

Fig. 130

230

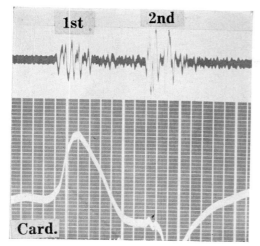

FIG. 131. Loud and split second pulmonic sound in mitral stenosis. Phonocardiogram and low frequency tracing over pulmonic area.

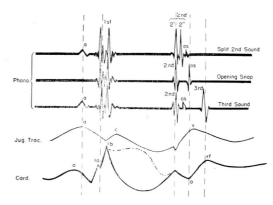

FIG. 132. Differential diagnosis between split second pulmonic sound (2nd), opening snap of the mitral valve (os), and third sound (ventricular type of triple rhythm). The jugular tracing and the low frequency tracing of the apex are used for identification of the additional sound in early diastole.

mitral regurgitation (p. 219) even in cases where no systolic murmur was heard or recorded. However, cases of pure mitral stenosis may not present it. The stenosis of the mitral valve is frequently revealed by a small, notched, or prolonged atrial wave in presystole. If there is atrial fibrillation, the presystolic atrial wave disappears.

Cardiomanometry

Catheterization of the right heart reveals that the pressure of the right ventricle, pulmonary artery, and pulmonary capillaries, is frequently increased. This is due to the narrowing of the mitral valve plus structural changes of the arterioles, and frequently also pulmonary vasoconstriction. Average values for the pulmonary artery are 30/16 in patients without heart failure and 69/34 in patients with failure. These values should be compared with the normal average figures of 20/9. Direct re-

cording of pressure in the left atrium before commissurotomy has revealed normal or slightly elevated diastolic pressures and systolic pressures of 25–30 mm. Hg resulting from the insufficiency of the mitral valve. Evaluation of the mitral area and of the regurgitant flow has been attempted on the basis of data supplied by cardiomanometry.

X-RAY

The typical aspect of the cardiac shadow is that of a silhouette with increased transverse diameter and a reduced length of the left ventricular arch. The right ventricle is broadened. The middle arch is bulging. The apex is rounded (fig. 133).

The anterior development of the right ventricle is apparent chiefly in the lateral positions. *The left atrium is very large* so that its shadow is confused with that of the spine in the oblique positions. *It may be-*

FIG. 130. Cases of mitral stenosis. a, Phonocardiogram at apex and electrocardiogram. Atrial fibrillation. Opening snap of the mitral valve (os); diastolic rumble. b, Phonocardiogram and low frequency tracing (Card.) at apex. Sinus rhythm. Opening snap of the mitral valve (os); diastolic-presystolic murmur. Slow filling of the left ventricle in early diastole. c, Phonocardiogram at apex and electrocardiogram. Sinus rhythm. Presystolic murmur (p.m.) and systolic murmur (s.m.). d, Phonocardiogram at apex and electrocardiogram. Atrial fibrillation. Systolic murmur (s.m.); opening snap (os); diastolic murmur (d.m.).

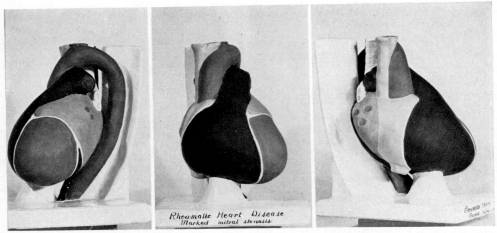

FIG. 133. X-ray model of the heart in mitral stenosis (from a model of the American Heart Association.)

come visible as a thicker shadow within that of the right atrium in the frontal position and may overlap the latter, forming a second border at the right of the right atrium. More rarely, the left atrial shadow creates a second image outside the left cardiac border (fig. 136).

The enlargement of the middle arch is due to two different factors: dilatation of the pulmonary artery and enlargement of the left appendage. The enlarged conus of the right ventricle usually does not reach the left border (23). The calcified mitral valve is visible in some cases (fig. 134).

The left bronchus is bent; the esophagus is compressed and displaced posteriorly and to the right by the left atrium (fig. 135). The hilar shadows are usually dilated and thick. The right hilum may show pulsations transmitted from the left atrium.

Roentgenkymography reveals a slow diastolic filling of the left ventricle and a slow contraction of the left atrium. The middle arch shows pulsations of a vascular type in the upper part, and of atrial type in the lower (22).

Angiocardiography has confirmed that the left atrium is the main factor in determining

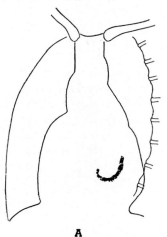
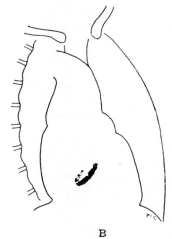

A   B

FIG. 134. Horseshoe calcification of the mitral valve in the left (A) and right (B) oblique positions. (From M. de Oliveira.)

a mitral configuration and in displacing the pulmonary artery (23) upwards and anteriorly.

In simple circulation models, the production of a severe mitral stenosis causes decreased systolic discharge, reduction in arterial pressure, accumulation of "blood" in the left atrium and its tributary veins, and increase of the mean pressure of the pulmonary artery (9a). Animal experimentation confirms these facts. The reduction of the mean aortic pressure and of the pulse pressure is then gradually compensated by higher atrial pressure and stronger atrial contractions as well as by prolonged ventricular filling.

The results of narrowing of the mitral valve are felt mainly in the left atrium, in the pulmonary circulation, and in the right ventricle. The chambers involved dilate and present a gradual hypertrophy of their walls. A similar process occurs in the pulmonary vessels.

As the normal filling of the ventricles takes place mainly during two phases, early diastole (passive rapid filling) and presystole (atrial contraction), blood passing through the narrow orifice will create both a thrill and a murmur in those two phases.

If atrial fibrillation exists, the presystolic murmur disappears.

When the efficiency of the heart muscle is good, the amount of blood reaching the left ventricle is normal or subnormal and the size of the other heart chambers is limited. Thus the murmur may be reduced to a few low-pitched vibrations or even disappear. This occurs at times after digitalization.

When a *systolic murmur* exists, it is due to associated mitral regurgitation and not to stenosis.

There are cases where, in spite of the existing atrial fibrillation, a presystolic murmur is heard. It is an acoustic illusion because the closure of the mitral valve is delayed (main vibration of the 1st sound) and the small initial vibrations of the 1st sound seem presystolic.

Hardening of the structures of the mitral valve and difficult ventricular filling explain the loud 1st sound (*closing snap of the mitral*) and its delay over the apical thrust. They also explain the apparent splitting of the 2nd sound (main vibration of the 2nd sound-complex followed by the *opening snap of the mitral*).

Actual splitting of the 2nd sound, when present, is due to a nonsimultaneous closing of the semilunar valves of the aorta and the

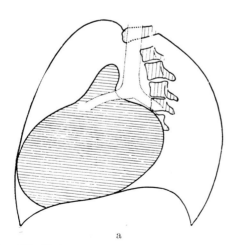 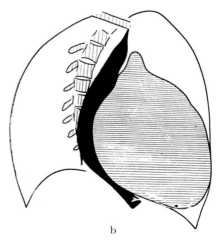

a   b

FIG. 135. Enlargement of the left atrium causing a bronchial angle above 70° with bending of the left bronchus (a), and indentation of the esophagus (b). (From Cossio.)

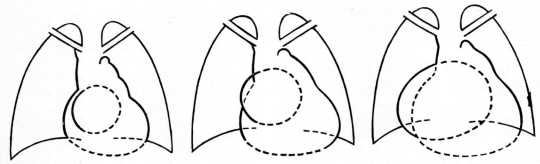

FIG. 136. Aneurysm of the left atrium in PA view. The rounded shadow, due to the left atrium, gradually emerges from the cardiac silhouette. (From Laubry.)

pulmonary artery. The high pressure of the latter causes an early and snapping closure of the leaflets. A soft diastolic murmur over the pulmonary artery (*Graham Steell murmur*) is usually due to relative insufficiency and is found rarely except when heart failure is also present (14, 24). If the murmur persists, it has a different significance and is due to anatomical changes (pages 301 and 304).

Precordial pain at times is due to coronary heart disease. However, it is more often due to anoxia with an overworked and hypertrophied myocardium (25).

Difficulty in swallowing and changes of the voice, as well as posterior pain, are caused by the enlarged left atrium. This organ displaces the esophagus (*dysphagia*), compresses the left recurrent nerve (*dysphonia*), and impinges on the spine (*pain*).

Percussion, x-ray, cardiography, and phonocardiography reveal data which are due to the already described changes in the shape and function of the heart. The longer course followed by the stimulus in the left atrial wall explains why the left P wave is often delayed or abnormal. *Prolongation of the P-R interval* may be caused by minute scars left in the conducting tissues by rheumatic disease.

Persistent distention of the pulmonary veins and the anastomoses between these and the bronchial veins explain why recurrent bronchitis and *chronic bronchial catarrh* are so frequent. The *hemorrhagic sputum* (hemoptysis) is explained both by

the high pressure in the lung capillaries and by the frequent occurrence of *varicosities* in the bronchial veins (26a) (fig. 127). A process of arteriosclerosis of the pulmonary vessels may occur, increasing the effects of the high pressure and further favoring the hemoptysis.

Cyanosis is partly of central type and is caused by the reduced size of the alveolar spaces (distended capillaries) and by the slower pulmonary circulation. If congestive failure occurs, an important peripheral element is added.

COURSE AND COMPLICATIONS

In some patients, mitral stenosis gradually becomes more and more severe. This is due at times to the progressive course of the fibrosis and occasionally to calcification of the valve. However, when many years have elapsed since the original acute stage, the mitral lesion has usually reached its maximum and any further change is due to recurrence of *rheumatic carditis* which may be unobserved.

Any deterioration in the functional state of the myocardium causes dilatation of the left ventricle and adds *relative stenosis* to the *anatomical stenosis* by increasing the disproportion between valvular opening and left ventricular chamber. The murmurs then become louder and the general condition deteriorates.

A common cause of functional deterioration is the gradual establishment of *new valvular lesions.* Mitral insufficiency frequently occurs. Tricuspid insufficiency and stenosis may develop. Aortic insufficiency and stenosis are not rare. In all such cases, the general outlook is poor. Another possibility is the occurrence of constrictive pericarditis which, however, is rare. This might have a certain influence in limiting the functional adaptation of the heart.

Subacute bacterial endocarditis is another dire occurrence which should be always considered.

Arteriosclerosis of the pulmonary vessels is a possible complication and is favored by the high pressure of the lesser circulation.

Pulmonary tuberculosis is unusual in its active type. However, torpid tuberculosis with exudative and fibrous evolution is not exceptional. As both mitral stenosis and tuberculosis may give similar auscultatory findings in the lungs, only x-ray evidence of cavities or positive finding of the Koch bacillus in the sputum will be accepted as a definite proof of tuberculosis.

Hemoptysis is usually moderate. However, in exceptional cases it may be so abundant as to be the cause of death.

Thrombosis of the atrial wall is a common complication. If limited in extent, it does not cause mechanical obstacle; otherwise it may obstruct the cavity or the valves. A ball thrombus of the left atrium may be the cause of acute episodes followed by death (page 214). The thrombi are also a common source of *embolism. Pulmonary infarction* is a frequent complication when the embolus starts from the right heart. *Cerebral embolism,* often followed by hemiplegia, is also frequent when the embolus starts from the left heart.

The mural thrombi may become *calcified* and be revealed by the x-ray. Slowing of the blood stream favors the formation of clots; acceleration of the blood stream tends to dislodge them. Once the thrombi are present in the atria, and especially in the appendages, they may remain silent for a long time.

Aneurysm of the left atrium is not un-common. It may occasionally reach an enormous size (page 393).

Atrial fibrillation, atrial flutter, and ventricular tachycardia are common complications. The first usually starts in coincidence with an episode of heart failure, then becomes habitual and persistent.

Attacks of dyspnea (cardiac asthma) are frequent. *Attacks of pulmonary edema* are less common but are not exceptional, especially in pregnant women (page 555).

Heart failure may start insidiously and may be revealed by slight pitting edema, small areas of chronic edema of the lungs, or enlargement of the liver. The complete picture of congestive failure is the most typical: engorgement of the large veins, peripheral edema, large liver, transudates in the serous cavities, cyanosis, dyspnea, and small irregular pulse.

Paralysis of the left recurrent nerve is a rare complication probably due to compression of the nerve by a large left atrium or a large pulmonary artery.

DIAGNOSIS

Mitral stenosis is the valvular defect which is easiest to diagnose yet may present the most difficult diagnostic problems.

The clinical diagnosis is based largely upon auscultation. No difficulty is present when a diastolic-presystolic rumble is heard. However, the physician should be cautioned about the following possibilities: a) The observer may hear a crescendo presystolic murmur while there is either *a crescendo-type,* or *a gradually increasing pitch, of the vibrations of the first sound.* b) *There are functional diastolic rumbles which simulate mitral stenosis* (page 237). In the first group of cases, a phonocardiogram easily disproves mitral stenosis. In the second group, the phonocardiogram may indicate the truth if attention is paid to certain graphic features indicated by the author (page 244).

When only the *opening snap* is audible, differential diagnosis should be made with: a) a physiological opening sound; b) a third sound or a ventricular type of triple rhythm; c) a split 2nd sound due to bundle branch block. The recognition is mainly graphic (fig. 132).

The physiological opening sound has a lower pitch and is usually nearer to the main vibration of the 2nd sound-complex. In the experience of the author, if the extra-sound is more than 0.08″ from the above-mentioned vibration, or is small and very rapid, and recorded on the whole precordium, it is definitely a pathological opening snap.

Cases where there is a loud 1st sound and cases having also pulmonary emphysema or pulmonary tuberculosis may be diagnosed with the help of the x-ray and of the phono-cardiograph.

The cases of "mute mitral stenosis," where no murmur is audible, are often obscure only because the correct diagnosis is not considered. In many of them, the graphic tracings and the x-ray permit a correct diagnosis. Sound records after exercise seldom fail to reveal the murmur. However, occasional cases, erroneously diagnosed as bronchial asthma or chronic cor pulmonale, are still described (72).

The finding of a dilated left atrium may be important in doubtful cases but not when the whole heart is enlarged or when mitral insufficiency is also present.

• *Patent ductus arteriosus* has a typical murmur at the base (page 290) but may have a diastolic rumble at the apex. However, the left atrium is normal or only slightly enlarged; there frequently is left axis deviation. The hilar shadows are dilated and pulsating but the lung fields are clearer than in mitral stenosis. Right axis deviation, prolonged P-R, or atrial fibrillation are in favor of mitral stenosis in doubtful cases.

Patients with arteriosclerotic or coronary heart disease or with aortic insufficiency having a large left ventricle may present a diastolic murmur due to *relative stenosis* of the mitral valve. The differential diagnosis is partly clinical and partly based on data of the phonocardiogram (page 244).

The prognosis should be based upon the severity of the lesion, the age of the patient, the existence of associated valvular and myocardial lesions, and the existence of signs of failure.

Mitral stenosis in children has a serious prognosis.

Prognosis in pregnant women will be discussed later (chapter 31). There is no doubt that maternity represents a risk in these patients, even if not to the extent considered in the past.

Infections, strenuous work, and irregular living, may shorten the lives of these patients by causing heart failure.

The possibility of a recurrence of rheumatic disease and of bacterial endocarditis should be taken into consideration.

TREATMENT

Patients with mitral stenosis and no signs of heart failure should not be digitalized. They should be cautioned against strenuous physical exertion and excess of food, drink, or stimulants. *Digitalization* may be used whenever exertion cannot be avoided or in the last stages of pregnancy (page 549).

The first signs of failure indicate the need for digitalis. Treatment will be started with the patient either in bed or at rest. When the maintenance dose of digitalis is reached and the symptoms of failure have disappeared, a gradually increasing activity will be permitted. When normal activity is resumed without causing trouble, digitalis may be interrupted tentatively (short periods of 1 week per month, at first) and then completely discontinued.

The patient should be instructed to report if any sign or symptom reappears and not to use digitalis without medical advice. Many failures of treatment are due to indiscriminate, erroneous, or excessive use of digitalis.

The general rules of *digitalization* should be followed (chapters **32** and **36**). *Mercurial diuretics* (**11, 12**), *ammonium chloride* (**13**), or both, can be used following the customary precautions and rules (chapters 32, 35, and 36) if there is peripheral edema or evidence of pulmonary congestion. *Quinidine* (**24**) or *pronestyl* (**27**) can be used if there is atrial fibrillation but not before obtaining improvement by means of digitalis. The danger of mobilizing emboli from the fibrillating atria should be considered but has been overemphasized in the past (page 592).

The *diet* during failure will be described later (chapter XXXV and appendix I).

Surgical treatment of mitral stenosis is one of the recent conquests of cardiac surgery. Candidates for surgery are patients with no evidence of left ventricular enlargement, moderate or absent mitral regurgitation, and no aortic or tricuspid defects. The best results are obtained in cases between 20 and 45 years of age who present paroxysmal attacks of dyspnea, pulmonary edema, or hemoptysis. Intractable right heart failure, rheumatic activity, bacterial endocarditis, and severe pulmonary arteriosclerosis, are definite contraindications. Catheterization of the right heart may supply evidence of right heart failure or pulmonary arteriosclerosis. Clinical and laboratory data usually indicate the existence of other valvular defects, rheumatic carditis, or bacterial endocarditis. It has been proven, however, that rheumatic myocarditis may not be revealed by general or laboratory data. Mitral regurgitation can be evaluated fairly well by means of electrokymography.

The best intervention is *commissurotomy* (**71, 77**); second best is *digital dilatation* or *finger fracture* of the *commissures*. The mitral valve is reached through the left atrial appendage. This structure should be ligated and resected at the end of the intervention, in order to limit the dangers of future embolizations. Cerebral embolism during surgery can be prevented by temporary occlusion of the carotids during digital exploration.

While other valvular defects were initially considered as a definite contraindication, reports of more complex surgical interventions suggest the possibility of operating cases with multiple valvular lesions (pages 255 and 275).

Patients presenting *multiple peripheral emboli* who are poor surgical risks can be treated by the use of *anticoagulants*. *Dicumarol* (**64**) has been given for several years in certain cases. The results seem good (**72, 86**).

Relative Mitral Stenosis

It has been proven that, whenever the left ventricle is severely dilated, the blood penetrating through the mitral valve creates whirlpools which cause a rumbling diastolic murmur. This murmur may be recorded by phonocardiography. It can be often differentiated from that of organic mitral stenosis because *composed of high and irregular vibrations which start rather late in diastole and are not preceded by an opening snap of the mitral valve*. These vibrations may be recorded in certain cases *over a wide surface of the precordium* (**83**) (fig. 143).

It should be kept in mind that, upon auscultation, the presystolic murmur of mitral stenosis may be simulated by a "crescendo-type" of the first sound and by triple rhythms or other abnormal cadences (**73, 83**).

Double Mitral Defect

The double mitral defect is the association of mitral insufficiency with mitral stenosis and is undoubtedly common. Theoretically, nearly all cases of mitral defects of rheumatic nature are double defects. However, in cases in which one of the two lesions is greatly predominant, the diagnosis of either mitral insufficiency or mitral stenosis should be made and not that of double mitral defect.

The heart with double mitral defect is increased in all its diameters as shown by percussion and fluoroscopy. The left atrium and

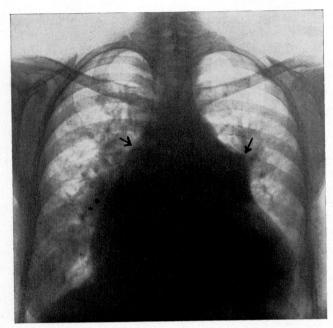

FIG. 137. Mitral stenosis and insufficiency. Arrow at right indicates the dilated pulmonary artery. Arrow at left indicates aneurysm of left atrium.

both ventricles are enlarged, usually with predominance of the right.

Auscultation and phonocardiography at the apex reveal a typical *diastolic rumble* and a loud first sound, followed by *a soft systolic murmur "in decrescendo"*.

Cyanosis and *dyspnea* occur earlier than in the single defects. The complications are those of mitral stenosis and the course is similar. The prognosis is the same as that of mitral stenosis but more severe.

Aortic Insufficiency

Aortic insufficiency exists when the semi-lunar leaflets of the aorta are incompetent. The regurgitation of blood takes place during diastole and causes compensatory changes of the left ventricle and of the arteries of the greater circulation.

CAUSE

The following lesions may cause aortic insufficiency.

a) *Congenital lesions.* These may consist of *fenestrations* of the leaflets (28) or a *bi-cuspid valve* (29, 30). The latter, however, seldom produces insufficiency by itself.

b) *Rheumatic endocarditis.*[52]

c) *Bacterial endocarditis.* Benign endocarditis caused by the Pneumococcus or the Gonococcus has been so far the most common cause but other bacterial forms are becoming more common through healing of acute and subacute bacterial endocarditis. The latter is not unusual when there is a bicuspid valve (28, 30).

d) *Syphilitic endocarditis.* It is common in the geographic areas where syphilis is diffuse and is usually associated with a lesion of the aorta (aortitis).[53]

e) *Arteriosclerosis* may cause aortic insufficiency (50, 85). The valvular defect of such patients may also be due to incomplete rupture of the aorta, being, therefore, of a special nature (page 525).

f) *Traumatic.* Strenuous physical effort

[52] Aortic insufficiency, caused by endocarditis, is also called *Corrigan's disease.*

[53] Aortic insufficiency, caused by syphilis, is also called *Hodgson's disease.*

may lead to *eversion* or *rupture* of the semi-lunar cusps. In practically all cases this happens when the valves have been damaged by one of the previously named processes.

LESIONS

Aortic insufficiency is a common valvular disease, although less frequent than the mitral defects. It is more frequent in males.

In *congenital cases*, the leaflets present small linear openings below the line of contact (fenestrations) or number only *two* instead of three. It may be observed that in many cases a bicuspid valve is due to endocarditis causing fusion of two leaflets and that, in others, insufficiency occurs only after rheumatic or bacterial endocarditis.

In cases due to *bacterial endocarditis*, the valves may show small openings or fissures caused by ulcerations, or small aneurysms of the sinuses of Valsalva.

Both in *rheumatic* and *syphilitic* cases the valves are thicker, harder, have fibrous or calcareous plaques, and are often fused at the commissures.[54] If the lesion is still developing, there is swelling of the leaflets and small vegetations are present.

In some cases, the valves form a semirigid funnel projecting into the aorta. In such cases, valvular stenosis is also present.

The *arteriosclerotic lesions* consist of: a) *calcareous infiltration* which starts at the base of the leaflets and extends toward the free margins; and b) yellow and opaque infiltration due to *atheromatous changes*.

Valve cusps may rupture or become everted.

The left ventricle is dilated and has a thick and hypertrophic wall. The rest of the heart is nearly normal but moderate displacement of the interventricular septum may cause a slight dilatation of the right ventricle. The heart has a typically elongated shape (*coeur en sabot*) (fig. 138).

[54] These lesions should not be confused with the *nodules of Arantius* which are normally found on the free margins of the valves and have no pathological importance.

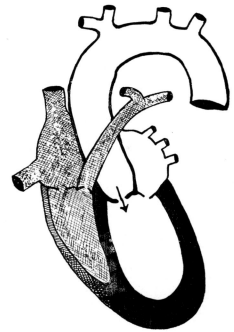

Fig. 138. Effect of the valvular lesion on the heart and aorta in aortic insufficiency.

The aorta may be slightly dilated in the rheumatic forms. It may show atherosclerosis in the forms associated with valvular sclerosis. In some cases, the lineal scar of an *incomplete rupture of the aorta* is present. The valvular leaflets are then normal or sclerotic but their line of insertion is dilated, resulting in poor support for the valves and valvular incompetence.

In *syphilitic* cases, the aorta presents a typical *aortitis* with localization in the ascending part. There usually is severe dilatation of this vessel which may be uniform or localized (aneurysm). The existence of *miliary gummata* may give the aspect of a *geographic map* to the aorta.

Syphilitic and atherosclerotic lesions of the valves and of the aorta may be associated.

The *coronary arteries* are often arteriosclerotic; the process is favored by the valvular defect. In syphilitic patients, the coronary lesion is localized at the mouths of the vessels.

Lesions of the kidneys, peripheral arteries (sclerosis), liver, lungs, and brain, are common as a result of the valvular defect and heart failure.

SIGNS AND SYMPTOMS

Aortic insufficiency frequently permits normal physical activity for a long time. This is chiefly true in the luetic form and accounts for the accidental finding of the disease in manual workers.

Patients may live for years with few complaints. If questioned, they admit that physical effort causes *dyspnea, precordial oppression*, or *precordial pain*. Occasional complaints of a *dry cough* and queer sensations in the chest due to *premature beats*, are encountered. The most frequent complaint is that of *heart palpitation* and of *pulsation of all organs*, occasionally associated with *pulsating headache*.

Some patients experience *giddiness, dizziness*, or *fainting spells;* some complain of *visual disturbances*.

The patients are usually *pale* and, even when heart failure occurs, the color is never frankly cyanotic but more often *grayish*.

A series of vascular signs is typical of this disease.

Arterial dance. All visible arteries show evidence of a quick and strong pulsation. This is apparent at the suprasternal notch and on the lateral regions of the neck, on different points of the arm and forearm, at the epigastrium, and at the groin. The pulsation of many secondary arteries, such as the temporal or the ulnar, becomes visible.

A particular manifestation of this vascular dance is shown by the following two signs: a) The first consists of a rhythmic backward movement of the head with every systole. b) The second consists of the abrupt, rhythmic extension of one leg when crossed over the other, coincident with systole.

The *pulse* is typical; it quickly distends the artery and quickly disappears (*pulsus celer* or *Corrigan's pulse* (31)). By palpating the forearm with appropriate pressure it is possible to feel a *thrill* which occurs at every pulsation. Tachycardia is common.

When the stethoscope is applied lightly over the brachial or femoral artery the observer hears either one snapping sound (*pistol shot sound*) or two (*double tone of Traube* (32)). When the stethoscope is applied so that it exerts a marked compression, a *double blowing murmur* is heard (*double murmur of Duroziez* (33)).

The small parenchymal arteries cause the pulsation of many organs: a) Rhythmic distention of the uvula and of the tonsils. b) Rhythmic narrowing of the pupils. c) Rhythmic *expansion of the fingertips*, which can be appreciated by palpation. d) Rhythmic expansion of the area of redness caused by rubbing the skin (forehead) and narrowing of an area of pallor made by compressing the skin by means of a glass or by compressing the nail (*capillary pulse; Quincke's sign* (34); *ungual pulse*).

The effects of the changed cardiac dynamics can be felt by auscultating at the mouth of the patient during slow expiration and noting a series of whiffs. These can be observed by the patient himself when smoking (*cog-wheel respiration*) (35).

Local Signs

The *apical thrust* is usually accentuated. There may be a *massive movement* of the precordial region to the left (bulging of the left section and depression of the right section in early systole) (1). If the late-systolic expansion of the 2nd and 3rd right interspaces, caused by the expansion of the aorta is marked, a *see-saw movement* takes place.

The site of the apical impulse is displaced to the 6th or 7th intercostal space, at the anterior or even at the mid-axillary line.

Palpation allows the observer to appreciate a quick pulsation at the suprasternal notch where a *systolic thrill* is also often present. The aortic arch may be palpable when the aorta is dilated.

The *cardiac dulness* is typically elongated

with a cap of dulness at the 2nd and 3rd right interspaces (if the aorta is dilated).

Auscultation reveals *a soft, blowing diastolic murmur*. This murmur starts immediately after the 2nd sound, then gradually fades like a jet of steam. It is of maximum intensity over the 2nd right interspace but may be heard best in the 2nd left (especially when aortic and mitral valvular disease are associated), along the left sternal border, and even over the epigastrium. When the aorta is dilated, this murmur is heard at the suprasternal notch (12) (fig. 139). If the murmur is faint, it may be heard better by having the patient exercise and then lean forward in forceful expiration (73).

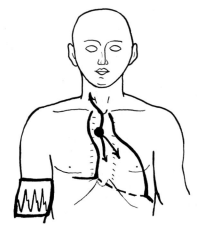

FIG. 139. Cardiac dulness and transmission of the diastolic murmur in aortic insufficiency.

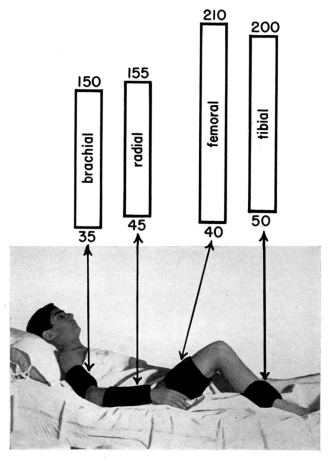

FIG. 140. Blood pressure in aortic insufficiency

242   HEART

In some cases, the murmur is *harsh, musical,* or *similar to the cry of a sea gull.* This usually occurs when the valves are broken, perforated, or everted.

A *systolic murmur,* heard best over the 2nd right interspace and the suprasternal notch (12), is often present. This may be due to associated aortic stenosis or relative stenosis.

Auscultation at the apex may reveal one of the following phenomena: a) Transmission of the murmurs from the base. b) A triple rhythm. c) A diastolic-presystolic murmur, simulating that of mitral stenosis (*Austin Flint* murmur (36, 38).

BLOOD PRESSURE

Blood pressure readings are important and have a diagnostic value. The fundamental change is represented by *a marked increase in the amplitude of the pulse pressure.* As the mean pressure may be increased, normal, or high, a high systolic with normal diastolic (210/80), or a normal systolic with a low diastolic (130/40) pressure can be observed (fig. 140).

Regional measurements of blood pressure show two changes which are part of the same phenomenon (fig. 140): a) The forearm has a slightly higher systolic pressure than the arm (39, 40). b) The leg has a much higher systolic pressure than the arm (39, 40).

GRAPHIC TRACINGS

Electrocardiogram

The most typical finding is *left axis deviation,* revealed by comparison of aVL with aVF, and lead 1 with lead 3 (fig. 141). Additional changes may consist of:

1) Prolongation of the P-R interval. 2) Evidence of left ventricular hypertrophy or "strain." The former consists of increased voltage; a slight prolongation of QRS (not exceeding 0.11 second); and high complexes in V6 and V7. The latter consists of lowering

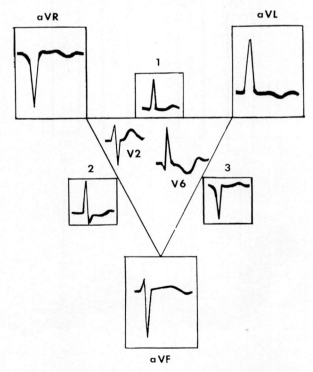

FIG. 141. The electrocardiogram in a case of aortic insufficiency. The tracings of the V-leads of the limbs are purposely made larger than those of the standard leads.

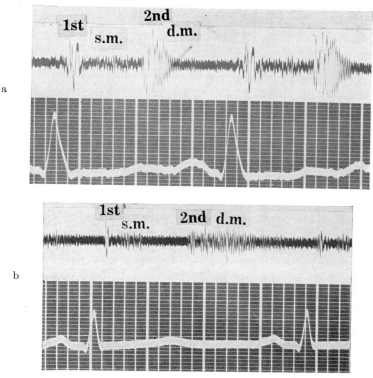

FIG. 142. Phonocardiograms in cases of aortic insufficiency. The tracings are recorded over the aortic area with a logarithmic microphone and are compared with the electrocardiogram. Case *a* had an everted aortic valve.

or inversion of T in aVL (and lead 1), and in the chest leads V4 to V6. 3) Left intraventricular block or bundle branch block. 4) Abnormalities of S-T and T, other than those related to "strain" or bundle branch block. These changes are connected with either rheumatic lesions (P-R) or coronary heart disease. The latter is favored by the hemodynamic changes caused by the valvular lesion. 5) Left ventricular premature beats are common. Ventricular tachycardia may occur.

Phonocardiogram

Tracings recorded over the aortic area show that the main vibration of the second sound-complex is followed by a series of other vibrations of high pitch (*diastolic murmur*). They are usually of limited amplitude in comparison with the auditory impression

and decrease gradually (fig. 142). When a broken or everted valve is the cause of regurgitation, the vibrations are higher and may be regular (*musical murmur*) (fig. 142a). The first sound may be *impure* (low, or prolonged) because of myocardial damage.

Vibrations due to a *systolic murmur* are common; they are similar to those encountered in organic aortic stenosis, "relative stenosis" of the aorta, and aortitis.

The characteristics of the *diastolic murmur* vary. In some cases, the vibrations follow each other with a "decrescendo" type. In other cases, the vibrations have a crescendo-decrescendo type (74). The murmur sometimes ends in early diastole. If the murmur is musical, as in cases with an everted aortic valve or calcification of one of the leaflets, the vibrations are regular and present a "concertina-like" appearance.

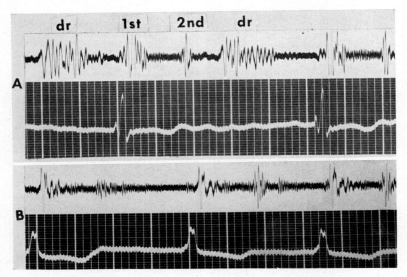

FIG. 143. Hypertensive and coronary heart disease, possible luetic heart disease. Aortic insufficiency. Loud diastolic rumble (dr) at apex (A) which disappeared 1 year later (B). This was caused by "relative" mitral stenosis.

Studies of the author and others on the *Austin Flint murmur* (38) have revealed the following facts:

1) In some cases, *a triple rhythm* is present (page 370). 2) In others, the low amplitude of the first phase of the first sound and a high vibration due to the opening of the aortic valve give *the impression of a presystolic murmur* to the unaided ear. A delay in the occurrence of the first sound may contribute to this. 3) In others, slow vibrations, arising in the aorta, are louder than the first sound and may be easily mistaken for it. Therefore, in most cases, either there is *a triple rhythm*, or the presystolic murmur is due to *an auscultatory illusion*.

Subsequent studies (75, 83) have shown that, in rare cases, the phonocardiogram reveals *a diastolic rumble which may be mistaken for that of mitral stenosis* (fig. 143). However, the following differential data may be observed in such cases: There is no opening snap of the mitral valve; the murmur starts rather late in diastole; *the vibrations are usually of large amplitude;* and they are recorded *over a large area*, sometimes over the entire precordium.

Phonoarteriogram

Arterial sound vibrations may present the following types:

1) There may be a single, extremely loud, sound during the expansion of the artery (*pistol-shot sound*). 2) There are two sounds. The first of them falls during the expansion of the artery while the second falls during arterial collapse and precedes the dicrotic wave (*double tone of Traube*). 3) There are two murmurs. These replace the two sounds and are favored by compression below the point of recording. They are more easily observed over the femoral artery (*double murmur of Duroziez.*)

Cardiogram

In most cases the low frequency tracing of the apex (apex cardiogram) shows a high, early systolic wave followed by a deep depression (fig. 144a). In certain cases, however, a high systolic plateau is present. If the record is taken outside the apex, a deep systolic depression represents the main aspect of the tracing.

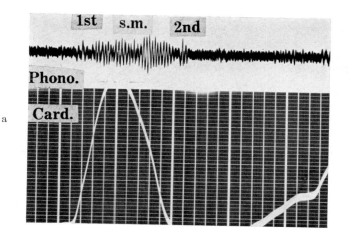

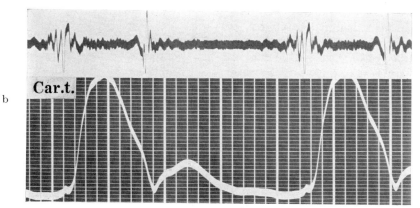

FIG. 144. Heaving apical thrust (a) and typical carotid pulse (b) in cases of aortic insufficiency

Pulse Tracing

The typical pulse curve presents *a rapid ascent, a rapid drop,* and a small dicrotic wave (fig. 144b). The rapid drop is systolic and therefore not directly connected with the regurgitation of blood. The comparison of various tracings at different sites shows that transmission of the pulse wave is rapid in all arteries.

Electrokymogram

The border tracing of the *aortic arch* reveals a rapidly expanding and rapidly collapsing pulse; the absolute magnitude of the pulse is increased. The border tracing of the *left ventricle* shows a pulsation made of a rapid and large drop (rapid ventricular contraction) and *a rise in early diastole which is*

faster than in normal subjects. The latter is due to the fact that the left ventricle is distended by two streams, the normal left atrial blood and the aortic regurgitant blood.

X-RAY

The most frequent findings are: dilatation of the ascending aorta, aortic arch, and left ventricle. The systolic contraction of the latter and the systolic expansion of the former are increased and rapid. The point of connection between the vascular peduncle and the right atrium on the right is lowered (6). The heart has the shape of *an egg* or *a shoe* but this is mostly due to the fact that the apex is partially masked by abdominal organs (fig. 145).

The *retrocardiac space is often obscured* in

CARDIOVASCULAR SYPHILIS
AORTIC REGURGITATION
ANEURYSM ASCEND. AORTA

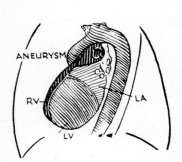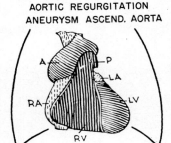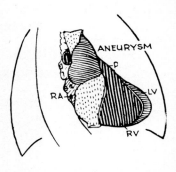

FIG. 145. The heart on x-ray in aortic insufficiency. (Courtesy of Dr. G. R. Herrmann and the C. V. Mosby Co.)

the left anterior oblique (enlarged left ventricle). The aorta is enlarged anteriorly, as demonstrated in the left anterior oblique.

Roentgenkymography. The systolic dilation of the aorta occurs very early but the pulse wave moves slowly at first, owing to the tonic reaction of the vessel (22).

MODE OF ORIGIN OF THE SIGNS

Experiments performed on circulation models show that aortic insufficiency causes a *drop of mean pressure and an increase of pulse pressure.* If cardiac output is increased, the original level of mean pressure is reestablished, but the pulse pressure increases further.

Insufficiency of the aortic valve results in regurgitation of blood into the left ventricle during diastole. Experimental studies have shown that the amount of regurgitating blood can range from 5 per cent with small leaks up to 50 per cent when the cusps are totally destroyed (43, 44). The tension period is extremely short *in cases having large leaks.* The aortic pressure rises very early, but drops sharply during late systole. *A further drop occurs in early diastole before mitral valve opening because of the regurgitation,* but little change of pressure takes place later (43, 44). *Small leaks* cause smaller changes but the pressure drop of the aorta takes place *rather later after the mitral valve has opened* (43, 44). This avoids any impair-

ment to the normal flow into the left ventricle.

Regurgitation of blood into the left ventricle causes *dilatation* of this chamber and *hypertrophy* of its wall. This causes an increased systolic discharge and a *dilatation of the aorta which is dynamic at first but may become permanent later.*

Dilatation of the left ventricle compensates for the increased volume of filling so that no increase of diastolic pressure takes place in the ventricle as long as there is no failure. This was proven by left heart catheterization in man (82).

The *low diastolic pressure* is caused directly by the reflux. It favors an *increased speed* of the pulse wave toward the periphery because the wave enters a poorly filled arterial system. Closure of the semilunar valves takes place while the pulse wave has not yet reached the small arteries and *continues its forward movement.*

The reflux into the left ventricle causes *a greater retraction of the aorta and of the large vessels* whenever the leak is small or medium. This retraction may suffice to avoid reflux from the more distant vessels.

The violent stimulation of the arterial wall by a large pulse wave necessarily causes a stronger elastic and muscular reaction. This is partly responsible for the typical *signs of vascular pulsation* which are similar to those caused by adrenalin and for the rapid progression of the pulse wave (46).

The so-called *capillary pulse* has been shown to be due, in most cases, to the intermittent shaking and pulsation of the small arterioles. The capillary flow, on the other hand, is *continuous*, as in normal people.

Intermittent stimulation of the carotid sinus and aortic receptors may account for a marked increase of tonus of the peripheral arteries. It may not account for the *tachycardia*.

The *soft diastolic murmur*, heard over the aortic area, is apparently due to a turbulent flow of blood which enters the left ventricle during the phase of regurgitation. It is louder, more musical, and more prolonged when the leak is small; it is soft and short in larger leaks where the 2nd sound practically disappears (43, 44).

The *aortic systolic murmur* may be due to either real stenosis (rheumatic or arteriosclerotic heart disease) or relative stenosis (syphilitic heart disease).

The mechanism of the *Austin Flint murmur* has caused several discussions (36). This murmur is due, in many cases, to an *auscultatory illusion* (page 244) which is clearly revealed by phonocardiography. The most likely mechanism in the other cases is that of a *relative mitral stenosis* (27, 37) and is, therefore, not typical of aortic regurgitation but common to all cases of extreme left ventricular enlargement (75).

Rapid rise and fall of the pulse wave are typical. The rapid collapse of the pulse occurs during systole (46); it is not due to the regurgitation but to the *great speed of the pulse toward the periphery*.

The *large pulse pressure and the high systolic pressure in the distant arteries* can be explained through simple mechanical phenomena.

The *deep systolic collapse* of the jugular vein tracing, of the cardiogram, and of the pneumocardiogram, are explained by the fact that *a large mass of blood leaves the thorax in systole*. A retraction of the inter-costal spaces and an aspiration both of air into the lungs and of blood into the right atrium is necessary in order to replace it in the relatively rigid thoracic chamber.

The *high wave of early diastolic filling* in the cardiogram, and *the rapid diastolic rise* of the left ventricular electrokymogram can be explained as the effect of regurgitation of blood into the left ventricle. The dicrotic wave observed in normal peripheral tracings is now considered as the result of an aortic "standing wave" reflected by branching. Failure of the aortic valve to close destroys the resonance and decreases the height of the dicrotic wave in these patients (84).

The arterial thrill, the double tone of Traube, and *the double murmur of Duroziez* have caused many discussions. Sound records of these phenomena led the author to the following conclusions (33d): a) The double tone is due to the rapid expansion and collapse of the arterial wall. b) The turbulent conditions of the blood in the pulse wave may lead to the formation of "breakers" and to the feeling of a systolic thrill and of a water-hammer quality of the pulse. c) The double murmur is due to a double centrifugal movement of the blood. This takes place when an adequate compression of the artery is made.

The *pallor* of these patients can be explained through the lower level of the mean pressure and the peripheral vasoconstriction.

The tendency to *fainting* is explained by the greater effect of the backflow on the cerebral circulation, especially in the standing position, and by frequent vasomotor reflexes. The increased stimulation and the continuous adjustments taking place through carotid sinus receptors may lead to a further decrease of pressure in the cerebral vessels.

COURSE AND COMPLICATIONS

Aortic insufficiency permits normal physical activity for long periods. Accidents may cause sudden death. They are directly related to the disease because automobile or airplane fatalities, sudden drownings, and work, accidents are often due to dizziness or fainting at critical moments.

Acute attacks often represent a danger signal. They are:

a) *Attacks of precordial pain* related to myocardial infarction or angina pectoris (page 431).

b) *Attacks of paroxysmal dyspnea* (page 555) *or pulmonary edema* (page 556).

These attacks may be followed by death or by progressive heart failure. Often, however, the patient recovers within a few hours and may lead a normal life for years before another attack occurs.

Subacute bacterial endocarditis is a possible complication, both in the rheumatic and the luetic types.

Rheumatic endocarditis may complicate the disease, not only as a recurrence of a previous rheumatic fever but also as a new disease in a luetic or arteriosclerotic patient.

Dissecting aneurysm of the aorta is a possible complication, especially in the arteriosclerotic and luetic patients. *Aortic aneurysm* is possible in luetic patients if they received incomplete treatment.

Renal complications are not unusual, especially in luetic and arteriosclerotic patients. They increase the severity of the disease through hypertension and increased load on

the heart. *Coronary heart disease* is frequent. It is favored by lesions of the coronary vessels due to the same cause as the valvular lesion (rheumatic coronaritis, coronary arteriosclerosis, narrowing of the coronary mouths by luetic aortitis). It is further increased by the hemodynamic effect of the valvular defect (poor diastolic flow) (fig. 146). *Myocardial infarction* is even more serious than in cases without valvular disease.

Disturbances of the heart rhythm are frequent. They may consist of *ventricular premature beats* or *ventricular paroxysmal tachycardia*. The load placed on the left ventricle explains why these occur. On the contrary, atrial fibrillation is rare.

Bundle branch block is common. *Pulsus alternans* may occur and is a sign of severe myocardial damage. A *triple rhythm* is frequent and is evidence of myocardial strain (page 370).

Cerebral complications may occur, caused by cerebral arteriosclerosis or embolism. The embolus may start from a thrombus of the left ventricle, usually following myocardial infarction, or from the aortic valve.

DIAGNOSIS

The diagnosis of aortic insufficiency is usually easy and can be made on the basis of physical examination alone. The basic signs are: elongated heart with a rapid apical thrust; soft diastolic murmur over the base; and increased pulse pressure with vascular signs.

Doubt can arise if: a) the murmur is heard over a different area; b) there is no murmur; c) there is a combined valvular defect; or d) there are no vascular signs.

In such cases, electro- and phonocardiograms and x-ray usually make the diagnosis possible; they reveal the existence of: left axis deviation, enlargement of the left ventricle, high-pitched diastolic murmur in decrescendo, increased amplitude of the aortic pulsations, and dilatation of the aorta.

Differential diagnosis with pulmonic insufficiency will be discussed in Chapter 12;

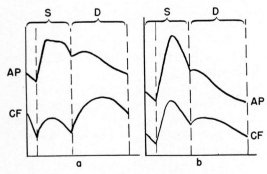

FIG. 146. Arterial pressure (AP) and coronary flow (CF) in the normal individual (a), and in aortic insufficiency (b), While normal coronary flow is mainly diastolic, in aortic insufficiency it is mainly systolic. S, systole; D, diastole. (Adapted from Wiggers.)

that with patent ductus, in Chapter 13. Differential diagnosis from *mitral insufficiency* is simple: mitral insufficiency gives a soft systolic; aortic insufficiency, a soft diastolic murmur. The former often has a reduced pulse pressure; the latter, an increased pulse pressure. The former has an enlarged left atrium and frequently an enlarged pulmonary artery; the latter, an enlarged aorta.

Differential diagnosis with *mitral stenosis* may be necessary whenever an apical diastolic rumble is heard in patients with aortic insufficiency. The diagnosis should ascertain whether or not there *also* is a mitral stenosis. As previously mentioned (pages 244 and 247), the phonocardiogram often permits a clear differentiation. X-ray will show enlargement of the left atrium, if there is mitral stenosis.

Aortitis, aortic atherosclerosis. They are often present together with the aortic insufficiency. If no diastolic murmur is present, the aortic lesion may explain the clinical picture without valvular insufficiency.

In exceptional cases, an *aneurysm of one of the sinuses of Valsalva* perforates into the right atrium. Then, the rough diastolic murmur, the congestion of the venous system, the sudden onset, and the brief course, permit a correct diagnosis.

TREATMENT

When the disease causes no symptoms, treatment is not necessary. The patient should be warned about the possibility of fainting and should not be allowed to drive.

Mild sedation by means of *phenobarbital* (**29**), *chloral hydrate* (**34**), and occasionally *tincture of opium*, may help in preventing paroxysmal attacks.

Papaverine (**43**) may be useful in hypertensive patients.

Potassium iodide (**73**) is often helpful in luetic and arteriosclerotic patients. Treatment of cardiovascular syphilis by means of either arsenicals or *penicillin* should be attempted only with caution because initial reactions may lead to increased severity of signs and to heart failure. It should not be attempted in the presence of failure.

Digitalis glycosides can be given whenever heart failure occurs.

Digitalization should be done gradually and extreme bradycardia should be avoided because it might increase the effects of regurgitation by prolonging diastole.

Strophanthin (**9**) has been advocated in preference to digitalis but there is no special indication. *Squill glycosides* (**10**) may be used for a mild and prolonged treatment.

The treatment of coronary attacks and of paroxysmal cardiorespiratory episodes will be indicated in chapters XIX and XXIX.

Grafting of an artificial valve in the aorta has been successfully tried in animals. It is possible that this method may be applied to clinical cases in the future. Surgical treatment by means of a flap of pericardium has been tried in rheumatic cases. The results are still not definite (77).

Relative Aortic Insufficiency

Relative insufficiency of the aortic valve is due to incomplete closure caused by weakness of the musculature of the left ventricle. This has been described in *heart failure*, after *myocardial infarction*, in *acute rheumatic disease*, and *thyrotoxicosis* (47). The possibility of a functional aortic insufficiency in *severe hypertension* has been demonstrated (48, 49). In all these cases the only sign is *the diastolic murmur*. The pulse pressure is not increased, and there may not be left axis deviation.

Valvular insufficiency due to *incomplete rupture of the aorta* is functional only in relation to the valve (page 485). It may give the complete clinical picture if the regurgitation is large.

In these cases, the only graphic findings are the vibrations of the diastolic murmur in the phonocardiogram. The murmur usually consists of three to five vibrations in decrescendo immediately after the second sound. The pulse and blood pressure tracings, the electrocardiogram, and the electrokymogram, usually fail to show typical data.

Aortic Stenosis

Aortic stenosis is the narrowing of the ostium leading from the left ventricle into the aorta. It hinders the flow of blood into the aorta and creates a typical clinical picture.

CAUSE

Several different causes for the stenosis are recognized:

a) *Congenital*. This may involve either *the valve* or the *infundibulum (subaortic or infundibular stenosis)*. Subaortic stenosis may be associated with hypoplasia of the aorta or interventricular septal defect; valvular stenosis, with patent ductus arteriosus.

b) *Rheumatic*. It is a fairly common valvular lesion, frequently associated with aortic insufficiency, mitral valve disease, or both. Calcification of the aortic valve occurs in a high percentage of cases.

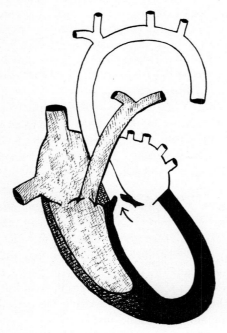

FIG. 147. Changes of the heart in aortic stenosis.

c) *Bacterial*. This is not common except during acute endocarditis. It may become more frequent in view of the fact that a larger number of patients are now saved by chemotherapy and antibiotics.

d) *Luetic*. It is unusual because syphilis causes dilatation of the aorta and the ostium. Still it may occur through fibrous healing of the valvular lesions, followed by calcification.

e) *Atherosclerotic*. It is a relatively frequent occurrence and is due to *calcification* of the valve. Actually, *calcific aortic stenosis* is an anatomical entity. The pathologist quite often is unable to recognize the cause of calcification or does it only through evaluation of associated lesions. It has been suggested that calcific aortic stenosis develops more often in cases with a bicuspid aortic valve (78). It has also been stated that rheumatic cases have adhesions between cusps while the others have calcareous masses within the sinuses of Valsalva.

LESIONS

Aortic stenosis is less frequent than other valvular defects of the left heart. However, if cases with combined valvular defects are included, it becomes more frequent.

Subaortic stenosis is a *congenital lesion*. It is the result of a slight displacement of the septum caused by disturbance in the torsion of the primitive heart. Therefore, it may be associated with a ventricular septal defect.

Valvular congenital stenosis is caused by fusion of the semilunar leaflets and is probably due to *fetal endocarditis*. If severe, it may be associated with a compensatory patency of the ductus.

Endocarditic stenosis is due to *fusion, shrinking, and deformation of the semilunar valves*. These may form a semirigid funnel projecting into the aorta. Subaortic stenosis, caused by septal endocarditis or retraction of the anterior mitral leaflet, has been described in unusual cases.

Partial fusion of the semilunar valves, followed by calcification, occurs in atherosclerotic cases.

The left ventricle is dilated and has a marked hypertrophy of its walls (fig. 147). In subaortic stenosis, a dilatation of the last part of the infundibulum is frequently encountered. In valvular stenosis, the first part of the aorta may be dilated.

SIGNS AND SYMPTOMS

The valvular defect often may be tolerated well for many years. The patients, however, may complain of *palpitation, oppression,* or *exertional dyspnea.*

Sudden attacks of *suffocating dyspnea* with *extreme pallor,* followed by cyanosis, are not uncommon when heart failure begins. At times, effort is followed by *syncope,* a fact which is unusual in other valvular defects (51). During syncope, the pulse may disappear while the heart rate is rapid.

The patients are usually *pale.* Moderate underdevelopment may exist in congenital cases.

The *pulse* may be normal but is frequently *small* and has a *slow rise (pulsus tardus)*; it is also frequently *slow* (52) being between 55 and 65 *(pulsus rarus)*. Even when the patient is in congestive failure, the pulse is slower than might be expected.

Local Signs

There may be a *precordial bulge.* The *apical impulse* is below and to the left of the normal site. The impulse is clearly visible but is *slow* and *prolonged.*

A *systolic thrill* can be palpated. It is of maximal intensity at the manubrium and in the 2nd and 3rd right interspaces. It may be present only in the right supraclavicular space.

The *cardiac dulness* is enlarged and elongated. The sternal manubrium is usually clear (fig. 148).

Auscultation reveals a *loud, harsh, systolic murmur* having maximal intensity over the 2nd or 3rd (subaortic stenosis) right in-

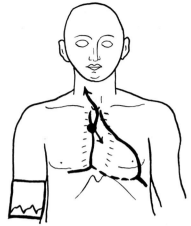

Fig. 148. Cardiac dulness and transmission of the systolic murmur in aortic stenosis.

terspace; this is well transmitted to the suprasternal notch (12) and along the carotid arteries. It may have a *musical* or *"sea-gull-cry"* quality; it is often heard over the back.

The 2nd aortic sound may be normal but is frequently *weak.* It may be weak *only in the first interspace,* where transmission from the pulmonic valve is minimal. In subaortic stenosis, both the systolic murmur and the weak 2nd sound are heard best *in the 3rd right,* and occasionally in the 3rd left, interspace.

BLOOD PRESSURE—BMR

The blood pressure is often normal or slightly low. Sometimes, however, there is a definite *hypotension* (systolic pressure between 80 and 90) or hypertension. *Instability of the blood pressure* has been described (53).

The observation of an *auscultatory gap* (57 a, b) (fig. 149) is frequent and typical. This phenomenon consists of the *absence of arterial sounds between systolic and diastolic pressure in spite of good pulsations of the vessel.*

Relative hypotension in the legs is frequent but moderate (8).

Increased BMR may occur and is not well explained.

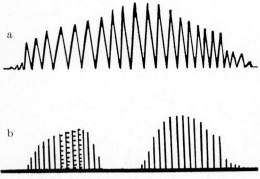

FIG. 149. Auscultatory gap in aortic stenosis. The oscillatory curve (a) fails to show any abnormality while the auditory curve (b) is interrupted by a gap between systolic and diastolic pressure.

GRAPHIC TRACINGS

Electrocardiogram

The data are similar to those caused by aortic insufficiency (page 242) because they are related to the enlargement of the left ventricle and to the possible association of coronary and myocardial lesions. *Sinus bradycardia* is frequently observed.

Phonocardiogram

The phonocardiogram gives evidence of the basal *systolic murmur*, which is revealed by a series of vibrations of both high and low pitches. The vibrations increase gradually and often take the shape of a wave having maximum intensity in the second half of systole (*diamond-shaped murmur*) (fig. 150). The second sound has a low amplitude and may disappear over the 1st or 2nd right interspaces. A loud fourth (atrial) sound is often recorded at the apex.

Cardiogram

The ascending part of the systolic impulse is either slow or double ("camel-back" or "staggered" profile). The systolic murmur may be accompanied by a series of vibrations which are the graphic expression of the thrill (fig. 150a).

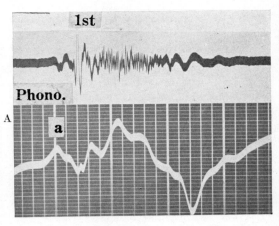
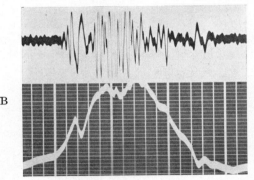

FIG. 150. Phonocardiograms of aortic stenosis. A, sound tracing and low frequency tracing (cardiogram) over 2nd right interspace; B, sound tracing and pulsations of suprasternal notch.

Arterial Pulse

The pulse tracing shows an ascending phase which is slower than normal. As this phase is often interrupted by a well-marked depression (anacrotic notch), the pulse is called *anacrotic pulse* (figs. 150b and 151). If recorded at the suprasternal notch or on the carotid arteries, the pulse tracing may show a series of vibrations which are simultaneous with the murmur (so-called *carotid shudder*).

Blood Pressure

Graphic tracings of blood pressure frequently reveal an *auscultatory gap*. This consists of the absence of arterial sounds in a zone between systolic and diastolic pres-

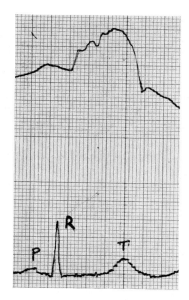

FIG. 151. Carotid tracing and ECG in a case of aortic stenosis: slow rise and anacrotic depression of the pulse.

sures. While the sound tracing reveals the "gap", the pulse tracing does not.

Electrokymogram

The border tracing of the aortic knob presents *an anacrotic depression* similar to that exhibited by the carotid pulse; the border tracing of the left ventricle reveals abnormalities of contraction similar to those exhibited by the apex cardiogram.

X-RAY

The aorta may be normal, small, or slightly dilated. The profile of the left ventricle shows an increase in size. The left atrium and the right ventricle are normal; the pulmonary artery is normal (fig. 152).

The systolic contraction of the left ventricle is slow and the systolic dilatation of the aorta is also slow. The aortic valve may be visible, if calcified.

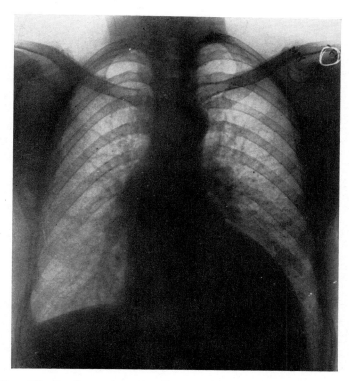

FIG. 152. Cardiac and aortic silhouette in a case of aortic stenosis

MODE OF ORIGIN OF THE SIGNS

It has been shown that the aortic opening must be reduced to one-fourth of its normal size in animals in order to decrease systolic discharge (43, 44). Then the initial pressure curve of the ventricle rises more quickly and to a higher level, reaching its maximum earlier than normal. The aortic pressure rises rapidly at first, slowing at the time of the anacrotic notch. The pulse pressure is reduced in proportion to the stenosis.

The obstacle to the emptying of the left ventricle causes a compensatory *dilatation* of this chamber followed by severe *hypertrophy*. If the stenosis is not too tight, this compensatory phenomenon is sufficient to raise blood pressure to a normal level again. Otherwise, hypotension is present.

A further compensation is represented by the *prolonged duration of systole*. This, together with the effect of the obstacle, causes the *double wave* of the cardiogram, and the *anacrotic pulse*.

The *auscultatory gap* has been attributed to anacrotism (57a, b) or to this plus arterial hypotonus (58). A slower vibration of the arterial wall fails to elicit the typical snapping arterial sound and it cannot be denied that the gap is usually present in that phase of pressure which corresponds to the anacrotic depression.

The *systolic murmur* is caused by the ed-

dies formed by the blood in passing through the narrow opening. It is present even in slight stenosis. The typical transmission toward the neck indicates that the sound vibrations are largely carried by the stream of blood. The *thrill* is merely the palpatory expression of the same phenomenon. The *weak 2nd sound* is due to the rigidity of the leaflets.

A *relative coronary insufficiency* is common (fig. 153).

Slight bradycardia is probably due to a vagal reflex starting from left ventricular receptors.

The *effort syncopes* are not due to bradycardia. On the contrary, tachycardia, which prevents efficient emptying of the left ventricle, has been advocated (51).

The eddies formed distal to the narrowing cause a moderate dilatation of either the last part of the infundibulum (subaortic stenosis) or the initial part of the ascending aorta.

COURSE AND COMPLICATIONS

Patients with aortic stenosis may suffer from *bacterial endocarditis*. Bacteria may attack the aortic valves in any type of lesion, even (though less frequently) in luetic and arteriosclerotic cases.

Heart block, caused by extension of the inflammatory process from the aortic valve to the septum with lesion of the bundle of His, is a possibility (59).

The onset of heart failure may be revealed by *relative mitral insufficiency, chronic pulmonary edema*, or *continuous dyspnea*. Acute pulmonary edema is not a frequent complication. Patients with aortic stenosis *may die suddenly* (60), a fact which has been attributed to sudden hooking of the hardened leaflets, so that they cannot open again (61). Apart from this, the usual outcome of the disease is chronic congestive failure.

DIAGNOSIS

The diagnosis of aortic stenosis is possible on the basis of the clinical signs: pallor,

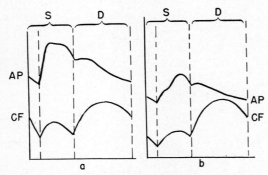

FIG. 153. Arterial pressure (AP) and coronary flow (CF) in the normal individual (a), and in aortic stenosis (b): that part of flow which takes place during systole is reduced. (Adapted from Wiggers.)

small and slow pulse, enlarged left ventricle, systolic thrill and murmur over the aortic area.

The diagnosis is undoubtedly more difficult when other valvular defects are also present. In such cases, the electro- and phonocardiographic tracings, the cardio- and sphygmogram, the x-ray, the aortic electrokymogram, and the blood pressure data will be of help. In particular, the anacrotic pulse, the auscultatory gap, the vibrations of the aortic tracing, and the lack of aortic dilatation, are valuable signs. The weak 2nd sound and the diamond-shaped murmur are also important.

Differential diagnosis should be made with *relative aortic stenosis*. This is usually accompanied by loud 2nd aortic sound, high blood pressure, and dilated aorta, and fails to show the other typical data (see below).

Mitral insufficiency can be excluded because the murmur of this valvular defect is softer, is apical, and is transmitted toward the left axilla. On phonocardiographic tracings, this murmur has a different aspect and never shows the diamond-shaped type of murmur of aortic stenosis.

Roger's disease. Interventricular septal defect gives an early-systolic murmur which is louder over the 3rd *left* interspace and is often transmitted toward the *right* side of the chest. Transmission toward the suprasternal notch is far less than with aortic stenosis. There is no left axis deviation. The pulse tracing fails to show the typical changes of aortic stenosis. The other signs of aortic stenosis are absent.

Pulmonary stenosis. The murmur is similar but is of maximal intensity over *the 2nd left* interspace and is not transmitted to the suprasternal notch (unless it is extremely loud). There is *right* axis deviation. The patient is slightly cyanotic, not pale.

Aneurysm of the ascending aorta. There is an area of dulness and a bulge with expansive pulsation at the right of the sternum. The 2nd aortic sound may be loud. Pulse

tracings and cardiograms give different findings from those of aortic stenosis.

Coarctation of the aorta. The murmur is less loud and better audible *at the left* of the sternum. The aortic arch is dilated. The blood pressure is higher at the arms, lower at the legs. There is an extensive arterial collateral circulation in the intercostal spaces.

Patent ductus arteriosus. The murmur has its maximal intensity over *the 1st and 2nd left* interspaces. It is a late-systolic-early-diastolic murmur (phonocardiogram) which is different from that of aortic stenosis. The pulmonary artery is dilated (percussion, x-ray). The pulse has no anacrotism. The pulse pressure is increased, not decreased as in aortic stenosis.

PROGNOSIS

The prognosis of aortic stenosis is always serious. Still, a long span of life is often possible, and the severity is proportional to the tightness of the narrowing, not to the loudness of the murmur. It is therefore more favorable in the arteriosclerotic than in the endocarditic and congenital types.

TREATMENT

The general rules concerning physical exercise, diet, and medical treatment are the same as in other valvular defects.

Surgical treatment is possible (87). The best intervention is *dilatation of the valve*, which can be performed through the ventricular wall.

Relative Aortic Stenosis

This name has been used for those cases where a *systolic murmur* is present over the 2nd right interspace without any other sign of stenosis. In some of these patients, the aorta is dilated owing to aortitis or atherosclerosis. A *relative stenosis*, namely a disproportion between normal aortic orifice and vessel, can be admitted in most of these cases. This causes formation of eddies and, therefore, a systolic murmur.

In other cases, the margins of the aortic valve are *irregular and roughened*. This may cause a slight systolic murmur even without hindering the blood flow.

In a third group of patients, the aorta is functionally dilated owing to an increased amount of circulating blood or to increased energy of the heart. This leads to stretching of the insertion of the valves and to *trigonoidation* of the opening (62) which is purely functional and barely causes any hindrance to the flow. This phenomenon is not uncommon in pregnancy, fever, and thyrotoxicosis. All functional signs of stenosis are missing and frequently a similar murmur is audible over the pulmonic area.

A systolic murmur, having its maximal intensity over the mid-precordium and well transmitted both toward the neck and the apex, has been described in *hypertensive patients* with a very large left ventricle. It has been explained by hypertrophy of the interventricular septum (63). This interpretation is still far from being accepted. If true, it would place the patients in the category of subaortic stenosis.

Double Aortic Defect

The double aortic defect consists of the association of aortic stenosis with aortic insufficiency.

The *congenital* and *luetic* cases are rare; pure stenosis is the rule in the former, pure insufficiency in the latter. Therefore, apart from a limited number of *arteriosclerotic* patients, the great majority of cases are due to *endocarditis*, either *rheumatic or bacterial*.

The existence of stenosis attenuates the peripheral signs of aortic insufficiency; the presence of insufficiency attenuates the type of *pulsus rarus* and *tardus* of aortic stenosis. There may be a *carotid shudder* (56).

Some of the typical signs may be more severe. The enlargement of the left ventricle and left axis deviation are among them.

Auscultation reveals a *double murmur* over the aortic area with typical irradiation: the systolic murmur more toward the carotid arteries; the diastolic, more toward the xiphoid process.

The patients are *pale*, have frequent *dizzy* and *fainting spells*, and complain of *weakness, dyspnea*, and *precordial pain*. Their *mean blood pressure* is *low*, with either a normal or a large pulse pressure.

Double aortic defect is tolerated less well than either of the pure defects.

Diagnosis is limited to the exclusion of relative stenosis in cases of aortic insufficiency.

BIBLIOGRAPHY

1. DRESSLER, W. a) *Die Brustwandpulsationen.* Wien, Maudrich, 1933.
   b) *Clinical Cardiology.* New York, Hoeber, 1942.
   c) Arch. Int. Med., 1937, **60,** 437 and 663.
2. COSSIO, P. Rev. Arg. Cardiol., 1943, **10,** 145.
3. TAQUINI, A. C., MASSELL, B. F., AND WALSH, B. J. Am. Heart J., 1940, **20,** 295.
4. a) WEITZ, W. Deut. Arch. klin. Med., 1918, **124,** 155.
   b) FRANK. Quoted by WEITZ.
5. TAQUINI, A. C. *Exploración del Corazón por Via Esofágica.* Buenos Aires, El Ateneo, 1936.
6. ROESLER, H. *Clinical Roentgenology of the Cardiovascular System.* Baltimore, Thomas, 1943.
7. COSSIO, P. Bull. Soc. Méd. Hôp., 1937, **53,** 215.
8. BASSI, M. Riv. Clin. Med., 1934, **35,** 823; and 1935, **36,** 29.
9. a) WIGGERS, C. J. 5th Ed. *Physiology in Health and Disease.* Philadelphia, Lea and Febiger, 1949.
   b) McDOWALL, R. J. S. Quart. J. Exper. Physiol., 1926, **16,** 1.
10. BAILEY, D. T., AND HICKHAM, J. B. Am. Heart J., 1944, **28,** 578.
11. BASS, M. H., AND CO-WORKERS. J. A. M. A., 1933, **101,** 17.
12. LUISADA, A. A. Rass. Int. Clin. Ter. (Naples), 1937, **18,** N. 16 and 17.
13. POTAIN, P. C. É. Clin. Méd. Pitié. Paris, Masson, 1844.
14. STEELL, G. Med. Chron., 1888–89, **9,** 182.
15. LUISADA, A. A. Am. Heart J., 1941, **22,** 245.
16. COSSIO, P., AND BERKONSKY. Rev. Arg. Cardiol., 1943, **10,** 162.
17. LUISADA, A. A. Cuore e Circ. (Rome), 1935, **19,** 77.

18. Luisada, A. A. J. Lab. & Clin. Med., 1940, **25**, 1146.
19. Laufer, S. Arch. Mal. Coeur, 1935, **28**, 98.
20. Laufer, S., and Rubino, A. Clin. Med. Ital., 1936, **67**, N. 6.
21. Sossai, A. Cuore e Circ. (Rome), 1938, **22**, 441.
22. Cignolini, P. *Roentgenchimografia Cardiaca e Regmografia.* Bologna, Cappelli, 1934.
23. Grishman, A., Sussman, M. L., and Steinberg, M. F. Am. J. Roentgenol., 1944, **51**, 33.
24. White, P. D. J. A. M. A., 1928, **90**, 603.
25. Burgess, A. M., and Ellis, L. B. New England J. Med., 1942, **226**, 937.
26. a) Ferguson, F. C., Kobilak, R. E., and Deitrick, J. E. Am. Heart J., 1944, **28**, 445.
    b) Harris, A. W., and Levine, S. A. Am. Int. Med., 1941, **15**, 637.
27. a) White, P. D. Boston Med. Surg. J., 1926, **195**, 1146.
    b) Bland, E. F., Jones, T. D., and White, P. D. Am. Heart J., 1935, **10**, 995.
28. Abbott, M. *Congenital Heart Disease. Nelson's Loose Leaf Medicine.* New York, Nelson 1943, vol. 4.
29. Herrmann, G. R. *Synopsis of Diseases of the Heart and Arteries.* St. Louis, Mosby, 1941.
30. Brown, J. W. *Congenital Heart Disease.* London, J. B. Med. Publ., 1939.
31. Corrigan, D. J. Edinburgh Med. & Surg. J., 1832, **37**, 225.
32. Traube, L. Berl. klin. Woch., 1872, **9**, 573.
33. a) Duroziez, P. D. Arch. Gen Méd., 1861, **17**, 417.
    b) Pasoli, E. Cuore e Circ. (Rome), 1930, **14**, 389.
    c) Blumgart, H. L., and Ernstene, A. C. J. A. M. A., 1933, **100**, 173.
    d) Luisada, A. A. Am. Heart J., 1943, **26**, 721.
34. Quincke, H. Berl. klin. Woch., 1868, **5**, 357.
35. a) Frugoni, C. Riv. Crit. Clin. Med. (Florence), 1914, **15**, 100.
    b) Luisada, A. A. Min. Med. (Turin), 1928, **8**, 1139.
    c) Luisada, A. A. Am. Heart J., 1942, **23**, 676.
36. Flint, A. Am. J. M. Sci., 1862, **44**, 29.
37. White, P. D. *Heart Disease.* New York, Macmillan, 1944.
38. a) Luisada, A. A. Am. Heart J., 1944, **28**, 156.
    b) Cossio, P., and Sotomayor, O. Rev. Arg. Cardiol., 1945, **12**, 70.
39. a) Hill, L., Flack, M., and Holtzman, W. Heart, 1909–1910, **1**, 73.
    b) Hill, L., and Flack, M. Brit. Med. J., 1909, **1**, 272.
    c) Murray, J. R. Brit. Med. J., 1914, **1**, 697.
40. Luisada, A. A. Cuore e Circ. (Rome), 1926, **10**, 221.
41. Wolferth, Ch., and Margolies. In *Stroud's Cardiovascular Disease.* Philadelphia, Davis, 1943.
42. Cossio, P., and co-workers. Rev. Arg. Cardiol., 1943, **10**, 21.
43. Wiggers, C. J., and Maltby, A. B. Am. J. Physiol., 1931, **97**, 689.
44. Wiggers, C. J. J. A. M. A., 1931, **97**, 1359.
45. Schneyer, K. Deut. Arch. klin. Med., 1934, **176**, 1.
46. Stewart, G. N. Arch. Int. Med., 1908, **1**, 102.
47. Vaquez, H. *Les Maladies du Coeur.* Paris, Baillière, 1928.
48. Garvin, C. F. Ann. Int. Med., 1940, **13**, 1799.
49. Loewenberg, S. A. Ann. Int. Med., 1940, **14**, 991.
50. Gouley, B. A., and Sickel, E. M. Am. Heart J., 1943, **26**, 24.
51. Gallavardin, L. Arch. Mal. Coeur, 1937, **30**, 745.
52. Schneyer, K. Zeit. Kreislauff., 1938, **30**, 161.
53. Gallavardin, L. *La Tension Artérielle en Clinique.* Paris, Masson, 1921.
54. De Heer, J. L. Pfluegers Arch., 1912, **148**, 1.
55. Allan, A. Heart, 1926, **12**, 181.
56. Evans, W., and Lewes, D. Brit. Heart J., 1945, **7**, 171.
57. a) Gallavardin, L., and Tixier, L. Arch. Mal. Coeur, 1919, **12**, 447.
    b) Barbier, J. *La Méthode Auscultatoire.* Paris, Baillière, 1921.
58. Laubry, C., Brosse, T., and van Bogaert, A. Arch. Mal. Coeur, 1931, **24**, 143.
59. a) Traube. Quoted by Lutembacher (b).
    b) Lutembacher, R. Rev. Méd., 1938, **46**, 436.
60. Marvin, H. M., and Sullivan, A. G. Am. Heart J., 1935, **10**, 705.
61. De Veer, A. J. Am. Heart J., 1938, **15**, 243.
62. Chisholm, D. R. Am. Heart J., 1937, **13**, 362.
63. Gallavardin, L. Quoted by Giraud (64).
64. Giraud, G. *Lesions de l'Orifice aortique, in Nouveau Traité de Médécine* by Roger, Widal, Teissier. Paris, Masson, 1933.
65. a) Parsonnet, A. F., Bernstein, A., and Martland, H. S. Am. Heart J., 1945, **31**, 438.
    b) Ashworth, H., and Morgan Jones, A. Brit. Heart J., 1946, **8**, 207.

66. RYTAND, D. A., AND LIPSITCH, L. S. Arch. INT. Med., 1946, **78**, 544.

67. a) SCHUR, M. Erg. inn. Med., 1934, **47**, 348.
b) HOLOWSKY, M. Klin. Med., 1947, **2**, 540.

68. MANTOVANI, A., AND LORENZONI, B. Folia Card. (Milan), 1947, **6**, 51.

69. a) BLOOMFIELD, R. A., AND CO-WORKERS. J. Clin. Investigation, 1946, **25**, 639.
b) McMICHAEL, J. Am. Rev. Physiol., 1948, **10**, 201.

70. LUISADA, A. A., AND FLEISCHNER, F. G. Am. J. Med., 1948, **4**, 791.

71. BAILEY, C. P. Dis. of Chest, 1949, **15**, 377.

72. COSGRIFF, S. W. J. A. M. A., 1950, **143**, 870.

73. ALIMURUNG, M. M., RAPPAPORT, M. B., AND SPRAGUE, H. B. New England J. Med., 1949, **241**, 631.

74. WELLS, B. G., RAPPAPORT, M. B., AND SPRAGUE, H. B. Am. Heart J., 1949, **37**, 586.

75. LUISADA, A. A., AND PERÉZ MONTES, L. Ann. Int. Med., 1950, **33**, 56.

76. O'NEILL, T. J. E., BAILEY, C. P., AND GLOVER, R. P. Acta Med. Scand., 1952, **142** (Suppl. 266), 817.

77. O'NEILL, T. J. E., GLOVER, R. P., AND BAILEY, C. P. J. A. M. A., 1951, **147**, 1032.

78. Case 33211 of Massachusetts General Hospital. New England J. Med., 1947, **236**, 806.

79. DAVISON, S. J. Mt. Sinai Hosp., 1948, **14**, 941.

80. LASSER, R. P., EPSTEIN, B., AND LOEWE, L. Am. Heart J., 1952, **44**, 681.

81. GEILL, T., AND KIAER, W. Acta Med. Scand., 1952, **142** (Supp. 266), 413.

82. ZIMMERMAN, H. A. J. Clin. Investigation, 1950, **29**, 1601.

83. LUISADA, A. A. Chicago Soc. Int. Med., 1952, **19**, 70.

84. ALEXANDER, R. S. Am. J. Physiol., 1949, **158**, 294.

85. FENICHEL, N. M. Am. Heart J., 1950, **40**, 117.

86. a) SPRAGUE, H. B., AND JACOBSEN, R. P. Med. Clin. North America, 1948, **32**, 1309.

87. BAILEY, C. P., AND RAMIREZ, R. J. A. M. A., 1952, **150**, 1647.

CHAPTER 12

The Valvular Defects of the Right Heart

Pulmonic Insufficiency

Pulmonic insufficiency occurs when the semilunar valves of the pulmonary artery become incompetent and permit regurgitation during diastole. This causes a typical clinical picture and a series of compensatory changes in both in the right heart and in the vessels of the lesser circulation.

CAUSE

Different causes may determine pulmonic insufficiency:

a) A *congenital lesion,* consisting of the absence or malformation of one of the valvular cusps (1b); it is often associated with other abnormalities.

b) A *rheumatic lesion.* Severe lesion is rare (51) while moderate alterations are probably common (50). The pulmonic is usually associated with a mitral defect.

c) A *bacterial lesion.* Pulmonic insufficiency during an acute streptococcic endocarditis is common. A healed gonococcic, pneumococcic, or streptococcic endocarditis may be the cause of the lesion.

d) A *luetic lesion* is rare but possible, especially if there is a luetic arteritis of the pulmonary artery (chapter 21). Pressure irritation from an aortic aneurysm is one of the mechanisms producing this type of lesion.

e) An *atherosclerotic lesion* may occur in cases with primary atherosclerosis of the pulmonary artery, chronic cor pulmonale (chapter 23), congenital defects, or mitral stenosis as a result of long lasting pulmonary hypertension.

f) Surgery of the pulmonic valve (page 267).

LESIONS

Pulmonic insufficiency is seldom pure. It is observed more commonly in combination with other valvular defects or lesions of the pulmonary artery.

The valvular lesions are those typical of the different forms and consist of deformation, retraction, or partial destruction of the leaflets. In lues and atherosclerosis, the process predominates in the artery and is transmitted to the cusps. Fibrotic changes of the leaflets as well as adhesions have been described in cases of aortic aneurysm, compressing the pulmonary artery.

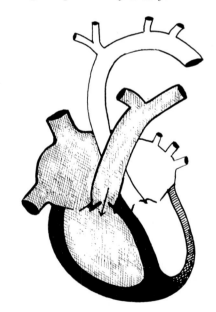

FIG. 154. Changes of the heart in pulmonic insufficiency.

The *right ventricle is dilated* and its wall is markedly hypertrophied. The right atrium

259

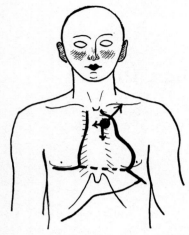

Fig. 155. Cardiac dulness and transmission of the diastolic murmur in pulmonic insufficiency.

is usually somewhat dilated. *The pulmonary artery and its branches are extremely dilated;* their walls are thickened and may become sclerotic.

SIGNS AND SYMPTOMS

The symptoms of these patients are seldom characteristic and are separated with difficulty from those of other cardiovascular lesions. Physical effort causes *dyspnea, palpitation, dizziness,* and, sometimes, *precordial pain.* The patient is *weak* and may present *nosebleeds, obstinate dry cough,* and, occasionally, *bloody sputum. Attacks of suffocation associated with cyanosis, cog-wheel respiration,* and *somnolence,* have been described.

The patients have *cyanosis* and frequently *clubbing* of the fingers and toes.

The pulse is *small* and *not* collapsing.

Local Signs[55]

There is a *diffuse systolic pulsation* between the sternum and the left midclavicular line. *Epigastric pulsation* is common. There is *no thrill.*

Percussion reveals that the heart is en-

[55] Owing to the rarity of cases, the description will be based mainly on the signs of a typical case studied by *Dressler* (2).

larged toward the right and that *there is a "cap" of dulness in the 2nd and 3rd left interspaces* (fig. 155).

Auscultation reveals a *long diastolic murmur,* having its maximum intensity over the 2nd or 3rd left interspace. This murmur starts immediately after the 2nd sound and gradually fades away. It may be *low-pitched* and *rumbling* (3) but more often is *soft.* The murmur is transmitted toward the left clavicle and toward the 3rd and 4th right interspaces. It is not transmitted toward the apex or the suprasternal notch (4). It usually becomes louder when the patient is raised to the erect position (5).

A *systolic murmur* of lesser intensity may also be present.

The *2nd pulmonic sound is loud* in the luetic and atherosclerotic forms; it *is weak and barely audible* in the others. Auscultation at the mouth may reveal *intermittent whiffs due to emission of air* (5).

BLOOD PRESSURE—GRAPHIC TRACINGS

The mean pressure is low, the pulse pressure is normal.

Pulse tracings fail to show the rapid rise and the rapid drop which are typical of aortic insufficiency.

The *electrocardiogram* shows *right axis deviation.*

The *phonocardiogram* reveals a murmur similar to that of aortic regurgitation, except for the area of best recording (2nd and 3rd *left* interspaces).

X-RAY

The cardiac shadow seems to rest on the diaphragm but the apex appears to be elevated. The pulmonary knob is dilated and shows ample and rapid pulsations. This is particularly evident in the right anterior oblique position.

The *hilar shadows present extremely powerful pulsations,* called the *"hilar dance"* (6).

The aortic knob is small and shows normal pulsations. *Roentgenkymography* and *electrokymography* reveal a typical tracing over the pulmonary knob (*collapsing pulse*). The electrokymographic study of the hilar shadows and of the pulmonary parenchyma reveals *high and collapsing pulsations*, and a rapidly progressing pulse wave, in the vessels of the lesser circulation.

MODE OF ORIGIN OF THE SIGNS

Valvular insufficiency causes a regurgitation of blood into the right ventricle during diastole, the results of which are similar to those occurring in the left ventricle and the aorta with aortic regurgitation (page 246).

There is enlargement of the right ventricle and the pulmonary artery. There is a violent pulsation of the pulmonary artery and of its branches, causing the *hilar dance* on fluoroscopy.

The *diastolic murmur* is due to the regurgitating blood. The *systolic murmur* is either caused by stenosis or is a murmur due to dilatation of the pulmonary artery and similar to that occurring in the aorta in aortic regurgitation (*relative pulmonic stenosis*) (page 267).

Cyanosis, hemoptysis, somnolence, and *clubbing* of the fingers, are all due to sclerosis of the pulmonary vessels which frequently accompanies pulmonic insufficiency.

COURSE AND COMPLICATIONS

The most frequent complications are: pulmonary embolism, profuse hemoptysis, acute or chronic bronchitis, and aneurysm of the pulmonary artery. Nothing definite can be stated about the course because of the rarity of the cases. It seems that periods of heart failure can alternate with periods of improvement. The picture of failure includes severe peripheral edema, very large liver, severe cyanosis, somnolence, and obstinate cough.

DIAGNOSIS

Owing to the rarity of cases of uncomplicated pulmonary insufficiency, the diagnosis will be made mostly in cases where a mitral stenosis is associated with organic insuffi-

ciency of the pulmonary valve (page 301), and in cases with relative insufficiency.

Relative Pulmonic Insufficiency

This condition is usually the result of high pressure in the pulmonary artery. It may be found in mitral stenosis (10), arteriosclerosis of the pulmonary circulation (11), septal defects (9), complex congenital malformations (Eisenmenger complex), and subacute bacterial endocarditis. It is revealed by a *diastolic murmur in decrescendo*.

In certain cases, the murmur is transitory because the high pulmonic pressure decreases with therapy (an example is the G. Steell murmur of mitral stenosis). *The murmur is usually soft* and seems caused by distention of the right ventricle.

Distention of the pulmonary artery itself usually causes a *systolic murmur*.

Pulmonary Stenosis

Pulmonary stenosis exists when a narrowing, either at or before the valvular opening of the pulmonary artery, is present. Deep changes in the structure and function of the right ventricle follow.

CAUSE

Different causes may be responsible for the stenosis.

a) *A congenital lesion.*

b) *A rheumatic lesion.* Extremely rare.

c) *A bacterial lesion* (pneumococcal, gonococcal, or streptococcal).

d) *A luetic lesion.* Rare (14).

LESIONS

There are several types of pulmonic stenosis:

a) *Pulmonary hypoplasia.* Unequal division of the common arterial trunk causes narrowing of the orifice and of the pulmonary artery. The pulmonic valve is often bicuspid.

b) *Valvular stenosis.* Thickening of the leaflets and fusion of the commissures reveal

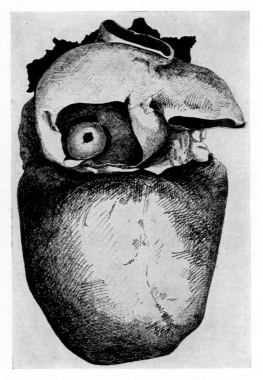

FIG. 156. Drawing from a specimen of pulmonic stenosis. Typical *fish-mouth shape of the valve*.

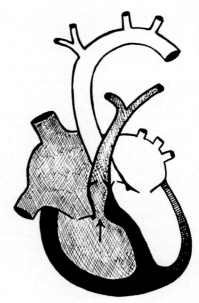

FIG. 157. Changes of the heart in pulmonic stenosis.

a previous inflammatory process. The pulmonary artery is frequently dilated.

c) *Diaphragmatic type of stenosis.* Complete fusion of the cusps forms a cone-shaped membrane protruding into the pulmonary artery and having a small central opening of 1 to 5 mm. This type is also probably due to endocarditis (fig. 156).

d) *Subpulmonic stenosis.* A horizontal fibrous membrane with a central perforation can be found below the valvular opening. This is a congenital malformation.

e) *"Conus separate chamber."* The outflow tract of the right ventricle is separated from the main cavity by muscular bands which leave only a small opening. The pulmonary orifice may be normal or hypoplastic.

The right ventricle presents severe dilatation and hypertrophic walls. This leads to a more horizontal position of the heart with the apex raised from the diaphragm.

If the foramen ovale is patent, the clinical signs are different (page 308).

SIGNS AND SYMPTOMS

There may be *exertional dyspnea* and *precordial oppression.* Pure pulmonic stenosis has been considered rare. However, if the milder forms are included, the defect becomes much more common. Severe pulmonic stenosis has been described in patients from birth to about 26 years. Occasional cases were older, and the longest survival is 78 years.

Cyanosis may be minimal or absent. When severe, it indicates the association with septal defects, or is caused by heart failure. A *greyish color* has been observed (13). *Attacks of dyspnea, dizziness, suffocation,* and *dry cough* may occur. *Periods of somnolence* have been described.

Cold and *bluish extremities* are frequent. A condition of *infantilism* may be present in the congenital cases. The *pulse* is *small* but not *tardus. Clubbing* of the fingers and toes and *squatting* may be occasionally noted but are not the rule.

Local Signs

A *precordial bulge* is frequent in the congenital cases. There is a *diffuse systolic pulsation* of a large median area (fig. 158).

Palpation reveals a *systolic thrill*, having its maximal intensity over the 2nd or 3rd left interspace and transmitted toward the left clavicle.

The *cardiac dulness is markedly enlarged to the right.* There usually is no dulness in the 2nd left interspace.

Auscultation shows the following data:

a) *The 1st sound is loud over the pulmonic area.* It may be followed by a *snapping sound* in early systole (*opening click of the pulmonic valve*).

b) The *2nd pulmonic sound is weak* in most of the cases. It may be loud in those caused by vascular alterations of the pulmonary artery.

c) There may be *an atrial type of triple rhythm* over the median region of the heart and at the epigastrium (page 370).

d) The most typical sign is *a loud and harsh systolic murmur.* This has a maximum loudness over either the 3rd or the 2nd left interspace. It is transmitted toward the left clavicle and may be heard over the left side of the neck if there is consolidation of the upper lobe of the left lung. It is poorly transmitted toward the cardiac apex and the suprasternal notch (4). It is heard well over the left scapula (14) and the left lung field (16) and is increased by inspiration or inspiratory apnea (45).

A presystolic sound over the femoral vein at the groin has been described (14).

BLOOD PRESSURE

The blood pressure is usually low; the pulse pressure is somewhat decreased.

BLOOD—BLOOD GASES

There may be moderate *polycythemia.* The *oxygen saturation of the arterial blood is decreased.*

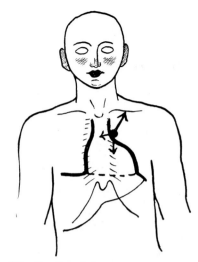

Fig. 158. Cardiac dulness and transmission of the systolic murmur in pulmonic stenosis.

While the oxygen saturation of the peripheral blood does not change after an exercise test, *the amount of oxygen consumed per liter of ventilation falls after exercise* (42).

CIRCULATION TIME

Circulation time is increased, both in the arm-to-lung and in the arm-to-periphery tests.

GRAPHIC METHODS

Electrocardiogram. There is marked *right axis deviation.* There is evidence of *right ventricular hypertrophy* (fig. 159) and there may be right bundle branch block. The P wave is often high in leads 2, 3, aVF, and especially in V1 (pattern of *right atrial hypertrophy*).

Phonocardiogram. The tracings recorded over the second left interspace may show a very high vibration. This is the *opening snap of the pulmonic valve.* It is followed by a series of both high- and low-pitched vibrations, presenting first an increase and then a decrease, and resembling the shape of a pulse wave. This is the so-called *diamond-shaped murmur* (fig. 160). However, the murmur is sometimes so loud that it includes all systole without any variation of intensity. The *second sound is weak*; however, if the murmur is loud and prolonged, it is difficult to state whether the latter is weak or covered by the murmur.

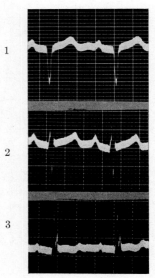

F<small>IG</small>. 159. Electrocardiogram in a child with pulmonic stenosis.

Jugular tracing, hepatic tracing. These tracings may show a high atrial wave.

Epigastric tracing. This tracing shows a high atrial wave and a high, but slow, initial ventricular wave.

Apex cardiogram. There frequently is a negative systolic wave.

Electrokymogram. The border tracing of the pulmonary knob frequently reveals *a decreased magnitude of pulsations.* However, these may be large in cases with valvular stenosis or associated aneurysm of the pulmonary artery. The *densograms of the hilar shadows, and especially those of the lungs, reveal small or absent pulsations in all cases.*

Cardiomanometry. The *pressure of the right ventricle is high.* Pressures of 65/5 (and even 190/0) have been encountered. On the other hand, the *pressure of the pulmonary artery is normal or low* with values of 12/0 to 20/14. Thus the *pressure gradient between right ventricle and pulmonary artery is increased.* This is the most significant fact which has diagnostic value in cases of mild and well-tolerated stenosis. Pressure tracings of the right atrium may show the existence of extremely *high atrial waves* due to strong contractions of the right atrium. Mild forms may present a normal pressure of the right ventricle and a low pressure of the pulmonary artery. The gradient is thus increased and is further increased by exercise.

X-RAY

The cardiac silhouette is enlarged and has no typical shape. *The right heart is large, the lungs are clear, and there is a variable size of the main pulmonary artery. This may be either small (18, 20, 21) or*

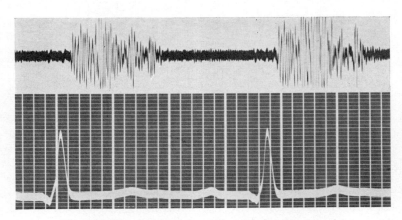

F<small>IG</small>. 160. Sound tracing in a case of pulmonic stenosis.

dilated (12, 22), the last being the most common occurrence.

The *hilar shadows* are small or normal but not pulsating. The *fine pulmonary network is poorly visible.*

Angiocardiography may give important data: *a narrow channel may reveal the area of stenosis in the subpulmonic type.* The right ventricle is enlarged; the pulmonary artery is either thin or dilated (9) (fig. 161). It is typical to observe a prolonged sojourn of the contrast medium in the right ventricle in comparison with normal hearts.

MODE OF ORIGIN OF THE SIGNS

The obstacle encountered by the blood flowing from the right ventricle causes dilatation of this chamber and hypertrophy of its wall.

Right ventricular contraction is often somewhat slow as revealed by different tracings. The effect of this will be visible in the higher atrial wave of the venous tracings (jugular, hepatic tracings) and of the electrocardiogram. The right ventricular enlargement is revealed by the ECG (right axis deviation) and the x-ray.

The eddies which originate at the point of narrowing cause the systolic murmur.

This has its maximum intensity at mid-systole, when the outflow is greatest. The diffusion of the murmur is explained by the transmission of the sound vibrations along the blood stream, unless its intensity is such that they are diffused by the bony structures.

The "opening click" is found mainly in cases following endocarditis. The weak 2nd pulmonic sound is caused by the rigidity of the leaflets of the pulmonary valve. Enlargement of the pulmonary artery is due to poststenotic dilatation because of the eddies which form beyond the narrowing.

Cyanosis, when present, is due either to low pressure and slow flow through the lungs or to peripheral factors (heart failure). As there is no mixture of blood between the right and left hearts, cyanosis, clubbing, and polycythemia are absent or moderate. Moderate failure causes *an increase of the residual blood and of the diastolic pressure of the right ventricle.* Right atrial pressure also rises.

VARIETIES

A primary distinction should be made between the *subpulmonic variety* and the others. In the former, the thrill and the

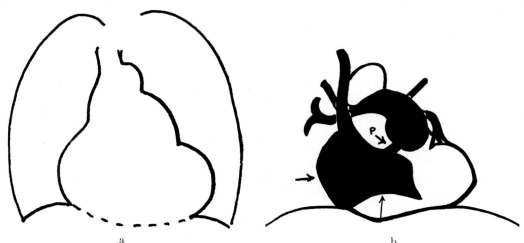

a   b

FIG. 161. Cardiac silhouette (a), and angiocardiogram of the right heart (b) in pulmonic stenosis. P, narrow pulmonary opening. (Section b is inspired by originals of Sussman and coworkers.)

murmur are lower (3rd left interspace), the pulmonary knob is smaller, and the 2nd pulmonic sound is weaker. There is frequently *infantilism*.

In another variety (12, 22, 23), the narrowing of the pulmonic orifice is moderate, the lesion is relatively well tolerated, and the diagnosis is purely clinical. The murmur is heard better when the patient is supine than when he is in the erect position. The T wave of the ECG is high. The pulmonary knob may be full but not prominent. There may be liver engorgement and, in the older individuals, ascitis and peripheral edema (46). The existence of this syndrome has been confirmed by *Dexter* through right heart catheterization. Many of these patients have no complaints and reach a normal physical development. However, their resistance to physical strain is below norm and they may succumb to bacterial endocarditis. While *Cournand* considers that normal right ventricular pressure with low pulmonic pressure is the result of a primary dilatation of the pulmonary artery, others believe that the increased gradient of pressure is the result of mild pulmonic stenosis. If the gradient is increased by exercise, the second interpretation is probably correct.

COURSE AND COMPLICATIONS

The most frequent complications are: pulmonary infarction, pulmonary tuberculosis, and subacute bacterial endocarditis.

The *infarction* is caused by an *embolus* starting from that dilated section which is immediately below the stenosis.

Pulmonary tuberculosis has been found in 36 per cent of the cases (13). It is, therefore, a frequent complication.

Subacute bacterial endocarditis is also fairly common (13). *Heart failure* is inevitable with the exception of the mild stenosis. *Liver cirrhosis* has been frequently found and is attributed to passive liver congestion which is favored by the effects of the valvular lesion (14b, 16) and is later increased by chronic heart failure.

A possible complication is aneurysm of the pulmonary artery.

DIAGNOSIS

Diagnosis should be based on the following data: heart enlarged to the right; systolic thrill and murmur with weak 2nd pulmonic sound; usually prominent pulmonic knob with decreased pulmonary markings; evidence of right ventricular and right atrial hypertrophy in the ECG; exertional dyspnea; frequent absence of clubbing and squatting; only slight cyanosis. In difficult cases, catheterization supplies essential data.

Relative stenosis of the pulmonary valve will be discussed later (see below).

A *functional systolic murmur* of the pulmonic area is not accompanied by right heart enlargement, or right axis deviation; these signs are present in pulmonary stenosis. In doubtful cases, the differential diagnosis between mild pulmonic stenosis and dilatation of the pulmonary artery due to other causes requires catheterization.

Patent ductus arteriosus. This lesion gives a cap of dulness in the 2nd left interspace. The murmur is of a different type (machinery murmur). It occurs in late systole and early diastole or both in systole and diastole (auscultation, phonocardiography). The ECG shows a left axis deviation. The pulse pressure is frequently increased. At x-ray there is marked dilatation of the pulmonary knob and the hilar shadows are large and pulsating. The patients are often pale.

Ventricular septal defect. The murmur is transmitted better toward the right side of the chest. The ECG has no axis deviation. The patient is pale. In some cases, however, differential diagnosis may be difficult.

Fallot's syndrome and other malformations of the heart. As most of these have a pulmonary stenosis, the problem is to exclude the associated lesion. In all of them, cyanosis is severe and circulation time is shortened by the shunt (chapter 15).

Pulmonary stenosis caused by adhesive

pericarditis will be discussed later (chapter 20).

The only effective treatment is surgery. Both the *Blalock-Taussig* and the *Potts-Gibson techniques* have been advocated but the results have been poor. However, *Brocq* (49) described a new method (*valvulotomy followed by dilatation*) which seems definitely superior. The instrument is introduced through the right ventricular wall; a double cut is made in the stenotic valve, then dilatation is made. Pulmonic insufficiency may result but is minimal and unimportant on account of the low level of diastolic pressure in the pulmonary artery. Cases with subpulmonic stenosis have also been operated upon. In them, the protruding portion of the septum was removed by means of a rongeur. This last intervention is undoubtedly more hazardous and is still under experimentation (49, 50).

If *pulmonary tuberculosis* develops, it is primarily the lung rather than the heart which should be treated. *Collapse therapy* is well tolerated if started early, and offers the best chance of preserving the life of these patients (24). *Thoracoplasty* is not contraindicated.

When heart failure starts, *oxygen* is very useful, together with drug therapy.

Relative Stenosis of the Pulmonary Valve

This occurs when the pulmonary artery is dilated, causing a trigonoidation of the valvular opening (25) or a relative disproportion between the opening and the vessel. The resulting systolic murmur is the only manifestation. Therefore, cyanosis, right heart enlargement, axis deviation, and thrill are absent. A dilatation of the pulmonary knob is often present at fluoroscopy.

Double Pulmonic Defect

A double pulmonic defect occurs when *pulmonary stenosis* is associated with *pul-*

monary insufficiency. It is rare and is always due to endocarditis. Most of the described cases were due to Pneumococcus or Streptococcus infections and the local signs were overshadowed by severe general symptoms. Rare cases are due to rheumatic fever; multiple valvular lesions are then present (51). A *double murmur over the pulmonic area* is the typical expression of the double defect.

Tricuspid Insufficiency

Tricuspid insufficiency is present when the leaflets of the right atrioventricular opening are incompetent and permit regurgitation of blood from the left ventricle into the right atrium during ventricular systole. Adaptations take place not only in the right heart but also in the venous system and in the liver.

Different causes may determine this lesion.

a) *Congenital.* It consists of the absence or the downward displacement of one leaflet, so that one part of the ventricle is not separated from the atrium (13). This is a rare lesion which is usually associated with patency of the foramen ovale (page 278).[56]

b) *Rheumatic.* This is the most common cause.

c) *Bacterial.* It is rare but not exceptional.

d) *An acute myocardial lesion* may lead to stretching of the right atrioventricular opening with irreversible changes and permanent insufficiency (27b).

Tricuspid insufficiency is extremely rare as a "pure" defect. It is much more frequent if in combination with tricuspid stenosis, mitral defects, or an atrial septal defect.

The valvular lesions may consist of

[56] Some authors call the syndrome caused by this lesion "Ebstein's syndrome". Actually, such a syndrome is due to the association of the malformation of the tricuspid valve *plus* the patency of the foramen ovale.

fenestrations or *retraction* of the valves. The shortening of one of the papillary muscles or chordae may cause insufficiency without stenosis.

The heart is enlarged with dilatation and hypertrophy of the right atrium and ventricle. Both venae cavae and the hepatic veins are extremely dilated (fig. 162). The liver is large. There frequently is ascites.

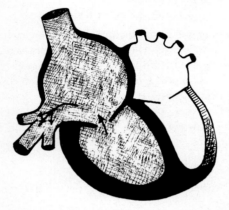

Fig. 162. Changes of the heart in tricuspid insufficiency.

SIGNS AND SYMPTOMS

The patients are *cyanotic*. They complain of *precordial* pain and *palpitation* after effort. Their *dypsnea* is moderate and not proportional to the cyanosis. *Digestive disturbances and sensation of fullness in the upper right abdominal quadrant* are early symptoms. The head of the patient may shake with rhythmic backward movements. This phenomenon is more apparent in the recumbent position and may disappear when sitting (38).

The *jugular veins are turgid and present intensive pulsations.* Occasionally, a visible pulsation of the veins of the forearm is present (41). Peripheral edema may be absent or moderate, in contrast with the increased size of the abdomen due to *early ascites.*

Local Signs

The precordial area presents a *massive displacement toward the right* at every sys-

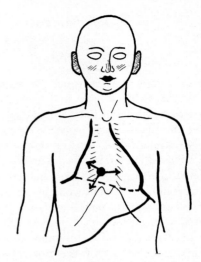

Fig. 163. Cardiac dulness and transmission of the systolic murmur in tricuspid insufficiency.

tole. The lower part of the right thorax and the upper right quadrant of the abdomen are thrust forward in systole while, at the same time, the region of the apex is depressed. Thus a *see-saw movement* takes place (2, 27).

There is *no thrill*. Palpation of *the liver* shows that *this organ pulsates strongly and expands in systole.*

Percussion reveals that cardiac dulness is enlarged toward the right where the right border often ends with an *obtuse cardiohepatic angle.*

Auscultation reveals a *long, soft, blowing systolic murmur,* having its maximum intensity at the 3rd or 4th right interspace near the sternum and transmitted toward the right clavicle but not toward the apex.

Auscultation of the mouth may reveal a *cog-wheel type of respiration* (26). If the systolic murmur over the tricuspid area is faint or absent, *deep inspiration followed by apnea increases its loudness or causes its appearance while other murmurs become less audible* (40). The short inspiratory apnea of crying children obtains the same result.

GRAPHIC TRACINGS

Electrocardiogram. There is a *right axis deviation.* Atrial fibrillation is common and occurs early. Ventricular premature beats and attacks of ventricular tachycardia are frequent in the later stages. A peaked and diphasic P wave in lead V1 is frequent in the early stages and reveals right atrial hypertrophy.

Phonocardiogram. This tracing records a *systolic murmur "in decrescendo"* or a *continuous systolic murmur*, over the tricuspid area and at the right of the sternum. This murmur is frequently high-pitched and becomes louder in inspiration (fig. 164). Thus, a comparison between tracings taken in inspiration and expiration permits differentiation from a mitral systolic murmur because the latter decreases or remains unchanged in inspiration. Moreover, this murmur is louder over the tricuspid area than at the apex; a comparison between the apical and the tricuspid phonocardiograms excludes a transmitted murmur.

Low frequency tracings. The region of the apex has a retraction or backward thrust during ventricular systole. On the other hand, there is a systolic, forward thrust of the epigastrium, the lower part of the sternum, and the right precordial area. This double motion creates a *see-saw movement*.

Jugular tracing, hepatic tracing. Both tracings show a high positive atrial wave (unless atrial fibrillation is present), and a high, positive, systolic wave. This wave becomes, in severe lesions, a positive, *systolic plateau*, similar to a tracing of intraventricular pressure (fig. 165). When regurgitation is associated with stenosis, both the ascending and the descending branch take place later. If the regurgitation is

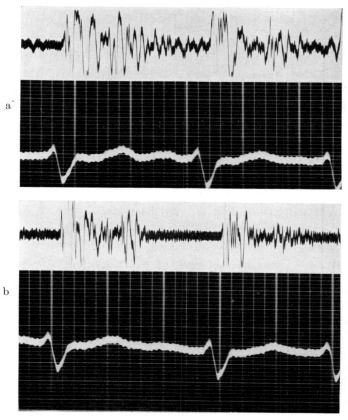

FIG. 164. Phonocardiogram recorded over the tricuspid area in a case of tricuspid insufficiency and stenosis. Murmurs louder in inspiration. a, inspiratory apnea. b, expiratory apnea.

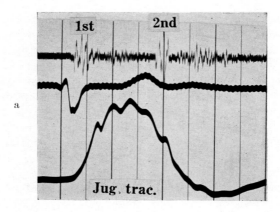

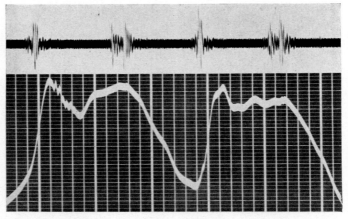

Fig. 165. Plateau-like positive wave in the jugular tracing (a), and hepatic tracing (b). Tricuspid insufficiency

moderate, the wave is more rounded, has a slow rise, a peak in late systole, and an abrupt descending limb in early diastole. The liver of these patients has been called "the systolic liver."

Venous pressure, cardiomanometry. Venous pressure is usually elevated.

The pressure of the right atrium is slightly elevated and presents a typical increase during ventricular systole. This has been demonstrated both in experimental defects and in clinical cases. The initial tension of the right ventricle is increased but the amplitude of the ventricular pulse pressure is decreased on account of the regurgitation. The pulmonary pulse pressure is decreased on account of reduced ejection of the right ventricle.

Pneumocardiogram. There is a deep negative systolic wave (fusion of *v1* with *v2*) followed by a positive, early-diastolic wave. The succession of the negative and positive waves may cause a very impressive movement of air (*cog-wheel respiration*).

Electrokymography. The border tracing of the right atrium in tricuspid insufficiency should present a typical pattern, identical to that of the left atrium in mitral insufficiency. Actually, the right atrial tracing is so influenced by the contraction of the right ventricle that *such a pattern is encountered only in severe regurgitation.* In many of the author's cases, the liver and the jugular tracing were typical while the electrokymogram was not. When typical, the EKY presents a deep, presystolic, negative wave caused by right atrial contraction. This is followed by *a large, square, positive, systolic plateau,* caused by the blood which flows back into the right atrium during ventricular systole. The plateau resembles a tracing of intraventricular pressure, as has been demonstrated by *Marchal.*

ARTERIAL PRESSURE—VENOUS PRESSURE

Arterial pressure is low; pulse pressure is normal; *venous pressure is usually increased.*

X-RAY

The cardiac shadow shows a dilatation of the right heart. The superior vena cava is dilated (20) and expands in systole (28). The *right atrium dilates in systole* (19). The upper margin of the liver shadow rises at every systole (29, 30). The pulmonary fields are clear, in contrast with the clinical picture of congestion and in contrast with the picture of mitral patients.

MODE OF ORIGIN OF THE SIGNS

The lesion of the tricuspid valve permits regurgitation of blood from the right ventricle into the right atrium during systole. This leads to distention of the right atrium and of the mouths of the venae cavae.

This regurgitation pushes the entire column of blood back into the veins during the phase of ejection. Since the proximity of the hepatic veins to the right atrium is greater than that of the veins of the neck, and gravity adds its effect, the backward flow is largely diverted into the liver. An enlargement of the tubercle of Lower seems to cause a dilatation of the lowest part of the right atrium by deflecting the flow; this is a further cause of dilatation of the hepatic veins (33).

The large veins, the liver, and the right atrium pulsate in systole like arteries. Their pulsation, however, is slower and takes place somewhat later than the arterial because of the damping due to the elasticity of the venoatrial system. This venous pulsation is the cause of the rhythmic movements of the head.

As soon as ventricular systole ends, a sudden inversion of the flow takes place in the veins; the stream stops, then rushes toward the right ventricle with greater speed than in normal subjects.

The fact that the blood leaves the thorax in systole, not only through the arteries, but also through the veins, leads to a tremendous suction (31) which causes the depression of the left side of the chest and the deep negative waves in the pneumocardiogram. The strong pulsation of the right ventricle and the systolic distention of the liver cause the systolic forward thrust of the right side of the chest and of the right upper abdominal quadrant.

Cyanosis is due to the increased venous pressure caused by the valvular lesion and not to heart failure or pulmonary damage.

The succession of a deep suction followed by emission of air is responsible for the cogwheel type of respiration.

The sudden onrush of blood into the thorax and the heart at the beginning of diastole is the cause of the positive wave of the pneumocardiogram.

The blood, regurgitating into the right atrium, forms eddies which are the cause of the soft systolic murmur.

The hypertrophy of the right atrium and ventricle is a compensatory element and is the cause of the strong contraction of these chambers. The extreme dilatation of the venae cavae permits regurgitation of blood during atrial contraction. Therefore, if sinus rhythm persists, a large atrial wave precedes the systolic plateau in the jugular and liver tracings.

Chronic congestion of the liver may exist without heart failure and is an element of compensation. On the other hand, it favors ascites and digestive disturbances.

Distention of the right atrium is a cause of functional disturbance of the myocardium which favors early atrial fibrillation.

COURSE AND COMPLICATIONS

The most frequent complications are: atrial fibrillation, ventricular tachycardia, pulmonary embolism, and aneurysm of the right atrium. Patients with tricuspid insufficiency have a clinical picture of congestion of the venous system which is similar to that of congestive failure. In the early stage, this is due to the dynamic effects of the valvular lesion and not to weakness of the myocardium. For this reason, the patients may sometimes attend to their usual occupations for a long period with infrequent attacks of dyspnea and no peripheral edema. On the other hand, digitalis has only a limited influence on the signs and symptoms, unless they are increased by heart failure and by relative insufficiency of the tricuspid. The latter increases the effects of the anatomical lesion.

DIAGNOSIS

The diagnosis is based upon right heart enlargement, see-saw movement of the chest, systolic pulsation of the jugular veins, possible ascites, and a large pulsating liver while there is no pulmonary stasis and no severe peripheral edema.

Differential diagnosis should exclude the following possibilities.

Relative tricuspid insufficiency. This will be considered below.

Tricuspid stenosis. In pure tricuspid stenosis, regurgitation of blood is limited or absent. Therefore, no systolic pulsation of the liver and veins is present. Enlargement of the right ventricle is moderate. Jaundice is more frequent.

Tricuspid insufficiency plus stenosis is revealed by a more oblique and delayed rise and fall of the systolic plateau in the jugular and hepatic tracings in comparison with the pure insufficiency.

Constrictive pericarditis. This picture will be described later (page 450).

Mitral valve defects. Coronary and arteriosclerotic heart disease. They may have a picture which is somewhat similar to that of tricuspid insufficiency but only if there is relative insufficiency of this valve (see below). Therefore, congestive failure is always present in such patients. Patients with tricuspid insufficiency have no congestion of the lungs unless they are in severe failure.

Prognosis and *treatment* will be described below (page 275).

Relative Tricuspid Insufficiency

A relative insufficiency of the tricuspid valve may be caused by marked dilatation of the right ventricle. This is frequent during congestive failure in patients with mitral valve defects, adhesive pericarditis, chronic cor pulmonale, coronary heart disease, congenital heart disease, and even hypertensive heart disease (32). The insufficiency is caused by *stretching of the papillary muscles* and *dilatation of the opening* because of myocardial weakness (figs. 103I and 126).

The movements of the precordium are seldom typical.

The main sign is a *soft, blowing, systolic murmur* over the tricuspid area but this is easily confused with a mitral or aortic murmur in the same phase. The hepatic and jugular tracings may present waves which are similar to those of organic insufficiency; this fact, however, is not constant because high pressure and high tension of the venous walls, which permit a rapid transmission of pressure in the organic lesion, are not always present here. In milder cases, a small and slow drop of the jugular tracing after the *c* wave may be the only graphic sign (19). Severe relative insufficiency may be accompanied by a typical systolic plateau (page 270).

Tricuspid Stenosis

Tricuspid stenosis is the narrowing of the right atrioventricular opening. The obstacle is *before* the right ventricle, and causes adaptations which are mainly outside the heart.

CAUSE

Two main causes originate tricuspid stenosis.

a) *A congenital lesion.* It is frequently associated with patency of the foramen ovale (page 302).

b) *A rheumatic lesion.* It usually occurs after recurrent attacks of rheumatic disease. Therefore the association of tricuspid stenosis with mitral stenosis is the rule.

LESIONS

Tricuspid stenosis is not rare because it occurs in 20 to 30 per cent of patients with rheumatic heart disease (32–35). However,

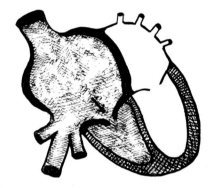

FIG. 166. Changes of the heart and large veins in tricuspid stenosis.

most authors call "tricuspid stenosis" any tricuspid lesions, even if it is a double defect with predominant insufficiency (36, 37). Therefore the actual frequency of the "stenosis" is lower than the above-quoted figures.

The tricuspid leaflets are usually shrunken and partly fused, resulting in the formation of a funnel which projects into the right ventricle.

The right atrium is dilated and has a thick wall. The rest of the heart shows no changes unless there are other defects (fig. 166).

Both venae cavae are tremendously dilated. *The liver is greatly enlarged* and *presents evidence of cardiac cirrhosis. Ascites is frequent.*

SYMPTOMS AND SIGNS

Cyanosis may be present. It may further increase in some periods. It is frequently accompanied by *slight jaundice (subicterus)*, often revealed only by a yellowish tinge of the sclerae. The *jugular veins* are distended; a high presystolic wave may be observed if there is no atrial fibrillation.

The *hearts* of these patients may have no typical signs except for *obtuseness of the cardiohepatic angle.*

There may be *no murmurs* caused by the valvular defect; on the other hand, a *diastolic rumble* is often present over the tricuspid area. This often escapes detection because it is confused with a similar murmur of the mitral valve (combined mitral and tricuspid stenosis). *It is increased by inspiration.*

The *lungs* are practically normal, even in the presence of slight congestive failure.

The *liver is large and firm.* It is not appreciably reduced by digitalis and even mercurial diuretics may not affect its size. *The liver may present an appreciable presystolic pulsation.* However, this is frequently absent either because of hepatic fibrosis or because there is atrial fibrillation.

There frequently is *ascites* with a pure

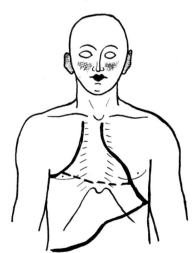

FIG. 167. Cardiac and hepatic dulness in tricuspid stenosis.

transudate in the abdominal cavity. *Peripheral edema* may occur but is usually slight and out of proportion to the abdominal signs.

GRAPHIC TRACINGS

Electrocardiogram. The electrocardiogram may present *high P waves*. However, atrial fibrillation is often present.

Phonocardiogram. The phonocardiogram may reveal the vibrations of a diastolic murmur over the tricuspid area. Comparative tracings show that this murmur is louder and has a lower pitch than the diastolic murmur recorded at the apex; moreover, it increases in inspiratory apnea.

Jugular and hepatic tracings. Both the jugular and the hepatic tracings show *a high atrial wave* if sinus rhythm is preserved. This large wave, however, has no diagnostic value because it may be present in patients having heart failure and right ventricular hypertension without tricuspid stenosis.

Cardiomanometry. The pressure of the right atrium is *high* but there is no increase during ventricular systole. Right ventricular pressure is normal or low.

VENOUS PRESSURE

Venous pressure is always elevated.

X-RAY

The *isolated increase in size of the right atrium* is a typical finding. The right atrial shadow becomes globular and convex (30). The cardiohepatic angle may become obtuse (20). The superior vena cava and the left innominate vein are dilated and opaque. The large right atrium may obscure the lower part of the retrocardiac space in right anterior oblique (30) and frequently *displaces the esophagus toward the left.*

The lungs are clear.

MODE OF ORIGIN OF THE SIGNS

The obstacle is placed so far toward the venous system that only the right atrium dilates while the rest of the heart tends to become smaller. As the efficiency of the right atrium is relatively poor and atrial fibrillation is frequent, no compensatory action of this chamber is possible. Therefore, distention of the large venous collectors and of the liver is early and severe. The scarcity of anastomoses between the portal system and the other venous systems is one of the causes of isolated liver enlargement.

The liver seems to act as a reservoir and to limit both the increase of venous pressure and the peripheral edema.

The ascites is caused by slow hepatic circulation, high portal pressure, and, later, by "cardiac" cirrhosis of the liver.

The frequent absence of a diastolic-presystolic murmur is due to the relative weakness of the musculature of the right atrium. A diastolic rumble would be noted more often if other cardiac murmurs would not mask it. However, *there frequently is a rumble* which has different graphic characteristics from those of the apical rumble due to mitral stenosis.

The infrequent congestion of the lungs and the moderate severity of the dyspnea are due to the fact that the right ventricle sends a limited amount of blood to the lungs because of difficult filling.

Cyanosis, if present, is a "peripheral cyanosis". It is favored by the high level of venous pressure.

The obtuseness of the cardiohepatic angle is caused by enlargement of the right atrium. This sign may be present only on percussion and not upon x-ray examination or it may occur also in the latter.

PROGNOSIS—COURSE—COMPLICATIONS

The patients usually seem to be in worse condition than they actually are. This is because, for many years, their signs are the result of a mechanical obstacle and not evidence of myocardial weakness. Therefore, these patients are capable of a greater activity than other cardiac patients with the same degree of cyanosis or ascites. However, they react poorly to digitalis, and only moderately to diuretics. They usually have a slow progressive course with a gradual downward condition. The course may last many years.

Usual complications are pulmonary embolism, aneurysm of the right atrium, thrombosis of the right atrium, and bacterial endocarditis.

DIAGNOSIS

The diagnosis is based upon the recognition of a large right atrium with a small or normal right ventricle and a large liver. Incorrect diagnosis of liver cirrhosis is often made. Therefore this possibility must be eliminated first.

Liver cirrhosis. The right atrium is small in liver cirrhosis. The veins are thin, venous pressure is low, and there is no cyanosis.

Patent foramen ovale. Both the right atrium and the right ventricle are large with patency of the foramen while only the right atrium is large in tricuspid stenosis. Usually the liver is not enlarged with patency of the foramen. The pulmonary artery and the hilar shadows appear large at x-ray with patent foramen ovale but not in tricuspid stenosis.

Tricuspid insufficiency. This lesion is accompanied by a large right ventricle, a high systolic wave of regurgitation in the jugular and liver tracings, and a typical movement of the precordial area.

Constrictive pericarditis. The only type which may simulate tricuspid stenosis is that consisting of localized adhesions around the venae cavae. In such cases, however, the right atrium is small (page 450) and not large as in tricuspid stenosis.

Pericarditis with effusion. The obtuseness of the cardiohepatic angle is present both in tricuspid stenosis and in pericarditis. The high venous pressure with absence of murmurs may be common to both. In tricuspid stenosis, a mitral lesion is nearly always present. Changes of cardiac dulness in different positions, x-ray (lack of pulsation of the cardiac border, changes of shape in different positions, etc.), and electrocardiographic (changes of S-T and T) data, are in favor of effusion.

TREATMENT OF TRICUSPID DEFECTS

Treatment with digitalis or other stimulants of the myocardium usually has little effect on the severity of the clinical signs. Far better results are obtained with *mercurial diuretics* (**11, 12**) and *ammonium chloride* (**13**) which promote diuresis. Stimulation of the heart by means of the *glycosides of squill* (**10**) has been suggested in order to use not only their cardiac action but also their diuretic effect which is greater than that of digitalis (page 589).

Restriction of sodium (or fluids) is often necessary. Periodic administration of *Mg sulfate* may be useful, because water is eliminated from the gastrointestinal tract through its action. *Periodic paracenteses* may be necessary when diuresis cannot be increased by means of drugs. *Venesection* may be useful when venous congestion is severe.

Tricuspid commissurotomy or *fracture of valvular adhesions* has been tried with success in certain cases.

Relative Tricuspid Stenosis

This condition is caused by severe enlargement of the right ventricle with a normal tricuspid valve. It may occur in cases with chronic cor pulmonale. The phonocardiogram reveals the existence of a diastolic rumble which becomes louder in inspiration and, therefore, simulates the rumble of organic tricuspid stenosis. This possibility is rare because the ostium of the tricuspid valve is usually dilated whenever there is severe right ventricular enlargement.

Double Tricuspid Defect

Double tricuspid defect is common. However, either the stenosis or the insufficiency predominates in most cases and the name of double tricuspid defect should be applied only to those cases in which the two defects are more or less equivalent.

The symptoms and signs are more severe than in the single defects as far as enlargement of the liver and ascites are concerned. On the contrary, the systolic murmur, the right ventricular enlargement, the jugular and hepatic pulsations, and the movements of the precordial area (all signs of tricuspid insufficiency), are less severe, being limited by the stenosis.

BIBLIOGRAPHY

1. a) Schwartz, S. P. Am. Heart J., 1927, **2**, 407.
   b) Schwartz, S. P., and Schelling, D. H. Am. Heart J., 1931, **6**, 568.
2. Dressler, W. Die Brustwandpulsationen. Wien, Maudrich, 1933.
3. Bryant. Quoted by Robinson, G. C. In Nelson's Loose Leaf Medicine. New York, Nelson, vol. IV.
4. Luisada, A. A. Rass. Internaz. Clin., Ter. (Naples), 1937, **18**, N. 16 and 17.
5. Gerhardt. Charité Ann., 1892, 92.
6. a) Pezzi, C., and Silingardi, S. Soc. Méd. Hôp., 1925, **49**, 117.
   b) Pezzi, C. Cuore e Circ. (Rome), 1927, **11**, 381.
7. Harvier, P., and co-workers. Paris Méd., 1937, **27**, 397.
8. White, P. D. J. A. M. A., 1928, **90**, 603.
9. Sussman, M. L., Grishman, A., and Sternberg, M. F. Am. J. Dis. Child., 1943, **65**, 922.
10. Steell, G. Med. Chron., 1888–89, **9**, 182.
11. Arrillaga, F. La Arteritis Pulmonar. Buenos Aires, Garcia, 1925.
12. Vaquez, H. Les Maladies du Coeur. Paris, Baillière, 1928.
13. Abbott, M. E. Nelson's Loose Leaf Medicine, vol. IV, 1943.
14. a) Giordano, C. Min. Med. (Turin), 1927, **8**, 1197.
    b) Currens, J. H., Kinney, T. D. and White, P. D. Am. Heart J., 1945, **30**, 491.
    c) Micheli. Quoted by Giordano.
15. Lian, C., and Welti, G. G. Arch. Mal. Coeur, 1937, **30**, 946.
16. Currens, J. H., Kinney, T. D., and White, P. D. Am. Heart J., 1945, **30**, 491.
17. Schnitker, M. A. Electrocardiography in Congenital Heart Disease. Cambridge, Harvard Univ. Press, 1940.
18. Groedel, F. M. Quoted by Attinger (21).
19. Groedel, F. M. Exper. Med. & Surg., 1945, **3**, 196.
20. Assmann, H. Die klinische Roentgendiagnostik der inneren Erkrankungen. Leipzig, Vogel, 1924.
21. Attinger, E. Schweiz. med. Woch., 1936, **66**, 1056.
22. Laubry, C., and Pezzi, C. Les Maladies Congenitales du Coeur. Paris, Baillière, 1921.
23. Bénard, R. Bull. Soc. Méd. Hôp. Paris, 1936, **52**, 643.
24. Auerbach, O., and Stemmerman, M. G. Am. J. M. Sci., 1944, **207**, 219.
25. Chisholm, D. R. Am. Heart J., 1937, **13**, 362.
26. Luisada, A. A. Arch. Pat. Clin. Med. (Turin), 1936, **16**, 404.
27. a) Fischer, R. Wien. klin. Woch., 1933, **46**, 1544.
    b) Dressler, W. Arch. Int. Med., 1937, **60**, 441.
28. Dietlen, H. Herz und Gefaesse im Roentgenbild, 1923.
29. Hitzenberger, K. Wien. Arch. inn. Med., 1924, **5**, 451; and 1924, **9**, 205.
30. Roesler, H. Clinical Roentgenology of the Cardiovascular System. Springfield, Thomas, 1943.
31. Lang, G. Deut. Arch. klin. Med., 1912, **108**, 35.
32. Cooke, W. T., and White, P. D. Brit. Heart J., 1941, **3**, 147.
33. Dressler, W., and Fischer, R. Klin. Woch., 1929, **8**, 1267 and 1316.
34. a) Altschule, M.D., and Blumgart, H. L. Am. Heart, J., 1937, **13**, 589.
    b) Altschule, M. D., and Budnitz, E. Arch. Path., 1940, **30**, 7.
35. Smith, J. A., and Levine, S. A. Am. Heart J., 1942, **23**, 739.
36. Tschilikin, I. Zeit. Kreislauff., 1930, **22**, 177.
37. Cataldi, G. M. Arch. Sci. Med., 1934, **58**, 205.
38. Cossio, P., and Marguery, E. E. El Dia Med. (Buenos Aires), 1945, **17**, N. 40.
39. Ellis, G. N., and Brown, N. W. Am. Heart J., 1946, **32**, 369.
40. Rivero Carvallo, J. M. Arch. Inst. Card. Mexico, 1946, **16**, 531. Also Am. Heart J., 1947, **34**, 114.
41. Levine, S. A. Clinical Heart Disease. Philadelphia, Saunders, 1937.
42. Bing, R. J., and co-workers. Mo. Conc. Cardiov. Dis., 1948, **17**, N. 3.

43. PARKER, R. L. Med. Clin. North America, 1948, July, 855.

44. POTTS, W. J., AND GIBSON, S. J. A. M. A., 1948, **137,** 343.

45. CHAVEZ, I., AND RIVERO CARVALLO, J. M. Arch. Lat. Amer. Card. y Hem., 1935, **5,** 115.

46. TAUSSIG, H. B. *Congenital Malformations of the Heart.* New York, Commonwealth Fund, 1947.

47. MESSER, A. L., HURST, J. W., RAPPAPORT, M. B., AND SPRAGUE, H. B. Circ., 1950, **1,** 388.

48. GLOVER, R. P., BAILEY, C. P., AND O'NEILL, T. J. E. J. A. M. A., 1950, **144,** 1049.

49. BROCK, R. C., AND CAMPBELL, M. Brit. Heart J., 1950, **12,** 377 and 403.

50. FRIEDBERG, C. K. *Diseases of the Heart.* Saunders, Philadelphia and London, 1949.

51. HYMAN, A. L., AND CO-WORKERS. Ann. Int. Med., 1951, **34,** 90.

CHAPTER 13

Simple Shunts Between the Greater and the Lesser Circulations

Simple shunts are those lesions which permit a more or less complete mixture of blood between the greater and lesser circulations without valvular lesions or complex malformations. The shunts are due to septal defects or communication between the aorta and the pulmonary artery.

Atrial Septal Defects[57]

The clinical picture is caused by the absence, incomplete closure, or secondary perforation of the septum. An abnormal communication between the atria, and in some cases their fusion into a single cavity, is the result.

CAUSE

a) There may be *lack of development* of the atrial septum.

b) The most common cause is a congenital abnormality consisting of the persistence of the *foramen primum* or of the *foramen secundum*, or of *various small openings* in the atrial septum.

c) Postnatal nonclosure, or subsequent reopening, of the *foramen ovale*.

d) Secondary perforation of the atrial septum following bacterial endocarditis has been described in rare cases.

The congenital types of septal defects are twice as frequent in females as in males (37).

LESIONS—MECHANISM

The following lesions may be present.

a) *A complete absence of the atrial septum;*

[57] Some authors exclude *patent foramen ovale* from the atrial septal defects. From a dynamic point of view, *it should be included.*

there is only one atrial cavity; sometimes rudimentary septal formations are present (*cor triloculare biventriculosum*).

b) *Large opening or multiple small defects* in the atrial septum.

c) *The foramen ovale is patent.*

Small openings in the septum have no clinical significance. Therefore, importance is attributed only to a foramen of at least 5 mm. in diameter open to blood flow in both directions. There may be a wide opening, or a hole which is surrounded by a thick ring or is bordered by a membrane in the upper part.

One type of lesion is due to changes taking place during early fetal life. In this, total or partial absence of the septum, or persistence of the foramen primum (page 9) at the base of the atrial septum, is present. There is severe dilatation of the right heart, involving both the atrium and the ventricle. There is *dilatation of the pulmonary artery* which may be of high degree. In contrast, *the aorta is often thin and poorly developed* (2).

A second type of lesion is actually *postnatal* because there is patency of the foramen ovale which normally closes soon after birth (page 9). In this group of cases usually the only abnormal finding is *a moderate dilatation of the right atrium* (fig. 168). Anatomically patent but functionally closed foramen ovale occurs in about 20 per cent of adults and is asymptomatic unless the pressure becomes higher in the right atrium.

Abnormalities of the mitral valve (2), the pulmonary veins, and the inferior vena cava (3), have been described. The pulmonary veins may open either into the right atrium or into the superior vena cava. The inferior vena cava may open at the level of the fora-men and, therefore, may be in communica-tion with both atria. Absence of the septum may be associated with *mongolism* (2) or *arachnodachtylia* (37).

SYMPTOMS AND SIGNS

Complete absence of the atrial septum is rarely compatible with life. However, there are cases, children as well as adults, where this severe abnormality is present without associated lesions and is relatively well tolerated. *All signs, including cyanosis, may be absent* in this severe lesion.

In all other atrial septal defects, the symptoms and signs are similar because the difference is purely structural. However, the size of the foramen is important; the larger it is, the more severe is the clinical picture. *These patients may have no symptoms whatsoever.* In many cases, the lesion is un-recognized during the greater part of life, and is revealed only accidentally or by autopsy. This, however, does not exclude the possibility of clinical signs. A *frail build* is frequent (gracile habitus). *Dwarfism* and *infantilism* are not exceptional. Onset of puberty is often delayed.

Pallor is often present, due to hypoplasia of the aorta or passage of blood from the left to the right atrium. *Cyanosis* is usually absent but may occur *late in life*. There may be intermittent cyanosis occurring in the form of *attacks*, which are not accompanied by the usual signs of congestive failure. In some cases, the cyanosis is due to a *late opening of the foramen ovale* because of right atrial hypertension (4).

Exertional dyspnea is an early symptom; *tracheal tug* is possible and caused by pres-sure of the large pulmonary artery on the bifurcation of the trachea or left bronchus. Upper respiratory infections are common. Chronic bronchitis is not unusual.

A well known sign is the so-called *para-doxical embolism* which is better defined as *crossed embolism*. Patients with phlebitis suddenly show a *cerebral embolism*. This oc-

currence, however, is proof of atrial septal defect only if other communications between the greater and lesser circulations can be excluded. As the blood usually goes from the left to the right atrium (fig. 168), crossed embolism is possible only when right atrial pressure is abnormally high. This may be caused by *acute cor pulmonale* after a pre-vious pulmonary embolism (5) or by *a transitory increase of venous return* (effort, straining, Valsalva).

It should be noted that transitory re-versals of the blood flow through the shunt are more common than in other septal de-fects (37).

Blood pressure may be low; pulse pressure, reduced.

Hemoptysis is a frequent symptom and *hoarseness* has been reported.

Local Signs

There may be *bulging* of the precordial region. The apex beat may be displaced toward the left. In severe cases, percussion reveals enlargement of the heart toward the right and an obtuse cardiohepatic angle. There may be a *thrill* over the 2nd and 3rd left interspaces.

There may be no *murmurs*. A *presystolic murmur* may be due, in rare cases, to blood passing through the foramen. However, its finding is unusual. A *systolic murmur* is commonly heard over the pulmonic area.

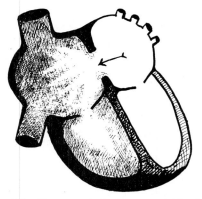

FIG. 168. Changes of the heart and blood flow in atrial septal defect.

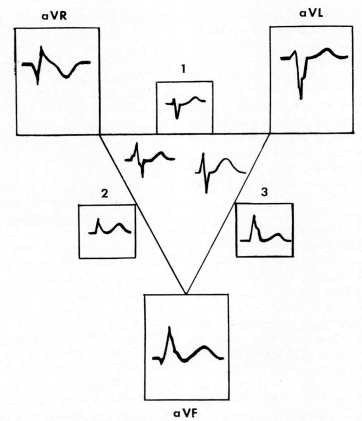

FIG. 169. Scheme of electrocardiogram in a case of large atrial septal defect

It seems due to the dilatation of the pulmonary artery (*relative stenosis*). *The 2nd pulmonic sound is loud and frequently split*, a fact which should be related to the existence of bundle branch block. There frequently is *a diastolic rumble at the apex* simulating mitral stenosis (relative mitral stenosis, page 237). There may be a short, early diastolic murmur over the pulmonic area due to either fibrosis of the leaflets or high pressure (45).

GRAPHIC TRACINGS

The *electrocardiogram* presents in a great majority of cases a *right bundle branch block* (47) (fig. 169). There may be right axis deviation (7, 8). The P wave is often high in leads 1 and 2 and has the type of *right atrial hypertrophy* in V_1-V_2 (47) (page 369). However, *atrial fibrillation* is frequent. The T wave may be inverted in leads 2 and 3. There may be a long P-R interval (37).

The *jugular and hepatic tracings* may show a high presystolic wave if there is sinus rhythm. The same is true for the *electrokymogram* of the right atrial border.

X-RAY

If the opening is large, the heart is markedly enlarged and has *a globular shape*; dilatation of the pulmonary knob and poor visibility of the aortic knob are apparent. If the opening is small, there is *dilatation of the right atrium* and *enlargement of the pulmonary knob*; this is in contrast to the small aortic knob (9, 10) (fig. 170). Enlargement of the heart toward the left, due to the fact that the enlarged right heart displaces the apex, is possible (6).

The hilar shadows are dilated and show a

strong pulsation. The vascular markings of the lungs are quite visible and are widespread.

Angiocardiography may show one of the two following possibilities: a) The contrast medium, upon reaching the right atrium, is diluted by the stream of blood due to the left-to-right shunt, and does not give a satisfactory visualization of the right heart. b) If the pressure of the right atrium is so increased by the injection as to cause an inversion of the stream through the shunt, the medium passes into the left atrium and causes early visualization of the aorta (11).

CATHETERIZATION

Catheterization of the right heart reveals that *the oxygen content of the right atrium is higher than that of the superior cava* (13, 36, 38). This increased saturation then continues into the right ventricle and pulmonary artery. Example:

	Oxygen (Vol. Per Cent)
Superior cava	11.5
Right atrium	13.8
Right ventricle	13.6
Pulmonary artery	13.7

The *pressure may be elevated* in the right atrium, right ventricle, and pulmonary artery, and may reach 140 mm. Hg in extreme cases, possibly on account of secondary changes in the pulmonary vessels (38). On the other hand, it may be normal. *Pulmonary flow usually exceeds systemic flow* but the opposite may occur (36).

Catheterization may give doubtful data as to whether the shunt is from right to left, whether the flow through the foramen is minimal, whether there is no effective mixture within the right atrium, or whether there are associated lesions.

CIRCULATION TIME—BLOOD GASES

The various tests usually give doubtful results. Ether, passing in minute amounts through the shunt, may give tingling or stinging sensations of the head and face of

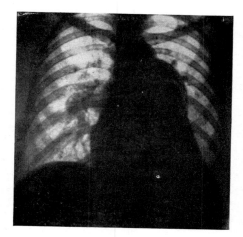

FIG. 170. X-ray silhouette of the heart in a case with atrial septal defect (frontal view). Large right heart and dilated pulmonary artery. (From Brumlik.)

a few seconds duration. This arm-to-face time may be as short as the arm-to-lung time (46).

Oxygen saturation of the arterial blood is usually normal. However, pulmonary complications, heart failure, or exertion (including the various exercise tests) may lead to inversion of the flow through the shunt. Then oxygen saturation falls (36).

MODE OF ORIGIN OF THE SIGNS

The left atrium has normally a slightly higher pressure than the right. This fact is due to greater distensibility of the right atrium and of the veins of the greater circulation (48–50). This gradient of pressure causes passage of a certain amount of blood saturated with oxygen from the left to the right atrium. The increase of flow leads to dilatation and hypertrophy of the chambers of the right heart (fig. 171). *The large pulmonary artery and the small aorta are due to the fact that pulmonary flow is greater than systemic flow.*

No cyanosis normally occurs. However, transitory conditions (attacks of laughing, crying, or coughing; straining at stool; increased inflow) or a lasting increase of pressure in the right heart (acute or chronic

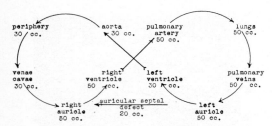

FIG. 171. Scheme of the blood flow in a case with atrial septal defect.

cor pulmonale) may cause an inversion of the stream with passage of blood, unsaturated with oxygen, from right to left. *Cyanosis* then appears.

The problem of whether a small amount of blood also passes from the right to the left atrium cannot be solved in general. *Some cases have a two-directional flow,* either because of nearly equal pressure within the two atria or because of a large opening.

The murmur which is present over the pulmonic area is probably *a murmur of relative stenosis* (page 267).

In the complete absence of the interatrial septum, a certain percentage of the blood coming from the venae cavae flows into the left atrium. But the proportion of the blood, not saturated with oxygen, which remains in the left atrium may not be sufficient to cause cyanosis. This shows that the two atria maintain a definite individuality even when the septum is lacking (1) unless the pressure is raised in the right atrium.

The occurrence of a *crossed embolism* is still a rather obscure phenomenon. It has been explained as the result of the *passage of blood from right to left during most of diastole* (excepting presystole). This fact, however, does not seem likely, as the difference in pressure between the two atria is not due to a difference in the strength of contraction. It is possible that *a pulmonary embolism occurs first.* This increases the pressure in the right heart and decreases the pressure in the left. A change in the normal gradient of atrial pressures may result, so that a subsequent embolus may pass through the septum from right to left (15, 5a).

The *right bundle branch block* is favored by the distention of the right ventricle with subsequent fibrosis. It explains the frequent splitting of the 2nd pulmonic sound (page 379).

COURSE AND COMPLICATIONS

If the atrial septal defect is uncomplicated, the course may be long, as proven by the fact that the lesion may be found in autopsies of old people. Sometimes short periods of cyanosis are separated by years of perfect health but usually the first symptoms appear in late middle age.

Severe disturbance may occur if pulmonary disease raises the pressure of the right heart. Congestive failure, favored by myocardial fibrosis, increases the pressure in both atria, chiefly in the right, favors an inversion of the stream passing through the shunt, and causes *severe cyanosis.*

Pulmonary congestion and chronic pulmonary edema occur frequently.

Rheumatic endocarditis develops in a high percentage of cases (37). The typical lesions may be localized, not only on the cardiac valves, but also on the ring of the congenital lesion. The association of a mitral valve lesion with an atrial septal defect gives a new syndrome with typical picture (*Lutembacher's syndrome,* page 304). Pneumonia and chronic pulmonary infections are frequent. *Thrombosis of the right atrium,* followed by pulmonary embolism, is a frequent complication (37).

Subacute bacterial endocarditis is not uncommon and the lesions are usually localized on the ring of the foramen.

Atrial fibrillation is a frequent and early complication. The return to normal rhythm is more difficult than in other diseases because of chronic distention of the right atrium, followed by fibrosis of the wall.

Atherosclerosis of the pulmonary artery and of its branches often occurs. *The dilatation of the pulmonary artery may become an aneurysm* and cause various signs and symptoms (page 484).

Atrial septal defect is a less severe lesion than other congenital heart diseases as shown by the fact that it is often encountered in old age. However, some patients suffer from infections and are generally less resistant than normal people. *When there is absence of, or a large opening in the atrial septum,* complications are more frequent and death occurs at a younger age.

DIAGNOSIS

The typical picture is the following: stunted growth, frequent bronchitis, right heart enlargement, systolic murmur and loud 2nd sound over pulmonic area, right bundle branch block and high P waves, large pulmonary knob with high pulsations of the hila, and increased pulmonary markings.

Crossed embolism is of diagnostic value only if there is no congestive failure and the patient has a phlebitis. Even then, it is only indicative of a septal defect in general.

Ventricular septal defect can be excluded only if there is no systolic thrill and no systolic murmur. Otherwise, catheterization is necessary. The heart is more rounded in this lesion than in atrial septal defect.

Pulmonary stenosis. This lesion can be excluded when no thrill and murmur over the second left interspace are noted. On the other hand, differential diagnosis is necessary when a *systolic murmur* is present over that area. Marked right ventricular hypertrophy is present in pulmonary stenosis and the second pulmonic sound is weak. In atrial septal defect, right bundle branch block is nearly constant; the second pulmonic sound is loud and frequently split. The hilar shadows have decreased pulsations and the vascular markings are poorly visible in pulmonary stenosis. The electrokymogram of the pulmonary artery reveals a late, slow, and frequently small pulsation in pulmonary stenosis; a large and rapid pulsation in atrial defect. Catheterization shows a higher content of oxygen in the right atrium than in the superior cava, in the atrial de-

fect; it shows an increased gradient of pressure between right ventricle and pulmonary artery, in pulmonary stenosis.

Patent ductus arteriosus. This lesion should be discussed only when the pulmonary artery is markedly dilated and the murmur is atypical. Phonocardiography usually permits the recording of a late-systolic-early-diastolic murmur in patency of the ductus. The pulmonic murmur, which may be present in atrial septal defects, is nearly always diamond-shaped and frankly systolic. The electrocardiogram reveals left axis deviation or normal axis in patent ductus, right axis deviation and nearly always right bundle branch block in atrial defects. Catheterization gives decisive data in doubtful cases.

Mitral stenosis. The absence of a diastolic rumble and of a presystolic murmur plus the presence of right atrial enlargement, are against this diagnosis. However, cases with *relative stenosis of the mitral valve* (page 237) and cases with *Lutembacher's syndrome* (page 304) are of more difficult exclusion. Here again, catheterization is needed.

Complex congenital heart diseases are at times excluded with difficulty. However, severe cyanosis, thrills, and murmurs, are usually present in them.

Constrictive pericarditis. This lesion causes an *early* enlargement of the liver, often with ascites. In atrial septal defects, the enlargement of the liver occurs *during* congestive failure and is not accompanied by ascites.

Tricuspid valve lesions. There is early engorgement of the liver, frequently accompanied by ascites; there is very little pulmonary congestion and no orthopnea. The opposite is true in atrial septal defects. Atrial fibrillation occurs earlier in atrial septal defects than in tricuspid lesions. A pulsating liver is a sign of tricuspid insufficiency.

Aberrant pulmonary veins opening into the right atrium may give findings similar to atrial septal defects. Catheterization and angiocardiography may not be helpful in these cases. It should be kept in mind that the association of this pulmonary abnormal-

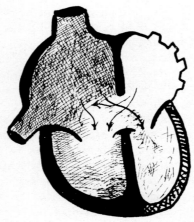

FIG. 172. Changes of the heart and blood flow in the *persistent common atrioventricular orifice*.

ity with the atrial defect is not unusual and complicates the diagnostic, roentgenological, and surgical problems. An accurate roentgenological study, however, usually reveals the aberrant insertion of the veins (51).

PROGNOSIS

If there is no cyanosis, the prognosis is good. If there is cyanosis while other signs of congestive failure are absent, the prognosis is fair. If congestive heart failure also occurs, the outlook is poor.

TREATMENT

Surgical closure of the atrial defect is possible. Anteroposterior compression by means of suture (52), direct closure through a rubber well temporarily connected with the left atrium (53), and suture by invagination of the redundant atrial wall (54) have been advocated. It should be kept in mind that patients with secondary arteriosclerosis of the pulmonary vessels and patients with aberrant insertion of a pulmonary vein may not benefit from the intervention.

Persistent Common Atrioventricular Orifice (37, 55)

CAUSE—LESIONS

This congenital abnormality is due to an early arrest of development of the heart, before the completion of the atrial and ventricular septa. As a result of the communication, the leaflets of the mitral and tricuspid valve are fused together to form *a single atrioventricular valve with four leaflets*. In rarer cases, two separate septal defects are present, one in the atrial septum, the other in the ventricular, and the valves are normal. Some admixture of blood occurs in both the atria and the ventricles but more in the former than in the latter, the atrial orifice being larger (fig. 172).

SIGNS AND SYMPTOMS

Almost invariably the patient is a *mongolian idiot*.

Cyanosis is usually slight and may be absent. There is no clubbing of the fingers and toes. The heart is slightly enlarged to the right. There are a *systolic thrill* and a *systolic murmur*, which are similar to those of ventricular septal defect as far as type and location.

X-ray reveals a slight enlargement of the right atrium and ventricle.

The *electrocardiogram* is not typical and presents right axis deviation.

Oxygen saturation of the arterial blood is low.

DIAGNOSIS

Differential diagnosis should be made chiefly with atrial and ventricular septal defects. Angiocardiography and catheterization of the heart seldom give decisive data. The association of the above described picture with mongolism should lead to suspicion of this malformation.

Ventricular Septal Defects

The clinical syndrome is caused by the *absence, incomplete closure, or rupture of the ventricular septum*. The communication between the two ventricles may be so large as to create a *single ventricular cavity*. If there is a small, low opening, the syndrome is called *Roger's disease* (16).

CAUSE—LESIONS

There are two types of septal defects: the congenital and the acquired.

1) *Congenital defects.* Different varieties are created by the location of the shunt, the size of the opening, and the associated lesions.

a) High septal defect (fig. 174).

b) Low septal defect.

c) Large septal defect.

d) Absence of the ventricular septum (*cor triloculare biatriatum*).

e) Septal defect plus incompetence of the tricuspid or the aortic valve.

f) Septal defect plus subaortic stenosis or aortic hypoplasia.

In many of the cases, the defect has a diameter of 10 to 15 mm. with a smooth border. The border, however, may be irregular, either because of subsequent rupture or as a result of secondary endocarditis. There may be a small perforation of the septum either in the lower part or near the base; this has usually a diameter of 3 to 10 mm. The aortic valve may be incompetent. The congenital defect is due to an abnormal development in the region of the bulbus cordis and is probably associated with a faulty torsion of the primitive cardiac tube (pages 9 and 310).

The *heart is globular*, with rounded apex and enlargement of both ventricles.

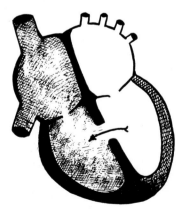

FIG. 173. Changes of the heart and cardiac dynamics in ventricular septal defect.

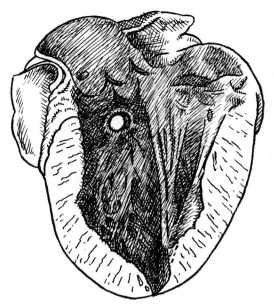

FIG. 174. View of the perforated septum in a case of high ventricular septal defect. (Inspired by originals of Paul D. White.)

2) *Acquired defects.* They may be due to the following causes:

a) *Rupture of an abscess* (acute purulent myocarditis, possibly during acute bacterial endocarditis) or *rupture of a fibrotic plaque.*

b) *Softening of a gumma* (subacute luetic myocarditis).

c) *Recent myocardial infarction.*

A special variety occurs when the rupture causes communication *between left ventricle and right atrium.*

SIGNS AND SYMPTOMS

Ventricular septal defect is usually well tolerated, in children as well as in adults, may cause no appreciable symptoms, and its discovery may be accidental. However, a certain mortality reduces the number of cases during childhood.

In general, *cyanosis, dyspnea, and clubbing*, are absent (18). However, this is not always true, especially in the case of a large septal defect.

Cyanosis is frequently present when the interventricular septum is absent but even then is not necessarily severe. *Hemoptysis* is not rare. The *pulse may be small. Crossed embolism* is possible.

Local Signs

An *epigastric pulsation* is sometimes visible.

Palpation reveals a *systolic thrill*, having its maximal intensity in the 3rd left interspace, *transmitted towards the right*. Percussion shows a slight increase of the transverse diameter so that the area of cardiac dulness becomes nearly round.

On auscultation, *a systolic murmur* is always heard. It is loud and harsh and may obscure the 1st heart sound. It has *its maximal intensity in the 3rd and 4th left interspaces near the sternum and is transmitted in all directions but chiefly toward the right* (fig. 175). Transmission toward the left axilla, the suprasternal notch (20), and along the carotid arteries (18) is poor, at least in adults. The murmur is loudest with defects of medium size and may be absent in the absence of the ventricular septum. The *Valsalva test* is said to decrease it (21). A *diastolic murmur*, due to associated aortic incompetence, is audible in some of the cases. The *2nd pulmonic sound* is usually loud and may be split. A *triple rhythm* is frequently heard at the apex.

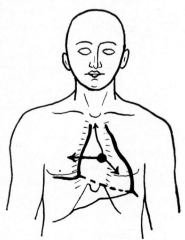

FIG. 175. Cardiac dulness and transmission of the murmur in ventricular septal defect.

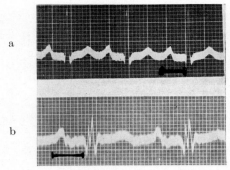

FIG. 176. Electrocardiograms in two cases of ventricular septal defect. In both cases, there is prolonged P-R. In case b there is intraventricular block.

BLOOD PRESSURE

Arterial pressure is usually normal. *Venous pressure* is also normal.

BLOOD

No polycythemia is present, except in some cases where there is complete absence of the septum. Oxygen saturation of the arterial blood is usually normal.

Circulation time. Both the *arm-to-lung* (ether) and the *arm-to-periphery tests* (decholin) give doubtful results or a double reaction. By *the lung-to-ear test* (*inert gas*), *circulation time is shorter* (page 157).

CATHETERIZATION

The pressure of the right ventricle is higher than normal, especially in the high septal defects. *The oxygen content in this chamber is significantly higher than in the right atrium* (13b, 36).[58] The flow of the pulmonary artery exceeds that of the systemic circulation.

GRAPHIC RECORDS

The *electrocardiogram* may be absolutely *normal* but *slight right axis deviation is common. Intraventricular block, changes of the S-T and T, prolongation of the P-R interval*, or *complete heart block* are frequently encountered (fig. 176). They are due, how-

[58] In high septal defects, the increased amount of oxygen may be found *only in the pulmonary artery.*

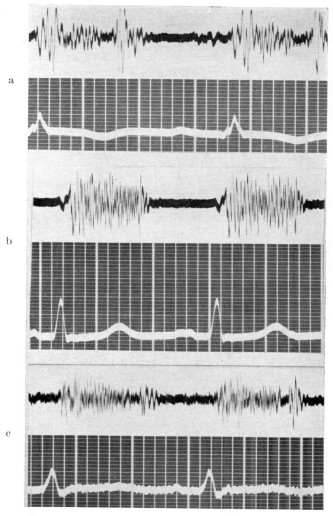

FIG. 177. The systolic murmur recorded by sound tracings in cases of ventricular septal defect. a, man of 30—congenital defect; b, woman of 25—congenital defect; c, woman of 67—perforation of the septum after myocardial infarction (p.m. control).

ever, to an association of lesions and may be absent.

The *phonocardiogram* shows a series of large and slightly irregular vibrations (fig. 177). The murmur may be *diamond-shaped* or *irregular*. It may be midsystolic, late-systolic, or all-systolic.[59] A *split 2nd pulmonic sound* and a *triple rhythm* at the apex are frequently recorded.

[59] Phonocardiography may permit an exact diagnosis even during fetal life (23).

X-RAY

The heart shadow is *globular* with increase of both diameters (fig. 178). In some cases, however, the heart is either normal or slightly dilated toward the right. There may be only an *increased amplitude of ventricular systole* (24) which is confirmed by *roentgenkymography* (25).

The left atrium is somewhat enlarged. The *pulmonary knob* is *normal* in the small perforation (Roger's syndrome) but is *dilated*

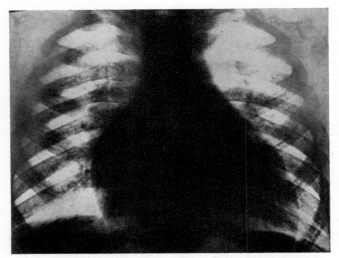

FIG. 178. Cardiac silhouette in a case of ventricular septal defect

if there is a large, high septal defect (37); this dilatation may even reach the size of an aneurysm and be accompanied by visible pulsations of the pulmonary parenchyma. The hilar shadows are large and pulsating and the pulmonary markings are increased in cases with severe increase of pulmonary flow and pulmonic hypertension.

Electrokymography. There is a pulse wave of the pulmonary arch which is higher than normal but not higher than the aortic wave; the hilar and pulmonary pulses are higher than normal. The speed of the pulse wave in the pulmonary circulation is normal or only slightly increased (40). The pulsations of both ventricles are increased.

Angiocardiography. In certain cases, angiocardiography reveals the shunt as a *clear spot within the right ventricular shadow* (11) (fig. 179).

MODE OF ORIGIN OF THE SIGNS

The higher systolic pressure of the left ventricle causes systolic passage of blood only from the left to the right ventricle. Only a minimal passage of blood takes place during diastole. As the blood passing through the septum is saturated with oxygen, the oxygen content of the blood in the right ventricle and pulmonary artery increases. In the high septal defect, the blood may

be shunted directly into the pulmonary artery, so that the changes are observed only in the latter.

The right ventricle is dilated and hypertrophied. Pulmonary arterial pressure is increased by flow through the shunt and by increased diastolic length of the fibers of the right ventricle (56). Active pulmonary congestion is caused by increased flow through the lesser circulation.

Both the systolic thrill and the systolic murmur are caused by the stream of blood through the septal defect and are typically transmitted toward the right side of the chest.

Hemoptysis is favored by high pressure of the pulmonary circulation. Dyspnea is favored by the same factor.

The alterations of conduction (long P-R, a-v block) are due to *associated abnormalities of the bundle of His* and are not secondary to the defect. This is proven by cases of complete absence of the septum and normal conduction, due to the fact that the bundle of His had developed along the posterior wall of the single ventricular chamber (27).

VARIETIES

In addition to the more typical cases, there are others in which the thrill is absent and the murmur is faint. In these cases,

even the x-ray and electrocardiographic signs
may not be typical. A-v block may lead one
to suspect a ventricular septal defect.

The acquired septal defects always have
a sudden onset and usually are accompanied
by a loud murmur with typical transmission.

*When the communication takes place be-
tween the left ventricle and right atrium, the
systolic may be followed by an early diastolic
and, possibly, by a presystolic murmur.*

From a roentgenological point of view,
two varieties can be observed:

a) That with a normal pulmonary artery.

b) That with a large pulmonary artery
(high septal defect).

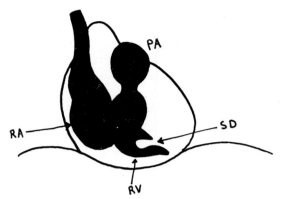

FIG. 179. Angiocardiogram of the right heart
in ventricular septal defect. The septal defect
(SD) is represented by a white gap. (Inspired by
originals of Sussman, Grishman and Steinberg.)

COURSE AND COMPLICATIONS

The disease is often silent and permits an
active life. In some cases, pregnancy and
labor may be normal except for the occasional occurrence of slight cyanosis. Therefore, the disease may be an accidental finding at any age.

If an increase in the pressure of the right
heart occurs, severe cyanosis may appear.
Inversion of the blood stream through the
septal defect is frequent during coughing
and may cause attacks of cyanosis.

Pulmonary diseases are favored by the
congestion of the pulmonary circulation
existing in this condition. They increase the
severity of cyanosis and dyspnea. Pneumonia causes a higher mortality.

Pulmonary arteriosclerosis, followed by
secondary chronic cor pulmonale, is a possible complication.

Endocarditis is a possible complication.
Rheumatic endocarditis may occur with
localization on the mitral valve, on the
valves of the right heart, or on the border
of the defect. *Acute or subacute bacterial
endocarditis is frequent.* The bacteria lodge
around the septal ring and in that part of
the right ventricle where the shunted blood
hits the cardiac wall, forming typical vegetations. If the septal defect is high, the vegetations may be located in the pulmonary conus,
just below the pulmonary orifice (37). *Pul-*

monary emboli are frequently caused by
these masses.

Congestive failure may occur causing
dyspnea, venous and hepatic engorgement,
severe cyanosis, or peripheral edema.

DIAGNOSIS

The diagnosis is based on the thrill, the
systolic murmur with typical transmission,
and the x-ray findings. The electrocardiogram is sometimes of help (prolonged P-R,
a-v block). The absence of cyanosis, clubbing, and polycythemia is important. In
the adult, the diagnosis of congenital heart
disease will be made only after exclusion of
acquired valvular defects.

In difficult cases, angiocardiography,
catheterization of the heart, and lung-to-
lung circulation tests give positive data.

Differential diagnosis should be made with
the following conditions.

Relative mitral stenosis. The thrill, the enlarged heart, and the localization of the murmur, are differential data. The murmur of
relative mitral stenosis can be frequently
recorded over a larger area of the precordium.

Mitral stenosis. In ventricular septal defect, a triple rhythm can be heard at times,
due to an additional diastolic sound. In
mitral stenosis, if there is a triple rhythm,
this is due to an opening snap of the mitral

valve (differentiation possible in graphic tracings, page 231). Otherwise, there is a low-pitched diastolic rumble, different from a triple rhythm. The left atrium is more dilated in mitral stenosis than in ventricular septal defect.

Mitral insufficiency. The murmur is loudest over the mid-precordium and is transmitted toward the right in Roger's disease; it is loudest at the apex and is transmitted toward the left axilla in mitral insufficiency. The murmur is louder and harsher in Roger's disease. *Enlargement of the left atrium may be present in both but its systolic dilatation (EKY) is typical of mitral insufficiency.*

Tricuspid insufficiency. Cyanosis, changes of the jugular and liver tracings, and x-ray data showing systolic distention of the right atrium and of the liver, are typical of tricuspid insufficiency and absent in ventricular septal defect.

Aortic stenosis. This lesion causes a systolic thrill and murmur which may be loudest at the 3rd left interspace. However, there is enlargement of the left ventricle, slow apex beat, *anacrotic pulse*, transmission of the thrill and murmur to the suprasternal notch and to the carotid arteries, and *left axis deviation*. The phonocardiogram shows the vibrations of a diamond-shaped murmur. The 2nd aortic sound is weak in aortic stenosis, loud in ventricular defects.

Pulmonary stenosis. Murmur and thrill may be localized over the 3rd left interspace but they are transmitted upwards to the left clavicle, not towards the right side. The shape of the heart, as visualized by x-ray, is different from that of ventricular septal defect. The ECG reveals right ventricular hypertrophy in pulmonary stenosis. The murmur frequently shows a different type of vibration in phonocardiograms. The lung markings are decreased in pulmonary stenosis, increased in ventricular septal defect. The 2nd sound is weak in pulmonary stenosis.

Patent ductus arteriosus. There frequently is a machinery murmur, loudest at the end of the systole and prolonged into early diastole. Electrokymography and angiocardiography may contribute to the diagnosis. However, cases with septal defect plus aortic insufficiency are difficult to distinguish from cases of patent ductus; only a retrograde aortogram, or passing of the catheter from the pulmonary artery to the aorta allows a definite diagnosis.

Atrial septal defects. Diagnosis is possible only through catheterization which reveals high oxygen content in the right atrium. Right bundle branch block is typical of atrial defect even though it may be found in ventricular septal defect.

In some cases of ventricular septal defect, hemoptysis, possible bronchial signs, slight cyanosis, and tachycardia may lead to confusion with *pulmonary tuberculosis*. A careful examination is sufficient for excluding the latter, and the x-ray data will be decisive.

In *acquired septal defects*, differential diagnosis shall be made chiefly between rupture of one of the chordae tendineae (page 214) and rupture of the interventricular septum.

TREATMENT

Treatment of the shunt consists of surgical closure of the opening. *Anteroposterior compression* by means of sutures (52) represents only a brilliant but inadequate solution. *Actual closure* by means of a graft is theoretically possible and should be possible in the near future with the help of an "artificial heart" or using body refrigeration.

Communications Between Aorta and Pulmonary Artery

The clinical picture of these cases is caused by an abnormal communication between the two largest arterial vessels.

CAUSES—LESIONS

Different types of communication may be present.

1) The communication is due to *persistance of the ductus arteriosus (patent ductus*

arteriosus) (fig. 180). This ductus has a special function which ends at birth when pulmonary respiration begins. If the ductus fails to obliterate, it causes a typical syndrome. Patency of the ductus may be associated with aortic lesions (aortic stenosis, coarctation of the aorta) but it may exist without them.

The ductus may be *incompletely patent* (occlusion of one of the openings); then it is an autopsy finding. On the other hand, it may be *completely patent*, either as a *conic canal* with the larger end toward the aorta, or as a *cylindric canal*, 1 to 3 cm. long. It may have the appearance of an *aneurysm*, communicating with both the aorta and the pulmonary artery. The diameter of the ductus may vary from a tiny channel to 15 mm. or more.

2) *A direct communication may exist between the aorta and pulmonary artery.* This may be due to:

a) *Incomplete closure of the septum which divides the common arterial trunk* (page 10), a congenital anomaly (*aorto-pulmonary fistula*).

b) *Rupture of an aneurysm of the ascending aorta into the pulmonary artery.* This is usually luetic.

c) *Rupture of a congenital aneurysm of* the right sinus of Valsalva into the pulmonary artery.

In all these eventualities, the two ventricles are enlarged but the left is more so than the right. In most cases, the pulmonary artery and its main branches are dilated and there may be aneurysm of the pulmonary artery.

Fibrosis, atherosclerosis, and calcification are frequently encountered in the wall of the ductus, even in young individuals.

The mechanism of closure of the ductus after birth is still debated and imperfectly understood (page 13). When the muscular spasm which causes functional closure fails to occur, thrombosis of the ductus and its subsequent transformation into a fibrous ligament do not take place. Therefore, a

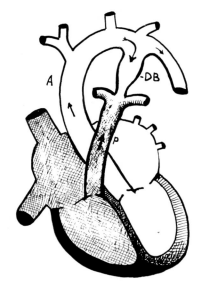

Fig. 180. Changes of the heart and large vessels in patent ductus arteriosus.

permanent communication between the aorta and pulmonary artery is maintained.

SYMPTOMS AND SIGNS

There may be infantilism but this is not common. *Cyanosis* and *clubbing* of the fingers are *absent*.

Dizziness and *fainting* are not unusual. The patients often complain of *oppression in the chest, palpitation,* and *shortness of breath* upon exertion.

Hemoptysis is frequent. *Hoarseness,* with sudden changes of the voice, is also common (18). All the above symptoms, however, may be absent.

Local Signs

The apex impulse is heaving and is often displaced to the left. Palpation may reveal a systolic *thrill* in the 2nd left interspace, transmitted both toward the left clavicle and the suprasternal notch.

Percussion reveals that cardiac dulness is increased chiefly towards the left. There is a *cap of dulness from the 1st to the 3rd left interspace* (fig. 181).

Auscultation reveals *a murmur with maximum intensity in the 2nd left interspace.* This

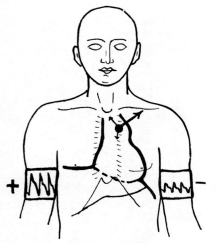

FIG. 181. Cardiac dulness and transmission of the murmur in patent ductus arteriosus.

murmur, caused by the blood passing through the ductus, is proportional to the pressure difference between aorta and pulmonary artery. In *infants*, the difference being less, the murmur is less loud and *may seem only systolic*. In *children* or *adults*, the difference is greater and there is a *grinding machinery murmur having its greatest intensity at the end of systole and at the beginning of diastole*.

Transmission of the murmur toward the suprasternal notch and along the carotid arteries has been recorded by the author. The murmur is loudest during inspiration but may disappear at the end of this phase (29). It may be heard best in the sitting position (30). The 2nd pulmonic sound is *loud*; it may be *split* or followed by a *loud snap*. There may be a *triple rhythm* at the apex and, occasionally, a *diastolic apical rumble* (42) due to relative mitral stenosis (page 237).

The pulse may be smaller in the left radial artery (31) and, occasionally, in the left carotid artery also (30). In typical cases, the pulse is *celer* and has a water-hammer quality. *Increase of the pulse pressure, low diastolic pressure, and double murmur of Duroziez,* are typical. These signs are similar to those of aortic insufficiency (page 240).

Diastolic pressure may fall to near zero after exertion.

GRAPHIC TRACINGS

The *electrocardiogram* may be normal. However, it usually shows a marked *left axis deviation*, and may present a Q3 and evidence of left bundle branch block (8). It may present a slight prolongation of P-R (fig. 182).

The *phonocardiogram* gives important data. *Coarse vibrations*, present in any phase, but *predominant in the last part of systole and in the first part of diastole*, are typical (32) (fig. 183). Sometimes the murmur occurs only in late systole and rides over the 2nd sound, ending with a loud series of vibrations in early diastole.

The *ballistocardiogram* may reveal a deep K wave and an L wave as high as J (58).

Electrokymography reveals that the pulsation of the pulmonary artery has the following characteristics (40). The systolic wave is far higher than normal and may exceed in height that of the aortic arch. The rise of the pulse is steep (*pulsus celer*). There may be a high dicrotic wave, a fact which probably gave rise to the roentgenkymographic finding of a double wave (33). *The*

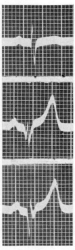

FIG. 182. Electrocardiogram of a case of patent ductus arteriosus. Leads 1, 2, 3. Left axis deviation.

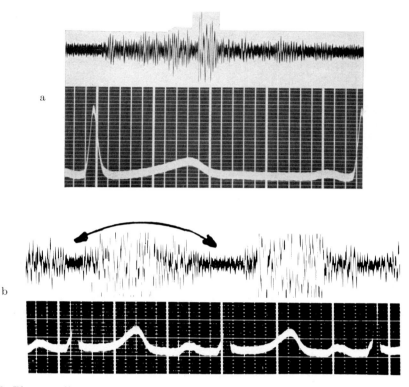

FIG. 183. Phonocardiograms in cases of patent ductus arteriosus. a, woman of 30; b, child of 1

speed of the pulse in the lesser circulation is increased and is far higher than in any other uncomplicated shunt (fig. 184). The hilar pulsations are increased in height (hilar dance) and may present a high dicrotic wave. The pulsations of the pulmonary parenchyma are also increased in height and present a steep rise and occasionally a very high, late peak.

X-RAY

The following changes may be found. a) *Enlargement of both the aortic and pulmonary knobs.* They pulsate violently but maintain their individualities. b) *Enlargement of the pulmonary knob* which shows strong pulsations and is visible chiefly in the right anterior oblique position. There may be a *hilar dance.* c) *Complete fusion of the aortic and pulmonary knobs,* with violent pulsation of the resulting cap (fig. 185).

Roentgenkymography may show the presence of a *double wave* in the pulmonary artery (33).

Calcification of the aortic wall near the opening of the ductus or of the ductus itself may be observed (2). This finding is very significant in children and young people.

CATHETERIZATION

This technique reveals normal pressures in the right atrium. The pressures of the right ventricle and pulmonary artery are also usually normal but *become higher whenever there is even a moderate increase of resistance in the pulmonary vessels.* A sudden increase in pressure with a typical profile of the pulse has been described in a limited section of the pulmonary artery, that corresponding to the opening of the ductus (57).

The blood of the pulmonary artery reveals a significant *increase in the oxygen content*

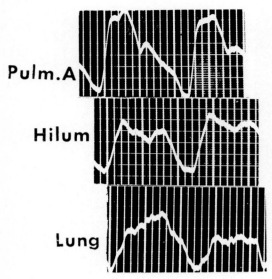

Pulm.A

Hilum

Lung

FIG. 184. Superimposed electrokymograms of the pulmonary artery, right hilum, and base of right lung, in a case of patent ductus arteriosus. High speed of the pulse wave, typical patterns.

both in comparison with that of the right ventricle and that of normal subjects (13, 36).

Pulmonary flow is higher than systemic flow on account of the shunt. The oxygen consumed per liter of ventilation rises with exercise while the oxygen saturation of the peripheral arterial blood is unchanged (36).

Passing of the catheter through the ductus supplies the ultimate proof of its existence.

Angiocardiography may reveal the patency either through a "filling defect" in the shadow of the pulmonary artery (penetration of blood without contrast medium from the aorta) or through reopacification of the pulmonary artery at the time in which only the left ventricle and the aorta are visualized (44). In questionable cases, *retrograde aortogram* shows the filling of the pulmonary artery through the ductus.

BLOOD—CARDIAC OUTPUT— CIRCULATION TIME

There is no polycythemia. The oxygen saturation of the arterial blood is normal.

Study of the *cardiac output* shows that a large part of the output of the left ventricle may be lost through the ductus. The actual per cent of loss was found to be as high as 45 and even 75 per cent (34). The average cases, however, have lower figures.

Circulation time tests usually give doubtful results.

MODE OF ORIGIN OF THE SIGNS

The existence of a large opening at the end of the aortic arch has been compared to an arteriovenous aneurysm. Actually, it is different. In the a-v aneurysm both ventricles increase their work; in patent ductus arteriosus the left ventricle alone increases its output; in extreme cases the left ventricle may pump as much as four times more blood than the right (34) (fig. 186).

High stroke volume, decreased peripheral resistance, and increased blood volume contribute to create strong pulsations in the peripheral vessels.

When the ductus is large, the blood passes from the aorta to the pulmonary artery during the entire cycle. However, the maximum passage occurs in the second half of systole, after the aortic pressure has reached its peak.

When the ductus is small, the passage of blood takes place only during the last part of systole and slightly afterwards. The diastolic murmur may be due, not only to passage of blood through the ductus, but also to *insufficient aortic or pulmonic valves* on account of valvular sclerosis. This is more common in the older age group. It is difficult to decide whether the loud snap which can be recorded in sound tracings is a vibration due to the wall of the ductus or is a split second sound.

Chronic pulmonary lesions may cause hypertrophy of the right ventricle and inversion of the blood stream through the ductus. It has been stated that increase of diastolic pressure of the pulmonary artery is revealed by the fact that the murmur, instead of being continuous, is only systolic (41).

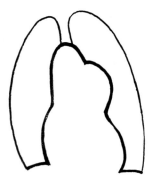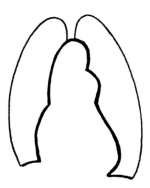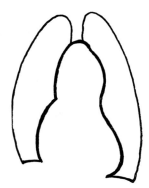

FIG. 185. Sketches of cardiac silhouette in different cases of patent ductus arteriosus

The dilatation of the pulmonary artery is constant and is in contrast to the predominant enlargement of the left ventricle.

The fact that the leakage of blood through the ductus occurs late in systole, when the pulse wave is already in the periphery, explains the possible occurrence of peripheral and functional signs similar to those encountered in aortic insufficiency. These, however, are not constant, as the leakage may be continuous or slight.

Ligation of the ductus usually gives a slower pulse. This is a reflex phenomenon due to greater distention of the carotid sinus when the leakage is stopped.

Hoarseness or dysphonia is due to paralysis of the left recurrent nerve, which surrounds the ductus and the aortic arch.

COURSE AND COMPLICATIONS

Patency of the ductus causes a decreased resistance toward fatigue, the strain of pregnancy, and infections. Pulmonary diseases are especially common. In spite of this, the patency is often well tolerated and life may be of normal duration.

Rheumatic valvular lesions cause severe disturbances by changing the normal ratio of pressure between aorta and pulmonary artery. Aortic stenosis may be compensated by the passage of blood from the pulmonary artery into the aorta but causes cyanosis and severe dyspnea.

Syphilis may cause serious manifestations because the aortitis is often followed by arteritis of the pulmonary artery, with resulting aneurysm of the pulmonary artery and of the ductus.

Subacute bacterial arteritis with localization on the ductus is a dreaded complication. It is, however, less frequent than originally thought.

Thrombosis of the ductus may occur. *Rupture of an aneurysm*, either of the ductus or of the pulmonary artery, has been described.

Complete aphonia may occur.

Heart failure is accompanied by a clinical picture resembling that of aortic insufficiency.

VARIETIES

The different varieties are due to:
a) The cause of the communication.
b) The size of the communication.
c) The seat of the communication.

The above-described clinical picture refers mainly to patency of the ductus arteriosus. When the ductus is large, the typical set of signs and symptoms occurs. However, if

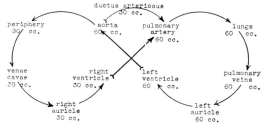

FIG. 186. Scheme of the blood flow in patent ductus arteriosus.

there is only a thin channel or a small hole connecting the two vessels, the only sign may be a late systolic murmur, barely prolonged beyond the 2nd sound.

When *the communication takes place immediately above the aortic valves*, both the murmur and the thrill are very intense and have their maximal intensity in the 3rd left interspace. The murmur starts earlier in systole. The heart is larger.

When the communication is due to *rupture of an aneurysm*, the onset of the signs and symptoms is *sudden*. The signs are similar to those caused by patency of the ductus but toleration is worse and failure sets in earlier. When an *aneurysm of the sinus of Valsalva* ruptures into the pulmonary artery, the murmur is in the 3rd interspace near the sternum and is transmitted toward the right side.

DIAGNOSIS

The diagnosis is not difficult when the typical sign is present: *the continuous machinery murmur*. The existence of left axis deviation is important because practically all other conditions associated with a large pulmonary artery have a right axis deviation[60]. The typical graphic aspect of the murmur (late systolic-early diastolic) is also important for the diagnosis.

Many conditions should be excluded in doubtful cases.

Mitral insufficiency. In the shunts, the murmur is located in the 2nd left interspace and has a different transmission from that of mitral insufficiency. The peripheral vascular signs favor the diagnosis of patent ductus. In mitral insufficiency, cyanosis is more frequent. The ECG is more often normal in patent ductus than in mitral insufficiency. The phonocardiogram shows an early systolic murmur in mitral insufficiency;

[60] Cases of patent ductus with pulmonary hypertension may not have left axis deviation and may even present right axis deviation. This is also true of coarctation of the aorta with ductus opening below the narrow section.

a late systolic and early diastolic in patent ductus. X-ray shows an increased size of the left atrium in mitral insufficiency; typical changes of the aorta and of the pulmonary artery in patent ductus. The vascular network of the lungs is more clearly visible in mitral insufficiency.

Aortic stenosis. The murmur and thrill are to the right of the sternum in aortic stenosis; to the left in patent ductus. They are transmitted more clearly to the carotid arteries in aortic stenosis. The pulse is slow and small in aortic stenosis; it is large and collapsing in patent ductus. The ECG shows a more marked left axis deviation in aortic stenosis. X-ray shows either normal large vessels or small aorta in aortic stenosis; it reveals dilated pulmonary artery and often also dilated aorta in patent ductus. The pulse pressure is increased in patent ductus; decreased in aortic stenosis.

Pulmonary stenosis. Slight cyanosis, frequent occurrence of clubbing, and enlarged transverse diameter of the heart are present in pulmonary stenosis. The murmur is not transmitted toward the carotid arteries. The ECG reveals right axis deviation in pulmonary stenosis; frequently a left axis deviation in patent ductus. The phonocardiogram shows that the murmur of pulmonary stenosis never goes into diastole.

Ventricular septal defect. There is no dulness in the 2nd left interspace; the murmur and thrill are located lower than in patent ductus and are transmitted more toward the right. The x-ray shows a more rounded heart in ventricular septal defect and less dilatation of the pulmonary artery. The phonocardiogram reveals a *systolic murmur* in ventricular septal defect; a *late-systolic-early-diastolic murmur* in patent ductus. Cases of patent ductus with high pulmonary pressure may have a murmur which *clinically* sounds like a pure systolic murmur. Upon reading of phonocardiographic tracing, however, most of these cases also have diastolic vibrations. Therefore, the question would arise only in a small percentage of them.

These cases have more complex lesions and can still be recognized because they have a lower arterial saturation in the femoral in comparison with the brachial arteries.

Venous hum. This is a continuous murmur, occasionally heard in children over the base of the heart. Pressure over the neck veins or movement of the head from side to side usually causes disappearance of the venous hum. The murmur is loudest on the right side of the neck, except in rare cases where it is caused by eddies in a left superior vena cava.

Atrial septal defects. The differential diagnosis has been already discussed (page 283).

PROGNOSIS

The prognosis of the congenital cases (patent ductus) is usually good, but the possibility of complications and of heart failure will be kept in mind. The prognosis of acquired cases (perforation) is always bad.

Treatment

Surgical closure of the ductus has been successfully accomplished in a large number of cases with no fatalities. The best indications for surgery are (37): stunting of growth, great cardiac enlargement, extremely low diastolic pressure (or its fall after exercise), initial heart failure, rheumatic or bacterial endocarditis or endarteritis. However, any patient below the age of 30 where there are no contraindications should be considered for surgery on account of possible dangers which may arise in the future if the ductus is not closed. Above the age of 30, surgery should be considered only in the presence of one of the above indications. Surgical closure is easier in younger patients; shortening, fibrosis, aneurysm, or calcification of the ductus may cause difficulty in adults.

Ligation of the ductus was made at first; then it was proven that *separation* of the ductus was a more effective procedure (34). Closure of an aorto-pulmonary fistula is possible (59); however, it is dangerous.

Closure of the ductus should be preceded

by penicillin treatment, especially in cases of bacterial endocarditis. It should be avoided whenever the patency is accompanied by other congenital lesions, as it may exclude a shunt which is essential for life. It should be kept in mind that surgery does not prevent completely subacute bacterial lesions.

Treatment of acquired lesions (communications between aorta and pulmonary artery through perforation) is limited to treatment of heart failure.

BIBLIOGRAPHY

1. COSTA, A. Cuore e Circ (Rome), 1931, **15**, 263.
2. ABBOTT, M. E. *Nelson Loose Leaf Medicine.* New York, Nelson, 1941, vol. 4.
3. BROWN, J. W. *Congenital Heart Disease.* London, J. B. Med. Publ., 1939.
4. VAQUEZ, H. *Les Maladies du Coeur.* Paris, Baillière, 1921.
5. a) WHITE, P. D. *Heart Disease.* New York, Macmillan, 1944.
   b) McGINN, S., AND WHITE, P. D. Am. Heart. J., 1933, **9**, 1. Also New England J. Med., 1936, **214**, 763.
   c) BURRETT, J. B., AND WHITE, P. D. Am. J. M. Sci., 1945, **209**, 355.
6. BEDFORD, E., PAPP, C., AND PARKINSON, J. Brit. Heart J., 1941, **3**, 37.
7. SCHNITKER, M. A. *The Electrocardiogram in Congenital Cardiac Disease.* Cambridge, Harvard Univ. Press, 1940.
8. BRUMLIK, J. Klinika Vrozenych poruch Srdce a cev., 1937, **5**, 109.
9. COSSIO, P. Bull. Soc. Med. Hôp., 1937, **153**, 215.
10. ROESLER, H. Arch. Int. Med., 1934, **54**, 339. Also *Clinical Roentgenology of the Cardiovascular System.* Springfield, Thomas, 1943.
11. a) CASTELLANOS, A., PEREIRAS, R., AND GARCIA, A. Presse Méd., 1938, **46**, 1474.
    b) SUSSMAN, M. L., GRISHMAN, A., AND STEINBERG, M. F. Am. J. Dis. Child., 1943, **65**, 92.
12. GROLLMAN, A. *Cardiac Output.* Baltimore, Thomas, 1932.
13. a) DEXTER AND BURWELL. New England Heart Assoc., Meeting of Nov. 1945.
    b) DEXTER, L. Radiology, 1947, **48**, 451.
    c) BRANNON, E. S., WEENS, H. S., AND WARREN, J. V. Am. J. M. Sci., 1945, **210**, 480.
    d) BALDWIN, E. DE F., MOORE, L. V., AND NOBLE, R. P. Am. Heart J., 1946, **32**, 152.
14. LAUBRY, C., ROUTIER, O., AND HEIM DE

BALZAC, R. Bull. Mem. Soc. Hôp. Paris, 1941, **56,** 847.

15. THOMSON, T., AND EVANS, W. Quart. J. Med., 1930, **23,** 135.

16. ROGER, H. Bull. Acad. Med. Paris, 1879, **8,** 1074.

17. KEITH, A. *Human Embryology and Morphology.* London, Arnold, 1921.

18. LAUBRY, CH., AND PEZZI, C. *Les Maladies Congenitales du Coeur.* Paris, Baillière, 1921.

19. BURRESI. Lo. Sperim. (Florence), 1880, n. 46, 480.

20. LUISADA, A. A. Rass. Intern. Clin. Ter. (Naples), 1937, **18,** 733 and 791.

21. GIUFFRÈ. Gazz. Osp., Clin. (Milan), 1906, **27,** 1385.

22. MORQUIO, M. L. Semaine Méd., 1901, **21,** 398; and Arch. Mal. Enf., 1901, August.

23. SMITH, A. L. Arch. Ped., 1941, **58,** 549.

24. DENEKE, TH. Deut. Arch. klin. Med., 1906, **89,** 39.

25. BORDET, E., AND FISCHGOLD, H. *La Radio-kymographie du Coeur et des Vaisseaux.* Paris, Masson, 1937.

26. ATTINGER, E. Schweiz. Med. Woch., 1936, **66,** 1056.

27. a) BATTRO, A., AND QUIRNO, N. Rev. Arg. Cardiol., 1936, **11,** 335.
   b) BATTRO, A., AND DE LA SERNA, A. Rev. Arg. Cardiol., 1927, **3,** 427.

28. GERHARDT, C. Verh. Congr. inn. Med.-Wiesbaden, 1892, **11,** 290.

29. FRANÇOIS-FRANK. Gaz. Hebd. Méd., Paris, 1878, **15,** 588.

30. DOMINICI, G., AND FERRERO, A. Min. Med. (Turin), 1929, **9,** (v. 2), 41.

31. SOKOLOFF, A. St. Petersb. med. Woch., 1910, **35,** 583.

32. a) ROUTIER, D. Arch. Mal. Coeur, 1937, **30,** 388.
   b) HUBBARD, J. P. J. Pediat., 1943, **22,** 50.
   c) GRAF, W., MOELLER, T., AND MANNHEIMER, E. Acta Med. Scand., 1947 suppl. 196, 167.

33. BITTORF, A. Muench. med. Woch., 1903, **1,** 1771.

34. a) GROSS, R. E., AND HUBBARD, J. P. J. A. M. A., 1939, **112,** 729.
   b) GROSS, R. E. Ann. Surg., 1939, **110,** 321; J. A. M. A., 1940, **115,** 1257; J. Thoracic Surg., 1947, **16,** 314.

c) KREUTZER, R. Rev. Arg. Card., 1944, **11,** 240.

35. CURTIS BAIN, C. W., AND PARKINSON, J. Brit. Heart J., 1943, **5,** 97.

36. BING, R. J., AND CO-WORKERS. Mo. Conc. Cardiov. Dis., 1948, **17,** N. 3.

37. TAUSSIG, H. B. *Congenital Malformations of the Heart.* New York, Commonwealth Fund, 1947.

38. MASSEE, J. Am. J. M. Sci., 1947, **214,** 248.

39. COURNAND, A., AND CO-WORKERS. Am. J. Physiol., 1947, **150,** 267.

40. LUISADA, A. A., AND FLEISCHNER, F. G. Am. J. Med., 1948, **4,** 791.

41. DOUGLAS, J. M., AND CO-WORKERS. Proc. Staff Meet., Mayo Clin., 1947, **22,** 413.

42. a) LEVINE, S. A., AND GEREMIA, A. E. Bull. New England Med. Center, 1946, **8,** 148.
   b) RAVIN, A., AND DARLEY, W. Ann. Int. Med., 1950, **33,** 903.

43. COHN, R. Am. Heart J., 1947, **33,** 453.

44. CHAVEZ, I., DORBECKER, N., AND CELIS, A. Arch. Inst. Card. Mexico, 1947, **17,** 121.

45. DRY, T. J. Med. Clin. North America, 1948, July, 895.

46. HITZIG, W. M. Mo. Conc Cardiov. Dis., 1947, **16,** N. 8.

47. ZUCKERMANN, R., CISNEROS, F., AND NOVELO, S. Arch. Card. de Mexico, 1951, **21,** 61.

48. OPDYKE, D. F., AND CO-WORKERS. Am. J. Physiol, 1948, **154,** 258; 1949, **158,** 241; and 1950, **160,** 556.

49. COURNAND, A., AND CO-WORKERS. Am. J. Physiol, 1947, **150,** 267.

50. LITTLE, R. C. Am. J. Physiol., 1949, **158,** 237.

51. GRISHMAN, A., AND CO-WORKERS. Am. J. Roentgenol., 1949, **62,** 500.

52. MURRAY, G. Ann. Surg., 1948, **128,** 4.

53. a) GROSS, R. J. A. M. A., 1953, **151,** 795.
   b) SWAN, H. J. A. M. A., 1953, **151,** 792.

54. BAILEY, C. P., AND CO-WORKERS: Ann. Surg. 1952, **136,** 919.

55. CURTIN, J. Q.: Am. Heart J., 1952, **44,** 884.

56. HAWLEY, J. G., LITTLE, R. C., AND FEIL, H. Circ., 1950, **1,** 321.

57. LEVINSON, D. C., AND CO-WORKERS. Am. J. M. Sci., 1951, **222,** 46.

58. DESOLDATI, L., AND CO-WORKERS. Rev. Arg. Card., 1951, **18,** 189.

59. GROSS, R. E. Circ., 1952, **5,** 858.

CHAPTER 14

Combined Defects of the Heart

Combined defects are lesions of two or more valves or those of one valve plus a shunt between the greater and lesser circulations. Any or all the lesions may be congenital in nature.

Combined Defects of the Mitral and Aortic Valves

This association is frequent because the mitral and aortic valves are frequently damaged by endocarditis, usually rheumatic. There almost always is a double defect of both valves but the clinical picture can vary on account of predominance of stenosis or insufficiency of either valve.

DOUBLE MITRAL DEFECT PLUS AORTIC INSUFFICIENCY

These patients have cyanosis, visible pulsations of both the arteries and veins of the neck, and *pulsus celer.*

The heart is tremendously enlarged (cor bovinum) (fig. 187). The apex impulse is violent; there are multiple pulsations in different intercostal spaces. There is a *diastolic thrill* over the midprecordium. Auscultation reveals a *diastolic-presystolic rumble* and a *soft systolic murmur* at the apex while a *soft blowing diastolic murmur* is present over the base. There may be an opening snap of the mitral valve.

The liver is often enlarged; there may be signs of chronic edema of the lung bases.

Attacks of paroxysmal dyspnea, acute pulmonary edema, and precordial pain, are typical of this syndrome.

The pulse pressure is somewhat increased but less than in pure aortic insufficiency. The blood pressure is higher at the leg than on the arm, a fact which is unusual in mitral defects (1).

If the mitral stenosis is slight, only a soft systolic apical and a soft diastolic basal murmur are present.

Combined insufficiency of the aortic and mitral valves may also be due to atherosclerosis or syphilis. In the first instance, arteriosclerosis, hypertension, and coronary heart disease are frequently present; in the second, hypertension and aortitis are often associated to the valvular lesions.

In many of these cases, differential diagnosis between the diastolic rumble caused by organic lesion of the mitral valve and that caused by relative stenosis or other functional mechanism (Austin Flint murmur, page 242) is necessary. X-ray, electrocardiography, electrokymography, and phonocardiography may be of help.

DOUBLE AORTIC DEFECT PLUS MITRAL INSUFFICIENCY

This association is not rare. It is frequently caused by rheumatic heart disease but may also be due to arteriosclerosis.

Aortic stenosis predominates in the clinical picture. Therefore, pallor, *pulsus tardus,* reduced pulse pressure, and low tibial pressure are usually present.

There is a systolic thrill at the base. A harsh systolic and a soft diastolic murmur are present over the aortic area; a softer systolic murmur, at the apex.

The vascular signs are seldom those of aortic insufficiency owing to the effect of both the aortic stenosis and the mitral insufficiency in neutralizing them.

In most cases, x-ray, electrocardiography,

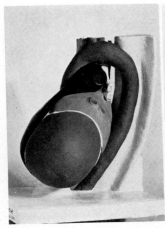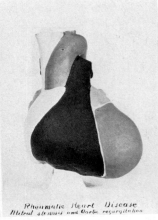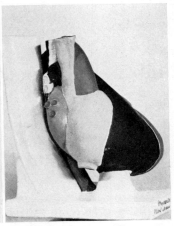

Fig. 187. Changes of the heart and large vessels in the combined lesion of the mitral and aortic valves. (From a model of the American Heart Association.)

electrokymography, and phonocardiography are of help. The prognosis is worse than in patients with lesions of only the mitral or the aortic valve.

MITRAL AND AORTIC STENOSIS

The combined stenosis of the mitral and aortic valves creates a syndrome which is not uncommon (30). This double lesion is always rheumatic and can be found in middle-age patients in over one-half of the cases. Attacks of precordial pain, paroxysmal dyspnea, pulmonary edema, and of syncope, are typical. The aortic systolic murmur may be typical, but it may be maximal over the 3rd left interspace, or may seem unimportant.

This syndrome may be well tolerated for a long time but frequently causes a short and irreversible episode of heart failure.

Combined Defects of the Mitral and Tricuspid Valves

This is a relatively frequent association, occurring in as many as 20 to 30 per cent of the valvular defects (2, 3). It is usually due to rheumatic disease and rarely to benign bacterial endocarditis.

Two clinical pictures can be recognized: a) *Double mitral defect plus tricuspid insufficiency*, and b) *double mitral defect plus tricuspid stenosis*. The eventuality of a *com-* *bined insufficiency of the two valves without stenosis* is a third possibility but is exceedingly rare (4).

In these cases, recognition of the mitral lesion is usually based upon the finding of diastolic thrill and murmur over the apex. However, the existence of large liver, ascites, no peripheral edema, no orthopnea, very large right atrium (x-ray, fig. 188), and no signs of pulmonary congestion, permit the diagnosis of an associated tricuspid lesion (fig. 189). If stenosis of the tricuspid valve predominates over the insufficiency, the liver is not pulsating. If, on the contrary, insufficiency of the tricuspid predominates, both the liver and the jugular veins expand in systole. Extreme distention of the right atrium or presence of liver cirrhosis may lessen these pulsations. Slight jaundice may occur.

The prognosis is worse than in cases with defects of the mitral valve alone. However, as the most apparent signs are caused by a mechanical obstacle and not by heart failure, the interval between the first signs of abdominal congestion and the patient's death is longer than where there are only mitral defects.

Differential diagnosis includes atrial septal defects, constrictive pericarditis, and Ebstein's syndrome.

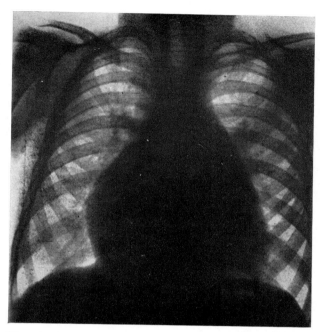

FIG. 188. Cardiac silhouette in a case of combined mitral and tricuspid defects (From Assmann.)

Combined Defects of the Aortic and Pulmonic Valves

The association of aortic and pulmonic lesions is rare. It may be caused by rheumatic disease (5), bacterial endocarditis, or lues (6). Either stenosis or insufficiency of the two valves may be predominant.

The clinical diagnosis is difficult because the murmurs of both lesions are similar in type and phase. However, the heart is more enlarged toward the right than where there are aortic defects alone, and some of the signs of pulmonic lesions may be recognized.

Electrokymography may be of help for the diagnosis; catheterization of the pulmonary artery and right ventricle may be resorted to, if necessary.

Mitral Stenosis Plus Pulmonic Insufficiency (24)

A certain number of patients with mitral stenosis or Lutembacher's syndrome present the clinical signs of an associated pulmonic insufficiency. These are: a) *loud, soft, blowing diastolic murmur over the 2nd or 3rd left* *interspace* (fig. 190). The murmur does not change with the changing functional conditions of the heart. It tends to increase with the years and has been observed and recorded even for 7 years without attenuation (24). b) The pulmonary vessels are very dilated and show a *hilar dance*. The aorta is small and shows small pulsations. c) *Cyanosis* is rather severe. Right axis deviation is constant and severe. d) All peripheral signs of aortic insufficiency (including blood pressure changes) are missing.

Organic pulmonic insufficiency may be due to a stretching of the artery, caused by *atherosclerosis* (17, 18, 19) or *lues* (20). In most of the reported cases an aneurysm of the pulmonary artery was present. A different cause may be *a rheumatic lesion*, because the pulmonary artery and the pulmonic ring are frequently damaged by rheumatic disease (21, 22, 23) and, in rare cases, the leaflets are also involved.

Clinical studies of the author led to recognition of the possible association of mitral stenosis with pulmonic insufficiency caused

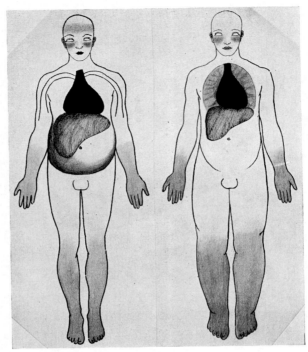

FIG. 189. Sketch of the congestion and edema: a, in mitral plus tricuspid defect, and b, in the common mitral defect.

by rheumatic lesions (24). So far, post-mortem examinations are rare (28, 34).

The diagnosis is based upon the persistence of the basal murmur, its independence from congestive failure, its loudness, and the typical transmission. As mitral

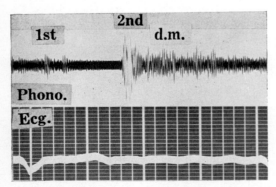

FIG. 190. Phonocardiogram over the pulmonic area in a case with combined lesion of the mitral and the pulmonic valves. Soft, early diastolic murmur in decrescendo.

stenosis is typical, these data will permit exclusion of a Graham Steell murmur.

Tri-Valve Defects

About 20 per cent of the patients with rheumatic heart disease have lesions of three valves, usually the mitral, aortic, and tricuspid (2, 3).

The mitral and aortic lesions are the main causes of the local signs. The aortic lesions mainly determine the arterial signs; the tricuspid lesions are more important in relation to the venous and hepatic signs.

This association of defects seldom is recogeznid during life but should be always kept in mind.

Four-Valve Defects

In a small percentage of cases with either rheumatic or bacterial endocarditis (2.5 to 10 per cent) (3, 6), all four valves are attacked and show similar lesions (28). An exact diagnosis is always difficult, especially if the lesions are due to an acute bacterial endocarditis.

Tricuspid Defect Plus Patent Foramen Ovale (Ebstein's Syndrome) (8, 9)

Most cases are congenital. However, a few exceptions are due to either fetal endocarditis or rheumatic lesion of the tricuspid valve in a patient with patent foramen ovale. The age of the described cases varies from 3 to 61 years.

LESIONS

Two main types of tricuspid lesion have been described (7):

a) An incomplete development of two cusps of the tricuspid valve (the anterior cusp is often normal).

b) The substitution of a membranous diaphragm for the tricuspid valve; this is displaced toward the apex of the right ventricle (8).

The first lesion causes regurgitation because of incompetence of the valves; the second does likewise, but the fact that *one part of the right ventricle is above the valves* adds a further cause of regurgitation. The contraction of this supravalvular section not only pushes the blood of the atrium backwards, but prevents a complete closure of the tricuspid.

Both the right atrium and the right ventricle are dilated. The foramen ovale is widely patent. The left atrium is either normal or enlarged. The pulmonary artery is hypoplasic, the superior cava is dilated (fig. 191).

Tricuspid insufficiency causes regurgitation of blood into the right atrium and into the cavae during ventricular systole. The septal defect shunts most of this regurgitant blood into the left atrium and decreases the evidence of regurgitation. Thus, the flow of blood of the greater circulation is greater than that of the lesser circulation. The mixture of bloods into the left atrium due to the right-to-left shunt is the cause of cyanosis.

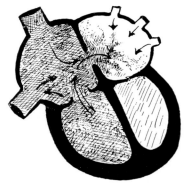

Fig. 191. Changes of the heart in *Ebstein's syndrome*.

SIGNS AND SYMPTOMS

There is *cyanosis* which may not be severe. *Clubfingers* may be present. *Attacks of dyspnea* may occur. *Palpitation* is frequent.

A *systolic thrill* and a blowing *systolic murmur* are present in most of the cases over the tricuspid area. A *diastolic murmur* may also be present (9). The *electrocardiogram* frequently shows *right bundle branch block* (27, 31). When spreading of the impulse is normal, *left axis deviation* may be present (increased flow through the left heart). *Giant P-waves* have been noted in the right precordial leads (31). Attacks of *atrial tachycardia* or frequent *premature beats* are common.

There is a *positive systolic pulsation* of the *jugular veins* and of the *liver*, clearly revealed by graphic tracings. The *electrokymogram* reveals a *positive, systolic plateau* over the border of the right atrium indicating regurgitation (31).

Circulation time tests reveal a shortening of the arm-to-tongue time.

X-ray reveals marked enlargement of the heart, especially of the right atrium and ventricle (10, 11). The left atrium is less enlarged. The superior cava is large and pulsating. There is a small pulmonary artery and the lungs are clear.

Angiocardiography may reveal passage of the radio-opaque substance through the atrial septum with early filling of the left atrium. However, the great volume of the right heart chambers frequently causes dilution of the contrast medium and poor visualization.

Diagnosis is possible if the clinical picture is known. However, pulsations of the veins may be prevented by excessive distention, and pulsations of the liver may be prevented by the same condition or by liver cirrhosis.

Differential diagnosis should exclude *a combined mitral and tricuspid defect* or the *uncomplicated atrial septal defect*. The first is accompanied by definite signs of mitral stenosis. The uncomplicated defect is not accompanied by such a large liver and has no cyanosis. *Circulation time is shortened in Ebstein's syndrome and prolonged in mitral plus tricuspid lesion*; doubtful results are obtained in atrial septal defects.

The Ebstein's syndrome may show an x-ray picture which simulates *pulmonic stenosis*. However, the latter presents more marked electrocardiographic evidence of right ventricular hypertrophy, a murmur which is usually louder and harsher, no venous or hepatic systolic waves, and no shorter circulation time (unless there also is a patent foramen ovale).

Mitral Defects Plus Patent Foramen Ovale (Lutembacher's Syndrome) (15, 16)

CAUSES

This syndrome was attributed at first to the combination of two congenital lesions (15). Later, cases with rheumatic mitral defects in patients having a patent foramen ovale were recognized. Therefore, either a *congenital* or a *congenital plus rheumatic lesion* may occur.

The syndrome is twice as frequent in females as in males (27).

LESIONS

The mitral valve shows a partial fusion of its cusps resulting in narrowing of the orifice. In some cases, retraction due to previous endocarditis has been found. *The foramen*

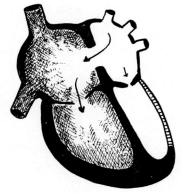

FIG. 192. Changes of the heart in *Lutembacher's syndrome.*

ovale is widely patent. Both the left atrium and ventricle are either normal or small. On the contrary, the right atrium and ventricle are greatly enlarged. The pulmonary artery and its main branches are remarkably dilated. There may be an aneurysm of the main trunk, frequently expanding into the left stem (fig. 192). These lesions of the mitral valve greatly increase left atrial pressure and a certain amount of blood goes through the shunt from the left to the right atrium. Therefore, the left atrium is not much enlarged while the right atrium and ventricle are dilated and have thick walls (fig. 192). The blood flow of the lesser circulation is far greater than that of the greater circulation.

SIGNS AND SYMPTOMS

Effort dyspnea, recurrent bronchitis, and *weakness* are usually present; *bloody sputum* and *dizziness* are frequently noted.

Cyanosis may be *slight* or substituted by *pallor. Chronic pulmonary edema* is frequent and occurs as an early sign.

A heaving systolic pulsation of the jugular veins may be observed in some cases. When present, it indicates *severe mitral insufficiency* which causes regurgitation of blood from the left ventricle to the left atrium, and thence to the right through the shunt.

There are multiple pulsations over the precordial area and a visible *epigastric pulsa-*

tion. The entire cardiac dulness is displaced to the right so that the heart rests in a median position. There is a *diastolic thrill* over the 4th left interspace and a *diastolic-presystolic rumble* is heard over the same area. *A presystolic murmur* has been heard behind the manubrium of the sternum. *A systolic murmur* is often present over the pulmonic area. *A soft diastolic murmur* may also be present over the same area (24). The liver may have a presystolic pulsation (13).

GRAPHIC RECORDS

The *electrocardiogram shows right axis deviation.* Changes of the P wave and of the P-R interval are similar to those of mitral stenosis. Atrial fibrillation is frequently observed.

Both the jugular and the hepatic tracings present high presystolic waves if sinus rhythm is preserved. A high systolic wave may be recorded if mitral insufficiency predominates (blood regurgitating through the shunt) or if relative tricuspid insufficiency is present.

The *phonocardiogram* records the typical vibrations of mitral stenosis. High-pitched vibrations may be recorded over the pulmonic area, after the 2nd sound.

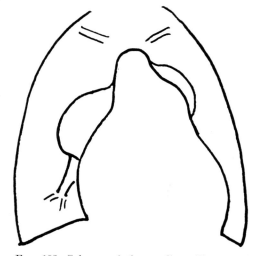

FIG. 193. Scheme of the cardiac silhouette in a case of *Lutembacher's syndrome.*

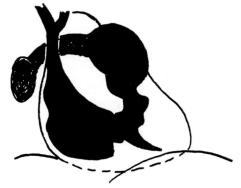

FIG. 194. Angiocardiogram in *Lutembacher's syndrome.* (Inspired by originals of Sussman, Grishman, and Steinberg.)

X-RAY

Both the left atrium and ventricle are normal or small. Both the right atrium and ventricle are enlarged. The aorta is small, the pulmonary artery is very large. The branches of the pulmonary artery are so distended that they may simulate a mediastinal tumor (fig. 193). *A hilar dance may be observed.*

Angiocardiography and *catheterization* of the heart give data of diagnostic value. The first reveals an important passage of blood from the left into the right atrium (fig. 194). The second reveals an increase of right atrial pressure which is unusual in uncomplicated patent foramen ovale.

Circulation time is prolonged; there is no polycythemia.

MODE OF ORIGIN OF THE SIGNS

The increased amount of blood in the pulmonary circulation causes distention of the pulmonary vessels. Typically, these pulsate strongly as in pulmonic insufficiency.

The mitral murmur and the enlargement of the left atrium may be moderate or even absent. This is due to the fact that the shunt prevents the establishment of high pressure in the left atrium and severe hypertrophy of the wall of this chamber.

When a presystolic murmur is heard over the base, it is due to blood passing through the septal defect.

The systolic murmur over the pulmonic area is due to relative stenosis because of distention of the vessel. If a soft diastolic murmur is also present over the same area, two possibilities exist: a) A transitory murmur due to temporary insufficiency of the pulmonic valve (*Graham Steell murmur*). b) A persistent murmur caused by an anatomical lesion (page 259).

Congestion of the pulmonary circulation is due both to increased inflow and greater resistance to outflow, but to the former more than to the latter. For this reason, cyanosis is less marked than in mitral stenosis and may be replaced by pallor.

COURSE AND COMPLICATIONS

The patients may live until old age. The severity of the syndrome is determined by the degree of mitral stenosis and by the size of the septal defect.

The complications are those of mitral stenosis. However, atrial fibrillation, pulmonary congestion, chronic bronchitis, and chronic pulmonary edema occur earlier and are more severe than in mitral stenosis alone. Aneurysm of the pulmonary artery may occur. Arteriosclerosis of the lesser circulation may increase the severity of the clinical picture. Pulmonic insufficiency is more frequent than with pure mitral stenosis. On the other hand, aneurysm of the left atrium and phenomena of compression by this chamber are the exception.

Crossed embolism is extremely rare because of the predominant left atrial pressure. Congestive failure occurs earlier and subacute bacterial endocarditis is slightly more frequent than in mitral stenosis with closed atrial septum.

DIAGNOSIS

Diagnosis is based on the typical findings of mitral stenosis, associated with a relatively small left atrium and with severely dilated pulmonary vessels (x-ray).

Uncomplicated mitral stenosis presents a larger left atrium. *Uncomplicated patent*

foramen ovale usually fails to show a diastolic rumble. However, if such rumble is present (relative mitral or tricuspid stenosis), diagnosis may be difficult.

The *tetralogy of Fallot* causes an entirely different picture. The same is true for the *association of aortic stenosis or coarctation with patent ductus.*

Patent ductus causes a typical murmur, has a left axis deviation, and gives typical data upon catheterization. However, *atypical cases with patent ductus* may simulate Lutembacher's syndrome. Catheterization reveals the atrial defect of Lutembacher's syndrome while retrograde aortography rules out the ductus.

PROGNOSIS

The prognosis of such cases is not favorable. However, duration of life seems to be only slightly shorter than in cases of mitral stenosis.

VARIETIES

A variety of the syndrome consists of *mitral atresia plus atrial and ventricular septal defects*. Cases with this congenital lesion are rare and survive only for a limited time.

Aortic Stenosis (or Coarctation) Plus Patent Ductus Arteriosus

This is a syndrome of congenital nature having a clinical picture which is entirely different from that caused by the single isolated lesions.

LESIONS

Two different lesions may be present:

a) Aortic stenosis plus patent ductus arteriosus (fig. 195).

b) Coarctation of the aorta plus patent ductus (fig. 278, page 468).

The stenosis is of the subaortic type (page 250); the coarctation is in the region of the isthmus (so-called infantile type) and will be discussed later at length (page 467).

The narrowing of the aortic opening causes

a drop of pressure in the arterial system or in the lower parts of the body; this is compensated by the blood of the pulmonary artery which enters the aorta *via* the ductus. However, this blood is poorly saturated with oxygen.

A mixture of blood, proportional to the severity of the aortic lesion, occurs in the first variety. The coarctation limits the blood supply only to the lower half of the body in the second variety so that the mixture of blood takes place mainly in the descending aorta. The flow of blood through the shunt takes place from the lesser to the greater circulation owing to the low pressure existing in the aorta. In extreme cases, the aortic ostium may be closed (*aortic atresia*). In such cases, the arteries of the head and upper extremities, as well as the coronaries, also receive the blood *via* the ductus.

SYMPTOMS AND SIGNS

Cyanosis, clubfingers, attacks of dizziness or syncope, effort dyspnea, bloody sputum, and *recurrent bronchitis,* are typical. In cases with coarctation, cyanosis is exclusive of the lower extremities and the lower part of the body (27).

No arterial collateral circulation is present on the thorax as with uncomplicated coarctation (page 467).

Blood pressure is low, but *not much lower in the legs than in the arms.*

In cases with aortic stenosis, the typical *thrill* and *murmur* of this lesion are present at the right of the sternum. In addition, the *prolonged thrill* and *murmur* of patent ductus are present *at the left* of the sternum.

In cases with coarctation of the aorta, the local signs of patent ductus arteriosus (page 291) are the only ones present.

The *electrocardiogram* has a marked right axis deviation and low T waves.

The *phonocardiogram* reveals the typical murmur of patent ductus arteriosus (fig. 183).

X-ray shows a rounded heart with prominent pulmonary knob and hilar dance.

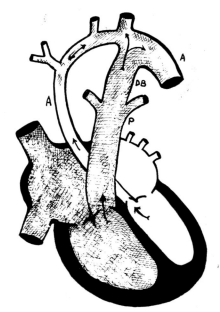

FIG. 195. Changes of the heart and large vessels in patent ductus arteriosus plus aortic stenosis.

Angiocardiography reveals that the contrast medium passes from the pulmonary artery into the descending aorta.

Circulation time tests show that the arm-to-tongue time is *shorter* than in normal individuals (but only in aortic stenosis plus ductus).

Blood. There is polycythemia.

COURSE AND COMPLICATIONS

In spite of the severity of the lesions, the disease may last for a long time. Some of the patients have reached adult age and even maturity. The complications are those of the associated defects. They include *subacute bacterial endocarditis, pulmonary infarction,* and (in the coarctation variety) *cerebral hemorrhage.*

VARIETY

Two main varieties have been already described. A third occurs when *aortic atresia is associated with patent ductus and patent foramen ovale* (7). In such cases, life is possible only for a few days after birth.

DIAGNOSIS

Diagnosis of these cases should be based on the finding of a large pulmonary knob (x-ray) together with cyanosis in the lower extremities (coarctation) or both in the left arm and the legs (aortic stenosis). Angiocardiography is helpful and may confirm the diagnosis.

Differential diagnosis should be made with the following diseases:

Uncomplicated patent ductus. The presence of cyanosis excludes this possibility.

Fallot's syndrome. The dilated pulmonary knob and the increased pulmonary markings exclude this syndrome.

Eisenmenger's syndrome. Exclusion is possible by means of catheterization or angiocardiography unless cyanosis of the lower extremities is present (coarctation plus ductus).

Uncomplicated aortic stenosis. The presence of cyanosis excludes this lesion.

Uncomplicated coarctation. The existence of cyanosis, the type of murmur, the lack of blood pressure difference between arms and legs, and of collateral circulation, exclude this lesion.

Pulmonary stenosis. The severely dilated pulmonary artery and the type of murmur are against this possibility. Cyanosis is more severe than in pulmonary stenosis.

Transposition of the large vessels. The thin vascular peduncle which is typical of the transposition is not present here. The murmur is different.

TREATMENT

Surgical treatment is difficult and has frequently met with unfavorable results. However, it is possible (33) and consists of the ligature of the ductus plus resection of the narrow portion of the aorta with graft of a new section in coarctation plus ductus. In aortic stenosis plus ductus, dilatation of the aortic ostium should precede ligation of the ductus.

Pulmonary Stenosis Plus Patent Foramen Ovale

This combination of congenital lesions is not rare but is less frequent than previously thought (25).

Narrowing of the pulmonary orifice leads to increased pressure in the right ventricle and, to a lesser extent, in the right atrium. This causes a passage of blood through the shunt from the right to the left atrium.

The patients have *severe cyanosis, clubbing of the fingers,* and *polycythemia.* The left section of the heart may enlarge even more than the right and there may be *dilatation of the aorta.* There is *a systolic murmur over the pulmonic area,* caused by the stenosis.

The *electrocardiogram* may show left axis deviation (26) but right axis deviation and right bundle branch block seem more common (25, 32).

X-ray reveals clear lung fields. Angiocardiography may reveal early visualization of the left atrium.

Circulation time tests show that the arm-to-tongue time is *shorter* than in normal individuals.

Diagnosis is always difficult.

Treatment is based on the *Brock operation* (page 267), possibly completed by closure of the atrial shunt (page 294).

Aortic Insufficiency with Patent Foramen Ovale (29)

This rare combination of lesions is due to the occurrence of luetic aortitis with aortic regurgitation in subjects having a patent foramen ovale.

The typical signs of aortic insufficiency are present, including the aortic diastolic murmur, the large pulse pressure, and the Corrigan pulse.

The *electrocardiogram* may present *right axis deviation* and, frequently, atrial fibrillation.

The *x-ray* reveals *dilatation of the pulmonary artery* and increased vascular markings of the lungs. Diagnosis is possible if attention is paid to the above described electrocardiographic and roentgenological signs associated with the physical signs of aortic regurgitation.

BIBLIOGRAPHY

1. BASSI, M. Riv. Clin. Med. (Florence). 1934 **35**, 823; and 1935, **36**, 29.
2. DRESSLER, W., AND FISCHER, R. Klin. Woch., 1929, **8**, 1267 and 1316.
3. COOKE, W. T., AND WHITE, P. D. Brit. Heart J., 1941, **3**, 147.
4. LUISADA, A. A. Arch. Pat. Clin. Med., 1936, **16**, 404.
5. DAGNINI, G. Cuore e Circ. (Rome), 1930, **14**, 15.
6. McGUIRE, J., AND McNAMARA, R. J. Am. Heart J., 1937, **14**, 562.
7. ABBOTT, M. E. In *Nelson Loose Leaf Medicine*. New York, Nelson, 1941, vol. 4.
8. EBSTEIN, W. Arch. Anat. Phys., 1866, **8**, 238.
9. ARNSTEIN, A. Virchows Arch. path. Anat., 1927, **266**, 247.
10. BAUER, D. DE F. Am. J. Roentgenol., 1945, **54**, 136.
11. BREKKE, V. G. Am. Heart J., 1945, **29**, 647.
12. YATER, W. M., AND SHAPIRO, M. J. Ann. Int. Med., 1937–38, **11**, 1043.
13. BROWN, J. B. *Congenital Heart Disease*. London, J. B. Med. Publ., 1939.
14. DRESSLER, W. *Clinical Cardiology*. New York, Hoeber, 1941.
15. LUTEMBACHER, R. Arch. Mal. Coeur, 1916, **9**, 235. Also Presse Méd., 1925, **33**, 236. Also Arch. Mal. Coeur, 1936, **29**, 229.
16. McGINN, S., AND WHITE, P. D. Am. Heart J., 1933, **9**, 1.
17. LAUBRY, C., AND THOMAS, M. Bull. Mem. Soc. Hôp. Paris, 1926, **50**, 639.
18. HARVIER, P., AND CO-WORKERS. Paris Méd., 1937, **27**, 397.
19. SCIMONE, V. Cuore e Circ. (Rome), 1927, **11**, 3.
20. LUISADA, A. A. Min. Med. (Turin), 1934, **25**, 421.
21. GOULEY, B. A., AND EIMAN, J. Am. J. M. Sci., 1932, **183**, 359.
22. VON GLAHN, W. C., AND PAPPENHEIMER, A. M. Am. J. Path., 1926, **2**, 235.
23. KUGEL, M. A., AND EPSTEIN, E. F. Arch. Path., 1928, **6**, 247.
24. LUISADA, A. A., AND WOLFF, L. Am. J. M. Sci., 1945, **209**, 204.
25. CURRENS, J. H., KINNEY, T. D., AND WHITE, P. D. Am. Heart J., 1945, **30**, 491.
26. WOOD, P. Brit. Heart J., 1942, **4**, 11.
27. TAUSSIG, H. B. *The Congenital Malformations of the Heart*. New York, Commonwealth Fund, 1947.
28. TREIGER, I. J. *Atlas of Cardiovascular Diseases*. St. Louis, C. V. Mosby, 1947, p. 54.
29. LIPSON, M. Am. Heart J., 1948, **35**, 497.
30. SOULIÉ, P., AND CHICHE, P. Bull., Mem., Soc. med. Hôp. de Paris, 1949, No. 25, 1040.
31. SOLOFF, L. A., STAUFFER, H. M., AND ZATUCHNI, J. Am. J. M. Sci., 1951, **222**, 554.
32. SELZER, A., AND CO-WORKERS. Am. J. Med., 1949, **6**, 3.
33. HAXTON, H. A., AND THOMPSON, M. L. Brit. M. J., 1948, (II), 1062.

CHAPTER 15

Complex Malformations of the Heart

The complex malformations of the heart are numerous if considered from a purely structural point of view. However, if the forms which do not permit survival are excluded and the mechanism of production outlined by Spitzer is considered, their number is greatly reduced.

Tetralogy of Fallot

This syndrome is the most common complex malformation of the heart and includes about 75 per cent of the cyanotic cases surviving beyond infancy.

LESIONS—MECHANISM

While certain lesions are basic and constantly present, a few others may be associated. The basic lesions are pulmonic stenosis, dextroposition of the aorta and ventricular septal defect; right ventricular hypertrophy is a necessary consequence.

Pulmonic stenosis. Contrary to older concepts, this may be due to various mechanisms (fig. 197):

a) *A valvular stenosis* (in approximately one-third of the cases).

b) *Hypoplasia of the pulmonary artery with bicuspid pulmonic valve and subpulmonic stenosis.*

c) *Infundibular stenosis.* This may be so low as to create what resembles a separate chamber leading to the ostium.

d) Both infundibular and valvular.

Dextroposition of the aorta. This abnormality should not be confused with the persistence of the right aortic arch (page 464), a possible associated lesion. *The aorta of these patients is a large vessel resulting from fusion of the two fetal aortae.* This vessel is far more to the right than a normal aorta and overrides the ventricular septum so that it may receive blood from both ventricles. It should be kept in mind that the displacement of the aorta may be of varying degrees; if minimal, it may be overlooked by the pathologist.

The third lesion, a *high ventricular septal defect*, is thus a necessary association, while the fourth, *right ventricular hypertrophy*, is an obligatory consequence of the communication between the two ventricles and of pulmonic stenosis.

Associated lesions may be: a) Quadricuspid aortic valve. b) Persistence of the right aortic arch. c) Some degree of transposition, so that the pulmonary artery is either behind or to the left of the aorta.

Large bronchial arteries usually supply anastomotic vessels which contribute to the blood supply of the lungs.

The complex abnormality of Fallot's syndrome is determined by an *incomplete torsion* of the primitive cardiac tube (*Spitzer's theory (2)*). If severe, this may cause occlusion of the left aorta (which normally develops into the definitive aorta) and persistence of the right aorta. If the faulty torsion is slight, on the other hand, the two fetal aortae fuse together and result in a large artery which rides squarely over the septum (fig. 196). The pulmonary artery is thin because it results from only one-third instead of one-half of the common arterial trunk on account of the fusion of the two primitive aortae into a larger vessel. These conditions somewhat resemble those which are normal in the reptilian heart.

In exceptional cases, inflammatory stenosis of the pulmonary valves occurs in patients with Eisenmenger's syndrome (page 318) and a partially acquired Fallot's syndrome is the result.

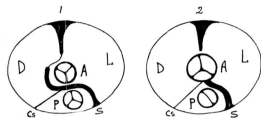

Fig. 196. Position of the aorta in the normal heart (1) and in the *tetralogy of Fallot* (2). D, right ventricle; L, left ventricle. (Adapted from Spitzer.)

SIGNS AND SYMPTOMS

A *stunting of growth* is common but not constant. *Cyanosis is usually present at birth* but may start later. It is of variable degree but is usually severe. It is increased by exertion or crying and is particularly evident in the extremities and on the mucosae.

Clubbing of the fingers and toes (occasionally of the nose) is constant and is associated with watch-glass nails.

Exertion is frequently followed by *dyspnea*. The children may try to relieve this by assuming a *squatting position* (31). *Paroxysmal dyspnea* at rest, accompanied by severe cyanosis, is common. These episodes are usually brief.

Attacks of dizziness, fainting, or *convulsions* are not unusual.

Pulsations of the epigastrium are visible. A *systolic thrill* is often present at the base of the heart with transmission toward the neck.

Percussion reveals a heart with marked enlargement toward the right. No dulness is present in the 2nd left interspace but there may be dulness in the *2nd right* interspace.

Auscultation reveals a *loud, harsh, systolic murmur* with maximal intensity over the 3rd left interspace. This murmur is well transmitted toward the 2nd right interspace, the suprasternal notch, and the carotid arteries (4). It may be heard over the left scapula (5) and continues throughout all systole. The intensity of the murmur is mostly related to the pulmonic stenosis and

is relatively less affected by the septal defect and the eddies which form in the ascending aorta. *The 2nd pulmonic sound is usually weak.*

A *systolic type* of *triple rhythm* may be present over the midprecordium.

The *pulse* is usually *full.* The *blood pressure* may be normal, low, or increased. Figures of 140 to 150 for the systolic pressure are not unusual.

GRAPHIC TRACINGS

The *cardiogram,* as well as the *jugular* and *hepatic tracings,* reveal a *high atrial wave.*

The *electrocardiogram* usually shows a *severe right axis deviation* and evidence of right ventricular hypertrophy (fig. 198). However, cases with moderate deviation have been described. Right atrial hypertrophy may be apparent. While *i.v. block* or *a-v block* may be present, both may be temporary (7). The chest leads reveal *hypertrophy of the right ventricle and of the right atrium* with a high, diphasic P in V_1–V_2. The rotation of the heart due to the hypertrophy of the right ventricle may be such that V_1 has a left ventricular pattern qR while RS patterns are present in V_5–V_6.

The *phonocardiogram* reveals a series of *coarse vibrations* during systole. In some cases, the systolic murmur is separated from the 1st sound by a short pause (7) (fig. 199). This is the cause of the triple rhythm. The murmur may end at midsystole or continue all through systole. Both the 3rd and the 4th sound may be loud.

Electrokymography reveals the following data: a) Lack of pulsations in the pulmonary window. b) Small or absent hilar pulsations. c) Absent pulsations of the pulmonary parenchyma.

CATHETERIZATION OF THE HEART

Catheterization of the right heart reveals three sets of phenomena:

a) *Pressure tracings reveal a high pressure in the right ventricle* (figures of 90 to 110 mm. Hg are not unusual) *while the pressure is*

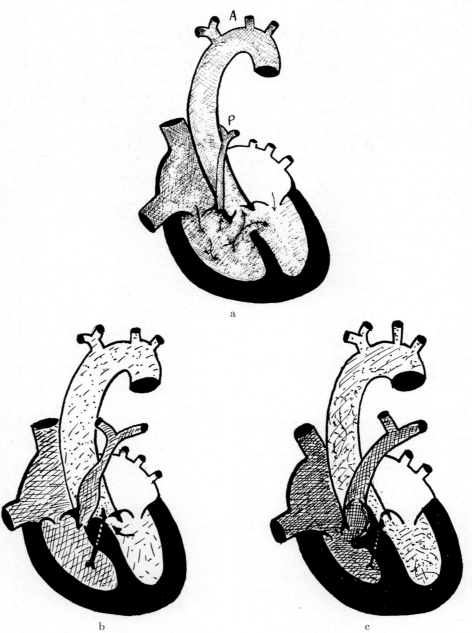

FIG. 197. Scheme of the changes of the heart and large vessels in the *tetralogy of Fallot*. a, Valvular stenosis, hypoplasia of the pulmonary artery. b, Subvalvular stenosis with poststenotic dilatation. c, Infundibular stenosis with formation of a separate chamber before the valve.

either normal or low in the pulmonary artery. Therefore, while there is a high gradient of pressure between right ventricle and pulmonary artery, right ventricular pressure is similar to systemic pressure.

b) *Oxymetry* usually reveals a normal oxygen content in the right atrium and *a high oxygen content in the right ventricle* (blood shunted from the left ventricle through the septum).

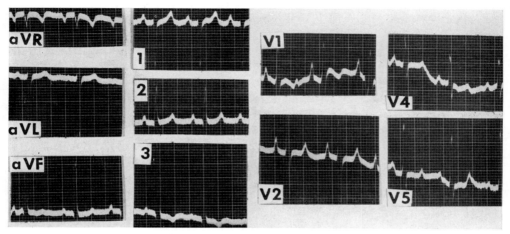

FIG. 198. Electrocardiogram in a case of *tetralogy of Fallot*

c) The catheter may fail to enter the pulmonary artery on account of the stenosis; it may pass from the right ventricle into the ascending aorta.

Calculations based on the oxymetric data indicate that systemic flow is higher than pulmonic flow.

X-RAY

The cardiac shadow is usually not enlarged. The apex may be raised from the diaphragm (*sheep-nose profile*) (fig. 200). There are different aspects according to the type of lesion and to the possible associations previously mentioned.

The following data can be considered as typical (9):

a) *The shadow of the ascending aorta is displaced to the right* and bulges from the cardiac shadow. It is easily visible in the left anterior oblique position; poorly, in the right (especially in adults).

b) *The pulmonary knob is small or substituted by a concavity* (fig. 201).

An exception is represented by cases with valvular stenosis where the pulmonary knob may be full. If there is *persistence of the right aortic arch*, the data of this lesion will be found including a typical notching of the esophagus, revealed by a barium swallow (page 464).

The pulmonary fields are abnormally clear but in older patients a thick network, due to the development of collateral circulation, may be visible in the hilar regions. When this happens, the hilar shadows do not present visible pulsations (31).

Angiocardiography. After filling of the right ventricle, the contrast medium penetrates simultaneously into both the aorta and the pulmonary artery; this is a strong indication of the existence of an overriding aorta. Sometimes the pulmonary artery fills only after the aorta (fig. 202).

BLOOD—BLOOD GASES

Severe *polycythemia* is constant. It may even reach 10 million RBC per mm.[3] Normal or decreased plasma volume and increased total blood volume have been found (11).

Increased oxygen capacity and *decreased oxygen saturation* of the arterial blood are typical. While extremely low figures of saturation have been recorded (60–65 per cent), there are cases with moderate decrease.

Exertion decreases the amount of oxygen consumed per liter of ventilation and the oxygen saturation of the arterial blood (19).

CIRCULATION TIME

There is a *shorter arm-to-tongue time*. The ether test frequently gives uncertain results but it may cause tingling sensations in the

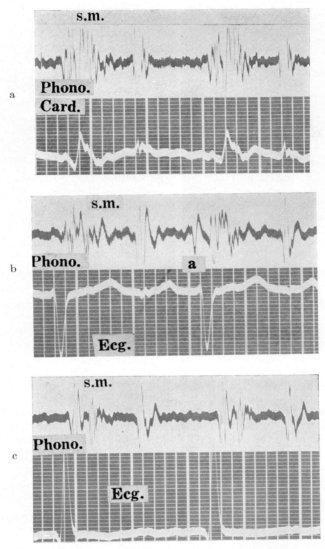

F<small>IG</small>. 199. Sound tracings of a child with *tetralogy of Fallot*. a, prolonged apical systolic murmur; b, fourth sound, short, split systolic murmur over the pulmonic area; c, systolic snap over the tricuspid area.

head and face if it is shunted into the systemic circulation (36).

The *eyegrounds* present thick-walled capillaries and violet color.

The *peripheral capillaries* are wide and tortuous. The velocity is rapid, and large bead-like formations, slowly moving in the direction of the blood stream, are visible.

MODE OF ORIGIN OF THE SIGNS

Stenosis of the pulmonary artery causes a poor blood supply to the lungs as well as dilatation and hypertrophy of the right ventricle. As the two ventricles communicate through the wide-open septum, the pressure is similar in both of them.

Blood from both ventricles enters the

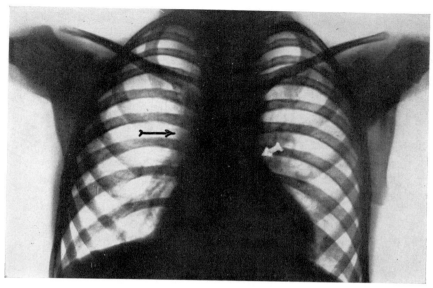

FIG. 200. Cardiac silhouette in a case of *tetralogy of Fallot* (young woman). The white arrow indicates the depression of the pulmonic knob; the black arrow indicates the displacement of the aortic shadow toward the right.

aorta because this vessel overrides the septum. This leads to a mixture of saturated and unsaturated bloods, so that the aorta contains a relatively large percentage of poorly oxygenated hemoglobin.

The systolic murmur is due to the pulmonary stenosis while the eddies formed by the meeting of two streams of blood, coming from the ventricles and entering the aorta seem to contribute very little to it (31). When both the pulmonary stenosis and the displacement of the aorta are slight (the two facts are connected), the cyanosis and the murmur may be slight. When, on the contrary, these changes are marked, the cyanosis is severe and the murmur is loud.

While the cyanosis and the polycythemia are mostly caused by the mixture of bloods within the aorta, pulmonic stenosis contributes to them in two ways: the first is through the decreased blood flow of the lungs; the second is through the increased pressure of the right ventricle which prevents a severe left-to-right shunt through the septum and causes penetration of right ventricular blood into the aorta.

The hypertrophy of the right ventricle is due to the stenosis of the pulmonary artery, to the communication between the two ventricles, and to the increased venous return to the right atrium (the flow of the aorta is greater than pulmonic flow).

The typical x-ray configuration of the heart is due to the existence of a small pulmonary artery which, furthermore, is displaced toward the right, together with the aorta. The resulting picture is a concavity of the pulmonary knob and a convexity of the right border of the ascending aorta.

COURSE AND COMPLICATIONS

In spite of the severe and multiple lesions, many of these patients reach adult, and even old, age (13).

The most frequent complication is subacute bacterial endocarditis or endarteritis. Rheumatic endocarditis is also common.

Pulmonary tuberculosis is fairly frequent. Myocardial fibrosis is frequent. Peripheral embolism, occasionally due to phlebitis of the leg (crossed embolism), may occur.

Thrombosis of capillaries or arterioles of

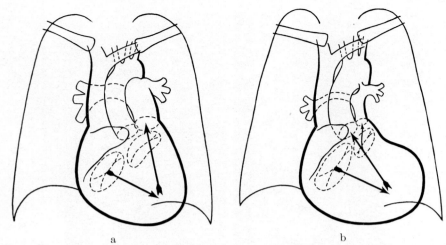

Fig. 201. Differential diagnosis on x-ray between mitral stenosis (a) and the tetralogy of Fallot (b). (From Dr. E. Zdansky. Courtesy of H. Roesler and Charles C Thomas, Publisher.)

pulmonary or cerebral circulation is frequently observed in patients with extreme polycythemia and this complication is favored by dehydration (31, 33). *Cerebral abscesses* are not unusual and are due to the fact that, on account of the shunt, bacteria occasionally present in the blood are not filtered out by the pulmonary capillaries (32). *Fainting attacks* upon exertion are due to cerebral anoxia because the oxygen saturation of the arterial blood, already low, further falls with exercise.

VARIETIES

Different clinical pictures may be due to the concurrence of various additional lesions. The existence of a right aorta, with or without a diverticulum (page 464), and that of transposition of the great vessels (page 321) may change the local and x-ray signs.

The severity of the pulmonary stenosis and the degree of intensity of the cyanosis also may influence the clinical picture. If there is *pulmonary atresia* instead of stenosis, life is possible if the *ductus arteriosus is patent*; then, pulmonary circulation occurs only through this vessel (31). However, extremely rare cases of atresia survive in spite of closure of the ductus through well-developed collateral circulation.

DIAGNOSIS

Squatting, severe cyanosis, and clubbing of fingers and toes, are sufficient for a general diagnosis of congenital malformation of the heart. The loud systolic murmur, right axis deviation, and shorter circulation time, are important contributory data. The x-ray signs (concavity of the pulmonary knob, convexity of the right aortic border, and raised apex), are decisive for the diagnosis.

Cases with moderate cyanosis and clubbing may occur. The x-ray data, however, are still typical.

The following diseases should be excluded:

Uncomplicated septal defects and *patent ductus arteriosus* are excluded by the cyanosis and the ischemia of the lungs of tetralogy of Fallot.

Pure pulmonic stenosis. Cyanosis is more severe in Fallot than in pulmonary stenosis. Circulation time is *longer* than normal in pure pulmonary stenosis; *shorter*, in tetralogy of Fallot. The murmur is louder and more limited to the left of the sternum in pure pulmonary stenosis. X-ray data are different in the two syndromes.

Lutembacher's syndrome. The type of murmur and the x-ray data are different. The pulmonary vessels are dilated in Lutembacher's syndrome, thin, in tetralogy of

Fallot. The circulation time is *shorter* in tetralogy of Fallot but not in Lutembacher's syndrome.

Aortic stenosis plus ductus arteriosus. The aorta is dilated and displaced in Fallot's syndrome; is thin and not displaced in aortic stenosis plus patent ductus. The murmur is different in the two syndromes.

Eisenmenger complex. The pulmonary artery is dilated in this clinical picture; it is small and displaced in tetralogy of Fallot. Hoarseness is frequent in Eisenmenger's syndrome but not in Fallot's. The fine network of the lungs is dilated in Eisenmenger's syndrome.

Tricuspid atresia plus shunts. The heart is elongated and has left axis deviation; the opposite is true in Fallot's syndrome.

Single ventricle with pulmonary stenosis may be confused with cases of Fallot. The electrocardiogram does not reveal evidence of right ventricular hypertrophy in single ventricle.

Transposition with pulmonary stenosis. The patient has a large heart with a narrow pedicle. Cyanosis is more severe and physical efficiency more impaired.

Pulmonary stenosis with patent foramen ovale. The differential diagnosis is very difficult, even with the help of catheterization. Angiocardiography may give definite clues.

PROGNOSIS

The immediate prognosis must be based on the condition of the patient. In general, the prognosis should be more favorable than in other congenital malformations of the heart. The localization of the narrow section is of great importance for surgery. Attacks of paroxysmal dyspnea at rest have a poor prognostic significance.

TREATMENT

The efficiency of patients with Fallot's syndrome is hampered by two main facts: a) the faulty blood supply to the lungs, and b) the mixture of blood in the aorta.

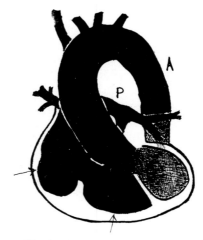

FIG. 202. Angiocardiogram in a case of tetralogy of Fallot. (Scheme; inspired by originals of Sussman, Grishman and Steinberg.)

This consideration led to several surgical interventions. The first and most widely used is the *Blalock-Taussig operation* (14) which is based on the creation of an artificial ductus by an anastomosis between subclavian artery and a pulmonary branch. The second intervention is the *Potts-Gibson operation* (34, 42) which consists of the creation of an aorto-pulmonic fistula. The third is *Brock's operation* (43), which can be done if there is pulmonic valvular stenosis. And the fourth is *resection of the protruding ridge* of septum attempted by *Bailey* and coworkers (44) in cases with infundibular stenosis.

The greatest indications for surgery are: 1) attacks of dyspnea at rest with severe cyanosis and loss of consciousness; 2) blood count above 8 million RBC. If there is no urgency, surgery should be postponed until the best age, e.g. between 6 and 14. However, surgery has been done even in infants who otherwise might not have reached childhood.

Surgery is usually followed by a striking transformation: cyanosis and polycythemia decrease and may disappear; physical efficiency increases; physical development is accelerated. This striking change is due to the fact that increased blood flow to the lungs leads to greater flow from the left ventricle into the aorta. Therefore, in addition to better oxygenation of the blood, a smaller amount of right ventricular blood enters the aorta and the greater circulation.

The overall surgical mortality is about 5 per cent.

In general, the Potts operation is preferred in infants or in cases where the Blalock intervention is impossible or was subsequently followed by thrombosis of the anastomosis. Resection of the septal ridge is a dangerous procedure which is still under experimentation. In case of necessity, a Blalock operation can be repeated on the opposite side.

In considering all the risks of surgery, one should keep in mind: a) that a certain percentage of fatalities is unavoidable; b) that the anastomosis increases the load of the left ventricle; c) that the newly-formed channel may be later the seat of bacterial arteritis; and d) that valvulotomy may be followed by an overloading of the pulmonary circulation. Surgery will be of no avail if

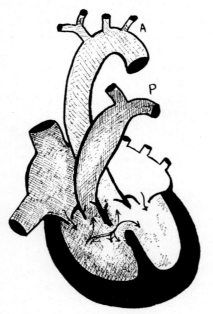

Fig. 203. Changes of the heart and large vessels in *Eisenmenger complex.*

the oxygen saturation in the peripheral blood is above 85 per cent (37); if the pressure of the pulmonary artery is higher than 22 to 25 mm. Hg (14b); or if the heart is too severely enlarged.

Pentalogy of Fallot (41)

This syndrome is due to the lesions already described under the name of "tetralogy" plus an atrial septal defect.

The clinical picture is similar to that of the tetralogy of Fallot but the heart is larger.

The *electrocardiogram* presents marked *left axis deviation* and tall, peaked P-waves.

The *x-ray* reveals a concavity in the region of the pulmonary artery; an enlargement of the inflow tract of the left ventricle; and an enlargement of both the right atrium and the right ventricle.

The differential diagnosis with the tetralogy of Fallot is largely based on electrocardiographic data since the pentalogy has a left axis deviation; that with tricuspid atresia is based on the evidence supplied by x-ray and angiocardiography.

Eisenmenger's Complex (15)

LESIONS

This syndrome, which is less frequent than the tetralogy of Fallot, is based on a similar disturbance of fetal development. The following lesions are typical (fig. 203):

a) Interventricular septal defect.

b) Displacement of the aorta to the right.

c) Dilatation and possible aneurysm of the pulmonary artery.

The *pulmonary valve is often bicuspid and may be incompetent.* The aortic cusp lying above the septal defect may be unusually large and may be placed lower than the others. The *aortic valve may be incompetent,* either because of scarring or on account of the above described abnormalities (31). *Hypertrophy of the right ventricle* is constant.

The lesions are caused by faulty torsion

of the primitive cardiac tube with fusion of the right with the left aorta.

The abnormality underlying the Eisenmenger's syndrome is probably identical to that called by Spitzer "mixed transposition type IV" (page 321). If this is so, the apparent septum is actually formed by the crista and trabecula of the fetal heart and is not the equivalent of the real septum of the normally developed heart. Whenever the pulmonary artery is displaced more to the right and overrides the so-called septum, *Taussig's syndrome* takes place (page 323). While the septal defect and the overriding aorta are truly congenital lesions, *changes of the pulmonary vessels gradually develop during life*. Their establishment (probably connected with the wide shunt between the ventricles in the absence of pulmonic stenosis) further increases the pressure in the right ventricle and, therefore, the amount of right ventricular blood penetrating the aorta. It should be kept in mind that pulmonary changes may develop early, during the first 10 years of life.

SYMPTOMS AND SIGNS

Cyanosis is usually absent at birth and develops gradually, either during adolescence or, more commonly, during the adult age. *Hoarseness* is very frequent. *Clubbing* may appear late in life. *Bloody sputum* is relatively common.

Cardiac dulness is enlarged toward the right. There is a *cap of dulness* in the 2nd left interspace.

Auscultation reveals a *loud systolic murmur* behind the sternum and frequently a *soft, blowing, diastolic murmur in decrescendo* over the 2nd right or left interspaces (aortic or pulmonic insufficiency).

The *electrocardiogram* reveals a *right axis deviation* which may be moderate; there may be right i.v. block and grade 1 a-v block.

CATHETERIZATION OF THE RIGHT HEART

The *pressure of the right ventricle is high and may be extremely high*. Figures of 100,

120, and even 150 mm. Hg have been recorded (35, 45, 46). *Systolic pressure of the right ventricle is identical with that of the pulmonary artery* indicating the absence of pulmonic stenosis. It should be identical with that of the aorta but pulmonary vascular lesions may explain cases where right ventricular pressure was higher than left ventricular pressure. The wedge pressure of the pulmonary arterioles (so-called pulmonary capillary pressure) may be normal, indicating *high pulmonary vascular resistance*.

Oxygen saturation is higher in the right ventricle than in the right atrium. It is normal in the pulmonary veins.

X-RAY

X-ray reveals a very marked dilatation of the pulmonary artery and its branches. The heart is globular in shape. *The aorta is dilated and displaced toward the right*. The hilar shadows are wide and strongly pulsating (*hilar dance*) (fig. 204).

Angiocardiography shows a direct passage of the radio-opaque dye from the right ventricle to the aorta (10b) (fig. 205).

BLOOD—CIRCULATION TIME

The blood presents *polycythemia*.

Oxygen saturation of the peripheral arterial blood is low and *falls* after exercise. The amount of oxygen consumed per liter of ventilation, on the contrary, *rises* after exercise (35).

Circulation time tests show that the arm-to-tongue time is *shorter* than in normal people.

MODE OF ORIGIN OF THE SIGNS

As no obstacle is placed against the blood entering the pulmonary artery, the main cause of right ventricular enlargement is the communication between the two ventricles. Therefore, right ventricular hypertrophy and right axis deviation are less than in tetralogy of Fallot. For the same reason, the mixture of blood in the aorta is moderate

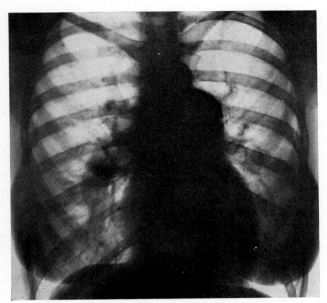

Fig. 204. Cardiac silhouette in a case of *Eisenmenger complex* (courtesy of Dr. S. C. Burwell.)

and less cyanosis, polycythemia, and clubbing are present.

Cyanosis is due to admixture of bloods in the aorta as proven by the fact that oxygen saturation of the pulmonary venous blood may be normal (46).

The frequent hoarseness is due to compression of the left recurrent nerve by the dilated pulmonary artery. Bloody sputum is caused by active congestion of the pulmonary vessels.

The soft diastolic murmur frequently observed at the base is due to either aortic or pulmonic insufficiency (incompetent bicuspid aortic valve; stretching of the pulmonic ring; or fibrosis of the pulmonic leaflets).

The dilatation of the pulmonary artery and of the hilar vessels is caused by the fact that there is high pressure in the right ventricle and no pulmonary stenosis. Moreover, on account of a high septal defect, blood is frequently shunted from the left ventricle into the opening of the pulmonary artery, thereby increasing pulmonary flow.

COURSE AND COMPLICATIONS

The syndrome is relatively well tolerated. Many cases have reached adult age and

some, old age. In some cases, repeated pregnancy caused no special disturbance. However, pulmonary congestion, chronic bronchitis, pulmonary infarction, or aneurysm of the pulmonary artery, may occur, in addition to other common complications.

DIAGNOSIS

Diagnosis is based on the systolic murmur and a loud P_2 in the presence of a wide pulmonary artery and a large aorta. The existence of cyanosis (started late in life), shortened circulation time, and hoarseness, are also important for the diagnosis.

Differential diagnosis should be made with the following syndromes:

Tetralogy of Fallot. Cyanosis is more severe and starts earlier in tetralogy of Fallot; hoarseness and hemoptysis are more common in Eisenmenger's complex. The x-ray signs are decisive because they reveal large, pulsating pulmonary vessels in Eisenmenger's complex.

Patent foramen ovale. There usually is no cyanosis and there may be no murmur. When this is present, the x-ray finding of a small aorta is in favor of the patent foramen ovale. Circulation time is normal or delayed in patent foramen ovale, shorter in Eisenmenger's complex. Angiocardiography and catheterization decide in doubtful cases. However, cases with cyanosis may present serious diagnostic problems.

Patent ductus arteriosus plus aortic stenosis or coarctation. The finding of a small aorta is against Eisenmenger's complex. However, cases with coarctation of the aorta may have a large ascending aorta at x-ray. In Eisenmenger's complex the aorta is displaced toward the right. Cyanosis is greater in patent ductus arteriosus plus aortic stenosis than in Eisenmenger's complex. The murmur is different in phonocardiograms. Angiocardiography may decide in doubtful cases whether the shunt is from right to left; otherwise, a retrograde aortogram may permit diagnosis.

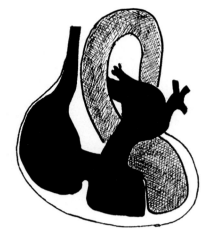

Fig. 205. Angiocardiogram in *Eisenmenger complex*. (Inspired by originals of Sussman, Grishman and Steinberg.)

PROGNOSIS

The heart usually presents a progressive enlargement. The difficulty of oxygen intake in the lungs becomes progressively greater. Therefore, patients with Eisenmenger's complex seldom live more than 10 to 15 years after cyanosis has become apparent (31). For this reason, cyanosis has a bad prognostic meaning in this syndrome.

THERAPY

No surgical therapy can be done at the present time. It is possible that, in the future, closure of the septal defect will be undertaken.

Transposition of the Great Vessels

LESIONS—MECHANISM

Each of the large arterial vessels, instead of arising from its respective ventricle, opens into that opposite. A large ventricular septal defect is always present and is necessary for survival. Diagnosis of transposition is sometimes difficult because there may be associated *dextrocardia* (page 548), *absence of the ventricular septum, persistence of the right aortic arch*, or any combination of them.

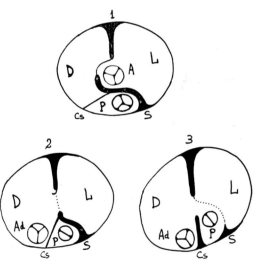

Fig. 206. Position of the septa and of the large vessels: 1, in a normal heart; 2, in partial transposition; 3, in complete transposition. (Adapted from Spitzer.)

Three main types have been recognized (2a) (fig. 206):

a) *Partial transposition:* both the aorta and the pulmonary artery open into the right ventricle, the aorta being at the right.

b) *Complete transposition:* the aorta opens into the right ventricle; the pulmonary artery, into the left.

c) *Mixed transposition:* the aorta opens

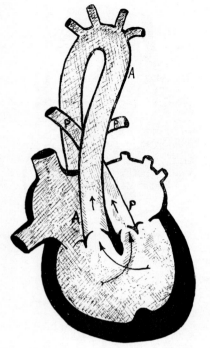

FIG. 207. Changes of the heart in the transposition of the large vessels.

into the right ventricle; the pulmonary artery, into the left; both the tricuspid and the mitral valves are in the left ventricle.

The so-called *corrected transposition* occurs when there is *complete transposition plus dextrocardia* or dextroposition of the heart.

In all these types, the ventricular septum has a large defect and may be absent (*cor biatriatum monoventriculare*) (fig. 207). In type c, the right ventricle receives blood from the left ventricle through the septum and sends it into the aorta.

The various types are different aspects of the same malformation. Faulty torsion of the primitive cardiac tube may be more or less severe and it often causes closure of the left fetal aorta with persistence of the right: *the so-called transposed aorta represents the persistence of the fetal right aorta.* Abnormality in the incorporation of the bulbus cordis has also been postulated (16). This, however, might be secondary to the above quoted anomaly.

When *a single ventricle is present*, there is a thorough mixture of the blood coming from the two atria before it enters both large vessels (17). In some cases, the interventricular shunt is absent and *the septum is closed.* Life is then possible only by the help of another shunt, patent ductus arteriosus or patent foramen ovale.

SIGNS AND SYMPTOMS

Cyanosis, polycythemia, and *clubbing* of the fingers and toes are constant and severe.

Osteoarthropathy is not unusual. *Squatting* is frequent. Cases having a patent ductus may present more severe cyanosis in the face and upper part of the trunk than in the rest of the body (31). This is due to the fact that the ductus carries oxygenated blood which comes from the left ventricle *via* the transposed pulmonary artery and that this blood flows mainly into the descending aorta. Attacks of *dyspnea, palpitation,* and *dizziness* are frequent after exercise. *Bloody sputum* is also common.

Different local signs may be present. The heart is enlarged and *globular.*

There may be a *systolic murmur* behind the sternum at the 3rd left cartilage (septal defect) and also a *diastolic murmur* (meeting of the two atrial blood streams in a single ventricle). The 2nd sound is often loud at the 2nd *right* interspace (actual pulmonary area). There may be a machinery murmur at the *right* of the sternum (actual seat of the ductus arteriosus). However, there may not be any murmur. A triple rhythm is frequently present.

ELECTROCARDIOGRAM

The electrocardiogram reveals right axis deviation, deep Q_3, and depressed S-T. There may be intraventricular block, long P-R, or a-v block. There may be a *mirror-type electrocardiogram* (even without dextrocardia) (18) (page 548).

High voltage, wide QRS waves with prominent R and S in leads 2 and 3, and slight intraventricular block have been suggested as being the signs of *cor biatriatum monoventriculare* (19).

X-RAY

The heart is rounded and vertical. It may resemble a "hot water bag," and therefore simulate pericardial effusion (20). The *aortic shadow is usually thin in the PA view while it becomes wide in LAO* (8, 19, 22, 23, 31). The pulmonary vessels are large and pulsating and there may be intensive mottling of the lungs (47).

Angiocardiography. The aorta fills with contrast medium directly from the right ventricle. The pulmonary artery either is not visible or fills after the aorta (passing of the dye through the ductus or a septal defect into the left heart). The aortic arch makes a wide sweep in LAO. The contrast medium leaves the heart rapidly and the pulmonary vessels are poorly visualized (41).

COURSE AND COMPLICATIONS

Many cases with transposition die during infancy or childhood. However, some cases with efficient shunts or a single ventricle have lived until maturity (17, 25). The complications are those of the complex malformations of the heart.

DIAGNOSIS

General diagnosis of congenital heart disease is simple. Exact diagnosis of the malformation is, on the contrary, difficult. The x-ray data are of decisive importance. Catheterization of the heart and angiocardiography may be needed. Electrocardiographic signs may be important in cases with a single ventricle.

PROGNOSIS

Prognosis is, in general, unfavorable but not absolutely negative. It is more favorable in cases with a high ventricular septal defect where a better distribution of blood is obtained (31).

VARIETIES

While three anatomical types have been described (partial, complete, and mixed transposition), the clinical varieties are largely influenced by the nature, location, and type of the shunt.

A special type of transposition should be called *Taussig's syndrome* (38). In this, the aorta arises from the right ventricle; the pulmonary artery is large, overrides the septum, and receives blood from both ventricles; there is a high ventricular septal defect. This syndrome is probably a variety of "mixed transposition". Its symptomatology resembles that of the Eisenmenger's complex and is compatible with life for a number of years. In this syndrome, cyanosis dates from birth. Exercise causes a fall of oxygen consumption per liter of ventilation. The pulmonary artery contains a higher content of oxygen than the femoral artery.

THERAPY

Surgery of this condition has been attempted in various ways: 1) by anastomosing the veins from the apical and cardiac lobes of the right lung either to the right atrium or to the superior cava (48); 2) by creating an atrial septal defect; 3) if pulmonary pressure is low on account of pulmonic stenosis, by means of the Blalock-Taussig operation. Recent attempts at reestablishing the normal connections of the two large arterial vessels are in an experimental stage.

Persistence of the Common Arterial Trunk Plus Shunts

LESIONS—MECHANISM

There are two main types (26).

a) There is a *short common arterial trunk* from which both the pulmonary artery and the aorta arise (partial persistence of the arterial trunk).

b) There is a *long common arterial trunk* from which all the branches of the pulmonary artery and of the aorta arise

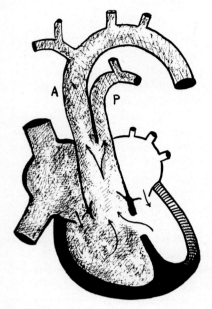

FIG. 208. Changes of the heart and large vessels in cases with persistence of the common arterial trunk.

(including the coronary arteries). The trunk continues as the descending aorta.

A third possibility is that of *pulmonic atresia* with *absence of the main pulmonary artery*; in such cases either a patent ductus or the bronchial arteries supply the lungs (31, 39). This type has been called *pseudotruncus*.

There usually is a *high ventricular septal defect* and the trunk overrides the defect (fig. 208). In some cases, however, the trunk arises *from the right ventricle* and circulation is maintained through an atrial septal defect, a patent ductus, or both. The left ventricle is atrophied.

The arterial trunk has *four semilunar valves* but two of them may be partially fused (5).

A singular malformation is a large arterial pouch from which all branches of the aorta and pulmonary artery arise and which communicates with both ventricles without being associated with shunts.

The cause of these malformations seems to be a faulty torsion of the primitive

cardiac tube which hinders atrophy of the bulbus cordis. This is then transformed into a large arterial vessel with a more or less advanced division. The four valves derive from the bulbus and would have given origin to both the aortic and pulmonic valves if the normal division had taken place (fig. 4).

SIGNS AND SYMPTOMS

Cyanosis is constant and severe. *Club-fingers, weakness,* and *dyspnea upon exertion* are constant. *Hematemesis* is frequent, caused by rupture of esophageal varices. On the other hand, *hemoptysis* is rare and attacks of suffocation are not frequent. The heart is enlarged and rounded. *The second sound at the base is loud and is never split.*

There may be a *diastolic thrill* behind the manubrium of the sternum and a *systolic thrill* over the mid-precordium. There may be dulness of the manubrium. Various murmurs may be heard; the most constant is a *continuous, rather soft murmur at the base and over the back. A soft, early diastolic murmur* in the 3rd left interspace may indicate insufficient valve of the trunk. There may be a *triple rhythm.* The cases with a *single ventricle* may have no thrills and no murmurs (31).

The *electrocardiogram* may reveal either right or left axis deviation (6, 39). High P in leads 1, 2, and V_1; depressed S-T and inverted T waves; and i.v. block, are frequent.

The *x-ray* shows a rounded heart of a "hot water bag" type. *The heart may be small or normal in size.* The right atrium may be large; the right ventricle shows increased pulsations. The hilar shadows are wide and present strong pulsations (27) unless the lungs are supplied by the bronchial arteries; in such cases, the hilar shadows may be absent or small (31). The shadow of the common trunk is not easily recognized. The upper left margin of the cardiac silhouette is concave (pulmonary conus and pulmonary knob are absent)

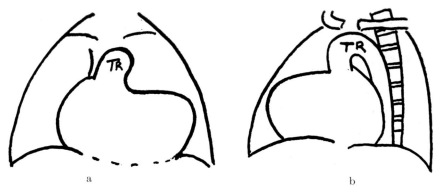

FIG. 209. Cardiovascular silhouette of a child with persistent common arterial trunk in the postero-anterior (a), and left oblique positions (b). TR, trunk. (Sketched after originals of Taussig.)

but the aortic knob is high and prominent at the left of the sternum. However, a right aortic arch is frequently present (page 464). There may be a subclavian artery posterior to the esophagus. The apex is upturned and the contour in left oblique is unique (31) (fig. 209).

Angiocardiography. Both in the PA and in the LAO portions, the contrast medium is seen filling a large trunk from the right ventricle. The pulmonary artery fills slightly later (41).

CATHETERIZATION

The data are similar to those of the tetralogy of Fallot, except that the pulmonary artery is usually not entered and that no pulmonic stenosis can be demonstrated.

Circulation time tests may reveal a shorter arm-to-tongue time.

COURSE AND COMPLICATIONS

The course is, in general, short because many complications invariably arise. They include rheumatic and bacterial endocarditis, pulmonary infarction, pneumonia, and congestive failure. However, the possibility that some exceptional case may reach maturity cannot be excluded.

DIAGNOSIS

Diagnosis of these cases is always difficult. However, circulation time tests, x-ray,

angiocardiography, and catheterization of the heart make diagnosis possible.

The differential diagnosis between a common trunk and a tetralogy of Fallot with wide aorta may be difficult, unless catheterization of the pulmonary artery is successful.

PROGNOSIS

Prognosis is always bad.

TREATMENT

If the pressure of the pulmonary artery is low, the Blalock-Taussig operation improves the outlook.

Tricuspid Atresia Plus Double Septal Defect (28)

LESIONS

The tricuspid orifice is closed; the right ventricle is extremely small; the right atrium is very large and sends the blood to the left through a septal defect. The mitral valve is normal. The blood of the left ventricle flows partly to the right ventricle through a septal defect. Some cases with closed ventricular septum have a patent ductus arteriosus instead of the septal defect. The left ventricle is greatly enlarged (fig. 210).

SIGNS AND SYMPTOMS

Cyanosis is constant and severe. *Clubbing* and *polycythemia* are also constant.

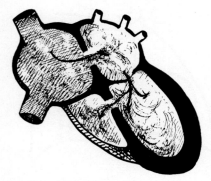

FIG. 210. Changes of the heart in tricuspid atresia associated with shunts.

Cardiac dulness is typically elongated, with an obtuse cardiohepatic angle and displacement of the apex to the left.

As a rule, there are no thrills and no murmurs. However, a midprecordial systolic murmur may exist.

The *electrocardiogram* reveals high P waves and *marked left axis deviation.*

The mechanical tracings show *high atrial waves.*

X-ray reveals an elongated heart with *enlargement of both the right atrium and the left ventricle.* The pulmonary window is empty on account of the thin pulmonary arch. The vascular markings are decreased.

Angiocardiography reveals that the contrast medium goes directly from the right atrium into the left. The aorta arises from the left ventricle and fills normally. The pulmonary artery is visualized after the aorta. The hypoplastic right ventricle may fill even later through the ventricular septal defect.

VARIETIES

If, instead of atresia, there is *tricuspid stenosis,* the clinical syndrome is less severe.

If there is *patent ductus arteriosus* instead of ventricular septal defect, both the right ventricle and the main pulmonary artery are atrophic. The x-ray indicates a *depression at the place of the pulmonary knob* but no enlargement or displacement of the aorta.

There are cases of tricuspid atresia plus transposition. The aorta arises from the underdeveloped right ventricle.

DIAGNOSIS

Diagnosis is possible if the clinical picture is known. The left axis deviation, the typical aspect of the cardiac shadow on x-ray, and the frequent absence of murmurs do not permit confusion with other syndromes.

On the other hand, it should be kept in mind that left axis deviation can be presented by other cyanotic congenital malformations so that it is not absolutely typical of this syndrome.

PROGNOSIS

Prognosis is always bad unless surgery is possible.

TREATMENT

Whenever catheterization reveals a low pressure in the pulmonary artery, surgery can be attempted. Surgery is indicated even in young infants (49) and should be attempted as early as possible. The best intervention is the Potts-Gibson aorto-pulmonary fistula.

Mitral Atresia Plus Double Septal Defect and Patent Ductus (40)

This rare malformation permits only a limited survival. There is *polycythemia, severe cyanosis,* and a *weak, slow pulse.* The heart is enormous and globular.

The *electrocardiogram* reveals a nodal or idioventricular rhythm; right axis deviation; and i.v. block.

The *x-ray* shows very large right atrium and ventricle.

Abnormal Number of Cardiac Chambers

Different possibilities exist:

A three-chambered heart with a single atrium (cor triloculare biventriculosum). This syndrome has been described with the atrial septal defects (page 278). The clinical picture is more severe than when there is only an atrial septal defect. Cyanosis is frequent but may not be severe. There may be no murmurs. However, an apical diastolic rumble due to relative mitral stenosis (page 267) may simulate an organic lesion of the mitral valve.

A three-chambered heart with a single ventricle (cor triloculare biatriatum). This syndrome has been described with the ventricular septal defects. The picture is more severe than in the limited ventricular septal defects; cyanosis is constant; there may be no murmurs. The lesion may be associated with a tetralogy of Fallot (page 310), transposition (page 321), or common trunk (page 323).

Three types have been described:

a) A normal-sized aorta springs from the common ventricle and a small pulmonary artery originates from a rudimentary chamber (a remnant of the bulbus).

b) There is transposition of the large vessels (page 321); a small aorta arises from the rudimentary chamber while a normal pulmonary artery arises from the common ventricle.

c) Both arterial vessels arise from the rudimentary chamber and are of a reduced size.

The absence of the interventricular septum does not necessarily increase the severity of the picture.

A two-chambered heart having a single atrium and a single ventricle (cor biloculare) (5, 29).

In one type, one defect at the lower part of the atrial septum (*persistent ostium primum*) is combined with another at the upper part of the ventricular septum. In a second type, complete absence of this septum occurs and there is a *common atrio-ventricular opening with five cusps* (page 284).

In all cases, the lesion is due to simultaneous arrest of growth during the 5th to 6th week of development.

Right axis deviation, intraventricular block, and "hot-water bag" heart at x-rays have been found.

These severe malformations seldom permit life but some cases in children and even in adolescents have been described.

d) *A five-chambered heart with three ventricles (cor triventriculare (30)).*

This curious malformation is due to the fact that *the right ventricle is divided into two cavities by an additional septum.* The blood goes through a small orifice of the latter from the tricuspid to the pulmonic opening. The malformation is due to a faulty incorporation of the bulbus cordis.

A loud systolic murmur over the midprecordium was found in a patient who died at the age of 23.

BIBLIOGRAPHY

1. FALLOT, A. Mars. Méd., 1888, 25, 77, 138, 207, 270 and 403.
2. a) SPITZER, A. Virch. Arch., 1923, **243**, 81.
   b) MAUTNER, H. Jahrb. Kinderheilk., 1921, **96,** 123. Also Med. Klin., 1933, **79,** 705.
3. FLEURY, J. Arch. Mal. Coeur, 1937, **30,** 121.
4. LAUBRY, C., AND PEZZI, C. *Traité des Maladies Congenitales du Coeur.* Paris, Baillière, 1921.
5. ABBOTT, M. E. In *Nelson Loose Leaf Medicine.* New York, Nelson, 1941.
6. SCHNITKER, M. A. *The Electrocardiogram in Congenital Cardiac Disease.* Cambridge, Harvard Univ. Press, 1940.
7. CALO, A. Arch. Mal. Coeur, 1937, **30,** 805. Also *Atlas de Phonocardiographie Clinique.* Paris, Masson, 1938.
8. ROESLER, H. *Clinical Roentgenology of the Cardiovascular System.* Baltimore, Thomas, 1943.
9. PAPP, C. Arch. Mal. Coeur, 1931, **24,** 249.
10. a) GRISHMAN, A., STEINBERG, M. F., AND SUSSMAN, M. L. Radiology, 1941, **37,** 178.
    b) SUSSMAN, M. L., GRISHMAN, A., AND STEINBERG, M. F. Am. J. Dis. Child., 1943, **65,** 922.
11. a) HALLOCK, P. Proc. Soc. Exper. Biol. & Med., 1940, **44,** 11.
    b) NELSON, W., AND CO-WORKERS. J. Clin. Investigation, 1947, **26,** 860.
12. SOLIS-COHEN, M., ZASLOW, J., AND ROLNICK, M. H. Am. Heart J., 1944, **28,** 115.
13. WHITE, P. D., AND SPRAGUE, H. B. J. A. M. A., 1929, **92,** 787.

14. a) BLALOCK, A., AND TAUSSIG, H. B. J. A.
    M. A., 1945, **128**, 189.
    b) BLALOCK, A. Ann. Surg., 1946, **124**, 879.
15. a) EISENMENGER, V. Zeit. klin. Med., 1897,
    32, Suppl. 1.
    b) TALLEY, J. H., AND FOWLER, K. Am. J.
    M. Sci., 1937, **191**, 618.
16. SAPHIR, O., AND LEV, M. Am. Heart J., 1941,
    21, 31.
17. BIZZARRI, A. Cuore e Circ., (Rome), 1929, **13**,
    492.
18. GRIESHABER, H. Schweiz. Med. Woch., 1936,
    66, 1307.
19. a) WHITE, P. D. Discussion of case 28532 of
    Mass. Gen. Hosp. New England J. Med.,
    1942, **227**, 1047.
    b) GLENDY, M. M., GLENDY, R. E., AND
    WHITE, P. D. Am. Heart J., 1944, **28**, 395.
20. McGINN, S., AND WHITE, P. D. New England
    J. Med., 1936, **214**, 763.
21. BLUMENFELDT, E. In *Spez. Path. und Ther.*,
    by Kraus and Brugsch. Berlin, Urban and
    Schwarzenberg, 1925.
22. ASSMANN, H. *Die klinische Roentgendiagnostik
    der inneren Erkrankungen.* Leipzig, Vogel,
    1924.
23. TAUSSIG, H. B. Am. Heart J., 1938, **16**, 728.
24. CASTELLANOS, A., PEREIRAS, R., AND GARCIA,
    A. Presse Méd., 1938, **46**, 1474.
25. CIUFFINI, P. Cuore e Circ., (Rome), 1938, **22**,
    125.
26. FELLER, A. Virchow's Arch., 1931, **279**, 869.
27. PEZZI, C., AND AGOSTONI, E. Arch. Mal.
    Coeur, 1928, **21**, 20.
28. TAUSSIG, H. B. Bull. Johns Hopkins Hosp.,
    1936, **59**, 435.
29. DRY, T. J. Am. Heart J., 1937, **14**, 135. Also
    Manual of Cardiology. Philadelphia, Saunders, 1933.
30. KOMVALER, B. E. Am. Heart J., 1944, **27**, 259.
31. TAUSSIG, H. B. *The Congenital Malformations
    of the Heart.* New York, Commonwealth
    Fund, 1947.
32. GATES, E. M., AND ROGERS, H. M.: Proc.
    Staff Meet., Mayo Clin., 1947, **22**, 401.
33. RICH, A. R. Bull. Johns Hopkins Hosp., 1948,
    82, 389.
34. POTTS, W. J., AND GIBSON, S. J.A.M.A., 1948,
    137, 343.
35. BING, R. J., AND CO-WORKERS. Mo. Conc.
    Cardiov. Dis., 1948, **17**, N. 3. Also BING,
    R. J., AND CARROLL, D. J. Lancet, 1951, **71**,
    444.
36. HITZIG, W. M. Mo. Conc. Cardiov. Dis., 1947,
    16, N. 8.
37. PARKER, R. L. Med. Clin. North America,
    1948, July, 875.
38. TAUSSIG, H. B. III Inter-American Congr.
    Cardiol., Chicago, June, 1948.
39. MARSHALL, R. Brit. Heart J., 1943, **5**, 194.
40. TAUSSIG, H. B. Bull. Johns Hopkins Hosp.,
    1945, **76**, 75.
41. GASUL, B. M., AND CO-WORKERS. J. Pediat.,
    1949, **35**, 413.
42. POTTS, W. J., SMITH, S., AND GIBSON, S.
    J. A. M. A., 1946, **132**, 627.
43. BROCK, R. C. Brit. M. J., 1948, **1**, 1121.
44. GLOVER, R. P., BAILEY, C. P., *et. al.* J.
    Thoracic Surg., 1952, **23**, 14.
45. COSBY, R. S., *et. al.* Am. J. Med., 1951, **11**, 31.
46. VOCI, G., JOLY, F., AND CARLOTTI, J. Bull.,
    Mem. Soc. Med. Hôp. Paris. 1952, 636
    (Nos. 18, 19).
47. CAMPBELL, M., AND SUZMAN, S. Circ., 1951, **4**,
    329.
48. HANLON, C. R., AND BLALOCK, A. Ann. Surg.,
    1948, **127**, 385.
49. GASUL, B. M., FALL, F. H., *et. al.* Am. J.
    Dis. Child., 1949, **78**, 16.

CHAPTER 16

Disturbances of the Heart Rate and of the Heart Rhythm

Disturbances of the heart rate and rhythm are caused by changes in the myocardial ability to create an impulse (automatism), to react to a stimulus (excitability), or to conduct a stimulus (conductivity). Either localized or diffuse changes of these functions may be responsible for the disturbance. These changes may be connected with intrinsic phenomena of the heart muscle (myogenic), with autonomic nerve impulses (neurogenic), or both.

The disturbances of rate can be divided into *rapid heart* (*tachycardia*) and slow heart (*bradycardia*). The disturbances of rhythm, or *arrhythmias*, may be associated with either rapid or slow heart. A simple classification separates the forms due to modified function of the S-A node (*sinus disturbances*) from the *ectopic rhythms*, and places into two different groups the forms due to *increased automatism or excitability* and those due to *decreased conductivity*.

I. Disturbances Due to Modified Function of the S-A Node

SINUS TACHYCARDIA

Cause and Types

The most common sinus tachycardia is caused by *exercise*. It lasts for a long time if the heart muscle is weak.

Digestion is often accompanied by increased heart rate. This occurs if the quantity of food and drink is too great or if the heart muscle is weak. The ingested fluid increases the volume of circulating blood, thus increasing cardiac strain. *Assuming the erect position* is accompanied by an increased heart rate because of decreased intensity of carotid sinus reflexes.

Emotion is accompanied by tachycardia. Many *drugs* and *poisons* also cause tachycardia. Among them, caffeine and nicotine are the most commonly used. *Fever* is usually accompanied by rapid heart action.

Endocrine disorders may be accompanied by rapid heart, the most frequent being hyperthyroidism (page 405).

Valvular defects, pericardial lesions, and *high* or *low blood pressure* may be accompanied by sinus tachycardia. This is due to the fact that they increase the work of the heart and, therefore, are the equivalent of exertion.

If the *myocardium is weak*, the heart maintains its output by reducing systolic discharge and increasing its rate.

Sympathetic stimuli or a *lesion of the vagus nerve* may be responsible for a rapid pulse.

Signs and Symptoms

The patient usually does not feel the tachycardia. However, if the latter is too high, he may complain of *palpitation*.

The *pulse* is regular and often small. It has no fixed rate; therefore exercise, change of position, and respiration may vary it. Spontaneous variations are also common (2). The *heart sounds* are regular and frequently have equal duration and loudness.

Graphic Methods

Electrocardiogram. The atrial and ventricular waves follow each other in a normal way. P-R may be slightly longer but not over 0.20 second. Diastole is short, so that the end of T is near the following P (fig. 211A). In the adult, the rate varies between 90 and 150 but is seldom above 100. Occasionally, higher figures have been described.

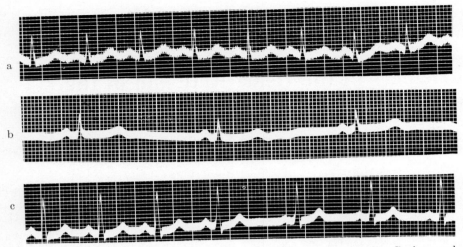

F<small>IG</small>. 211. Electrocardiograms of: A, sinus tachycardia; B, sinus bradycardia; C, sinus arrhythmia

Jugular tracing. There may be fusion of *v* with the following *a* wave.

Phonocardiogram. The heart sounds are short and loud. A triple rhythm is not unusual because of tumultuous ventricular filling (p. 370).

Diagnosis

Sinus tachycardia can usually be recognized because: a) it is connected with a definite cause; b) it does not start suddenly; c) it is well tolerated; d) very seldom does the rate exceed 150; e) the rate frequently changes; and f) there is a normal electrocardiogram.

Paroxysmal tachycardia gives an abnormal electrocardiogram, starts suddenly, and is less well tolerated.

Treatment

Treatment is directed, whenever possible, to removal of the cause. Whenever high excitability of the sympathetic system is involved, *ergotamine* or *hydergine* (**36**) may be used.

Digitalis (**5**) or *quinidine* (**24**) are indicated in some cases. *Coramine* (**61**) may be used with low blood pressure.

Rest, sedatives, and treatment of the thyroid, are necessary in some cases. In particularly severe and intractable cases, removal of the upper thoracic sympathetic ganglia (2nd to 5th) may be necessary (111).

SINUS BRADYCARDIA

Cause and Mechanism

Sinus bradycardia may result from *poisoning* or *infection.* Poisoning from biliary salts (jaundice), products of metabolism (uremia), or digitalis, are the most common. Typhoid, diphtheria, rheumatic disease, mumps, pneumonia, and cholera, may cause relative or absolute sinus bradycardia.

Convalescence is frequently accompanied by slow pulse due to sinus bradycardia.

Increased intracranial pressure is revealed by a slow pulse. *Visceral colicky pain* also is usually accompanied by slow pulse.

Patients with *myocardial fibrosis* may have a slow pulse which is persistent and only slightly affected by the position of the patient.

Hypothyroidism is frequently associated with bradycardia.

Patients with *abnormal sensitivity of the carotid sinus* have a sudden slowing of the pulse when a change of position or an external action stimulates the carotid receptors.

Lastly, some *normal individuals* have a constantly slow pulse; their condition has been called *vagotonia*. *Athletes* frequently have a slow pulse.

In all these cases, three possible mechanisms may exist:

a) There is a continuous reflex action which slows down the heart by way of the vagus nerve.

b) There is a high tonus and excitability of the medullary center of the vagus, so that normal stimuli are sufficient for maintaining the slow pulse.

c) The sinoatrial node itself is affected.

The reflex mechanism is involved in the cases with visceral pain or hypersensitive carotid sinus and may be involved in cases of myocarditis. A high excitability of the vagus occurs in patients with high intracranial pressure, in hypothyroidism, and in normal individuals with slow pulse. Direct change of the function of the S-A node is involved in myocardial fibrosis, in severe myocarditis, and in cases of poisoning. However, in many cases, a double mechanism (action on the cardiac muscle and on the vagus nerves) is involved. This is also true for digitalis (page 583).

A paralysis of the accelerans is possible in some cases, as a result of a central or peripheral lesion but this is the least frequent mechanism.

Signs and Symptoms

Symptoms are usually absent but a further strong stimulation of the vagus (sudden immersion in cold water, emotion, or pain) may cause *fainting*. In such a case, a vascular collapse is frequently associated with the bradycardia.

The *pulse* is slow and regular, but may present marked respiratory arrhythmia (page 332). The heart sounds and the pulsations of the jugular veins are normal.

The *systolic blood pressure* may be normal or slightly low and is usually accompanied by a large pulse pressure.

Graphic Methods

Electrocardiogram. The electrocardiogram is normal and shows a long diastole. P-R is normal. The rate is usually between 65 and 50, and only exceptionally between 50 and 40 (fig. 211B).

Pharmacologic and functional tests. The most important is the *atropine test.* Injection of 1 mg. of atropine sulfate hinders the action of the vagus nerve and accelerates the heart rate. Another pharmacologic test is represented by the *inhalation of amyl nitrite.* This is particularly effective in patients with coronary heart disease and bradycardia caused by functional depression of the S-A node.

Changes of position, exertion, and deep respiration are usually sufficient to accelerate the pulse in persons with sinus bradycardia. Compression of the carotid sinus may arrest the heart in patients with bradycardia due to hypersensitive carotid receptors. Both this maneuver and the compression of the eyeballs may arrest the heart in patients with an excitable vagus nerve.

Diagnosis

Diagnosis is not difficult in most of the cases. Clinical data are usually sufficient and may be supplemented by the functional and pharmacologic tests. The electrocardiogram may be needed in doubtful cases or when the rate is very slow.

Differential diagnosis should be made from *nodal rhythm*, A-V or S-A *block type 2 to 1*, and *complete A-V block.* The latter usually has a slower pulse but cases of congenital A-V block may have a pulse between 40 and 60. Differential diagnosis will be discussed in the respective paragraphs.

Treatment

No treatment is required in most cases. If possible, the cause of the bradycardia should be corrected.

In some cases, *atropine* (**21**), *ephedrine* (**57**), *benzedrine* (**58**), *caffeine* (**60**), or *mannitol* (**51**) will be required. The last is useful only in coronary heart patients.

SINUS ARRHYTHMIA

Cause

This common irregularity of the pulse is usually associated with respiration. It is particularly evident in children, convalescents, or people with unusually high excitability of the vagus nerve. It is also frequently present when pleuropericardial adhesions are stretched by respiratory movements. It may occur in old people with arteriosclerotic lesions and coronary heart disease.

Signs

The pulse is periodically and alternately rapid and slow. Slowing down of the pulse may be abrupt but is usually gradual in onset. The pulse may seem intermittent in the first case.

These changes of the heart rate are connected with respiration, the phase of rapid pulse occurring in the second half of inspiration and that of slow pulse in the second half of expiration.

Deep breathing accentuates the phenomenon; *suspension of respiration* causes its disappearance. *Atropine* usually abolishes sinus arrhythmia.

Graphic Tracings

Electrocardiogram. The electrocardiogram has normal waves; it shows, in general, gradual changes in the length of diastole (fig. 211C). If there are sudden changes and the long diastole is equal to twice the P-P interval, the cause is S-A block.

Arterial tracing. The pulse waves become gradually larger and have a lower starting point, then become smaller again, with a higher starting point. This indicates higher systolic and lower diastolic pressures during the phase of slower pulse, usually during the second half of expiration.

Mechanism

The various mechanisms of sinus arrhythmia are illustrated by the following scheme (134):

Vagal	Myocardial
respiratory	incomplete S-A block
anoxic (bulbar)	type I (periodic)
independent	type II (intermittent)
	S-A standstill

Diagnosis

The diagnosis can be made by means of the simple tests already described. Suspension of respiration causes a disappearance of the phenomenon. Atropine can be used in doubtful cases.

Differential diagnosis should be made with the following conditions.

Periodic S-A block may be connected with respiration and may be affected in the manner of respiratory arrhythmia by the functional tests. However, in S-A block *the long pause is equal to twice the short one;* in respiratory arrhythmia the long pause is *less than double;* the increase is gradual in the latter.

Sinus premature beats. These will be discussed later (page 349).

Prognosis—Treatment

Prognosis is favorable except in those cases where the irregularity reveals an initial cardiac failure (coronary heart disease). Therefore, correlation between sinus arrhythmia and all other clinical data is necessary.

No treatment is necessary. Atropine may cause disappearance of the disturbance.

II. Disturbances of Rate and Rhythm Caused by Increased Excitability of the Myocardium

ATRIAL AND NODAL TACHYCARDIA (15)

Cause and Mechanism

This paroxysmal syndrome is common and may occur at any age. It may be present at birth (109). Endocrine disorders (hyperthyroidism; disorders associated with uterine myoma, puberty, menopause, or pregnancy) favor it. Normal individuals with the Wolff-Parkinson-White syndrome are prone to such attacks of tachycardia. Nervous reflexes, due to cardiac or extracardiac stimulation and reaching the heart along the sympathetic pathways, may be involved.

Paroxysmal tachycardia is due to the rapid and regular production of stimuli in some area of the atrial or septal myocardium. Two different theories have been advanced: 1) that of circus movement, and 2) that of an abnormal pacemaker in the atrial wall (parasystole). Present evidence confirms the second theory because multiple studies prove that there is no circus movement in the atrial walls (116, 146). As the new rhythm is due to increased excitability of a new atrial or nodal focus, it has been called a new rhythm "by usurpation" (118).

Signs and Symptoms

The patients are usually in good health, with no other cardiac disturbance or lesion. They complain that *suddenly*, without any apparent cause (or after a minor excitement or effort), *they feel a shock in their chest* and have the impression that their hearts start beating at a tremendous rate. Some patients state that there seems to be "a sudden shifting of gears in their heart". Once the attack is started, it lasts from some minutes to some hours and exceptionally days.

During the attack the patient is somewhat *pale*. The *pulse* is small, regular, and has a rate of 160 to 180. A slower (120 to 160) or faster rate (180 to 240) may be found occasionally. Infants may attain the extreme rate of 300 or slightly more (1).

The patient usually abstains from exertion during an attack but, if necessary, can exert remarkable effort. A condition of *collapse* may occur if the rate is above 200.

In addition to *palpitation*, the patients complain of *precordial oppression* or *ache* and frequently of *anginal pain*.

The *jugular veins* are distended and pulsate. The apex impulse is so rapid that it may be felt like a vibration.

The heart sounds are loud and regular. The 1st sound may seem split on account of a *loud atrial rumble* (112).

Graphic Tracings

Electrocardiogram. During the attack, the ventricular complexes are regular and have a rate of 160–180 (occasionally higher or lower). The atrial waves have the same rate and are either upright with abnormal contour or inverted. The abnormal P may precede, follow, or be masked by QRS; it may fuse with the preceding T (fig. 212A). When P precedes QRS, there is *atrial tachycardia*; when P is inverted and is near QRS, there is *nodal tachycardia*.

Cases having a faster atrial rate and A-V block have been described (1, 10). As the mechanism of production of atrial tachycardia and atrial flutter is similar, it is preferable to diagnose such cases as atrial flutter (page 339).

After the attack, the ECG becomes perfectly normal. However, in some cases, a persistent inversion of T, lasting for 3 to 20 days, has been described (17).

Jugular tracing. There is only one wave, due to the fusion of the normal waves. When the atrial and the ventricular contractions occur at the same time, this wave may become very high (18).

Arterial pulse. The pulse becomes small during the attack. The dicrotic wave may be high and its fusion with the following pulse wave may simulate an anacrotic wave (18).

The speed of the pulse wave is often reduced.

Phonocardiogram. The heart sounds are of short duration. The interval between 1st and 2nd sounds during the attack is shorter than between the attacks. The sounds are louder than before the attack, especially the first (20).

In nodal tachycardia, the tracing may simulate splitting of the 1st sound due to additional atrial vibrations (112).

The vibrations of a systolic murmur may be recorded during the attack.

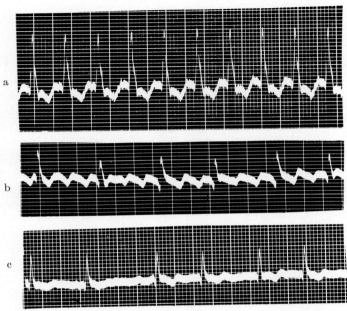

FIG. 212. Electrocardiograms of: A, atrial tachycardia; B, atrial flutter; C, atrial fibrillation.

Mode of Origin of the Signs

A severe atrial or nodal tachycardia has important effects which are common to most types of rapid heart action. The occurrence of more than one pulse wave in the arterial system is one; the possible simultaneous occurrence of atrial and ventricular contractions (nodal tachycardia) is another. It is apparent that the latter may cause insufficiency of the A-V valves and slight regurgitation into both atria. The high venous wave occurring in such cases is probably due to this mechanism.

The extremely short diastole may severely impair the coronary blood supply, which is so dependent upon diastolic filling of the coronaries (page 55, fig. 42).

Moreover, cardiac output may drop considerably while, at the same time, the demand for coronary flow is increased. This causes a relative myocardial ischemia (fig. 215).

The critical ventricular rate for the causation of anginal pain seems to be about 150 per minute (21a). When the ventricles beat at a lower rate, no pain occurs unless there is myocardial infarction.

The critical rate for the occurrence of vascular collapse seems to be about 200 per minute, (more than half of the cases) (21b).

Varieties

Different types are determined by the different ventricular rates and by the length of the attack. *Prolonged attacks* are more serious than short ones. *Chronic atrial tachycardia* is possible (22) and consists of recurring attacks, influenced by posture and often initiated by a premature beat.

Diagnosis

The diagnosis of atrial tachycardia is often possible on the simple basis of the history if attention is paid to sudden onset, sudden cessation, and nearly constant absence of heart disease. The electrocardiogram, taken between the attacks, is important by revealing a normal tracing. During the attack, the ECG shows the simultaneous increase of both atrial and ventricular rates.

Differential diagnosis should be made with the following conditions.

Atrial flutter. The pulse, during the attack of atrial flutter, has a definite ratio to the pulse between the attacks. Attacks of atrial flutter are frequently very long, those of paroxysmal tachycardia rarely so. The ECG between attacks reveals the flutter in atrial flutter and is normal in atrial tachycardia.

Ventricular tachycardia. This condition will be discussed later (page 336).

Sinus tachycardia. This condition is influenced by different stimuli and the pulse has no fixed rate. The pulse of sinus tachycardia is seldom above 120 but is always above 120 in atrial tachycardia.

Differential diagnosis with *myocardial infarction* is necessary when precordial pain is severe and inverted T waves are found in the ECG. When lasting changes are noted two possibilities should be considered:

a) Ischemia of the myocardium due to poor blood supply and increased strain (tachycardia) caused necrosis or injury.

b) The attack of tachycardia was reflexly caused by stimuli arising in an area of infarction.

Differentiation between the two is not always possible but the first more frequently gives signs of diffuse damage while the second more frequently gives a typical picture of either anterior or posterior infarction including Q waves (page 417).

Early evolution (about 1 week) of the electrocardiographic changes and prolonged Q-T interval with bizarre and prolonged T waves, are observed in cases without infarction (110) (so-called *post-tachycardial syndrome*).

Differential diagnosis between atrial tachycardia and *infection* is necessary in infants who present vomiting, diarrhea, abdominal pain, convulsions, and fever. The extremely high cardiac rate seems to cause this syndrome which is related to intoxication (23).

Prognosis

In general, the prognosis is good. A more guarded prognosis is necessary, however, in very long or recurrent attacks and in those cases presenting lasting changes of the ECG.

Treatment

During the attack, treatment is based on either *intense stimulation of the vagus nerves* or *inhibition of the sympathetic nerves*. For this purpose, many different maneuvers have been tried and some of them are discovered by the patients themselves. They are:

a) Deep inspirations; swallowing of a mouthful of food; or stimulation of the pharynx until vomiting occurs, are the most common. Some patients lie on a couch with the head at a lower level than the rest of the body.

b) A *strong compression of the eyeballs*.

c) A *compression of the carotid sinus of one side*.

In the author's experience, the most effective, although painful, maneuver is compression of the eyeballs.

When these measures are not effective, intravenous therapy with *cedilanid* (**6**) or *digoxin* can be tried (**24**) or subcutaneous administration of *prostigmin* (**72**) or i.v. injection of *pronestyl* (**26**). If these are ineffective, *hydergine* (**36**) or *quinidine* (**24**) may be tried. In infants, subcutaneous *prostigmin* (**72**) in dose of ⅛ mg. may be life-saving (**104**).

Prevention of the attacks is difficult. Possible factors which may initiate the attacks should be removed. Among them, abuse of stimulants and tobacco, constipation, indigestion, overexertion, and mental strain, are the most common. When a source of autonomic reflexes is present (gall stones, adhesions, etc.) it should be removed, if possible. Sympathetic depression with hydergine (**36**) may be tried. Prolonged treatment with *quinidine* or *digoxin* (24) is helpful in certain cases.

In some cases, surgical treatment of a thyroid condition has been successful. Perhaps the use of *thiouracil* may be helpful in poor surgical risks.

Surgical removal of the stellate ganglion on one side or of the upper left dorsal ganglion, has been advocated (6).

VENTRICULAR TACHYCARDIA

Cause and Mechanism

Ventricular tachycardia is a serious disturbance due to the existence of an abnormal pacemaker in one of the ventricles.

All factors responsible for increased excitability of the myocardium may be involved. Among them, stimulants, nicotine, fatigue, acute infections, hyperthyroidism, and digitalis poisoning, are common. However, coronary heart disease, acute myocarditis, and heart failure are the most frequent causes. For this reason, it can be stated that *ventricular tachycardia is often found in organic heart disease.*

Symptoms and Signs

When ventricular tachycardia occurs in persons with a normal heart, it produces the same symptoms as an attack of atrial tachycardia. When, on the contrary, it occurs in patients with heart disease, *the patient may be completely unaware of the attack.*

When the attack is brief, the patient's face suddenly becomes *pale*, then normally red again after the end of the paroxysm. When the attack is long, the patient may feel *dizzy* and complain of *buzzing of the ears*. The end of the attack is frequently marked by the impression of a sudden rush of blood to the head. *Precordial pain* and *fainting* are not unusual.

The *pulse* is rapid and regular. However, slight irregularities, with occasional larger pulses, are sometimes found (25, 106). The first sound has frequently a *variable intensity* being louder when the ventricular is preceded by an atrial contraction (25).

Graphic Tracings

Electrocardiogram. Two main varieties have been recognized:

a) *Salvo of ventricular premature beats* (26, 27). During sinus rhythm or atrial fibrillation, the usual rhythm is interrupted by a salvo of from 10 to 100 ventricular premature beats.

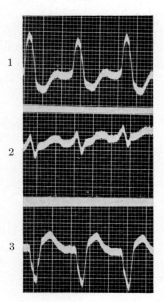

FIG. 213. Electrocardiogram of ventricular tachycardia.

b) *Real ventricular tachycardia.* It is similar to type a, except that the attack lasts for many hours or days. The beginning of the attack is sudden but it may be preceded by a few scattered premature beats having the same electrical appearance as the complexes during the attack. These are broad, have a high voltage, are notched, and are followed by a T wave which is in the opposite direction of the main complex (fig. 213). Occasional P waves, having a much slower rate than the ventricular complexes, may be seen.

Recognition of the focus of origin of the attack is similar to that of ventricular premature beats (fig. 223). After *the attack*, depression of S-T and inversion of T in

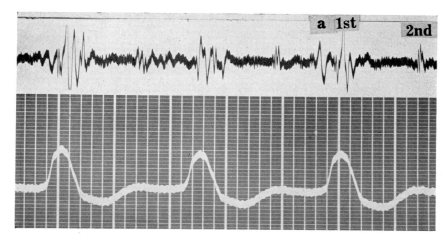

a 1st 2nd

Fig. 214. Electro- and phonocardiogram in a case of *ventricular tachycardia*. Atrial waves (a) appear at long intervals.

either lead 1 or lead 3, may be recognized. It is also possible to note a prolongation of Q-T (31).

Arterial tracing. The pulse waves are small and may show a phenomenon which has been considered typical: *variability of height of the different pulse waves*. There may be *pulsus alternans* (page 373).

Jugular tracing. High atrial waves are recorded, at a rate which is slower than that of the arterial pulse. However, this sign is missing is there is associated atrial fibrillation. The waves may be slightly irregular.

Phonocardiogram. The heart sounds, especially the first, *are loud and clear*. There may be no murmurs and no triple rhythm. On the other hand, the atrial contraction, which has a slower rate than the ventricular, may cause an *atrial sound* either in systole or in diastole according to the casual coincidence of the two rhythms (fig. 214). Splitting of the first sound has been erroneously reported; this splitting cannot occur because the interval separating the contractions of the two ventricles is shorter than the duration of the main phase of the first sound (136).

Mode of Origin of the Signs

Ventricular tachycardia is a serious disturbance, caused by the presence of an abnormal focus of excitability in one of the ventricles (either in one of the branches of the bundle of His or in the ventricular wall). This sends frequent, abnormal stimuli which determine the ventricular rate. In other words, there is an *abnormal ventricular pacemaker*. The stimuli reach the opposite ventricle only after a detour. This explains many common electrocardiographic points between ventricular tachycardia, bundle branch block, and ventricular premature beats.

The atria may behave differently during ventricular tachycardia:

a) They have a *slower* rate than the ventricles since they are ruled by the S-A pacemaker (27).

b) They have *irregularities of rhythm* due to occasional premature contractions caused by a *retrograde stimulus* coming from the ventricular pacemaker (28).

c) They beat regularly and *rapidly* at the same rate as the ventricles. This last occurrence is due to the fact that no blockage protects the atria from the frequent ventricular stimuli (*retrograde stimulation*) with the result that the ventricular pacemaker regulates both the ventricles and the atria. In such cases, the atrial contraction always follows the ventricular.

The delayed changes of the ECG, which

338 HEART

may simulate myocardial infarction, have been explained as being caused by a functional disturbance of the focus of stimulation persisting after the attack (16a). However, the possibility of a myocardial infarction causing the attack should not be overlooked and extensive damage caused by the tachycardia is also to be considered.

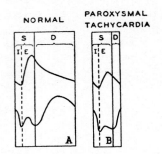

FIG. 215. Comparison between the normal blood flow in the coronary system (A) and that during an attack of paroxysmal tachycardia (B). S, systole; D, diastole; I, isometric phase: E, ejection phase; upper tracing, aortic pressure; lower tracing, coronary flow. (Sketched after Wiggers.)

The changes of the blood pressure, cardiac output, venous pressure, and circulation time (29) are determined by the rapid ventricular rate. This also causes precordial pain and vascular collapse, as in atrial tachycardia (21) (page 334).

Course, Complications, and Prognosis

Attacks of ventricular tachycardia are often a complication of different heart diseases. They increase the severity of the clinical picture and require a more guarded prognosis. The attacks may last from a few minutes to many weeks. In the latter case, they may be followed by *heart failure, ventricular anarchy* (page 395), or *ventricular flutter* (page 396).

The existence of ventricular complexes of the opposite type, *alternately originating from each ventricle*, implies a poor prognosis (1).

A certain number of cases, usually young people without cardiac lesions, present ventricular tachycardia with reversible cardiac enlargement. Following the attack, electrocardiographic changes may be observed consisting of depression of S-T in one lead with raising in another; symmetrical, deeply inverted T in one or more leads; and prolongation of Q-T. This electrocardiographic picture, which usually lasts about a week, has been called *post-tachycardial syndrome* (107, 108). Sudden death or heart failure occurred in a certain number of these cases and post-mortem failed to reveal myocardial or coronary lesions (108).

Diagnosis

When the rate of the heart is over 150, general diagnosis of paroxysmal tachycardia is imperative.

Clinical diagnosis may be tried on the basis of: a) visibility of slow atrial pulsations of the jugular veins contrasting with the rapid radial pulse; b) slight differences in the loudness of the 1st sound; c) occasional stronger arterial pulses recognized upon palpation and during blood pressure measurements. In general, however, the exact recognition of the nature and type of the attack requires the electrocardiograph. Broad and tall ventricular complexes, succeeding each other with regularity and not preceded by a P wave, are typical.

In difficult cases, esophageal electrocardiograms reveal large P waves with a rate which is slower than that of the ventricles (132).

The post-tachycardial syndrome should be differentiated from the *pattern of coronary insufficiency* which is chiefly observed in older people and is present both during and after the attacks. This pattern lasts for only a few days (138).

Between the attacks, the finding of abnormal electrocardiographic tracings or any other sign of heart disease is a point in favor of the diagnosis of ventricular tachycardia.

Cases where differential diagnosis between atrial and ventricular tachycardia is difficult are occasionally found.

Treatment

Stimulation of the vagus nerve by measures which are useful in atrial tachycardia is seldom effective. Moreover, it is contraindicated because it may favor ischemia of the myocardium and ventricular fibrillation. This is particularly true in cases with myocardial infarction.

The intravenous injection of *digoxin* has been used in the prevention of the attacks with some success (24). Intravenous *morphine* in dose of 15 mg., repeated if necessary ½ to 2 hours later, may be effective in the therapy of the attacks (103). It is possible that *atropine* in dose of 1 mg. is also useful and should be used in subjects with coronary lesions, and especially after myocardial infarction (105).

Pronestyl (**26**) in dose of 60 to 800 mg. by intravenous injection is definitely beneficial (140). It should not be given in cases of a-v block or bundle branch block. *Magnesium sulfate* may also be useful.

Oral *quinidine* (**24**) or *pronestyl* (**27**) are useful both in the therapy and in the prevention of such attacks. *Peritrate* (**50**) may be helpful in cases of coronary heart disease.

ATRIAL FLUTTER

Atrial flutter is a persistent and abnormal condition of the atria which is revealed to the patient by acute attacks of rapid ventricular action.

Cause and Mechanism

The atria of these patients contract at a very rapid rate, ranging from 200 to 400 per minute. The ventricular rate is usually much slower, a fraction of that of the atria, and may be either regular or irregular. This is due to the existence of an *a-v block* which may be 4 to 1, 3 to 1, or 2 to 1, and may be irregular. The paroxysms are due to the fact that the block disappears or changes in type so that the ventricles suddenly start contracting at a very rapid rate (1 to 1, if the atrial rate is relatively slow, or 2 to 1).

According to a common expression, the ventricles get "hooked up" to the atria.

Atrial flutter is found more commonly with heart disease than in its absence. It may be associated with valvular defects (especially mitral stenosis), hypertension, thyrotoxicosis, or coronary heart disease. Healthy people may, on the other hand, suffer from atrial flutter. The disturbance may be found at any age, even in infancy.

Sudden effort, excitement, trauma, and surgical intervention, may precipitate the occurrence of atrial flutter.

The mechanism of the disturbance is based upon:

a) An abnormal production of stimuli from an ectopic atrial pacemaker causing regular and rapid atrial contractions.

b) A protective block (constant or variable) between atria and ventricles.

c) Sudden disappearance of the block, causing paroxysms of rapid ventricular contractions.

The abnormal production of the stimuli was formerly attributed to a *circus movement* involving the S-A node (4). However, multiple experimental (116, 146) and clinical studies (146) seem to indicate that *a single atrial focus*, sending rapid stimuli at a rate of 150 to 400, is responsible for the disturbance.

Signs and Symptoms

The patients complain of *acute paroxysms of palpitation* during which they feel weak. These may be of variable duration, even lasting for weeks.

Precordial oppression or ache is frequent and *precordial pain* is possible. *Dizziness* or *fainting* may occur in some patients.

Observation of the patient *between attacks* usually reveals a *normal pulse* and a *normal blood pressure*. Inspection of the jugular veins, on the other hand, may reveal a series of rapid undulations. These pulsations are a multiple of the radial pulse.

Auscultation may reveal a series of frequent sounds which coincide with the atrial contractions and may have a clicking character (7, 10, 139).

Observation of the patient *during an attack* reveals a rapid and small radial pulse. *It is typical for the pulse to have a definite ratio to that between attacks* (like 160 to 80). The pulse is either regular or grossly irregular.

Auscultation frequently reveals an *additional sound* or *rumble* during the short ventricular diastole; this may simulate the rumble of mitral stenosis. If a slight irregularity of the ventricular rate occurs, a changing intensity of the 1st sound may be observed (117).

The patient usually avoids strain or effort and may show signs of heart failure which were not present before the attack.

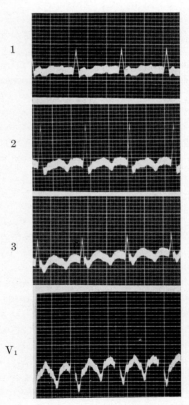

FIG. 216. Electrocardiogram during an attack of *atrial flutter*. Lead V₁ shows the most apparent atrial waves.

Compression of the eyeballs or *of the carotid sinus* may slow the radial pulse; this becomes a fraction of the previous pulse (160 to 80, 150 to 75). However, the favorable result of these maneuvers is less constant than in atrial tachycardia.

Blood Pressure

Systolic pressure is low (100 or less) and the pulse pressure is small (20 or less), during the attack.

Graphic Tracings

Electrocardiogram. Between attacks of rapid pulse, when the patient, however, still has atrial flutter, the ECG shows regular ventricular complexes of normal appearance. Between these are three or more P waves of normal shape, separated by regular intervals. The rate of the atria is from 200 to 400 per minute.

During an attack, there are three, two, or even only one P wave between ventricular complexes. In one type, the number of P waves is constant; in another, there may be a variable number in various cycles. *The P wave is frequently inverted* (figs. 212B and 216). When the P waves are diphasic, the negative phase corresponds to an inverted P; the positive phase, to a T wave (146). The T waves may be deformed by fusion with the P waves. Tracings recorded in V1 and V2 usually give the best evidence of the atrial waves. In certain cases, leads 3 and aVF are the best (135).

Cardiogram. Atrial waves may be recorded in the intervals between the ventricular waves of the cardiogram (6, 135).

Jugular tracing. Regular atrial waves, proving coordinated contractions of the atria, can be recorded (6, 135) (fig. 218A).

Phonocardiogram. The phonocardiogram may reveal the existence of *sounds of atrial origin*, not only during ventricular diastole but also during ventricular systole (7–10, 115, 135). When the ventricular rate is rapid, a *diastolic rumble* may appear at the apex simulating that of mitral stenosis

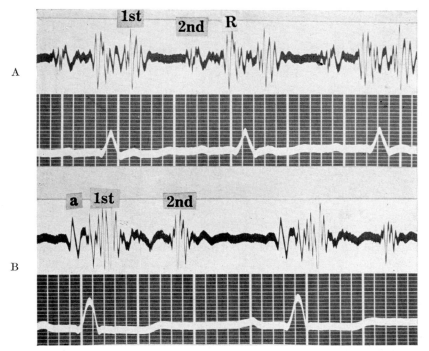

FIG. 217. Electro and phonocardiogram of a case during an attack of *atrial flutter* (A), and 2 weeks later (B). A diastolic rumble (R) simulating that of mitral stenosis is present during the attack; an atrial sound (a) and a prolonged 1st sound are present later.

(fig. 217). If slight irregularities of the ventricular rate occur, a *changing intensity of the first heart sound* may be observed (147).

Electrokymogram. If the slit of the pickup is placed across the border of either atrium, good evidence of atrial contractions can be secured (135) (fig. 218B). The atrial waves are usually of large amplitude and are significant in cases where the electrocardiographic tracing had led to admission of "flutter-fibrillation."

X-Ray

Fluoroscopic examination, with or without the help of a barium swallow, demonstrates regular, co-ordinated contractions of the atria (11, 12). The same demonstration is given by roentgenkymography (13).

Mode of Origin of the Signs

The atrial sounds have been attributed to tension of adhesions or to the same mecha-

nism as the 4th (atrial) sound (page 42). When they occur during systole, they may be due to vibration of the closed A-V valves.

Critical levels of ventricular rate for precordial pain and vascular collapse are the same as in atrial tachycardia (page 334).

Course and Complications

Atrial flutter is a persistent condition. There have been cases where the atrial disturbance continued for many years. On the other hand, rapid action of the ventricles may occur in attacks of variable duration. *They may last hours, days, and even weeks.* When they last for a long time, *congestive heart failure* may result.

Atrial thrombosis followed by peripheral embolism may occur but is not common.

Diagnosis

Sudden onset of attacks of rapid pulse, long duration of the attacks, ratio of the

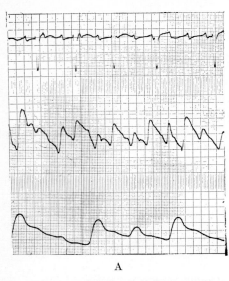
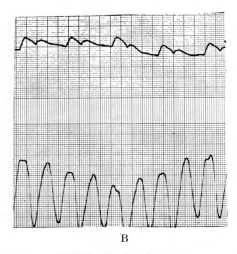

FIG. 218. Tracings in cases of *atrial flutter*. A. From above: ECG in V₂, jugular tracing, carotid tracing in a case with irregular pulse; the jugular tracing clearly reveals the atrial waves. B. From above: carotid tracing, electrokymogram of right atrium in a case with regular pulse; the atrium is contracting at a rate twice that of the ventricles.

pulse rate during the attack to that between attacks: these are the main data on which a clinical diagnosis of atrial flutter may be made. Rapid undulations of the jugular veins and rapid sounds over the precordium in the intervals between the radial pulses may permit diagnosis in the periods between attacks. The electrocardiogram gives important data. In difficult cases, an electrokymogram of the atria may be decisive. This is particularly important in cases with irregular pulse where differential diagnosis with atrial fibrillation is necessary.

Differential diagnosis should be made in order to eliminate the following conditions:

Atrial fibrillation. The atrial waves of the ECG are irregular and differ from each other. The ventricular rate is never absolutely regular. The pulse during attacks has no ratio to that between attacks. In general, diagnosis of atrial flutter is made by electrocardiography. Special attention should be paid to leads aVF and V1–V2 for recognition of atrial waves. In doubtful cases, demonstration of atrial sounds (phonocardiogram) and of atrial waves (jugular

tracing or electrokymogram), helps in excluding atrial fibrillation.

Atrial tachycardia. The attacks are usually short. Between attacks, the ECG is normal. The pulse during attacks has no ratio to that between attacks.

Sinus tachycardia. The pulse has no fixed rate and may be increased or slowed by various conditions. The ECG is normal.

Stokes-Adams. The electrocardiograms of S-A and of flutter may be confused by beginners because in both conditions the atrial are more frequent than the ventricular complexes. The main difference is that in atrial flutter the atrial rate is fast and the ventricular rate rapid or normal; in Stokes-Adams, on the contrary, the atrial rate is normal and the ventricular is slow.

Mitral stenosis. The atrial sound or rumble of atrial flutter may simulate that of mitral stenosis. As atrial flutter may occur in patients with mitral stenosis, only a careful study of the patient *after* the end of the attack may decide whether or not there also is a valvular lesion.

Treatment

Treatment of atrial flutter can be outlined as follows:

1) A large dose of digitalis (**1, 2**) (109) is given. The toxic effect of the drug causes an increased excitability of the myocardium and a shortening of the refractory period (page 583). This permits the transformation of atrial flutter into atrial fibrillation.

2) After obtaining the initial result, *quinidine* (**24**) is given (114). This drug prolongs the refractory period (page 592) and re-establishes the sinus rhythm.

3) Further use of digitalis is determined by the basal conditions of the heart and not by the knowledge that there has been atrial flutter (109).

If digitalis fails, quinidine usually does not help. There is no harm, however, in trying it.

ATRIAL FIBRILLATION (73, 74)

Atrial fibrillation is a common disturbance which is revealed clinically by total and complete irregularity of the ventricular contractions and of the pulse.

Cause and Mechanism—Lesions

Atrial fibrillation may occur in any type of heart disease. However, two are the most common:

a) Atrial fibrillation in patients with valvular diseases or atrial septal defect, and chronic distention of the atria. This is frequently seen in patients with mitral stenosis and even more often in those having combined lesions of the mitral and tricuspid valves. *The fibrillation is frequently associated with heart failure.*

b) Atrial fibrillation in patients with coronary heart disease and fibrosis of the myocardium. In these patients, *the fibrillation often is present without any sign of congestive failure.*

Atrial fibrillation is frequently encountered in *thyrotoxicosis* and may be found in patients with *acute myocarditis* (scarlet fever, pneumonia, diphtheria, rheumatic disease).

Experimental conditions favoring atrial fibrillation are:

a) Distention or anoxia of the atrial wall (96).

b) Acute lesion of the atrial myocardium.

c) Direct or reflex stimulation of the vagus nerve (97, 98, 100).

d) Digitalis toxicity.

Anoxia of the atria is frequent in congestive failure where it is associated with distention of the chambers. Vagal reflexes are important in digitalis poisoning, thyrotoxicosis, and rheumatic disease. In the latter, they are usually associated with lesions of the atrial myocardium and, possibly, with anoxia.

Paroxysmal atrial fibrillation may be caused by myocardial infarction, gall bladder colic, high tension electric discharge, or surgery.

Excitement, fear, alcohol, tobacco, and gas or food poisoning may favor either the acute or the chronic form of fibrillation.

Atrial fibrillation is usually encountered in old age. However, it may occur in young people and even in children.

There is no pathological change that is typical of atrial fibrillation. Organic heart disease may be present but frequently the only findings are hypertrophy of the ventricles and distention of the atria with irregular areas of fibrosis and degeneration.

Atrial fibrillation was attributed to the establishment of *a wave of excitation (and contraction), constantly circulating at a very rapid rate in the atria (circus movement)* (75). In most clinical cases, the "ring" where the stimulus was supposed to circulate would surround the venae cavae. From this ring, stimuli were said to go off irregularly into the rest of the atrial myocardium, causing fibrillary contractions. The ventricles were supposed to respond as rapidly as possible but with an irregular rhythm. The rate of circulation of the stimulus in the muscular ring was supposed to be between 300 and 500 per minute in man. However, recent evidence has accumulated in favor of the *theory of a single focus.* The disturbance seems to be initiated by rapid impulse formation in a single center and is favored by islands of refractory tissue causing the typical weaving and interweaving of the contraction (116). *Multifocal types* may also occur (80). Clinical electrocardiograms and experimental cinematograms (146) definitely proved the nonexistence of a circus movement.

It is interesting to note that experimental studies proved the possibility of fibrillation of only one atrium, usually the right (76, 144). Clinical cases with this partial disturbance or having flutter and fibrillation, respectively, in the two atria, have been described (14, 77–79, 145); however the clinical evidence is less convincing.

Signs and Symptoms

The pulse is *absolutely irregular* so that each pulse wave has different amplitude and duration.

Auscultation of the heart reveals a similar, complete irregularity of the heart sounds. If valvular defects are present, the murmurs vary from one cardiac cycle to the next. Some cardiac contractions are not followed by a radial pulse, expecially if there is heart failure.

Graphic Methods

Electrocardiogram. The following data are typical: there is no P wave; the intervals between the various ventricular complexes are never alike, having different lengths; even when at first glance the ventricular rhythm seems regular, careful measurements reveal the arrhythmia (fig. 212C).

There are two varieties:

1) There are fine and irregular waves at a rate of 300–600 per minute. This is typical atrial fibrillation.

2) There are coarse and somewhat irregular waves. This has been called *coarse fibrillation* or *flutter fibrillation.*

Jugular tracing. The c and v waves follow each other with complete irregularity. There are no *a* waves.

Low frequency tracing. The waves caused by ventricular contraction are of various height and configuration. When diastole is short, the subsequent period of systolic tension is longer. The height of the waves varies somewhat but is not proportional to the length of the preceding diastole.

Arterial tracings, hemodynamics. The pulse waves are typically irregular, having various height, length, and configuration. Patients in congestive failure often have a pulse deficit because some of the ventricular contractions are not followed by a pulse wave. Moreover, some waves may be present in the arteries nearer the heart and absent in those more distant. When failure is severe, a high pulse wave may be followed by gradually smaller ones (fig. 219). As long as the conditions of the myocardium are good, the stroke volume is directly proportional to the length of the preceding diastole and inversely proportional to the stroke volume of the preceding cycle. If, however, there is cardiac failure, no rule can be established. The speed of the small pulse waves is always greater than that of the large waves (121).

Phonocardiogram. The heart sounds have vibrations of similar amplitudes. The inter-

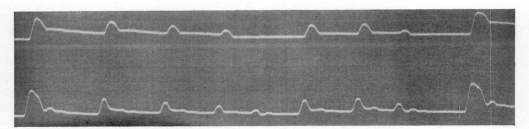

Fig. 219. The *pulse of Galenus* in atrial fibrillation. Tibial and brachial tracings.

val between QRS and the first sound may vary, being longer after a short diastole, as has been shown by the author (86) and confirmed by others (87, 137). This is more often the case in patients with mitral stenosis; the longer interval seems due to delayed closing of the mitral valve and delayed beginning of the sound on account of smaller atrioventricular gradient of pressure.

Electrokymogram. The atrial tracing shows the absence of atrial waves. The waves of the ventricular and arterial tracings (aortic and pulmonic) have a variable amplitude which is roughly proportional to the length of the previous diastole.

Cardiac Output

It has been demonstrated that cardiac output is reduced by atrial fibrillation (149). The effect is even more striking in cases with mitral stenosis where the strong compensatory contraction of the left atrium is abolished by fibrillation.

Varieties

According to the onset and duration, atrial fibrillation can be divided into the *paroxysmal* and *chronic* types. According to the ventricular rate, it can be divided into *rapid* and *slow*. According to the electrocardiographic aspect, into *coarse* and *fine*. It is possible that *partial fibrillation* may take place.

The initial stage of fibrillation may be preceded by a *prefibrillatory condition* and may be followed by an abnormal function of the atrial myocardium. This is revealed by the following electrocardiographic data (88, 120):

a) Atrial premature contractions with or without block.

b) Atrial paroxysmal tachycardia or flutter.

c) Polimorphous P waves.

A further type takes place when both *atrial fibrillation and a-v block* are present. This is recognized by the absolute regularity of the ventricular rhythm while fine "fibril-

lary waves" exclude a more common type of nodal rhythm (page 354). If this variety is not caused by digitalis, it has a poor prognosis (123).

Course and Complications

Atrial fibrillation prevents co-ordinated contraction of the atrial myocardium and favors the formation of *mural thrombi*. Sooner or later, these may cause an *embolism*.

Diagnosis

The clinical diagnosis of atrial fibrillation is usually possible. However, this disturbance may be confused with frequent and nonperiodic premature beats. Then, diagnosis is electrocardiographic.

Differential diagnosis between atrial flutter and fibrillation is based on finding of atrial waves between the ventricular complexes in the former. Moreover, many cases with atrial flutter have a regular ventricular rate. In doubtful cases, jugular tracings, phonocardiograms, and especially electrokymograms, will be of help by revealing evidence of co-ordinated atrial activity (page 342).

Differential diagnosis from *atrial standstill* is based on the absolute regularity of the ventricular rate in this condition and on complete irregularity in atrial fibrillation.

Inasmuch as the ventricular rate may be nearly regular, especially after digitalization, the electrocardiographic diagnosis can be done with certainty only if artefacts, especially muscular currents, are excluded. Therefore, complete relaxation of the patient in the recumbent or semirecumbent position during the taking of the ECG is indicated. However, even artefacts seldom obscure the existence of the P wave in cases having no fibrillation.

Prognosis

Prognosis is based on: conditions of the heart muscle, ventricular rate (rapid rate indicates more serious prognosis), and age and sex (worse in older patients and in males) (127).

Prognosis of atrial fibrillation in itself is usually good. Patients have lived even 15 or 20 years with this condition. However, the efficiency of a heart with fibrillating atria is lower than that of a normal heart. In particular, one of the compensatory mechanisms of mitral stenosis (the strong contraction of the left atrium) is not possible whenever there is atrial fibrillation.

Atrial fibrillation has a bad prognosis in children because it is usually associated with myocarditis and heart failure (89).

Treatment

a) *Atrial fibrillation and congestive failure.* When signs of failure are present, treatment with *digitalis glycosides* should be employed first. It may lead to return of sinus rhythm. However, a large number of patients still fibrillate when dyspnea, hepatic and pulmonary congestion, and peripheral edema, have disappeared. Then fibrillation will be treated by the same measures which are employed in patients without congestive failure.

b) *Atrial fibrillation without congestive failure.* In these cases, *quinidine* (24) should be used. It prolongs the refractory period of the atrial myocardium. By depressing the excitability of the cardiac fibers, it may inhibit stimuli arising in abnormal foci. The danger of mobilizing an atrial thrombus by means of quinidine has been overemphasized (122): embolism may occur with or without quinidine. The *initial dose* of quinidine is 0.2 gm. every 4 hours (day and night) and is increased by 0.2 gm. every 12 hours until normalization occurs, toxic phenomena appear, or the dose of 0.8 has been reached (122). When normal rhythm has been attained, an average *maintenance dose* of 0.3 gm. every 6 hours (though with important individual variations) is given for a long time.

The intramuscular injection of one single dose of *fagarine* of 0.05 to 0.1 gm. (113a) seems to be superior to quinidine (113b) but is not exempt from dangers in its clinical use.

c) *Atrial fibrillation after myocardial in-* *farction.* Early control of the fibrillation is advisable because its persistence increases the danger of embolism (99). Quinidine should not be used if there are conduction disturbances or congestive failure. The indications are as follows: *quinidine alone, if fibrillation is present without congestive failure; digitalis plus quinidine, if there is fibrillation and congestive failure* (99).

PREMATURE BEATS (PREMATURE SYSTOLES— EXTRA-SYSTOLES)

Premature beats or *premature contractions* represent a common disturbance due to early contraction of the heart. The name "extrasystole" is inaccurate, except in the case of an interpolated premature beat, where there really is an additional contraction.

Cause and Mechanism

An abnormal stimulus may arise in the heart, spreading from a point which is usually outside the normal pacemaker, and cause a premature contraction. In order to be effective, the stimulus must occur at a time when the heart muscle is not in the absolute refractory period (page 30). However, *increased excitability may permit a premature beat during the relative refractory period*, namely very soon after the end of a normal contraction and even during the T wave.

Certain factors are responsible for the abnormal production of stimuli. *Electrical, mechanical,* or *chemical stimulation* of the heart causes premature beats in experimental animals and man, if above a certain threshold. *Vagus nerve stimulation,* either direct or reflex, may elicit premature beats. This is true whether the carotid sinus is compressed, the stomach distended, or the gall bladder submitted to traction.

Forced respiration, overexertion, or *excitement,* may induce premature beats through autonomic stimuli. These frequently appear *after* and not during effort.

Fatigue, indigestion, cerebral lesions, and

hypertension, are frequently associated with premature beats.

Coffee, tea, alcohol, and *tobacco* favor premature beats, and so does *hyperthyroidism*.

Distention of the heart chambers, acute myocarditis, and *scars* left by this process or by coronary occlusion, favor the occurrence of premature beats. The same is true whenever there is *poor blood supply* to a given area of the cardiac muscle.

Among the drugs commonly used, *thyroid extract, digitalis,* and *epinephrine* favor the occurrence of premature beats.

Premature beats may occur at any age. They are frequent in newborn infants and even in the fetus (63), common in children or young people, and frequent in adults and in the aged.

The mechanism of premature beats is thought to be the following:

a) *When the abnormal stimulus arises in one of the atria*, it spreads in all directions, reaching both the S-A node and the A-V node. By so doing, it *discharges* the normal impulse which is forming in the S-A node and may disturb its activity. The pause following the premature beat is equivalent to the time interval required for the stimulus to reach the S-A node plus the time between two normal contractions. As this interval plus that preceding the premature beat is not double that of a normal interval, *the pause is not compensatory*. This means that the dominant rhythm is modified by the premature beat and that all the following contractions are somewhat advanced (fig. 220).

b) *When the abnormal stimulus arises in one of the ventricles*, it spreads in all directions, usually reaching the A-V node. It is often prevented from reaching the atria either because these are already contracting or because of a "protection block". The stimulus reaches the other ventricle in a roundabout way, similar to the course followed in bundle branch block (page 376). Therefore, the ventricle where the stimulus has arisen contracts first and is followed by the other.

The premature beat does not disturb the regular development of the sinus rhythm. The pause following the premature beat is therefore such that the interval between the last normal contraction before the premature beat and the first after it equals the double of a normal interval (*compensatory pause*) (fig. 221). This is not true in the

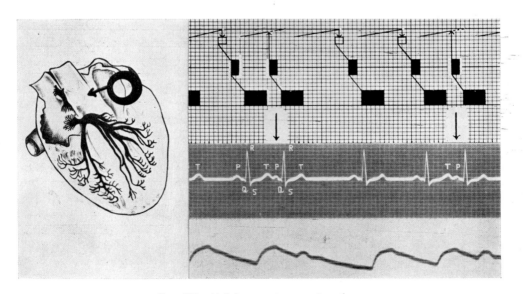

Fig. 220. Atrial premature contractions

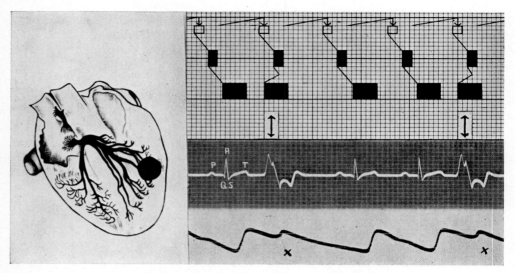

FIG. 221. Ventricular premature contractions

case of an *interpolated premature beat* which is not followed by a pause and is actually *an additional contraction* or *extrasystole*.

Among the different theories, that of "re-entry" should be mentioned. According to this, an area of muscle, refractory to normal stimulation, might contract later when reached in a roundabout way. This would cause a new stimulation of the rest of the heart.

Many premature beats bear a firm time relation to the normal preceding beat. This led to the belief that the abnormal stimulus is released by the normal contraction (64). It is possible that an abnormal focus is constantly building up stimuli at a different rate from that of the normal pacemaker. The normal contraction might release a "protection block" and permit the abnormal stimulus to excite the myocardium. It is also possible that the excitability of an abnormal focus is increased mechanically by the normal contraction so that its stimuli are able to overcome the threshold of the surrounding tissue.

It is admitted by many that stimuli, causing premature beats, arise only in the specific tissue of the atria or ventricles and not in the common myocardial tissue.

Signs and Symptoms

The patient may feel that premature beat in two ways:

a) A sensation of *shock, a tightness* in the throat or the chest, a *sticking pain*, or simply an *abnormal movement* in the precordial area or over the epigastrium taking place *at the time* of the abnormal beat.

b) A sensation of *falling* or a *sudden dizziness* taking place *after* the abnormal beat.

When multiple premature beats occur, different sensations are described, such as *palpitation, anginal pain*, or even fluttery, *bizarre movements* within the chest.

Palpation of the radial artery usually reveals the premature beat as a *missing pulse* or *intermittence*.[61] At times, however, a small pulse wave, nearer to the preceding than to the following pulse, is felt.

The premature beat is often revealed by a *sudden, high apical thrust* and by a *high wave in the jugular veins*.

Auscultation reveals the premature beat in the following ways:

After several normal couples of heart

[61] It is actually a *pseudo-intermittence* because the pulse is not missing, though so small as not to be felt.

sounds, there is *a sudden loud sound* (the 1st sound of the premature beat), followed by *a weak or split 2nd sound* (the 2nd sound of the premature beat); the latter may even be absent. Afterwards, a long pause follows. More complex phenomena may occur, because the premature beat may be followed by either a loud 3rd sound or a murmur (in cases of valvular defects).

When a *bigeminal rhythm* is present, it is common to hear two normal sounds followed by another (the 1st sound of the premature beat); then a pause; and then the same sequence again. In such cases, the premature beat may simulate a triple rhythm.

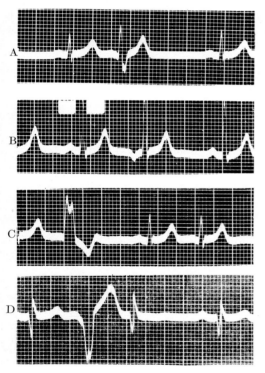

FIG. 222. ECG in cases of premature contractions (extrasystoles). A, The second complex is an *infranodal premature contraction with aberrant conduction*; B, the second complex is a *nodal premature contraction*; C, the first complex is a *ventricular premature contraction*; the third is an *atrial premature contraction*; D, the second complex is a *ventricular, interpolated premature contraction*.

Varieties

The premature beats may be of different types.

a) They are *isolated and occasional*; therefore, they are frequently absent during the examination. The premature beat may be situated between two normal cycles (interpolated premature beat).

b) They have a *periodic* connection with the normal contraction (periodic premature beat). The most common is *bigeminal rhythm* (normal contraction, premature beat, pause) (fig. 311B) which is frequently caused by digitalis. A *trigeminal rhythm* may also occur (normal contraction followed by two premature beats (70)).

c) There may be a *salvo of premature beats* which represents a short attack of tachycardia (page **III**).

d) There may be *frequent premature beats* without any fixed cycle, originating from different foci (fig. 222).

Graphic Tracings

Electrocardiogram. Several different types of tracings are observed, according to the rhythm, frequency, and point of origin of the premature beat (fig. 223).

a) *Atrial premature beats.* A normal P-QRS is followed by a short diastole, then by a slightly abnormal P-QRS. This has a slightly deformed (higher, broader, or lower) P wave and a slightly longer P-R interval. The QRS usually is normal, but may be slightly changed (*aberrant*). The premature beat is followed by a long diastole. However, *this pause is not compensatory* and causes a certain advancement of the following complexes (*occasionally, the pause may be compensatory.*) The first P wave after the premature beat may be higher and sharper than the others (64).

Among the atrial premature beats, some authors admit a separate class, that of *sinus premature beats*. These are said to have a normal P wave and a normal P-R and to be followed by a normal interval (1, 65). Slight

Position of heart	Origin of Stimulus							
Vertical	right base	right middle	right apex	—	left apex	left middle	left base	—
Oblique	—	right base	right middle	right apex	—	left apex	left middle	left base
Transverse	left base	—	right base	right middle	right apex	—	left apex	left middle

I

II

III

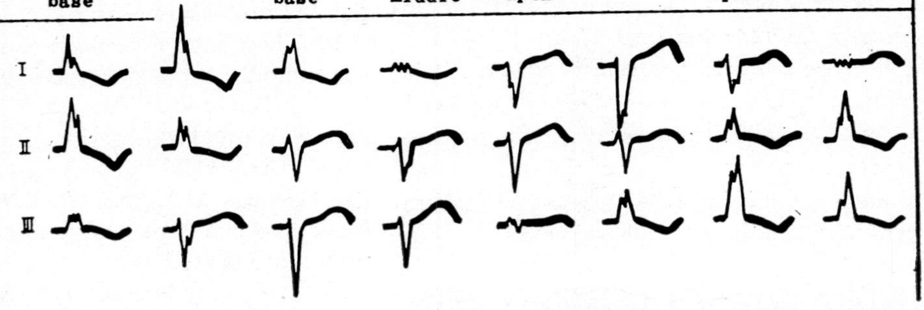

FIG. 223. Origin of ventricular premature contractions in the various positions of the heart. (After Holzmann.)

variations in the shape of the P wave should not rule out this type of premature contractions (133).

Blocked atrial premature beats are possible but uncommon. A P wave occurs very near the end of a normal or premature complex; it is *not* followed by a QRS; a small, flat, sluggish wave may follow the P representing the terminal deflection of the atrial complex (*Ta*, page 37).

When an atrial premature beat originates from a point near the A-V node, it is called a *nodal premature beat*. Its characteristics are: frequently inverted or deformed P wave; short P-R; P either preceding QRS or following it; normal QRS. The pause is seldom compensatory.

Atrial premature beats are seldom *interpolated*.

b) *Ventricular premature beats.* A ventricular premature beat is easily recognized because of the following characteristics: absence of the P wave; high voltage; long duration and splintering of the ventricular complex; raised S-T; T wave in the opposite direction from the main complex. It has been stated that right ventricular premature beats have an upright complex in lead 1; left ventricular premature beats, an inverted complex in lead 1 (66–68). However, *the position of the heart causes important modifications in the direction of the complexes.* Figure 227 shows the various patterns resulting from premature contractions occurring in the vertical, average, and horizontal hearts.

A ventricular premature beat may send its stimulus backwards to the atria, thereby causing a "retrograde" atrial contraction (150). Recognition of the fact is largely based on esophageal electrocardiograms. When this happens, the pause following the premature beat may be "noncompensatory".

A ventricular premature beat may occur as an *interpolated extrasystole*. This is more commonly, but not exclusively, found in the slow heart.

A *ventricular escape* can be easily differentiated from a premature beat because it occurs after a long pause, has a normal ventricular complex, is not preceded by an atrial wave, and is not followed by a compensatory pause.

Jugular tracing. Atrial premature beats have *a*, *c* and *v* waves which are similar to those of a normal tracing. Nodal and ven-

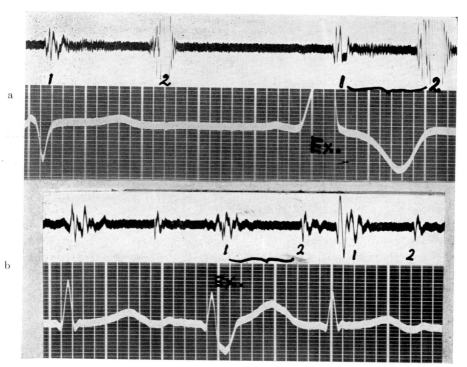

FIG. 224. In (a) the two heart sounds of the extrasystole are louder; in (b) both sounds are lower than in the normal contractions. ECG and sound tracings.

tricular premature beats, on the other hand, frequently have high *a* waves.

A left ventricular premature beat may show a delay of *v* over the second sound (earlier contraction of the left ventricle (68).

Phonocardiogram. Several entirely different phenomena can be recorded (fig. 224). *The first sound is usually normal or louder than in the normal contractions.* This seems due to the fact that, while in normal contractions the A-V valves are nearly closed before ventricular systole, in premature beats these valves are closed *from an open position* by a regurgitant flow of blood. For this reason, the beginning of the sound is delayed over that of QRS in ventricular premature beats. The two valvular phases of the first sound may be widely separated on account of the prolongation of the tension period and this may simulate splitting of the sound. *The second sound of the premature beat is normal or weaker than the others and may be absent. It may be split.*

A premature beat may be followed by either a diastolic murmur (69) or a diastolic sound which does not occur after normal contractions.

Arterial tracing, hemodynamics. The pulse wave of the premature beat may be as high as a normal wave and occasionally higher. It is usually smaller and may be absent. Records taken over different arteries show that the pulse wave of the premature beat may be present in the arteries near the aorta and absent in those distant. A drop in pressure occurs during the compensatory pause. The following wave is higher than normal, and is followed by a smaller wave; this may start a pulsus alternans.

The pulse of the premature contraction has *a low systolic and a high diastolic pressure* while the following pulse is much larger on account of high systolic and low diastolic pressure. From two to three pulse waves are necessary for reaching again a normal and stable level of blood pressure. On the other hand, the first normal contraction following an interpolated premature beat frequently yields a smaller pulse wave in the peripheral arteries (72).

The pulse wave of a right ventricular premature beat may be *delayed* over the beginning of the corresponding first sound (earlier contraction of the right ventricle) (67).

The *stroke volume* varies greatly, being inversely proportional to the length of the preceding diastole. Therefore, the earlier the contraction, the smaller the stroke volume. The compensatory pause is followed by a contraction with proportionally larger stroke volume if the myocardium is normal (121).

The *speed of the pulse wave* is directly proportional to the level of diastolic pressure; therefore the weak pulse of the premature contraction has a greater velocity than the others (121).

Electrokymogram. Premature contractions are easily studied by means of border tracings of the left ventricle, the pulmonary artery, or the aortic arch. If simultaneous tracings of the left ventricle and one of the arteries (aorta or pulmonary artery) are taken, conclusions may be drawn about the site of origin of a ventricular premature beat. The aspect of the tracing is dependent upon the time of the cardiac cycle at which the premature contraction occurs and the phase of ventricular filling.

If the contraction starts early in diastole, its amplitude is small, isometric contraction is prolonged, and the curve has a more peaked aspect. The prolongation of tension time, due to both the high level of arterial pressure and the small amount of ventricular blood, may last more than 0.06 second. If the contraction takes place immediately after the T wave, no pulsations of the aorta can be recorded. During the compensatory pause, an abnormally large filling of the ventricles takes place. This, plus the lower level of arterial pressure, causes a shortening of the isometric contraction period of the following contraction.

Blood Pressure

Different levels of blood pressure can be obtained if the premature beats occur periodically: 1) those corresponding to the systolic and diastolic pressure of the normal pulse waves; 2) those corresponding to the pulse waves of the premature beats (low systolic, high diastolic); and 3) those corresponding to the pulse waves immediately subsequent to the premature beats (high systolic, low diastolic).

X-Ray

The premature beats can be recognized on fluoroscopy. Ventricular premature beats may be revealed by the contraction, first of one ventricle and then of the other, with a slight delay between the two.

Mode of Origin of the Signs

The different signs are determined by the possible occurrence of three phenomena:

a) The atrial and ventricular contractions may *occur at the same time*, both in the nodal and in the ventricular premature beats. This causes a *backflow of blood into the veins*, either because the A-V valves are closed by the stronger ventricular contraction and the atria push the blood backwards, or because the simultaneous contraction causes a slight insufficiency of the A-V valves with regurgitation of blood from the ventricles.

b) Ventricular premature beats have a *nonsimultaneous contraction of the ventricles* which causes phenomena similar to those of bundle branch block (page 376). The delayed contraction of the right ventricle (left ventricular premature beat) is mainly apparent in the venous system, while delayed contraction of the left ventricle (right ventricular premature beat) is mainly apparent in the arterial system.

c) Premature beats occur at a time when the aortic pressure is still high. The contraction takes place when the ventricles are incompletely filled. This accounts for a *long tension period* and a *small pulse wave*. However, the possible absence of the pulse wave in the arteries may be due to peripheral factors.

The various symptoms described by the patients are due to the long tension period, accompanied by a strong shock against the chest wall, or to the drop in pressure which follows the premature beat.

Diagnosis—Prognosis

Diagnosis of premature beats is frequently possible on the basis of the history alone. Physical examination easily permits recognition of premature beats when they occur occasionally or periodically. In such cases, simultaneous auscultation of the heart and palpation of the radial artery reveals that every missing pulse is accompanied by two (occasionally only one) heart sounds (*false intermittence*).

Differential diagnosis from an *occasional* or *periodic heart block* is possible because in such cases the missing pulse is not accompanied by heart sounds (*real intermittence*).

Differential diagnosis from *atrial fibrillation* is easy when the premature beats occur occasionally or periodically but may be difficult when they are frequent and irregular.

The electrocardiograph is helpful in doubtful cases revealing typical broad complexes in cases of ventricular premature beats and normal complexes in cases of fibrillation. In atrial fibrillation, moreover, the P waves are missing from all complexes.

Differential diagnosis between atrial premature beats and *sinus arrhythmia* is based on the existence of a slight difference in the shape of the P wave and in the length of the P-R of the premature contraction.

Differential diagnosis between *bigeminal pulse* and *pulsus alternans* can be made by means of a pulse tracing or an electrocardiogram. In bigeminal pulse, the small wave is nearer the preceding large wave; in pulsus alternans, the small wave is at equal distance from the larger pulse waves. During pulsus alternans, the QRS complexes of the ECG are perfectly regular.

Once the diagnosis of premature beats is made, *evaluation of its clinical significance* is necessary. This can be done only after taking into account all clinical data of the patient, including x-ray and electrocardiogram.

Premature beats may be the forerunners of paroxysmal tachycardia, coronary occlusion, or heart failure. On the other hand, they may be absolutely harmless. The results of abstention from stimulants or drugs, the action of digitalis (if such drug has not already been taken), or the use of vasodilators, at times permit a better evaluation.

The fact that digitalis frequently causes ventricular premature beats, often bigeminal in type, should not be forgotten because the premature contractions are then evidence of toxicity. Atrial premature beats with continually changing P waves are evidence of *organic myocardial lesion*. The same is true for ventricular premature beats originating from several different foci.

Treatment

When the patient does not feel the premature beats, it is not advisable to tell him about them. If the patient is acquiring the habit of taking his pulse and counting its irregularities, he should be advised not to do so because a neurosis may be the result.

Harmless premature contractions need no treatment. Limitation in the use of coffee, tobacco, or alcohol; avoidance of certain foods, and sufficient night rest, are frequently helpful in limiting premature beats. It may be necessary to discontinue digitalis in some cases and administer it in others.

The use of drugs which depress the autonomic nervous system is indicated whenever reflexes are involved (**36, 37, 38**). *Atropine* is especially useful in ventricular premature contractions of coronary and hypertensive patients (105) and whenever reflex elements are involved.

Quinidine (**24**) or *pronestyl* (**37**) may be employed and their use may be prolonged even for months.

The association of *papaverine, quinidine,* and *atropine* is useful in patients with coronary heart disease. *Papaverine* alone has been described as effective, both by mouth (**43**) and by injection (**44**).

Bromides and *barbiturates* may be useful.

Magnesium sulfate (intravenous injection of 15 to 20 cc. of a 20 per cent solution) seems effective in the therapy of premature beats caused by digitalis; so is *potassium chloride* in a single oral dose of 2 to 10 gm. (142).

ESCAPES

Escapes (or escaped beats) occur whenever the activity of the A-V node or one of the ventricles reveals itself during a long pause; they are, therefore, due to a phenomenon of "default." Escapes may occur in the following conditions: 1) in pronounced sinus arrhythmia; 2) in partial A-V block or atrial fibrillation; 3) in cases with ventricular premature beats; 4) during cardiac standstill caused by strong vagal stimulation (compression of the eyeballs) with inhibition of both the S-A node and the A-V node.

Escapes are recognized in the electrocardiogram by the normal configuration of the ventricular complex.

Treatment should be directed toward removing the basic cause.

III. Disturbances of Rate and Rhythm Due to Decreased Conductivity

NODAL RHYTHM

Cause and Mechanism

Nodal rhythm is a regular and slow rhythm of the heart set up by impulses from the A-V node. The activity of the node becomes apparent in three conditions:

1) When an interruption of the conducting system prevents the stimuli of the normal pacemaker from reaching the A-V node. In such cases, the atria are controlled by the S-A node; the ventricles, by the A-V node: there is a *double rhythm.*

2) When there is *atrial fibrillation* or *atrial standstill.* In such cases, the atria are immobile and ventricular contraction is controlled by the A-V node.

3) When the activity of the S-A node is *suspended* or *depressed.* This is the typical *A-V nodal rhythm* and occurs mostly in aged people.

Clinical observations in young people have proven that strong reflex stimulation of the vagus may suppress the S-A activity and cause the appearance of nodal rhythm (141).

The disappearance of the sinus rhythm is not felt by the patients, because the A-V node takes over the function of the pacemaker. However, the new "center" is less efficient because its rate is slower, the normal succession of atrial and ventricular contractions is not preserved, and the influence of the cardiac nerves is nearly absent.

In typical nodal rhythm, the atria are stimulated in a retrograde direction by the A-V node. If the stimulus starts from the upper part of the node, the atrial contraction slightly precedes the ventricular. If, on the other hand, the stimulus starts from the lower part of the node, the ventricles contract first.

In all the above-mentioned conditions, there is a "nodal rhythm by default"; only the lack of a descending impulse enables the A-V node to take over the pacemaking function. A different type of nodal rhythm occurs when there is such an increase of A-V node excitability that this center becomes the pacemaker even when the S-A node is normal. This form has been called "nodal rhythm by usurpation" (118) and has been already described (p. 332).

Signs and Symptoms

The patients are usually unaware of the disturbance but they may complain of limited physical efficiency or occasional dizziness.

The *pulse* is regular and slow, between 40 and 50.

Exertion, fever, changes in position, atropine, and epinephrine, may accelerate the pulse only to a very limited extent.

Graphic Tracings

Electrocardiogram. The electrocardiogram reveals a series of normal ventricular complexes. *The P wave is usually inverted and very near QRS,* a fact which is most apparent in leads 2, aVR, and aVL. The P wave may precede or follow QRS by about 0.05 second. Unusual course of the stimulus in the atrial walls (or coincidence of two independent rhythms) may cause the less common occurrence of *an upright P wave.* If the atrial contraction follows the ventricular by more than 0.2 second, a second ventricular contraction may follow, producing a *bigeminal rhythm* with one atrial wave between the two ventricular.

Phonocardiogram. The phonocardiogram shows that the atrial sound is missing and the first sound is prolonged.

X-Ray

Fluoroscopy may show large pulsations of the superior vena cava due to coincidence of the atrial and ventricular contractions (1).

Diagnosis

The diagnosis cannot be made with certainty without the ECG. The finding of an inverted P in leads 1 or 2 and of P-R which is below 0.15, is decisive.

Prognosis

No special prognosis can be made on the basis of nodal rhythm alone. This disturbance, however, frequently reveals the existence of myocardial lesions and should be considered together with the other signs of cardiac disturbance.

Treatment

No special treatment is necessary. In digitalis poisoning, the drug should be discontinued.

CORONARY SINUS RHYTHM

A special type of ectopic rhythm is *the coronary sinus rhythm* (148). This is originated in an area which is adjacent to and above the upper part of the A-V node. It is revealed by a normal or slightly short P-R interval and by P waves which are low in lead 1 and deeply inverted in leads 2 and 3. This rhythm is mostly exhibited by patients with organic heart lesions. The vagus nerve has an important action on the "coronary sinus center."

HEART BLOCK

Heart block is due to delay or interruption of the stimulus in the conducting system. There are two main types, the S-A block and the A-V block.[62]

SINOATRIAL BLOCK

Sinoatrial block may be incomplete or complete. Incomplete S-A block may present: 1) prolongation of the S-A conduction time; 2) progressive increase of S-A conduction followed by absence of a complete atrioventricular cycle; or 3) sudden absence of an atrioventricular cycle.

Complete S-A block may cause diastolic standstill of the whole heart or cause the shift of the pacemaker to a lower center (nodal rhythm, page 354).

Graphic Tracings

Electrocardiogram. Occasional S-A block. A regular series of normal P-QRS complexes is occasionally followed by a long diastolic

---

[62] Block occurring below the bifurcation of the bundle of His (bundle branch block) will not be included in this chapter as it causes *no change of pulse rate or rhythm.*

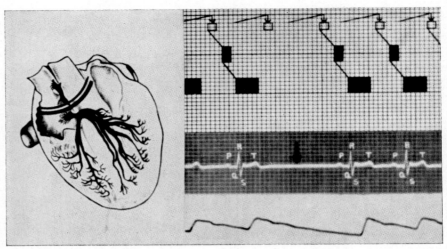

FIG. 225. *S-a block*. The arrow indicates the position of the missing atrioventricular sequence in the electrocardiogram.

pause. The length of the cycle, including this pause, is twice that of either the preceding or the following cycle (fig. 225).

Periodic S-A block: The P-QRS complexes are gradually more and more distant, being separated by gradually increasing diastolic pauses. After a certain number of them, a short diastole follows; the length of the short interval between Q and the following Q is equivalent to one-half of that of the immediately preceding interval and represents the only normal distance on which measurement should be based.

If the block occurs every second beat, the ECG simulates that of sinus bradycardia because no wave reveals the sinus impulses and the rate of the atria and ventricles is from 30 to 40. The disturbance is revealed only by the fact that, either spontaneously or after atropine, the rate suddenly doubles (from 40 to 80, from 35 to 70).

In certain tracings of S-A block, a second rhythm occurs during the long pause (*double rhythm type Rothberger*); this is revealed by complexes of a different shape, following each other at a more rapid rate.

Mechanism

Sinoatrial block is usually due to a functional disturbance. The view that this type of disturbance might be due to *periodic suspension* of the activity of the S-A node (48) and not to *periodic block* at the emergence of the stimulus (18) has been advocated. Animal experiments from the author's laboratory, however, have confirmed the second theory (49).

ATRIOVENTRICULAR BLOCK

Impaired conduction (block) of the stimulus between the S-A node and the A-V node; within the A-V node; or in the bundle of His, is the cause of this disturbance.

When the conducting tissues fail to transmit the excitation from the S-A node to the ventricles, a new pacemaker takes over the automatic functions; this may be located in the A-V node (nodal rhythm), in the bundle of His (septal rhythm), or in one of the ventricles (idioventricular rhythm). The block may be caused by: 1) a congenital lesion; 2) an inflammatory or degenerative lesion; 3) metastatic nodules; 4) areas of fibrosis (coronary heart disease); or 5) a functional or vascular disturbance of the conducting tissues.

Graphic Methods

Electrocardiogram. There are different types of tracings:

1) *Latent A-V block*, revealed by prolonga-

tion of the P-R interval up to 0.30 second (so-called *grade 1 A-V block*).

2) *Occasional A-V block*. Sporadically, a P wave is not followed by a ventricular complex.

3) *Periodic A-V block (type 1 of Wenckebach)* (18). The P waves have a regular succession; the P-R intervals gradually become longer until one P wave is not followed by a ventricular complex (*blocked P*). The entire cycle, from one normal P-QRS to the following normal, is called *the Luciani-Wenckebach period* (from the names of the authors who described it in animals and man) (fig. 226).

A curious type of tracing occurs at times in partial block; it has been called *interference dissociation*. The P and QRS waves have similar rates but no fixed relationship, so that P may either precede or follow QRS. From time to time, a seemingly normal P-QRS takes place through casual coincidence of the waves.

4) *Intermittent A-V block (type II of Wenckebach*, also known as *Mobitz type* of a-v block) (19, 101). Following two or three normal complexes, one P wave is blocked and there is no ventricular complex. In other words, there is the sudden occurrence of A-V block every two or three complete cycles but without the gradual changes of periodic A-V block.

5) *Complete A-V block*. While the previous types are also called *partial A-V block*, in other cases the block may be complete. The atrial waves have a normal rate (60 to 90) while the ventricular have a slow rate (10 to 40) and there is no relationship between the two. Two to five P waves may be present in the intervals between the QRS while some of them are superimposed on, or masked by, the ventricular complex. The blocked P waves often are followed by an afterdeflection called the T-atrial wave (*Ta wave*) which has the same meaning as the T wave of the ventricular complex (page 37). In *congenital block* the rate of

the ventricles may be faster (from 40 to 60) (44).

It is commonly stated that "bundle branch block frequently complicates A-V block". Actually, the idioventricular rhythm arises in one of the branches of the bundle of His so that the stimulus spreads first to the ipsilateral, then to the contralateral ventricle. The ventricular complexes resemble those of bundle branch block or paroxysmal ventricular tachycardia. There is some resemblance with ventricular tachycardia, except that, in A-V block, the phenomenon is caused "by default" and the rate is slow.

A *Stokes-Adams attack* is preceded by either increase or decrease of the atrial rate. During the attack, the ventricular rate may slow down further. On the other hand, there may be ventricular standstill, ventricular tachycardia, or ventricular flutter.

If the atrial rate is very slow and that of the ventricles is relatively rapid, the number of P waves becomes equivalent to that of the QRS complexes. Small, independent changes in rate of the two pacemakers modify the lengths of the P-R intervals. This singular phenomenon is called *isorhythmic dissociation*. This type of dissociation should be distinguished from the *A-V block with retrograde V-A conduction*. The latter presents atrial rate faster than the ventricular; absent or defective A-V conduction; and V-A conduction only after a short P-R interval (125).

Some patients present *occasional retrograde conduction* which is easily recognized because the retrograde P waves are inverted (143).

Phonocardiogram. Atrial sounds may be present during diastole. In general, *one dull sound* follows each P wave (fig. 227). In exceptional cases, an atrial contraction is followed by *two sounds* (45a, 50, 34); the second may be due to a vibration of the A-V valves (46). In an unusual case, three groups of vibrations were found for each

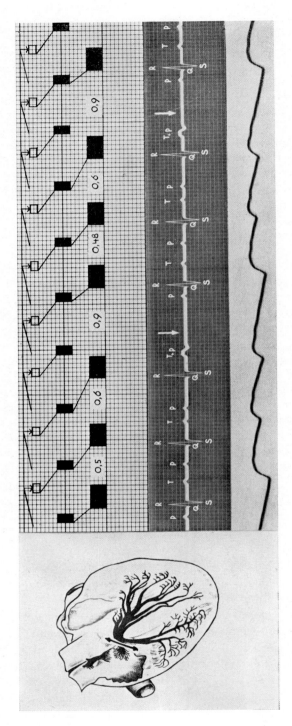

FIG. 226. Irregular pulse caused by *partial a-v block* with periodical absence of a ventricular contraction (arrow).

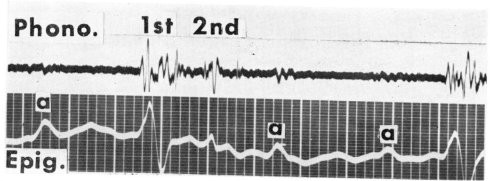

FIG. 227. *Complete A-V block.* Atrial sounds and atrial pulses (*a*), recorded between the ventricular contractions. Phonocardiogram and epigastric tracing.

P wave. The atrial sounds are louder in children and old people.

The vibrations of an *apical systolic murmur* are frequently recorded. Those of a *blowing apical diastolic murmur* coincident with the atrial contractions are recorded at times in elderly patients with a calcified mitral valve (102).

In cases of latent block, the first sound complex is of lower intensity (50). When atria and ventricles contract at the same time, a louder first sound is recorded (*cannon sound*).

Jugular tracing. The *a* waves are normal in shape and rate; and *c* and *v* waves occur at regular, but longer, intervals. Therefore, more than one *a* wave is found between a *v* wave and the next *c* wave. Occasional coincidence of an *a* wave with a *c* or *v* may occur, with a resulting higher wave.

Arterial tracing. A high and slow pulse is recorded. An anacrotic depression is fre-

quently present in the ascending branch of the curve (19). Multiple undulations follow the dicrotic wave. In occasional block, the tracings reveal the occasional absence of a pulse wave (*intermittence*). In periodic block, the series of pulse waves shows a periodic increase in the pause separating two pulses, then a longer pause with a deeper pressure drop. Interference dissociation may cause bigeminal rhythm, the second wave being paradoxically higher than the first.

Electrokymography. If atrial contraction falls during the ventricular systole, the atria decrease in volume as in normal subjects. If the atrial contraction falls during ventricular diastole, the pattern consists of an oblique descending line during atrial contraction, and a less steep rise subsequent to it (fig. 228).

X-Ray

The normal rate of the atria and the slow rate of the ventricles are apparent both on

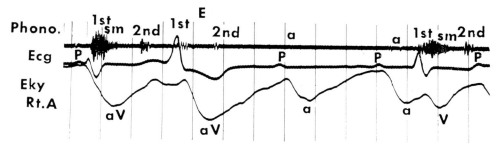

FIG. 228. Phonocardiogram and electrokymogram of the right atrial border in a case of *complete a-v block* with premature ventricular contractions.

fluoroscopy and roentgenkymography (41, 42). The ventricles dilate in successive steps coincident with the atrial contractions, then empty at once when ventricular systole takes place.

Blood Pressure—Cardiac Output

The systolic pressure is usually increased; the diastolic pressure is low; a high pulse pressure is the result.

Cardiac output is normal when the patient is at rest but its increase during exercise is far below average (128).

Cause and Mechanism—Lesions

Impaired conduction (block) of the stimulus between the sinoatrial node and the bundle of His or in the latter is the cause of this syndrome. This failure of the conducting tissues would cause death if a new pacemaker would not take over the automatic functions: this pacemaker is located in the A-V node (nodal rhythm), in the bundle of His (septal rhythm), or in one of the ventricles (idioventricular rhythm).

Different causes may initiate the block:

a) A *congenital lesion* (35, 107b). In these cases, there usually is a complete block, due to imperfect development of the bundle of His, and there is a frequent association with a ventricular septal defect. However, extremely rare cases of partial block have been reported.

b) *An inflammatory or degenerative lesion*, due to rheumatic disease, syphilis, tuberculosis, diphtheria, typhoid fever or pneumonia. Aschoff's nodules, gummata, tubercles, or nonspecific inflammatory areas may be present.

c) *Metastatic nodules*.

d) *Areas of fibrosis*. These may be found in patients with coronary heart disease (vascular lesions) or in patients with congenital heart disease (nutritional disorders).

e) *No visible lesion*. In such cases a functional disturbance of the conducting tissue or the supplying arterioles is admitted.

All the above-mentioned lesions may be located in the region of the A-V node or immediately above it, as well as in the bundle of His. However, they are occasionally located in a widespread area of the atria. Functional disorders may be favored by *digitalis poisoning*.

Even when there is a myocardial lesion, functional elements contribute to the occurrence of the block. This is proven by disappearance of a block following administration of drugs or change of position of the patient.

The hearts of these patients are, as a rule, *dilated* and *hypertrophied* as a result of the long-lasting low rate (128).

Signs and Symptoms

There may be no symptoms. However, the patients usually complain of *weakness*, *exertional dyspnea*, and *dizziness*. They may also suffer from *nausea*.

Certain patients complain of *sudden attacks of vertigo or syncope* and occasionally of *convulsive seizures*. These are called *Stokes-Adams attacks*.

The patients are *pale*. Their *pulse* is regular but *extremely slow*. It has been called *pulsus solemnis* because the interval between one pulse and the next is extremely long and the volume of the pulse wave is proportionately large. *The pulse rate is between 15 and 40* in typical cases.

In cases with *occasional block*, palpation of the radial artery reveals that, once in a while, one pulsation is missing (*pulsus intermittens*). In *periodic block*, the same phenomenon occurs but its recurrence is regular, once every 3, 4, or 5 pulses.

The *jugular veins* show rapid pulsations in the interval between one radial pulsation and the next.

Auscultation of the heart often reveals normal heart sounds. However, *phasic variations of the sounds* have been described. When the atria and ventricles contract simultaneously, a louder and sharper 1st sound is heart (*cannon sound*). A *soft blowing systolic murmur* is frequently heard at the apex. *Multiple sounds of poor intensity* may be heard during the long diastole. However, this finding is rare. *Blowing, apical diastolic murmurs,* coincident with the atrial contractions, have been described.

During the attacks, different phenomena may occur:

a) The pulse *slows down further* to 15, or even 10 per minute (1, 39). Rare cases where the pulse slows down temporarily to 1 or 2 per minute have been described (1).

b) There is a complete absence of the pulse because of either *ventricular standstill* or *ventricular flutter* (39, 40).

c) The pulse continues *at the same rate* as before the attack (39).

Mode of Origin of the Signs

The A-V block is frequently due to anatomical interruption of the conducting tissues. Microscopic studies often reveal a lesion which, in spite of its limited extension, causes severe results because of its location across the essential pathway connecting the atria with the ventricles. This is true chiefly in cases of *complete A-V block*. When the block is *partial,* a functional disturbance is involved, even if anatomical lesions also occur. In such cases, decreased excitability and longer refractory period of the conducting tissues are present. This may cause the lack of response to every 2nd (or 2nd and 3rd) stimulus, thus resulting in the regular absence of ventricular responses.

The site of the lesion is important in the determination of the ventricular rate. A pacemaker located in the bundle of His is able to maintain a rate of 25 to 35. A pacemaker located in the upper part of the stems is able only to maintain rates of 15 to 25. Lesions of the stems cause the occurrence of a lower pacemaker with a rate of 7 to 15 per minute.

Knowledge that stimulation of the vagus may cause A-V block in experimental animals led to *emphasis on vagal stimulation* as a factor favoring A-V block and causing Stokes-Adams attacks. There is no doubt that vagal stimulation should be avoided in these patients. However, the attacks may be preceded by either *a faster* (sympathetic stimulation) or a *slower atrial rate* (vagal stimulation) (52). The former may favor the attack by shortening diastole; the latter by directly impairing the conduction.

In complete block, the cardiac nerves are undoubtedly less effective but they can still influence the A-V node either directly or through the coronary arteries.

In certain cases, the attack is precipitated by *ventricular tachycardia, ventricular fibrillation,* or *ventricular standstill* (129).

In most cases, the attacks are more frequent and severe during the stage of incomplete block. Once complete block is established, the attacks are usually less frequent (54). In the former stage, the pacemaking function of the A-V node (or of lower areas) is suddenly required; in the latter, such function has already developed.

The fact that the hearts of these patients cannot increase their ventricular rates when called to increase their output represents a definite burden. Both this fact and the poor coronary flow caused by low diastolic pressure, favor heart failure.

The frequent occurrence of rhythms 1:1, 2:1 or 3:1 in complete heart block, a phenomenon which may temporarily disappear after exertion, indicates a series of mechanical and electrical interreactions between atria and ventricles which influences the two independent pacemakers (130). On the other hand, it has been shown that a slight irregularity of the atrial rate is not uncommon. This seems to be due to the fact that the increase of arterial pressure connected with ventricular systole acts on carotid sinus and aortic receptors and causes a reflex slowing of the atrial rate (131).

Varieties—Course and Complications

Latent block. This type, revealed only by the ECG, may be congenital, rheumatic, toxic (digitalis), or arteriosclerotic. It may gradually become more serious until A-V block develops.

Congenital block is usually complete, and is associated in two-thirds of the cases with ventricular septal defect (55). It is present from birth and is usually benign and well tolerated. The ventricular rate is faster than in acquired cases (44).

Block due to acute myocarditis is more serious than other types. Patients with acute rheumatic disease often present A-V block and occasional S-A block. They are liable to die suddenly because the inflammatory process inhibits the automatic properties of the A-V node and bundle of His.

A-V block may start after a *myocardial infarction*. It may cause death.

Unstable block is a type of block which frequently changes from partial to complete and vice versa (56).

Paroxysmal heart block is that occurring in attacks (57, 58); between them, the electrocardiogram is normal, having either a normal or a prolonged P-R (*latent block*).

Postural block. Certain patients with either incomplete or complete block in the supine position present a normal ventricular rate with prolonged A-V conduction when sitting (124).

Zeri's syndrome (59). This is a curious variety where the slow ventricular contractions and the respiratory movements occur at the same time (fig. 229). Exertion temporarily increases the respiratory rate but soon afterwards the synchronism is re-established (602). The syndrome seems more common than previously thought.

Diagnosis

Diagnosis is easy when the pulse is below 40 per minute. It may be difficult when the pulse is faster, as in many congenital cases. Then only the ECG permits an exact diagnosis. Recognition of the cause is important but not always possible. The localization is revealed by the ventricular rate because the lower the lesion, the slower the rate.

The cause and mechanism of the attacks may be studied by the following tests: atropine test, amyl nitrite test, exertion test, position test, and vagal stimulation (compression of the eyeballs or of the carotid sinus). The electrocardiogram should be recorded during these tests and also during an attack, if possible. The results of the tests and the changes of atrial rate *before* an attack indicate whether a coronary or a neurogenic cause is involved, also which autonomic stimuli are responsible for the attack.

Congenital heart block occasionally has been recognized during fetal life on the basis of slow fetal heart sounds (95). Phonocardiographic tracings may give a proof of this disturbance which can only be suspected upon fetal auscultation.

Prognosis

Heart block is always a serious condition but some patients may live for many years

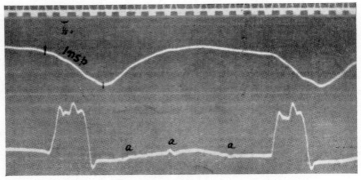

FIG. 229. *Complete A-V block* with cardiorespiratory synchronism. Respiratory tracing, apex cardiogram

in fairly good health. Stokes-Adams attacks are present in about one-half of the cases with complete block, and indicate a more severe prognosis, especially if they are of long duration. About one-half of the patients having Stokes-Adams attacks *die suddenly*; the other usually expire in *congestive failure*.

Treatment

Prevention of the attacks is important. If they are due to vagal stimuli, *atropine* (**21**) is indicated; if the vagus acts through a vascular mechanism, *atropine plus ephedrine* or *atropine plus papaverine* may be helpful. If they are due to sympathetic stimuli, *digitalis* or *barium chloride* may be used.

When frequent premature beats occur and ventricular flutter is feared, *pronestyl* (**27**) should be given.

Cases with coronary heart disease may benefit from the use of *atropine plus aminophylline* or *atropine plus papaverine*. These drugs act more by preventing sudden attacks than by changing the usual ventricular rate.

Rhythmic percussion of the precordial area can be tried during Stokes-Adams attacks. When ventricular flutter occurs, *intracardiac adrenalin* may be tried but only at the time of the standstill which follows the attack. Otherwise the flutter would become a fibrillation with a rapidly fatal result (page 396).

BIBLIOGRAPHY

1. WHITE, P. D. *Heart Disease*. New York, Macmillan, 1944.
2. GALLAVARDIN, L. *La Tension Artérielle en Clinique*. Paris, Masson, 1921.
3. MacWILLIAM, J. A. J. Physiol., 1887, **8**, 296.
4. BARKER, P. S., WILSON, F. N., AND JOHNSTON, F. D. Am. Heart J., 1943, **26**, 455.
5. DECHERD, G. M., AND co-workers. Am. Heart J., 1945, **29**, 20.
6. BATTRO, A. *Las Arritmias en Clinica*. Buenos Aires, El Ateneo, 1937.
7. BENNETT, D. W., AND KERR, W. J. Heart, 1932, **16**, 109.
8. LIAN, C., AND WELTI, J. J. Arch. Mal. Coeur, 1938, **31**, 518.
9. CALO, A. Cardiol., 1939, **3**, 203.
10. HECHT, H. H., AND MYERS, G. B. Am. Heart J., 1945, **29**, 610.
11. HOLZMANN, M., AND co-workers. *Lehrbuch der Roentgendiagnostik*. Leipzig, Thieme, 1932.
12. ROESLER, H. *Clinical Roentgenology of the Cardiovascular System*. Springfield, Thomas, 1943.
13. LUDWIG, H. Roentgenpraxis, 1936, **8**, 731.
14. LUISADA, A. A. Cuore e Circ. (Rome), 1935, **19**, 77. Also J. Lab. & Clin. Med., 1940, **25**, 1146.
15. a) BRISTOWE, J. S. Brain, 1887, **10**, 164.
    b) BOUVERET, L. Rév. de Méd., 1889, **9**, 753.
16. a) HUBBARD, J. P. Am. J. Dis. Child., 1941, **61**, 687.
    b) COSSIO, P., VEDOYA, R., AND BERCONSKY, I. Rev. Arg. Card., 1944, **11**, 149.
    c) GEIGER, A. J. Am. Heart J., 1943, **26**, 555.
17. a) CAMPBELL, M. Brit. Heart J., 1942, **4**, 49.
    b) CURRIE, C. M. Brit. Heart J., 1942, **4**, 149.
    c) EISAMAN, J. L. Am. Heart J., 1945, **30**, 401.
18. WENCKEBACH, K. F., AND WINTERBERG, H. *Die Unregelmaessige Herztaetigkeit*. Leipzig, Engelmann, 1927.
19. LUISADA, A. A. Arch. Mal. Coeur, 1927, **20**, 65.
20. WEYLER, H., AND DUSTIN, C. C. New England J. Med., 1942, **227**, 733.
21. a) WOLFF, L. New England J. Med., 1945, **232**, 491.
    b) WOLFF, L. New England J. Med., 1945, **232**, 527.
22. MILLER, R., AND PERLMAN, J. S. Am. Heart J., 1945, **29**, 555.
23. LEYS, D. Arch. Dis. Child., 1945, **20**, 44.
24. a) TANDOWSKY, R. M. Am. Heart J., 1945, **29**, 71.
    b) WEISBERGER, A. A., AND FEIL, H. Am. Heart J., 1947, **34**, 871.
25. LEVINE, S. A. Am. Heart J., 1927, **3**, 177.
26. GALLAVARDIN, L. Arch. Mal. Coeur, 1920, **13**, 207; and 1922, **15**, 298.
27. FROMENT, R. *Les Tachycardies Paroxystiques Ventriculaires*. Paris, Masson, 1932.
28. FISCHER, R. Wien. Arch. inn. Med., 1934, **25**, 469.
29. DOGLIOTTI, G. C., MONTUSCHI, E., AND BERETTA, A. Cuore e Circ., 1937, **21**, 265.
30. CALABRESI, M. Atti e Mem. Soc. Lomb. Med. (Milan), 1934, **2**, N. 12.
31. HEPBURN, J., AND RYKERT, H. E. Am. Heart J., 1937, **14**, 620.
32. CHAPMAN, D. W. Am. Heart J., 1945, **30**, 276.

33. SCHERF, D., AND BOYD, L. J. Am. J. M. Sci., 1943, **206,** 43.

34. CONDORELLI, L. Min. Med., 1928, **8,** (pt. 1) 1343 and (pt. 2) 343.

35. MORQUIO, M. L. Semaine Méd., 1901, **21,** 398.

36. MORGAGNI, G. B. *De Sedibus et Causis Morborum,* 1761; translated in *Cardiac Classics,* St. Louis, Mosby, 1941.

37. ADAMS, R. Dublin Hosp. Reports, 1827; reprinted in *Cardiac Classics,* St. Louis, Mosby, 1941.

38. STOKES, W. *The Diseases of the Heart and the Aorta.* Dublin, Hodges and Smith, 1854.

39. CALABRESI, M. Clin. Med. Ital., 1931, **62,** 331 and 646; and 1932, **63,** 27.

40. CONDORELLI, L. Arch. Sci. Med., 1932, **56**:

41. PERONA, P. Cuore e Circ., 1935, **19,** 2.

42. BATTRO, A., AND BRAUN MÉNANDEZ, E. Rev. Arg. Card., 1934, **3,** 199.

43. CAMPBELL, M. Brit. Heart J., 1943, **5,** 163.

44. CAMPBELL, M. Brit. Heart J., 1943, **5,** 15.

45. LEWIS, TH. a) *Lectures on the Heart.* New York, Hoeber, 1915. b) *The Mechanism and Graphic Registration of the Heart Beat.* London, Shaw, 1925.

46. COSSIO, P., BERCONSKY, I., AND TRIMANI, A. Rev. Arg. Card., 1942, **9,** 238.

47. LUISADA, A. A., AND MAUTNER, H. Exper. Med., Surg., 1943, **1,** 282.

48. LEWIS, TH. Quart. J. Med., 1921, **14,** 339.

49. RUBINO, A. Cuore e Circ. (Rome), 1935, **19,** 701.

50. WOLFERTH, C. C., AND MARGOLIES, A. In *Stroud's Cardiovascular Disease.* Philadelphia, Davis, 1945.

51. a) SCHERF, D. Wien. Arch. inn. Med., 1926, **12,** 327; and 1929, **18,** 403.
    b) SCHELLONG, F. Deut. med. Woch., 1926, **52,** 862.

52. CONDORELLI, L. *Patogenesi e Terapia della Sindrome di Morgagni-Adams-Stokes.* Naples, Idelson, 1933.

53. VAQUEZ, H. *Les Maladies du Coeur.* Paris, Baillière, 1928.

54. GALLAVARDIN, L. Arch. Mal. Coeur, 1914, **7,** 171.

55. JALESKI, C., AND MORRISON, E. T. Am. J. M. Sci., 1943, **206,** 449.

56. SABATHIÉ, L. G., AND GASPARI, F. V. Rev. Arg. Card., 1944, **11,** 215.

57. COMEAU, W. J. Am. J. M. Sci., 1937, **194,** 43.

58. CAMPBELL, M. Brit. Heart J., 1944, **6,** 69.

59. ZERI, A. Rif. Med., 1903, **19,** 701.

60. a) LUISADA, A. A. Min. Med., 1928 (p. 2), **8,** 913.

b) RASARIO, G. M. Cuore e Circ., 1940, **24,** 217.

61. CONDORELLI, L. Rass. Ter., Pat. Clin., 1930, **2,** 422.

62. LUCIANI, L. *Fisiologia dell' Uomo.* Milano, S. E. L., 1923.

63. ANTOINE, T. Zeit. Geburtsch., Gynaek., 1926, **90,** 112.

64. SCHERF, D., AND BOYD, L. J. *Clinical Electrocardiography.* St. Louis, Mosby, 1940.

65. CALABRESI, M. *Elettrocardiografia Clinica.* Bologna, Cappelli, 1935.

66. BARKER, P. S., MACLEOD, A. G., ALEXANDER, J., AND WILSON, F. N. Am. Heart J., 1930, **5,** 720.

67. BATTRO, A. *Las Arritmias en Clinica.* Buenos Aires, El Ateneo, 1937.

68. CASTEX, M. R., BATTRO, A., AND GONZÁLES, R. Arch. Int. Med., 1941, **67,** 76.

69. WEYLER, H. Am. Heart J., 1944, **27,** 409.

70. KISCH, B. Exper. Med., Surg., 1945, **3,** 191.

71. COSSIO, P. *Semeiologia del Apáráto Circulatorio.* Buenos Aires, El Ateneo, 1946.

72. LIAN, C., AND GOMES, V. Arch. Mal. Coeur, 1931, **24,** 721.

73. LEWIS, T. Brit. M. J., 1909, **2,** 1528.

74. ROTHBERGER, C. J., AND WINTERBERG, H. Wien. klin. Woch., 1909, **22,** 839.

75. LEWIS, T., DRURY, A. N., AND ILIESEN, C. C. Heart, 1921, **8,** 361.

76. a) SCHERF, D., AND SIEDECK, H. Zeit. exp. Med., 1935, **96,** 311.
    b) SCHERF, D. Zeit. Kreislauff., 1928, **20,** 432.

77. a) LAUFER, S. Arch. Mal. Coeur, 1935, **28,** 98.
    b) LAUFER, S., AND RUBINO, A. Clin. Med. Ital. (Milan), 1936, **67,** 365.

78. SOSSAI, A. Cuore e Circ. (Rome), 1938, **22,** 441.

79. CONDORELLI, L. Minerva Med., 1935, **26** (pt. 1), 73.

80. GARREY, W. E., AND KING, C. E. Am. J. Physiol., 1941, **133,** 288.

81. NYBOER, J., AND HAMILTON, J. G. M. Brit. Heart J., 1940, **2,** 263.

82. DE CASTRO, O. Arch. Mal. Coeur, 1934, **27,** 282.

83. FERREIRA, O. Presse Méd., 1935, **43,** 260.

84. PICCHINI, G. Cuore e Circ., 1934, **18,** 713.

85. DAGNINI, G. Cuore e Circ., 1937, **21,** 571.

86. LUISADA, A. A. Am. Heart J., 1941, **22,** 245.

87. COSSIO, P., AND BERCONSKY, I. Rev. Arg. Card., 1943, **10,** 162.

88. PAZZANESE, D. *Modificaçoes de Forma do Electrocardiograma.* Saõ Paulo, Gráfica de Prefeitura, 1942.

89. Gibson, S. J. A. M. A., 1941, **117,** 96.
90. Rosenbaum, F. F., and Levine, S. A. Am. J. M. Sci., 1939, **198,** 774.
91. White, P. D. Arch. Int. Med., 1916, **18,** 244.
92. Mobitz, W. Deut. Arch. klin. Med., 1923, **141,** 257.
93. Rothberger, C. J., and Winterberg, H. Pflueger's Arch., 1912, **146,** 385.
94. Fischer, R. Wien. Arch. inn. Med., 1934, **25,** 469.
95. Geiger, C. J., and Hines, L. E. J. A. M. A., 1940, **115,** 2272.
96. Smith, J. R., and Wilson, K. S. Am. Heart J., 1944, **27,** 176.
97. Altschule, M. D. New England J. Med., 1945, **233,** 265.
98. Nahum, L. H., and Hoff, H. E. J. A. M. A., 1935, **105,** 254.
99. Askey, J. M., and Neurath, O. Am. Heart J., 1945, **30,** 253.
100. Hoff, H. E. In *Howell's Textbook of Physiology.* Philadelphia, Saunders, 1946.
101. Mobitz, W. Zeit. exp. Med., 1924, **41,** 180; and Zeit. klin. Med., 1928, **107,** 456.
102. Rytand, D. A. Am. Heart J., 1946, **32,** 579.
103. Gonzales Sabathié, L. Am. Heart J., 1947, **33,** 719.
104. Mannheimer, E. Acta Ped., 1946, **33,** 383.
105. Wilburne, M., Surtshin, A., Rodbard, S., and Katz, L. N. Am. Heart J., 1947, **34,** 860.
106. Lian, C., Welti, J. J., and co-workers. Paris Méd., 1947, **37,** 191; and Arch. Mal. Coeur, 1947, **40,** 140.
107. a) Graybiel, A., and White, P. D. Am. Heart J., 1935, **10,** 345.
    b) Campbell, M., and Elliott, S. A. Brit. Heart J., 1939, **1,** 122.
108. a) Cossio, P., and co-workers. Rev. Arg. Card., 1941, **8,** 168; and 1944, **9,** 164.
    b) Etala, F., and Berreta, J. M. Rev. Arg. Card., 1948, **15,** 133.
109. Garvin, J. A., and Kline, E. M. Am. Heart J., 1947, **33,** 362.
110. Solarz, S. A. Ann. Int. Med., 1947, **27,** 447.
111. Chapman, E. M., and co-workers: J. A. M. A., 1948, **137,** 580.
112. Cossio, P. Rev. Arg. Card., 1938, **5,** 242.
113. a) Taquini, A. C. Am. Heart J., 1947, **33,** 719.
    b) Scherf, D. Proc. Soc. Exper. Biol. & Med., 1948, **67,** 59.
114. Tandowsky, R. M., and co-workers. Am. Heart J., 1946, **32,** 617.
115. Gonzales, M. M. Rev. Exp. Card., 1947, **1,** 143.

116. a) Scherf, D. Ztschr. exp. Med., 1926, **51,** 816; 1928, **61,** 30; and 1929, **65,** 198.
    b) Scherf, D., Romano, F. J., and Terranova, R. Am. Heart J., 1948, **36,** 241. Also Am. J. Physiol., 1949, **159,** 137.
    c) Scherf, D. Am. Heart J., 1949, **37,** 1069.
    d) Scherf, D. Arch. Int. Med., 1953, **91,** 333.
117. Harvey, W. P., and Levine, S. A. Am. Heart J., 1948, **35,** 924.
118. Ashman, R., and Hull, E. *Essentials of Electrocardiography.* New York, Macmillan, 1944.
119. a) Rosenbaum, F. F., and Levine, S. A. Am. J. M. Sci., 1939, **198,** 774.
    b) Chavez, I., Brumlik, J., and Sodi Pallares, D. Arch. Inst. Card. Mexico, 1946, **16,** 159.
120. Gonzales Sabathié, L., and Gaspary, F. Am. Heart J., 1947, **33,** 720.
121. Altana, G. Folia Card. (Milan), 1947, **6,** 1.
122. McMillan, W. L., and Welfare, C. R. J. A. M. A., 1947, **135,** 1132.
123. Haunz, E. A., and Smith, H. L. Am. J. Med., 1948, **4,** 237.
124. Stein, I. Am. J. M. Sci., 1946, **212,** 604.
125. Winternitz, M., and Langendorf, R. Am. Heart J., 1944, **27,** 301.
126. Cossio, P. Am. Heart J., 1947, **33,** 707.
127. Pánek, J. Časopis Lékařu Ceských (Prague), 1947, **86,** 423.
128. Stollbreiter, H. Klin. Woch., 1947, **24/25,** 257.
129. Schnur, S. Am. Heart J., 1948, **35,** 298.
130. Seghers, M., Lequime, J., and Denolin, H. Am. Heart J., 1947, **33,** 685.
131. Roth, I. R., and Kisch, B. Am. Heart J., 1948, **36,** 257.
132. Butterworth, S., and Poindexter, C. A. Am. Heart J., 1946, **32,** 681.
133. Langendorf, R., and Mintz, S. A. Brit. Heart J., 1946, **8,** 178.
134. Froment, R., and Gallavardin, L. Arch. Mal. Coeur, 1948, **41,** 113.
135. Contro, S. Cuore e Circ., 1953, **37,** 1.
136. Contro, S., and Luisada, A. A. J. Mount Sinai Hosp. of New York, 1952, **19,** 70.
137. Messer, A. L., Counihan, T. B., Rappaport, M. B., and Sprague, H. B. Circ., 1951, **4,** 576.
138. Vedoya, R., *et al.* Rev. Arg. Card., 1951, **18,** 77.
139. Rattigan, J. P., *et al.* New England J. Med., 1952, **246,** 150.
140. Brodie, B. B., *et al.* J. Pharmacol. & Exper. Therap., 1948, **94,** 359; and 1950, **98,** 21.

141. Daines, M. C., and Hecht, H. H. Am. Federation Clin. Research (Am. J. Med., 1951, **11**).

142. a) Enselberg, C. D., *et al.* Am. Heart J., 1950, **39,** 703 and 713.
   b) Szekely, P., and Wynne, N. A. Clin. Sci., 1951, **10,** 241.

143. Gallavardin, L., *et al.* Arch. Mal coeur, 1950, **43,** 114.

144. Lenzi, F., and Lenzi, S. Cardiol. (Basel), 1949, **14,** 21.

145. Rasario, G. M. Rif. Med. (Naples), 1948 (No. 27).

146. Prinzmetal, M., *et al.* J. A. M. A., 1951. **146,** 1275.

147. Luisada, A. A., and Pérez Montés, L. Ann. Int. Med., 1950, **33,** 56.

148. Scherf, D., and Harris, R. Am. Heart J., 1946, **32,** 443.

149. Hansen, W. R. Am. Heart J., 1952, **44,** 499.

150. Kistin, A. D., and Landowne, M. Circ., 1951, **3,** 738.

CHAPTER 17

Clinical Syndromes Due to Diffuse Myocardial Lesions

Atrophy of the Heart (131)

Atrophy of the heart is encountered in clinical cases with extreme wasting due to neoplasms, chronic infections, degenerative and metabolic diseases, or starvation. Prolonged illness, long permanence in bed, surgical procedures and chronic digestive disturbances are considered as predisposing conditions.

Atrophy may be *simple*, with an average cardiac weight of 200 grams. One-half of the cases, however, present a *brown atrophy* with deposition of pigment in the muscle fibers, and a slightly higher average weight.

The atrophic heart is normal or small in size; has a *regular rhythm* and a *slow rate*; and may present a faint, short, apical or midprecordial *systolic murmur*. Blood pressure is frequently low, but it may be normal or even high.

The *electrocardiogram* presents decreased voltage of all waves and a prolonged Q-T interval. Congestive failure is uncommon, possibly on account of the reduced metabolism.

An atrophic heart should be differentiated from a normal "small heart". The latter is found in asthenic but otherwise normal persons; it is associated with a narrow chest, and is usually a "vertical" heart. On the contrary, the atrophic heart is more horizontal (124).

Cardiac Enlargement—Ventricular Strain

Cardiac enlargement is a common finding in heart disease and may be due to one of the following causes:

a) *A valvular lesion or malformation* placing strain on one, two, or more cardiac chambers (rheumatic or bacterial valvular lesions, congenital heart disease).

b) *A persistent increase of resistance* in the vessels of either the lesser or the greater circulation, placing a strain on one of the ventricles (hypertensive heart disease, pulmonary heart disease).

c) *A diffuse structural lesion or functional disturbance* of the cardiac muscle due to inflammation or degeneration, metabolic or endocrine disturbance, or vitamin deficiency.

d) *A diffuse lesion of the coronary system* causing impairment of the blood supply to the heart (coronary heart disease).

In the above mentioned possibilities, cardiac enlargement is due to both *dilatation* and *hypertrophy*.

Cardiac hypertrophy may be an indirect cause of failure because the hypertrophic myocardium has a smaller number of capillaries per cubic mm. (84). This ultimately leads to *ischemia*, decreased nutrition, and anoxia of the muscle fibers. In advanced cardiac hypertrophy, all values of essential chemical components of the cardiac muscle (creatine, phosphorus, and potassium) have been found decreased, a fact which may be conducive to heart failure (85). Ischemia favors *fibrosis of the cardiac muscle* and this is usually accompanied by lesion of the intraventricular conducting tissues.

The following sequence is frequently observed: hypertrophy, ischemia, diffuse fibrosis, i. v. block or bundle branch block (especially on the left side).

The term *ventricular strain*, first coined as an electrocardiographic expression, has been replaced in ECG interpretation by the term "ischemia" while it still has a definite mechanical connotation.

ELECTROCARDIOGRAM

General data indicating ventricular hypertrophy are (128, 129):

1) High voltage in the limb leads (unipolar and standard), due to increased thickness of the ventricular wall.

2) Marked axis deviation, due to increased surface and thickness of one ventricle.

3) Increased duration of QRS (0.10–0.11 second) because longer time is required for the stimulus to reach the epicardial surface of the thickened ventricular wall.

4) Delay between beginning of the complex and intrinsicoid deflection in the chest leads of the hypertrophied side due to same mechanism.

5) Secondary changes of S-T and T. Following an altered course of depolarization, ventricular repolarization of the hypertrophied ventricle begins after that of the normal ventricle. However, measurements of the ventricular gradient indicate that there may also be primary changes of T due to relative ischemia.

Left ventricular hypertrophy is usually

TABLE 18A. *Left ventricular hypertrophy with vertical heart**

LEAD	PATTERN OF ECG
V1–V4	rS; slightly elevated ST segment; upright T waves
V5–V6	qR; depressed ST segment; *inverted T waves*; slight delay of the intrinsicoid deflection
aVR	QS or rS deflection with *diphasic or inverted T waves*
aVL	QS or rR and upright T waves
aVF	qR with depressed ST segment and *downward T*

* In these cases, the standard leads may show right axis deviation with depressed ST and downward T waves in 2 and 3.

TABLE 18B. *Left ventricular hypertrophy with horizontal position and counterclockwise rotation of the heart*

LEAD	PATTERN OF ECG
V1–V2	rS or QS; slightly elevated ST segment; upright T
V3–V6	qR; depressed ST segment; *downward T waves*; slight delay of the intrinsicoid deflection
aVR	rS or AS; downward T waves
aVL	qR; depressed ST segment; *downward T waves*
aVF	rS; upright T waves

TABLE 18C. *Left ventricular hypertrophy with horizontal position and marked clockwise rotation of the heart*

LEAD	PATTERN OF ECG
V1–V6	rS deflection; slightly elevated ST segment; upright T waves
aVR	QR, downward T waves
aVL	Qr, depressed ST segment, *downward T waves*
aVF	rS, upright T waves

accompanied by a marked left axis deviation;[63] this is easily evaluated by the White-Bock index which is above +17 mm.[64] If there is hypertrophy of the septum, there may be a deep Q wave in the chest leads (fig. 230).

The ECG details vary with the position of the heart and are summarized in table 18.

The pattern of *right ventricular hypertrophy* is not easily schematized because it may be caused by various clinical conditions. Several pictures have been described:

1) Normal electrocardiogram, due to the predominance of the left ventricle in spite of a moderate right ventricular hypertrophy.

2) There is right axis deviation, revealed

[63] This deviation is absent in the "vertical" heart.

[64] The *White-Bock index* is found by using the formula: (R1 + S3) − (S1 + R3).

by the fact that the White-Bock index is less than −14. R has a high voltage in V1–V2 (7 mm. or more) while there is an S with a high voltage in V5–V6 (7 mm. or more). Thus the ratio $\dfrac{(\text{R–S}) \text{ in V5}}{(\text{R–S}) \text{ in V1}} = 0.4$ or less. There may be evidence of associated right atrial hypertrophy.

(3 An average picture of right ventricular hypertrophy is summarized in table 18D and is schematized in figure 231.

4) There is an additional focal block of the right side (pages 376 and 379). The right chest leads have an rSR′ or rsR′ pattern and an inverted T. There are no further changes of the limb leads due to the focal block.

Atrial hypertrophy is revealed by changes of the axis of P, as well as by changes of its duration and configuration. Two patterns have been recognized: 1) Pattern of *right atrial hypertrophy*, encountered in chronic cor pulmonale and in congenital heart disease. There is *high voltage of P in 2, 3,* and aVF while V1 and V2 present a P wave made of a high positive phase followed by a brief and pointed negative phase.

2) Pattern of *left atrial hypertrophy,* encountered in mitral valve lesions. There is a notched P in 1 and aVL and a *diphasic* P with deep and broad negative phase, in 3 and aVF. V1 and V2 present a P wave having *a deep and broad negative phase.*

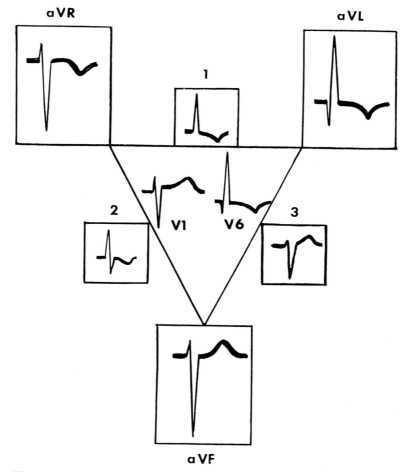

FIG. 230. Electrocardiograms in left ventricular hypertrophy with anterolateral ischemia (hypertensive heart disease).

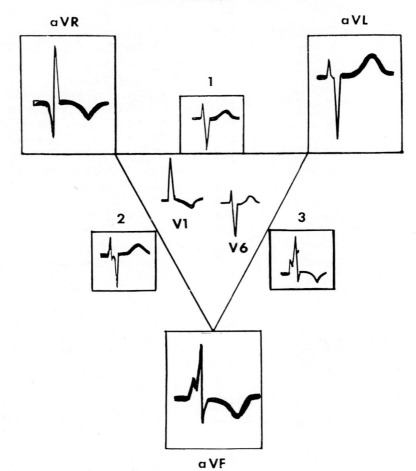

Fig. 231. Electrocardiograms in right ventricular hypertrophy (chronic cor pulmonale)

In both patterns, P lasts more than 0.10 second.

Low frequency tracings. Enlargement of one of the ventricles may be revealed by low frequency tracings (122).

TABLE 18D. *Marked right ventricular hypertrophy*

LEAD	PATTERN OF ECG
V4R, V1 (possibly V2)	R or Rs; depressed ST segment; inverted T waves
V5–V6	RS; normal ST segment: upright T waves
aVR	QR or qR; inverted T wave
aVL	rS, upright T wave; or QR, *inverted* T waves
aVF	rS or QR; *inverted* T *waves*

1) Left ventricular hypertrophy is revealed by a high, often plateau-like, positive thrust *at the apex*; at the same time, the epigastric tracing has a negative thrust.

2) Right ventricular hypertrophy is revealed by a high, early systolic thrust *at the epigastrium* while the apical tracing has a negative thrust.

3) A *large atrial wave* may be observed in either of the above two tracings and is evidence of increased atrial pressure.

Triple and Quadruple Rhythms of the Heart

The names *triple rhythm* and *quadruple rhythm* have been suggested (120) to indicate those cadences which are due to addition of one or two diastolic sounds to the more commonly heard two heart sounds. Older and well-known names were *gallop rhythm* (5) and *train-wheel rhythm* (6). The new definition is more comprehensive and includes several possibilities which were not considered in the older ones.

As already mentioned (pages 41 and 90), the normal heart may have four sounds. The two loudest are the first and second sounds, at the beginning and end of ventricular systole (*systolic sounds*); the other two, of less intensity, occur during ventricular diastole in coincidence with the phases of rapid filling of the ventricles. They are the third sound and the fourth, or atrial sound (*diastolic sounds*). They are usually inaudible in adults with the exceptions of persons with a flat, thin chest, who may have an audible third sound.

Until recently, a *triple rhythm* (gallop) was considered as a purely auditory phenomenon (152). However, phonocardiography has revealed that, in certain cases with a triple rhythm, the diastolic sound is inaudible because it is weak, low-pitched, or near the first sound (123). It has been suggested to consider "more pathological" any case having a diastolic sound with the following graphic characteristics: 1) frequency of vibrations of 30 or more per second, irrespective of its amplitude; 2) amplitude greater than two-thirds of the loudest of the two main sounds at the apex; or 3) both (123).

PHONOCARDIOGRAM, LOW FREQUENCY TRACING

Three main types of triple rhythm and one of quadruple rhythm have been recognized (fig. 232).

1) *Atrial type.* The additional sound occurs at the time of atrial contraction and represents the accentuation of the fourth sound. It usually falls in late diastole but, if the P-R interval is long and diastole is short, it may fall in early diastole.

2) *Ventricular type.* The additional sound falls in early diastole at the time of rapid filling and represents the accentuation of

the third sound. It occurs from 0.14 to 0.18 second after the second sound.

3) *Summation (or "nondescript") type.* There is an additional sound or a short rumbling murmur in mid-diastole. This is due to more or less simultaneous occurrence of rapid passive filling and atrial contraction causing the rapid succession, or fusion, of the third with the fourth sound (fig. 233).

4) *Quadruple rhythm.* There are two additional sounds in diastole representing the accentuation of both the third and fourth sound.

The diastolic sound is made of a high diphasic or triphasic vibration. It is simultaneous with a high wave in the low frequency tracings (cardiogram or epigastric tracing). In the summation type, two distinct waves may be present in the low frequency tracing even if a prolonged sound or short rumble is revealed by the sound tracing (122).

Phonocardiograms recorded first over the apex and then at the epigastrium reveal whether the triple rhythm originates in the left or in the right ventricle. A triple rhythm recorded only at the apex usually reveals left ventricular strain; a triple rhythm recorded only at the epigastrium usually reveals right ventricular strain. Other types of triple rhythms are recorded over both areas.

The following conditions increase the loudness of the diastolic sounds:

1) *Rapid heart action.* The short diastole causes a tumultuous filling of the ventricles.

2) *Prolonged interval between atrial and ventricular contractions.* The increased interval permits a better audition but does not change the graphic characteristics of the atrial sound.

3) *Hypertrophy of the left atrium,* as observed in mitral insufficiency without severe mitral stenosis, gives a powerful contraction displacing a large amount of blood. The same is true for the *right atrium* in cor pulmonale or mitral stenosis. This increases the loudness of the fourth sound.

4) *Dilated and weak myocardium.* The

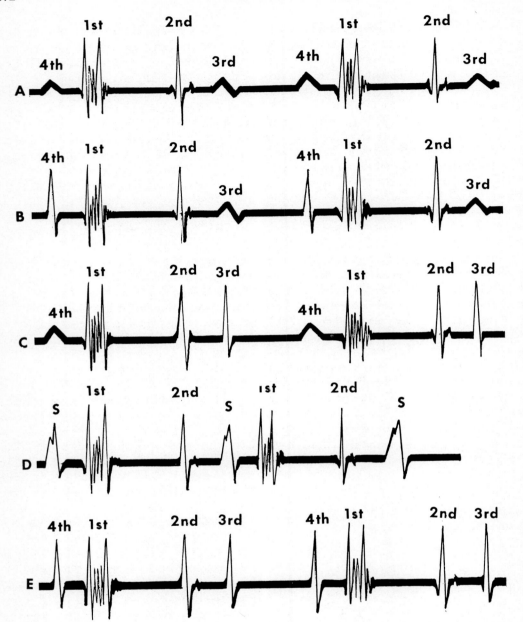

Fig. 232. Graphic diagnosis of the *triple and quadruple rhythms* (gallop or train-wheel rhythms). A, normal sounds; B, *atrial type* of triple rhythm (loud fourth sound); C, *ventricular type* of triple rhythm (loud third sound); D, *summation* (or nondescript) type of triple rhythm (fusion of loud third and fourth sounds); E, *quadruple rhythm* (loud and separated third and fourth sounds).

ventricular wall vibrates more when hit by the fluid wave. This is common in congestive failure and in coronary heart disease.

5) *Ventricular strain favors triple rhythms*

through increase of atrial pressure; this is typical of hypertensive heart disease.

These rhythms are commonly encountered in pregnancy, thyrotoxicosis, fever, anemia,

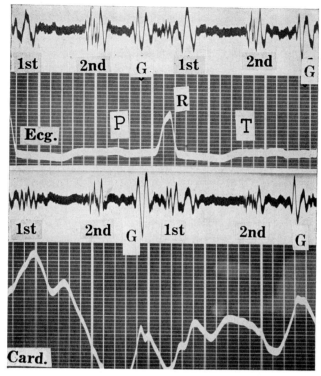

FIG. 233. *Triple rhythm. Summation (or nondescript) type.* G, additional sound. Case of coronary heart disease. Comparison of the sound tracing, first with the ECG, then with a low frequency tracing (Card.) of the precordium.

rheumatic or congenital heart diseases, and hypertensive or coronary heart diseases. The abnormal rhythm is caused by functional phenomena which may disappear (delivery of pregnant women, calming down of excited children, digitalization of valvular patients, sympathectomy or venesection of hypertensive patients) leading to normalization of the auscultatory phenomena.

While a triple rhythm is more frequent in cardiac patients than in normal subjects, it may be found occasionally in the latter because its production is favored by functional elements which may be present without heart disease.

A triple or quadruple rhythm is often evidence of *ventricular strain.* This is frequently observed in acute or subacute myocarditis, coronary heart disease (especially after myocardial infarction), and hyperten-

sive heart disease (especially malignant hypertension). However, no unduly severe prognosis should be based on this sign alone, because many reversible phenomena, especially tachycardia, may be causing it.

Pulsus Alternans

Pulsus alternans occurs when every other pulse wave is weak although there is no irregularity of the heart (fig. 234).

Pulsus alternans may appear during attacks of paroxysmal tachycardia. It is typical of hypertension, coronary heart disease (especially after myocardial infarction), and congestive failure.

Pulsus alternans is recognized by palpation of the radial pulse only when exceptionally severe. Manual compression of the brachial artery may cause halving of the pulse, and reveal less marked alternation.

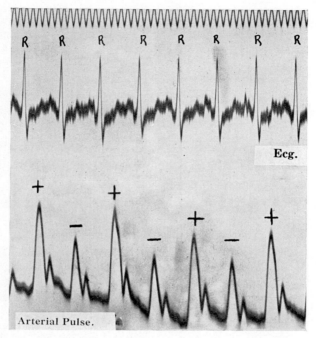

FIG. 234. Pulsus alternans

Blood pressure tracings easily reveal the alternans. If the patient has a heart rate of 60, decompression first shows the sounds due to the large waves (rate of 30), then those due to all waves (rate of 60). A new halving of the rate may be observed near the level of diastolic pressure.

There are four types of alternating pulse: 1) alternation of the peak (systolic alternation), 2) alternation of the foot (diastolic alternation), 3) alternation of both (systolic and diastolic alternation), and 4) alternation of the dicrotic wave. In exceptional cases, the tibial tracing fails to reveal an alternation which is present in the brachial tracing.

Several phenomena may alternate in cases of pulsus alternans: 1) The intensity of the cardiac sounds (13, 14) or the force of the apex beat (21). 2) The intensity of a murmur (15–18). 3) The amplitude of the ventricular contractions as recorded by the electrokymograph or the roentgenkymograph (20, 21). At times, the electrocardiogram reveals an alternation of P, R, T, or S-T, which may be concordant or discordant in relation to the pulse (3, 12, 14, 25). Exertion usually increases the alternation. A premature beat may start the alternation, which usually continues for some time thereafter.

MECHANISM

Alternation of various cardiac functions has been described. *Alternating conductivity* leads to periodic changes of the P-R interval or to periodic A-V block every second beat, and may cause an alternating bundle branch block. *Alternating automatism* has been advocated as the cause of bradycardia, similar to that of periodic S-A block type 2:1 (12). Similarly, *alternation of the strength of ventricular systole* is the cause of pulsus alternans.

The most likely explanation is the following. A certain area of the ventricular myocardium possesses a *longer refractory period* than the rest of the heart, either because it has been damaged or because its blood supply is poor. When a stimulus reaches the ventricle after a long pause (respiratory arrhythmia, compensatory pause after a premature beat, or during a slow rate caused by vagal reflex) *all fibers contract, causing a large blood wave to enter the aorta.* However, this contraction is followed by a shorter diastole which is not sufficient to restore the fibers of the damaged area. The following stimulus causes the contraction of all fibers except those damaged (which are still in a relative refractory period) whereupon a *small blood wave enters the aorta.* Then a large and a small wave alternate again until a change occurs in the heart rate or in the conditions of the myocardium. In

pulse with alternately smaller and larger waves. Recognition of the phenomenon can be made by the above mentioned maneuvers (manual compression of the brachial artery, inflated blood pressure cuff, exertion).

Differential diagnosis from a *bigeminal pulse* is easy with an electrocardiogram and a pulse tracing. The ventricular complexes are identical in pulsus alternans while the complex of a premature contraction periodically follows a normal complex in bigeminal pulse. The small wave is *nearer the following large wave* (or is at an equal distance) in pulsus alternans; it is *nearer the preceding large wave* in bigeminal pulse.

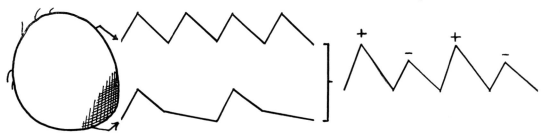

FIG. 235 Mechanism of pulsus alternans

other words, a difference in the length of the refractory period of some fibers makes it possible that they contract only every other stimulus while all other fibers contract with every stimulus (fig. 235). Pulsus alternans indicates that large numbers of fibers are in an abnormal functional condition. However, if the damaged fibers are in an area which has little or no influence on the size of the pulse, other manifestations of cardiac activity may reveal the disturbance or this may not be apparent.

It is possible that pulsus alternans is caused occasionally by alternating changes in the tonus of the aorta and even in the tonus of one or more peripheral arteries. Proof of this, however, is not altogether convincing.

DIAGNOSIS

Diagnosis of pulsus alternans is simple if it is remembered that this is a *regular*

In certain cases, if respiration is rapid, the cardiac rate may be one-half of the respiratory rate. This may cause a nonpathologic alternation of the pulse. Inviting the patient to "hold his breath" for a few seconds reestablishes equal pulses.

PROGNOSIS

The pulsus alternans of paroxysmal tachycardia, and that occurring for only 5 to 6 contractions after a premature beat, are of limited importance. Nevertheless, they add severity to the syndrome. The pulsus alternans of all other conditions has a very serious prognosis. Its importance should be evaluated together with all other clinical data but there is no doubt that pulsus alternans is an ominous sign.

Disappearance of pulsus alternans in a hypertensive patient after surgery of the sympathetic system has been observed by the author.

Bundle Branch Block

DEFINITION—MECHANISM

Impairment in the transmission of the stimulus is not limited to the bundle of His (page 355). If it occurs below the bifurcation of the bundle, it may delay or block the conduction toward one ventricle. When the delayed conduction is in one of the stems of the bundle, there is *bundle branch block* (B.B.B.). When there is diffuse impairment in the more distal subdivision, there is an *intraventricular block* (I.V. block). When there is localized impairment in one of the distal branches, there is a *focal block.*

These disturbances fail to cause any apparent change of the heart action because the affected ventricle is stimulated in a devious way through the septum (fig. 236). On the other hand, this process causes delay of both stimulation and contraction of one ventricle in comparison with the other.

CAUSE

Bundle branch block and I.V. block are caused by inflammation, ischemia, or fibrosis of the conducting bundles. Inflammation may be due to myocarditis (rheu-

matic, diphtheritic, or other). Ischemia is usually due to coronary heart disease but may be the result of long-lasting hypertrophy of one ventricle, like that occurring in hypertensive heart disease or cor pulmonale, or in congenital or rheumatic heart disease. Fibrosis may be the result of myocarditis, myocardial hemorrhage, or coronary arteriosclerosis. Rarer conditions (trauma, tumor, bacterial myocarditis) may also cause B.B.B. or I.V. block.

An extremely rare condition is the absence of conduction on one side due to *congenital* lack of one of the stems of the bundle of His (162).

Right bundle branch block may be due to an extremely minute lesion because the right stem is long and thin. On the contrary, left bundle branch block is usually the result of a more diffuse lesion because the left stem branches nearly immediately below the bifurcation (page 22). Intraventricular block is always caused by widespread lesion of either side.

In coronary arteriosclerosis, B.B.B. is usually due to a *bilateral lesion* which predominates on one side. In the other cases, unilateral lesion is the rule.

PHYSICAL DATA—X-RAY

Physical data are few. There may be a *faint* and *prolonged first sound*; a *split second pulmonic sound* is common (over one-half of the cases).

The apical impulse may be prolonged.

Fluoroscopy and *roentgenkymography* may reveal a delay in contraction of the ventricle on the side of the block.

GRAPHIC TRACINGS

Electrocardiogram

The electrocardiogram, recorded in the limb leads, shows that QRS is broader and lasts more than 0.12 second in adults (more than 0.10 second in children) and is notched or slurred.

Left bundle branch block. There is no S

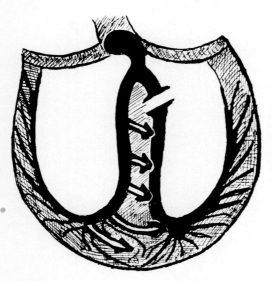

Fig. 236. Propagation of stimulus in *left bundle branch block.*

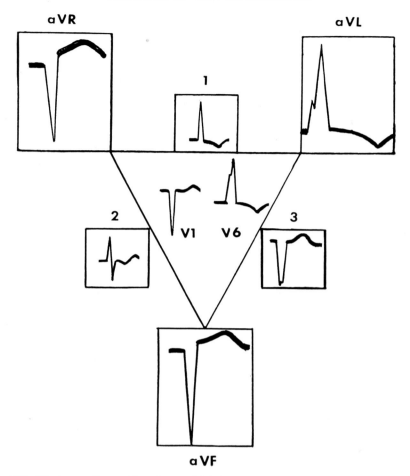

FIG. 237. Electrocardiographic scheme of *left bundle branch block* in a horizontal heart

wave in lead 1.[65] The T wave may be in either the same or the opposite direction of the main QRS complex. The direction of the main wave in leads 1 and 3 fails to give a clue; it may be of either the concordant or the discordant type (left axis deviation) according to the position of the heart. However, the last is more frequent. the precordial leads give basic data: there is a small R wave followed by a deep and broad S (rS) in leads V1 and V2; on the other hand, the R wave is tall and late in leads V5 and V6 (rR' or M); *there is no Q*

[65] A small and broad S1 (and S in V6) can be observed in cases of intraventricular block of the left base (S-type of left i.v. block).

wave in V5 to V6 because the septum is stimulated from right to left (fig. 237).

The data supplied by the unipolar limb and precordial leads are summarized in table 19.

In left ventricular hypertrophy, leads facing the epicardial surface of the left ventricle have a wide qR pattern. In left bundle branch block, leads facing the epicardial surface of the left ventricle show a wide R and no Q.

Right bundle branch block. The T wave is usually in the opposite direction of the main wave of QRS. The main wave in leads 1 and 3 is usually of the *concordant type* (right axis deviation). However, if the

TABLE 19. *Electrocardiographic changes in left bundle branch block*

POSITION OF THE HEART	UNIPOLAR LEAD	PATTERN OF ECG
Vertical heart (less common)........	Rt. arm	QS, raised S-T, upright T
	Lt. arm	QS or rS, small upright T
	Lt. leg	R, depressed S-T, inverted T
	V1–V4	QS or rS, upward T
	V5–V6	R, depressed S-T, inverted T
Horizontal heart.......	Rt. arm	QS, upward T
	Lt. arm	R, inverted T
	Lt. leg	QS, upward T
	V1	QS, upward T
	V2–V3	rS, upward T
	V5–V6	rR', inverted T

heart is horizontal, it is possible to observe a discordant type of electrocardiogram and no S wave. The precordial leads give basic data: the R wave is of great amplitude and is delayed 0.06 to 0.08 second over the beginning of the complex in lead V1 and V2 (like rSR' or M); it is of high voltage and occurs early in leads V5 and V6 (like qRS or RS) (fig. 238 and table 20).

A special variety of right bundle branch block is called *Wilson type of block*. Lead 1 has a tall R followed by *a deep and wide* S and by an upright T wave. Lead 3 has a qR type of complex and an inverted T. The chest leads V5 to V6 have a slurred, wide S and R' wave.

Bilateral bundle branch block. Cases with a QRS exceeding 0.12 second may not show

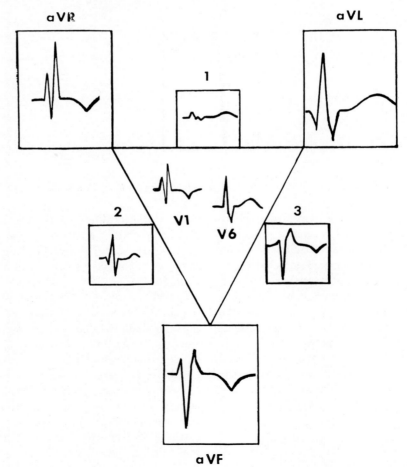

FIG. 238. Electrocardiographic scheme of *right bundle branch block* in a horizontal heart

evidence of unilateral block in the precordial leads (99). Unless there is an alternating type of block, it is apparent that in bilateral i. v. block the two ventricles contract more or less at the same time. On the other hand, if the block spreads upwards to the bifurcation, A-V block will become apparent.

Diffuse intraventricular block. QRS is severely prolonged and may last more than 0.15 second. Bundle branch block or ventricular hypertrophy may be contributory factors. In *left* intraventricular block a small Q may be observed in the chest leads V5 to V6. This is particularly significant because the delay of conduction in the left branch of the bundle should cause disappearance of a septal Q. Septal infarction should be excluded before explaining this Q as caused by intraventricular block.

It has been suggested that certain changes of the electrocardiogram indicate block of the stimulus in some definite layers of the ventricular wall: notchings of the ascending branch of QRS have been interpreted as due to block in the *subendocardial layers* while notchings of the descending branch of QRS have been explained as due to block in the *subepicardial layers.*

Focal block is revealed by a broadening of QRS in only one or two chest leads and not in the others. This is explained as due to local conduction disturbances.

TABLE 20. *Electrocardiographic changes in right bundle branch block*

POSITION OF THE HEART	UNIPOLAR LEAD	PATTERN OF ECG
Vertical heart (less common)	Rt. arm	rSR', inverted T
	Lt. arm	rSR', inverted T
	Lt. leg	qRS, upright T
	V1–V2	rsR', inverted T
	V4–V6	qRS, upward T
Horizontal heart	Rt. arm	rsR', inverted T
	Lt. arm	qRS, upward T
	Lt. leg	rSr' or rSR', upward T
	V1–V2	rsR' or M, inverted T
	V4–V6	qRS, upward T

Phonocardiogram

The *first sound is prolonged* and lasts more than 0.16 second. It is frequently of *low amplitude.* Splitting of this sound has been described by several authors. However, this observation is not confirmed by stethoscopic phonocardiograms (153) and should be attributed to inadequate technic. Ventricular asynchronism results in the delay of contraction of one ventricle of about 0.04 to 0.05 second. This is too short for causing a splitting of that central phase of the first sound which is clearly visible and which lasts from 0.06 to 0.08 second (page 91). However, *it causes prolongation of the first sound* in both the right and the left types of bundle branch block. *The second sound, being shorter, is frequently split;* the interval between the two phases of the split sound is from 0.03 to 0.04 (153).

Carotid Tracing, Jugular Tracing

The delay between beginning of first sound complex and rise of the carotid pulse (usually about 0.05 second) is increased and lasts from 0.07 to 0.08 second in *left bundle branch block.* The incisura of the carotid pulse coincides in normal subjects with the main vibration of the second sound. In left bundle branch block, *it coincides with the second phase of the split second sound* (8, 9, 10) (fig. 239).

The rise of the carotid pulse has a normal relationship to the beginning of the first sound in *right bundle branch block;* the incisura has a normal relationship to the first phase of the split second sound in this type of block.

In *right bundle branch block,* the study of the jugular tracing is of importance: *the peak of v is markedly delayed and occurs 0.08 to 0.14 second after the end of the second sound* (or after the second phase of the second sound, if this is split). In other words *v,* which usually occurs 0.08 to 0.14 second after the second sound, has the same relationship to the second phase of that sound, when this is split.

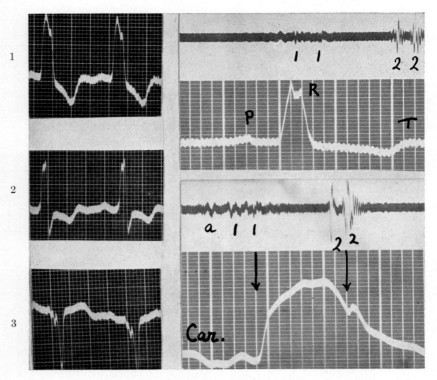

FIG. 239. Case of *left bundle branch block*. ECG in the three limb leads. Phonocardiogram compared first with lead 1 of the ECG, then with the carotid tracing. Prolonged and faint 1st sound. Split 2nd sound. The incisura of the pulse coincides with the 2nd phase of the split 2nd sound.

Electrokymogram

This method may be applied to the study of pulmonic or aortic expansions and to right and left ventricular contraction. The two ventricles and the two large arteries present pulsations which are either simultaneous or succeed each other within 0.01 second. The most common is the precedence of the right ventricle and of the pulmonic pulse by 0.003 second (154).

In about 30 per cent of the cases of *left bundle branch block*, left ventricular contraction and the aortic pulse were found delayed over the right ventricular and the pulmonic pulse by about 0.03 second (155). If there is hypertrophy or intraventricular block of the left side, the delay is greater. Hypertension of the greater circulation increases the delay revealed by the rise of the pulse, decreases that revealed by the incisura.

In about 30 per cent of the cases of *right bundle branch block*, the right ventricular contraction and the pulmonic pulse were found delayed over the left ventricular and the aortic pulse by about 0.03 second (155). If there is hypertrophy of the right ventricle or intraventricular block of the right side, the delay is greater. Hypertension of the lesser circulation increases the delay revealed by the rise of the pulse, decreases that revealed by the incisura. Systemic hypertension may partly neutralize the effect of right bundle branch block, so that the delay is less apparent.

In both types of block, a prolongation of the phase of isometric relaxation was observed. A large percentage of cases of bundle branch block, whatever the side, seem to present a *bilateral delay of contraction* upon EKY studies. However, studies conducted with mechanical and sound tracings reveal a much larger percentage of asynchronism.

VARIETIES

Incomplete bundle branch block. In this type of block, the stimulus is merely slowed in its course toward one of the ventricles. The heart sounds are somewhat prolonged; the QRS is between 0.10 and 0.12 in duration; both the precordial leads and the mechanical tracings give borderline data.

Unstable or intermittent bundle branch block (32). In this type, the block appears and disappears suddenly. This probably is due to initial vascular disturbances. When the blood supply improves, the block disappears.

Paroxysmal bundle branch block (33). It may be caused by acute infections (diphtheria, rheumatic disease) but usually is due to coronary heart disease. The failure of one branch of the bundle may be apparent during sudden changes of heart rate.

Bundle branch block with short P-R interval. This variety will be described below.

Alternating bundle branch block. This consists of the alternated appearance of ventricular complexes with the aspect of bundle branch block from either side. It is of rare observation; less rare, however, in the course of A-V block (page 357)

DIAGNOSIS

At first, the diagnosis of B.B.B. was based on peripheral ECG's alone and the importance of axis deviation was overemphasized. However, recognition of the fact that a) the common terminology was wrong, b) the two opposite types of B.B.B. may have a similar aspect on the peripheral ECG (34, 35), and c) the position of the heart is more important than the block in determining the electric axis (36), led to a change in the basic criteria for diagnosis.

Broadening of QRS, notching of the complex, and prolongation or splitting of the heart sounds are general signs of bundle branch block. Increased voltage, inversion of T, and axis deviation are secondary data. The diagnosis of side is based a) on precordial electrocardiographic leads and b) on demonstration that the contraction of one ventricle is delayed in comparison with the other (sound and carotid tracings, EKY).

Differential diagnosis should be made at times with *mitral stenosis*. The latter may give an "opening snap" which may simulate a split 2nd sound, and may be accompanied by broadening of QRS. As the jugular tracing of such cases may not be reliable (28), the diagnosis will be based mainly on the precordial leads.

Differential diagnosis between bundle branch block of the usual type and that *with short P-R interval* will be described below.

COURSE—PROGNOSIS

Incomplete bundle branch block may be a comparatively unimportant finding or may appear after severe disturbances of the heart, such as myocardial infarction. It may exist unchanged for many years permitting a normal activity but may, on the contrary, increase in severity within a few weeks or months as a result of progressive lesions of the myocardium.

Occasional cases do occur where B.B.B. is an isolated finding and has no special significance. This is relatively more common if the B.B.B. is on the right side (37). However, when B.B.B. is associated with other signs of heart disease, it definitely adds to the severity of the prognosis which, therefore, will be based on all data concerning the heart. Whenever there is coronary heart disease, considerable cardiac enlargement, and B.B.B., the prognosis shall be guarded.

The Wolff-Parkinson-White Syndrome (43)

This syndrome should be kept apart from that of intraventricular block because it is due to *preexcitation* of the ventricles and not to delay of ventricular excitation. It

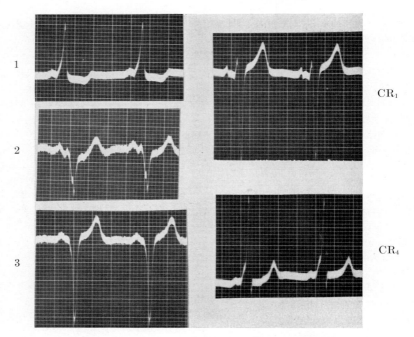

F<small>IG</small>. 240. Electrocardiogram in a case of *Wolff-Parkinson-White syndrome*

occurs mostly in young males who have attacks of paroxysmal tachycardia but are otherwise apparently normal.

The only physical evidence of the syndrome is a possible prolongation of the heart sounds.

GRAPHIC TRACINGS

Electrocardiogram

The electrocardiogram presents a *short P-R interval* (0.08–0.10 sec.); *QRS is increased in duration* (0.10–0.12) *and is slurred* (fig. 240). It is typical that *the first limb of QRS is slurred and slow while the second limb is rapid and normal.* The precordial leads usually fail to show those changes which are common in B.B.B. (page 357).

During the attacks of tachycardia, the ECG often presents normal PR and QRS intervals. However, attacks of ventricular tachycardia or atrial fibrillation may also occur (44). Cases where this syndrome is associated with rheumatic or congenital heart disease have been described.

Phonocardiogram

In general, the phonocardiogram fails to show prolongation of the first sound, as in bundle branch block. A case observed by the author presented a crescendo-type of first sound which had been erroneously interpreted as a presystolic murmur. Only rare cases present a split second sound.

Electrokymogram

The most common finding is that of delayed contraction of both ventricles, as revealed by simultaneous aortic and pulmonic tracings with an electrocardiogram. Less common finding is that of ventricular asynchronism.

MECHANISM

Among the different possible mechanisms suggested to explain this eventuality, the most likely is the following (45, 46): these patients have a *congenital abnormality* which consists of the existence of an accessory pathway of atrioventricular conduction; this may be similar to the *bundle of Kent* (47) and to the structures described by *Paladino* (48). The sinoatrial stimulus proceeds along both the abnormal and the normal pathways. The stimulus following the abnormal pathway reaches the ventricles more rapidly (short P-R) and causes *early activation* of the latter; the stimulus following the normal pathway reaches the ventricles slightly later and contributes to the second part of the QRS complex (49).

The abnormal pathway may be blocked by exercise, atropine, or amyl nitrite (50), following which, normal complexes appear.

The paroxysmal attacks have been explained in the following way:

a) A stimulus which has reached the ventricles along the bundle of His may re-enter the atria following the bundle of Kent in a retrograde direction and cause atrial tachycardia.

b) A ventricular premature stimulus may follow the bundle of Kent in a retrograde way and then re-enter the ventricles through the bundle of His, causing ventricular tachycardia.

The existence of an anomalous bundle connecting the right atrium with the right ventricle has been demonstrated already in several cases (51) while, in others, an anomalous bundle connected the left atrium with the left ventricle (143). The possibility that either the left or the right side of the heart receives an early activation is confirmed by the unipolar chest leads (144). Interference with QRS of a slow *Ta* wave (page 37) or the results of high A-V node excitability (145) may simulate a true Wolff-Parkinson-White syndrome.

PROGNOSIS

This condition is relatively harmless and should, therefore, be sharply differentiated from the common types of intraventricular block. It should not be ignored, however, because the attacks of tachycardia may cause giddiness or syncope and, in rare cases, heart failure.

Inter- and Intra-Atrial Disturbances

Extensive lesions of the atrial myocardium may cause abnormalities in the spreading of the stimulus which may be recognized by changes of the P wave.

Evidence of enlargement of either atrium can be found in the *electrocardiogram* (page 369). The finding of P waves of varying form with normal atrial rhythm and constant P-R is in favor of an *intra-atrial disturbance of conduction* (53, 54). Apart from broadening and splintering, the P wave may present *increased voltage, decreased voltage, diphasic shape, or inversion*. As the normal P wave represents the sum of the currents of both atria, these changes may be due to abnormal spread of the stimulus in either one of them.

A *negative P wave* may be caused by intra-atrial disturbances (55) (page 369). Isolated disturbances of this type are rare; more frequently they are found in patients having also A-V or intraventricular disturbances.

Special leads (esophageal leads, right precordial lead) permit differentiation between the currents of the two atria (page 128). Through their use, different disturbances have been recognized: a) delay in activation of the left atrium (56, 6, 161), b) delay in activation of the right atrium (6, 57, 161), and c) atrial dissociation with double pacemaker or inter-atrial block (55, 59, 60, 61, 119).

Acute and Subacute Myocarditis

The term "myocarditis" is applied in a broad sense to both the inflammatory and the degenerative lesions of the cardiac muscle. Chronic conditions with cardiac failure should not be labeled as "myocarditis" unless there is some evidence for it. Usually the diagnosis of "coronary heart disease with myocardial fibrosis" is the correct one. On the other hand, true myocarditis is not uncommon and is responsible for many cardiovascular disturbances, sometimes followed by death.

CAUSE

Numerous diseases may be associated with myocarditis.

a) *Rheumatic disease.*

b) *Multiple bacterial agents*; among them, the Streptococcus hemolyticus, the Gonococcus, the Pneumococcus, the Typhoid bacillus, and Bacillus diphtheriae, the Tubercle bacillus, and Brucella melitensis.

c) *Several spirocheta, trypanosomata,* and *rickettsiae,* including the agent of syphilis, the agent of Chagas disease, and that of yellow fever; also larger parasites including Trichinella spiralis, Ankylostoma duodenale, and the plasmodia of malaria.

d) *Certain viruses*; they include the agents of influenza, measles, parotitis, and poliomyelitis.

Several types of myocarditis are of unknown etiology, like *Fiedler's isolated myocarditis* (80a, 81). Others are connected with *hemolytic anemias* (64) or with *systemic diseases of the central nervous system* (65) or *the skeletal muscles* (66). Some of them, however, may be the result of vitamin deficiencies and will be considered later (page 402).

Another type of myocarditis is due to *allergy to drugs,* usually sulfonamides (62). This raises the question of possible other, less severe, allergic reactions of the myocardium.

Purely degenerative lesions of the heart muscle are caused by *acute poisoning* with phosphorus, arsenic, and other substances.

LESIONS

The old division in *parenchymatous* and *interstitial myocarditis* has not proven very useful because of the frequent association of the two types of lesions. On the other hand, the division of the myocardial lesions in a) *chiefly inflammatory* (*myocarditis*) and b) *chiefly degenerative* (*myocardosis*) still seems useful (62, 159).

The *chiefly inflammatory form* is found following most bacterial and viral infections or in the course of allergic diseases.

a) *Simple myocarditis.* The connective tissue is infiltrated with lymphocytes, plasma cells, and polymorphonuclears. Foci of fibroblastic proliferation are common in later stages as well as slight degeneration of the muscular elements. Streptococcal myocarditis is found also in cases with subacute bacterial endocarditis (page 208). The frequency of myocardial involvement has been demonstrated by patients cured with penicillin who died in congestive failure.

A typical aspect of *patchy myocarditis* has been described after *common upper respiratory infections.* A delay between the primary infection and the cardiac lesion may prevent a correct diagnosis (137a). On the other hand, the myocarditis which is associated with *glomerulonephritis* presents a widespread serous effusion into the interstitial spaces, and the myocardial damage seems to be related to increased capillary permeability (137c).

b) *Purulent myocarditis.* It may be due to extension of a purulent inflammation (purulent pericarditis, ulcerative endocarditis) or localization of germs during sepsis. Gross examination reveals *abscesses* in different stages of evolution. These are *multiple* in the hematogenous type; on the contrary, there is often only *one abscess* in the form caused by extension. The abscess is surrounded by an area of infiltration with necrosis of the myofibrils.

Typical lesions are found in cases of streptococcal, gonococcal, pneumococcal, or typhoid infections, and even in subacute bacterial endocarditis (78). Healing of both types of lesions results in *fibrosis* and *scarring* with occasional calcification.

The *chiefly degenerative* form can be found in chronic diseases of the kidneys (nephrosis) or the liver (cirrhosis); in comatose states (diabetes, uremia); in malignant diseases (multiple myeloma); during certain infections (sepsis and diphtheria); in chronic alcoholism; and in Addison's disease. The cases described by French authors with the name of "myocardie" (92) probably presented this type of lesion. A common factor seems to be hyproteinemia of the blood.

Gross examination shows that the heart is enlarged and flabby. The myocardium is variegated in color because of alternating reddish-brown and yellowish-gray areas. The latter indicate a degenerative process, even in the gross. Microscopic examination reveals diffuse or focal lesions, consisting of cloudy swelling and fatty or hyaline degeneration and resulting in obliteration of the myofibril striations. Small foci of inflammatory cell infiltrations are concomitant findings. "Healing" of these forms may occur only by *scarring*, as replacement hyperplasia of the myofibrils has not been proven.

Myocardial hypertrophy, sometimes severe, may be the result of subacute myocarditis in the absence of valvular lesions (133). Even *aneurysm of the ventricular wall* may be the result of isolated myocarditis (134). In rare cases, there may be *rupture of the ventricular wall* even without the formation of an aneurysm.

A certain number of subacute forms deserve further brief description.

Rheumatic myocarditis. Typical *Aschoff nodules* can be observed. These are tiny perivascular or interstitial nodules, usually invisible to the naked eye, most frequent in the left ventricle (page 190, fig. 108).

Syphilitic myocarditis. It may be *acute* (68, 69) with interstitial cellular infiltration which is either diffuse or patchy. However, the most common type is a *subacute* reaction consisting of perivascular inflammatory foci. Syphilis may cause entirely different lesions with the formation of *multiple small gummata, larger nodules, infarctions*, or *aneurysms of the wall. Sclerosis* may follow rapidly or slowly and frequently predominates in the right heart (64). The finding of spirochetes in the foci is not unusual. Another type spreads by continuity from the aorta and is associated with *aortitis* (140) (pages 201 and 475). The myocardial lesion originates from inflammatory foci in the media and spreads first to areas adjacent to the sinuses of Valsalva. Endoangiitis obliterans and perivascular infiltration with lymphocytes and plasmacytes are found.

Tubercular myocarditis. The myocardium has proven to be resistant to the localization of tubercle bacilli. However, several different lesions have been found occasionally such as: simple toxic myocardosis (70), nodular tuberculosis of the heart (71), miliary tuberculosis, and diffuse tuberculosis with scattered Langhans cells (72).

Myocardial lesions have been repeatedly described in *scleroderma* (135). It has been suggested that scleroderma, dermatomyositis and periarteritis nodosa, have something in common being "collagen diseases" (135b); the part played by an allergic mechanism is still hypothetical.

In *allergic* or *eosinophilic myocarditis*, gross examination reveals many pin-point, grayish-pink, areas. These are due to cellular infiltration, mostly consisting of eosinophils and monocytes in the interstitial tissue, especially around the blood vessels. These perivascular cellular infiltrates are also present in other organs and have been thought to represent an early stage of frank periarteritis (79).

Fiedler's or isolated myocarditis (80a). There is an isolated involvement of the myocardium with outspoken necrosis of the myofibrils without any endocardial or pericardial lesion (80b). There frequently are granulomata with necrosis and giant cells (81). This condition is seldom diagnosed during life and may cause sudden death.

"Neurogenic" and *"myogenic" heart lesions* consist of subendocardial hemorrhages, usually located in the interventricular septum, softness and flabbiness of the myocardium, and interstitial edema (65). Hyaline and fatty degeneration of the fibers, vacuolization, and, later, disappearance of the nuclei and fibrils, have been observed in cases of brain tumor, poliomyelitis, and Friedreich's ataxia (65). Myocardial fibrosis has been found after prolonged disease. *Fragmentation* or *segmentation* of the cardiac

fibers has also been observed (82, 83). On critical analysis of these findings, one cannot rule out the possibility of asphyxic, preagonic changes, or of an association with various other pathological conditions which were present in some of the published cases.

Diphtheria is one of the causes of myocarditis and is followed rather frequently by *calcification of the myocardium* (119).

Malaria. This disease is a frequent cause of both myocardosis and myocarditis, of subendocardial hemorrhages, and occlusive coronaritis (73, 1, 141).

Yellow fever, typhus, trichinosis, and *hookworm infestation* may be accompanied by diffuse myocardosis with parenchymatous hemorrhages (74). *Trypanosomas* may accumulate in the myocardium, causing severe disturbances (75). *Chagas disease* is frequently accompanied by A-V block, and cardiac lesions are found in one-half of the cases.

Actinomycosis may present multiple myocardial abscesses which often heal by *calcification.*

Echinococcal disease may be accompanied by cardiac cysts: dead (fibrosed or calcified); living; cysts which rupture into the cardiac chambers or into the pericardium (76, 77). The majority of cysts are in the right heart, more often in the right ventricle (77).

Virus myocarditis. Clinical signs and histologic evidence show that myocarditis may follow virus influenza. As the same process may follow upper respiratory infections (137a) or bronchopneumonia (137b), it is open to question whether the virus or the associated germs are responsible for the cardiac lesion. Another type of virus myocarditis is that which follows *poliomyelitis* (138). Widespread coagulation necrosis of the cardiac fibers and infiltration of cells, mainly polymorphonuclear leucocytes, seems to be typical. Perivascular and interstititial infiltration of macrophages has been observed also. Virus myocarditis was described in connection with *epidemic infectious hepatitis, infectious mononucleosis, yellow fever, varicella, dengue, atypical pneumonia, rubeola, measles, mumps, acute epidemic encephalitis.* In general, the myocardial lesion is mild and consists mainly of lymphocytic infiltration with only occasional polymorphonuclears, plasma cells, and fibroblasts.

SYMPTOMS AND SIGNS

The signs and symptoms are extremely variable because, on the one hand they are dependent upon the extension, severity, and location of the myocardial lesions, and, on the other, they may be obscured by disturbances caused by a generalized infection.

Precordial pain, dyspnea, rapid pulse, and *low blood pressure* are common.

Cyanosis is frequent. Peripheral signs of congestive failure soon occur.

Abnormalities of cardiac action are frequent and vary with the site of lesion. They may consist of *premature beats, paroxysmal tachycardia, atrial flutter,* or *heart block.* The combination of multiple premature beats from various foci, wandering pacemaker, and A-V block (occasionally also S-A block) is typical of myocarditis, if coronary occlusion can be excluded.

Cardiac dulness is usually enlarged and obtuseness of the cardiohepatic angle is not unusual.

Auscultation reveals that the *cardiac sounds* become *dull, soft, and prolonged.* The first sound frequently is altered more than the second. There may be *splitting of the second sound* because of bundle branch block. *Triple rhythm* and various *murmurs* are frequent. The most common is a *systolic apical murmur* which is frequently soft but may be harsh. A *diastolic rumble* simulating that of mitral stenosis, may occur. Differentiation is frequently possible because this murmur (due to relative stenosis of both A-V valves) is usually audible over a wide area of the precordium.

There is an *absolute or relative hypoten-*

sion[66] which usually is persistent. *Acute collapse*, on the contrary, is more often of vascular origin.

GRAPHIC TRACINGS

Electrocardiogram

The findings vary according to the more or less widespread type of lesion. They consist of:

1) Changes of rate.

2) Disturbances of the rhythm due to increased excitability (premature contractions; atrial flutter or fibrillation; atrial or ventricular tachycardia).

3) Disturbances of the rhythm due to altered spreading of the stimulus (prolong P-R; S-A or A-V block; B.B.B., I.V. block).

4) Abnormality of repolarization (changes of S-T and T) and prolongation of the Q-T interval. In certain cases the electrical pattern may simulate myocardial infarct.

The following changes may be found in the different diseases:

a) *Rheumatic disease* (1st attack). Prolonged P-R; changes of P, QRS, S-T, and T; A-V block; premature beats.

b) *Diphtheria*. Premature beats, A-V block, notching and broadening of QRS, low or inverted T, prolonged Q-T, raised or depressed S-T.

c) *Acute tonsillitis*. Changes of P, prolonged P-R, raised S-T, low or inverted T, broadened QRS, prolonged Q-T. These changes are usually of short duration.

d) *Typhoid*. Prolonged P-R, A-V block, low or inverted T.

e) *Scarlet fever*. Changes similar to tonsil infections. Occasional A-V block.

f) *Malaria*. Changes of S-T and T, occasional inversion of T.

g) *Pneumonia*. Displaced S-T, small QRS, deformed T_1, inverted T_2 and T_3, occa-

sional isolated changes of T_4. Changes simulating myocardial infarction have been described (3).

h) *Influenza*. Notched QRS, abnormal T for 3 to 4 months.

i) *Chagas disease* (South American tripanosomiasis). *Complete A-V block* is present in one-third of the cases, while right bundle branch block was observed in 40 per cent of the patients (139). *Ventricular extrasystoles* or *paroxysmal tachycardia* are not unusual. Changes of S-T and T revealing anterior wall ischemia have been observed.

j) *Syphilis*. Intraventricular block, diphasic or inverted T, prolonged P-R.

k) *Hemolytic anemias*. Prolonged P-R in a large percentage of cases (64).

l) *Parotitis*. Prolonged P-R, altered T wave (86).

m) *Myotonia atrophica*. Prolonged P-R, A-V block, notching of QRS, left axis deviation (66b).

n) *Friedreich's ataxia*. A-V block, intraventricular block, premature beats. In some cases, tracings simulating either anterior or posterior infarction have been described (93). These are not secondary to coronary disturbance but are caused by a primitive myocardial lesion.

o) *Trichinosis*. Changes of S-T and T; prolonged duration of QRS; less frequently, prolonged P-R.

p) *Scrub typhus* (*tsutsugamushi fever*). Deviation of S-T; prolonged P; low voltage; left axis deviation.

Phonocardiogram

The most common findings are: 1) Apical systolic murmur. 2) Triple or quadruple rhythm. 3) Prolonged, faint, and low-pitched first sound. 4) Split second pulmonic sound. 5) A diastolic rumble made of large vibrations.

Arterial Tracing

There may be either pulsus alternans or irregularities of the pulse caused by cardiac arrhythmias.

---

[66] The term *relative hypotension* is applied to a relative drop in blood pressure. A hypertensive patient, having a drop of pressure from 200/100 to 170/95, has a relative hypotension.

Electrokymogram

Certain cases having a severe but circum-scribed lesion of the left ventricle may pre-sent the pattern of *dynamic aneurysm* (page 425) over the border of the left ventricle. Patients with myasthenia gravis may also present this pattern which may disappear after treatment.

X-RAY

X-ray reveals an enlarged heart, fre-quently with a "hot-water bottle" shape. As the movements of the cardiac margins are weak, differential diagnosis from pericardial effusion is not always possible.

Serial observations of the heart size are a helpful guide. It should be noted that cardiac dilatation may persist for a considerable time after the acute stage of myocarditis.

The *Valsalva* and *Mueller tests* may also be of help because the dilated heart shows a greater change in size than either the normal heart or the heart with pericardial affusion. Further data will be given later (page 449).

Echinococcal cysts of the heart may be revealed by the x-ray.

COURSE AND VARIETIES

There is an *acute fulminating type* which rapidly causes cyanosis and death. The frequent clinical diagnosis of coronary oc-clusion then is disproven by post-mortem findings (87). This may occur in systemic diseases of the nervous system and of the muscles, as well as in cases of isolated myo-carditis.

There is a *subacute type* which lasts from a few days to a few weeks and may be accom-panied by general signs which simulate in-fection even when none is present; there is dyspnea, tachycardia, cyanosis, irregular pulse, low blood pressure, leucocytosis, and fever (88). It may occur in young or mature individuals and is usually seen in cases of *isolated myocarditis*, sometimes associated with myocardial infarction. The latter may complicate both the clinical and anatomical diagnoses.

The different infections which are associ-ated with myocarditis have various clinical pictures. Therefore, the picture of myo-carditis lacks unity and is variable.

DIAGNOSIS

The diagnosis of acute or subacute myo-carditis is usually not difficult if electro-cardiographic data are available. These will be of greater value if comparison can be made with tracings preceding the onset of the disease or between tracings recorded at regular intervals. Premature beats originat-ing in multiple foci, A-V block, or severe changes of P and T, have a definite value in the diagnosis of myocarditis. Bundle branch block or tachycardia not justified by fever are also valuable signs. Etiological diagnosis can be made only by taking all clinical data into account.

Differential diagnosis should be made with the following conditions.

Pericarditis with effusion. The shape and extension of cardiac dulness varies in differ-ent positions. Arterial pressure is frequently lower and venous pressure higher, in myo-carditis than in pericarditis. The pulsations of the veins are more apparent in the former. The ECG may show typical changes (page 445), and there frequently is a friction rub in pericarditis.

Hemorrhagic and vascular collapse. In these conditions, the heart usually becomes small; in myocarditis it is larger. Pallor is typical of collapse; livid color or cyanosis, of myo-carditis. The 1st sound is still distinct and at times loud in collapse but is dull and muffled in myocarditis. Pulse pressure is re-duced less in collapse than in myocarditis.

Mitral stenosis. Some cases of myocarditis may have a diastolic murmur simulating that of mitral stenosis. Usually phono-cardiography permits differentiation (page 237).

Myocardial infarction. This may be sus-pected in acute cases, and electrocardiograms assist correct diagnosis (page 416). However, an infarction may occur during acute or sub-acute myocarditis, complicating the problem.

Prognosis is not possible on the basis of the myocardial lesion alone because the signs of general infection should be taken into consideration. The existence of myocarditis makes the prognosis of any infection definitely more serious. Occurrence of A-V block is a more serious event than other abnormalities of the cardiac rhythm and may be a cause of death.

TREATMENT

The treatment varies with the different infections and is based on causal therapy. However, all drugs should be used with extreme care in order to avoid untoward reactions which may be followed by heart failure or even death. *Digitalis* should be given only if there is evidence of heart failure. The affected myocardium is very excitable and may react with tachycardia, arrhythmia, or block to average doses of the drug. On the other hand, the degenerated fibers of the cardiac muscle cannot be stimulated by drugs so that the results of digitalis treatment are less apparent than in heart failure without myocarditis. *Gitalin* (7) is the best tolerated digitalis glycoside.

Prolonged oxygen therapy with 40 to 50 per cent oxygen affects favorably the course of rheumatic carditis (101) and may be helpful in other myocardial diseases. Beneficial effects have been reported after intravenous or intramuscular injection of 100 to 200 cc. of 10 per cent *glucose solution* (102). These can be repeated but care should be taken not to overload the cardiovascular system.

Prolonged rest is needed. The patient should be kept immobile, but turned in bed every half-hour in order to avoid hypostasis; exertion is forbidden as long as the pulse rate is above normal.

Saline infusions and *blood transfusion* are unnecessary and may cause acute or subacute pulmonary edema (page 555). Only moderate doses of fluid should be introduced either by mouth or by vein (see above).

Antibiotics may be extremely helpful if the agent of the disease is known. *Emetine* is dangerous because of its action on the heart muscle.

Cortisone may be necessary, especially in rheumatic fever or in "collagen diseases." As it may lead to retention of sodium, the customary precautions (salt-poor diet, mercurials, high potassium intake, etc.) should be followed when giving this drug.

Amyloid Heart (160)

Amyloidosis is an uncommon systemic disease which may cause cardiac failure through involvement of the heart. In this disease, a foreign substance, *amyloid*, is produced and deposited in various tissues and organs including the heart. *Primary amyloidosis* is accompanied by maximal deposition of amyloid in the heart and lungs with formation of *nodular amyloid tumors*. *Secondary amyloidosis* may follow syphilis, tuberculosis, or chronic suppurations; it causes less extensive involvement of the heart. The same can be said for the *amyloidosis associated with multiple myeloma* and for the *tumors forming amyloid*.

Amyloidosis may cause different effects on the cardiovascular system by means of several mechanisms:

a) By infiltration of the pulmonary vessels causing chronic cor pulmonale.

b) By deposition in the coronary vessels.

c) By diffuse or localized nodular infiltration in the myocardium with or without degeneration of the cardiac fibers.

d) By deposition in the endocardium or pericardium.

e) By deposition in the cardiac valves resulting in valvular defects (insufficiency, stenosis, or both).

f) By multiple involvement of the cardiac tissues.

The signs and symptoms of primary amyloidosis are those of myocardial ischemia and of chronic irreversible cardiac failure. Since the majority of patients are old or middle-aged people, they may be erroneously diagnosed as arteriosclerotic.

Cutaneous or mucosal lesions accessible to biopsy; enlargement of lymph nodes; muscular, neurological, gastrointestinal, or arthritic involvement, may help for the diagnosis.

The clinical picture may be that of chronic irreversible heart failure. The *electrocardiogram* presents a wide variety of changes including prolonged P-R and QRS intervals, low voltage, and T wave changes. There may be a pattern of myocardial infarct even without infarction or fibrosis.

The clinical course is long and may last many years from the onset of symptoms.

No causal therapy is possible.

Myocardial Fibrosis and Calcification

Myocardial fibrosis is a structural lesion which is frequently associated with other cardiac syndromes and may be completely silent. When severe and extensive, this lesion may cause different clinical pictures, including that of cardiac failure.

CAUSE

a) It may be the result of a *myocarditis* (page 383) and present small, scattered areas of fibrosis. This is frequent after rheumatic fever or other acute diseases.

b) It may be the result of *coronary heart disease* because of systemic narrowing of the arterial vessels or as the result of myocardial infarction.

c) It may be found in *myocardial hypertrophy* and *dilatation*, often predominating in the wall of one chamber.

d) It may be due to *chronic congestion of the coronary venous system*, as frequently encountered in those conditions which raise the pressure in the right atrium.

e) *Trauma* may be a cause of localized scarring.

f) *Vitamin-B deficiency* causes myocardial fibrosis with edema.

From a practical viewpoint, several causes are frequently associated: hypertrophy of the left ventricle and coronary heart disease are frequent in systemic hyper-tension; hypertrophy of the right ventricle and high pressure of the coronary sinus are present in tricuspid and atrial defects; results of myocarditis, possible coronary lesions, effects of hypertrophy and of recurrent high venous pressure, are important factors in rheumatic heart disease with mitral lesions.

LESIONS

Two different types of lesions are apparent at gross examination: focal fibrosis (scarring) and diffuse fibrosis.

Gross scarring may follow trauma or myocardial infarction, the latter being the most common. On external examination, it frequently appears as a grayish-pink, or grayish, glistening, area from which radial bands of connective tissue spread like spokes of a wheel. In such areas, a dense connective tissue is present with a rich supply of blood vessels and, sometimes, a high amount of blood-derived pigment.

Diffuse fibrosis may represent the end result of various mechanisms. Once the process is set up, recognition of the cause may be difficult. The degenerative and necrotizing lesions may be followed by *calcification* but the latter is usually the result of coronary occlusion (119). The infarcted area may be replaced by calcific, bone-like material (*ossification of the heart*).

The following types can be recognized:

a) *Myocardial fibrosis caused by acute or subacute myocarditis or myocardosis*. It is usually scattered and shows small areas of connective tissue, surrounded by normal myofibrils. This type may be associated with one of the two others.

b) *Myocardial fibrosis caused by lesion of the coronary arteries*. It is frequently present in coronary heart disease and has been called *arterial cirrhosis* (89). Even if diffuse, there is more fibrosis in focal areas where occlusion has taken place. At times, however, the same lesions occur without occlusion because of coronary insufficiency due to structural (coronary narrowing) plus functional (coronary insufficiency) causes. *This type of fibrosis predominates in the ventricles, chiefly in the left.*

c) *Myocardial fibrosis caused by lesion of the coronary veins* (89, 90). This type has been called *venous cirrhosis* (89a). There is dilatation of the coronary sinus with insufficiency of its valve and dilatation of the secondary venous collectors. Regressive changes of the venous walls, fibrosis of the venules, and formation of connective tissue, starting from the veins and diffusing into the myocardium, are typical. The importance of this type of fibrosis which predominates in the atria, chiefly in the right, is under debate (91).

SIGNS AND SYMPTOMS

There are no specific signs or symptoms of myocardial fibrosis but myocardial fibrosis increases the severity of symptoms caused by other lesions and may be one of the causes of failure. In particular, the myocardium of hypertensive patients and of patients with mitral stenosis gradually becomes less efficient because of the development of fibrosis. This is usually caused by lesions of the coronary arteries in the former and of the coronary veins in the latter. Atrial fibrillation is favored by fibrosis of the atrial walls.

Myocardial Edema

Myocardial edema may occur in the following conditions: a) Vitamin-B deficiency (page 402). b) Myxedema (page 407). c) Patients with diffuse anasarca caused by congestive failure (page 563). d) Patients with diffuse anasarca caused by nephrosis.

These subjects present evidence of cardiac enlargement upon percussion and x-ray.

While the existence of *myocardial edema* may be suspected (94, 95), it is difficult to exclude enlargement of the heart connected with increased residual blood or transudative pericardial effusion. Actually, myocardial edema is often associated with either of the above conditions.

Myocardial Tumors

Myocardial tumors may be *primary* or *secondary*. The former are more common in the left heart; the latter, in the right. The most frequent primary tumors are *rhabdomyomata* and *sarcomata*. *Carcinoma* is the most common of the secondary tumors. A primary tumor usually consists of a single nodule or mass; a secondary tumor usually consists of multiple nodules (96).

SIGNS AND SYMPTOMS

There may be no signs or symptoms for a long time until the destruction of myocardial tissue causes *heart failure*. If the tumor is superficial, it may cause *pericardial effusion*. If it is in contact with the main coronary arteries, it may cause *angina pectoris*.

X-ray often reveals an enlarged cardiac silhouette because of pericardial effusion or actual enlargement of the heart. When one section of the ventricular wall fails to show pulsations (so-called *rigidity of the wall*), the finding may be of diagnostic importance.

The *electrocardiogram* may show A-V block (involvement of the A-V conduction system by a lesion of the septum) or changes of T and S-T (compression of the coronary vessels). There may be premature beats. A normal ECG, however, is not unusual.

Diagnosis is easier when there is a history of tumors in other organs. However, diagnosis during life is seldom made because of the absence of signs and symptoms or because the latter are atypical.

Treatment with radiation may be attempted whenever diagnosis is made.

Aneurysms of the Heart

Aneurysm of the heart is the name given to the dilatation of one part of the ventricular wall. The same name is improperly applied to the extreme and diffuse dilatation of one of the atria.

Parietal Aneurysm (98, 107)

This type of aneurysm is found exclusively in the ventricles, nearly always in the left ventricle, involving either the *anterior* or the *posterior wall*.

CAUSE

Cardiac aneurysms are usually caused by myocardial infarction. More rarely they are due to syphilitic (gummata), bacterial (abscess or embolus), rheumatic, or isolated myocarditis. They also may follow a congenital (aneurysm of the septum) or a traumatic lesion. A congenital diverticulum of the left ventricle is a rare possibility.

LESIONS

The aneurysm varies in size from that of a walnut to that of a large egg. Rare cases where the pouch was larger than a normal heart have been described. A *congenital diverticulum* may reach a large size and extend into the abdominal cavity (163).

There is a circumscribed dilatation which may be sharply limited from, or gradually fuse with, the rest of the ventricles. An internal *niche* without external bulging is called an aneurysm only by pathologists (98).

The wall of the aneurysm usually consists of thin fibrous tissue with occasional myofibrils. The cavity of the pouch is usually full of *thrombi* which may be organized and are occasionally *calcified*. The pericardium over the sac is usually adherent.

Aneurysm, due to occlusion of the anterior descending artery, is situated at the apex and involves the anterior wall of the left ventricle.

In some cases, the aneurysm forms early (even within 48 hours) after a coronary occlusion (page 417). In these cases, instead of a fibrous wall, an area of necrosis and hemorrhage is present at the site of the lesion. The most common occurrence is, however, a slow formation of the sac through scarring, leading to dilatation of the infarcted area.

SIGNS AND SYMPTOMS

There are no typical symptoms. Dyspnea, precordial pain, and palpitation are common.

Some patients complain of a *sharp pain*, limited to the cardiac apex, which is increased by pressure.

Different physical signs have been described in individual cases:

a) *Strong and extensive systolic impulse*, simulating the apical thrust (110). This is visible at times in the 3rd or 4th left interspace *above the apical thrust*, appearing like a separate pulsation (100). There may be a heaving pulsation of the entire precordium (3).

b) A *systolic click* due to traction of the sac on one of the papillary muscles (102).

c) A *rough, short, systolic murmur* and a *soft, high-pitched diastolic murmur* above the apex (100, 158).

d) *Different disturbances of the heart rate and rhythm:* paroxysmal atrial or ventricular tachycardia, or atrial flutter or fibrillation (101).

GRAPHIC TRACINGS

Electrocardiogram

It usually presents evidence of coronary heart disease and of previous infarcts. It has been stated that *persistent changes of S-T and T*, similar to those of myocardial infarct, are typical of ventricular aneurysm (103, 156, 157). However, they can be found even in cases without aneurysms.

Cardiogram—Phonocardiogram

The tracing of the pulsating area reveals slow movements, both at the beginning of systole and at the time of rapid filling. The cardiac sounds also may be represented by *very slow vibrations of the sound tracing*. The various murmurs are clearly recorded. The diastolic murmur may present a presystolic phase and simulate the murmur of mitral stenosis (157).

X-RAY

The *x-ray* reveals a typical aspect of the profile of the left ventricle. The dilated area is *immobile* or *expands in systole*. The localized bulge is inseparable from the cardiac shadow on rotation of the patient (fig. 241).

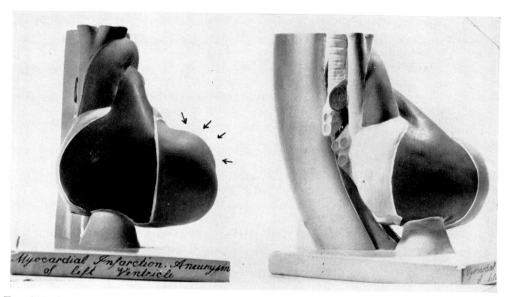

FIG. 241. Aneurysm of the left ventricle. X-ray model in P-A and right oblique (collection of the American Heart Association.)

There may be evidence of adhesions between the heart and the chest wall or the diaphragm. There may be *calcification of the sac or of its content.*

Aneurysms of the *anterior* wall are easily visible in the *right* anterior oblique position; aneurysms of the posterior wall, in the *left.* Posterior aneurysms may displace the esophagus. An aneurysm of the septum may be revealed by extreme enlargement of the heart to the right.

Roentgenkymography and *electrokymography* confirm the absence of pulsations or the systolic expansion. The latter is the most common occurrence and the pattern is similar to that of a dynamic aneurysm (page 425).

COURSE AND PROGNOSIS

A ventricular aneurysm may rupture suddenly, causing *hemopericardium* and *cardiac tamponade.* This fact is not unusual in aneurysms caused by recent infarctions (page 427) but is extremely rare when the sac is made of fibrous tissue (104–106).

Usually, progressive *congestive failure* is the outcome. *Peripheral embolism,* caused by mobilization of a small clot from the cavity of the sac, is a possible complication.

The *prognosis* of this lesion is, therefore, always serious.

DIAGNOSIS

In spite of the possible existence of physical and graphic signs, like expansive and apparently strong cardiac pulsation in contrast with low blood pressure, double apical murmur of a bizarre type, and slow pulsations of cardiograms, the diagnosis is usually made with the x-ray.

Differential diagnosis should exclude an enlarged right ventricular conus, aortic aneurysm, calcified pericardium, loculated pericardial exudate or cyst, and extracardiac tumors or cysts including tumors of the lung.

Surgical removal of a congenital diverticulum has been successfully effected (163). Removal of acquired aneurysms has been suggested but is hardly advisable if there is diffuse coronary heart disease.

Diffuse Aneurysm

A diffuse aneurysm is due to generalized fibrosis of the atrial wall caused by occlusion of small coronary vessels of the atria, or by myocarditis, usually rheumatic (120). High pressure in the chamber, absence of contraction (atrial fibrillation), and weakness of the myocardium (heart failure), are favoring elements. The regurgitation of blood under high pressure with each ventricular systole is an important element (120).

Aneurysm of the left atrium may be found in *mitral stenosis* (107) and, even more often, in *mitral insufficiency* (120). *Aneurysm of the right atrium* has been described in *tricuspid stenosis* and *tricuspid insufficiency* (108).

LESIONS

The wall of the distended atrium consists of fibrous tissue. The degree of enlargement is sometimes astounding as the dilated chamber may contain even one to two liters of blood (113) and cause compression of the surrounding organs. The rest of the heart is also enlarged but may seem like an appendage of the aneurysm.

SIGNS

Pain in the right chest or in the back is not unusual.

Different physical signs have been described in aneurysm of the left atrium. Among them are: a) A *systolic pulsation* of the posterolateral wall of the chest (109). b) A *systolic thrust* in the 4th interspace at the right midclavicular line, which may extend as far right as the axilla, upward to the 2nd rib, and downward to the 6th (110). c) A *systolic pulsation of the jugular veins*, transmitted from the left atrium (expanding in systole because of mitral regurgitation) to the right (110). These signs occur only if severe mitral insufficiency is present.

When the left atrium is extremely enlarged, different phenomena, caused by compression of the lungs, bronchi, veins, and nerves, may occur. Among them are: hoarseness, difficulty in swallowing, faint breath sounds over the right lung, and cough. In rare cases, erosion of the spine may take place (142).

X-RAY

The retrocardiac space is occupied entirely by the shadow of the left atrium. This is also visible in the frontal position as *a shadow which forms the right border of the heart* (fig. 246a). Within this is a second, lower, shadow which is the border of the right atrium (107a, 110, 112). In cases of severe mitral regurgitation, the two shadows may move in opposite directions, the left atrial border expanding in systole toward the right, the right atrial border moving toward the left (110) (fig. 242a).

In rare cases, the shadow of the left atrium creates *a second image at the outside of the left cardiac border* because of "migration" toward the left rather than toward the right (111).

In cases of *right atrial aneurysm*, the shadow of the right atrium nearly reaches the right chest wall (fig. 242b).

Electrokymography of the dilated atrium reveals a systolic distention of the chamber. There is a plateau-like curve which reproduces a tracing of intraventricular pressure (page 219, fig. 121). This is typical of mitral (or tricuspid) insufficiency but the systolic wave is much higher than in cases of valvular defect without aneurysm.

COURSE AND COMPLICATIONS

An atrial aneurysm is not likely to rupture. However, it may increase the symptoms of congestive failure and add new ones because of compression of the mediastinal organs. Should it attain an enormous size, it would cause a mechanical obstacle which is comparable to that of a large mediastinal tumor.

Atrial thrombosis is frequently present in cases of atrial aneurysm and may be the cause of dangerous embolisms. Regression of an atrial aneurysm to an average size and, in exceptional cases, return of the heart to normal sinus rhythm, may occur; such phenomena have been observed by the author.

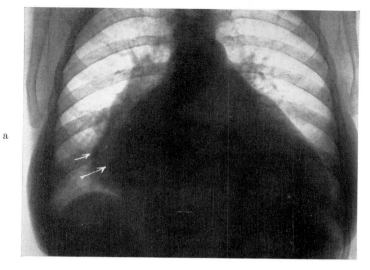

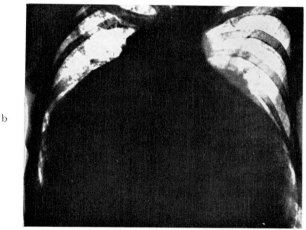

FIG. 242. a, *Aneurysm of the left atrium* in a case of mitral stenosis. The two arrows indicate the borders of the left (outward) and right (inward) atrium, respectively. b, *Aneurysm of the right atrium* in a case of tricuspid stenosis. (Courtesy of Dr. Taussig and the C. V. Mosby Co.)

The Last Manifestations of Cardiac Activity and Cardiac Death

Ventricular Anarchy—The Chaotic Heart (115)

The electrocardiogram presents: a) atrial fibrillation and extreme irregularity of the ventricular complexes; b) low voltage, multiple notchings, and irregular shape of the ventricular complexes; c) multiple ventricular premature contractions arising from different foci; episodes of ventricular tachy-cardia. There frequently is congestive failure; triple rhythm and murmurs are constant. This syndrome has a bad prognosis and may precede ventricular fibrillation by only a few days. Digitalis frequently increases the severity of the cardiac signs.

Ventricular or Total Standstill

If, for any reason, the S-A node fails to initiate the cardiac impulse or if a sudden block stops the progress of the stimulus, *standstill* occurs. This includes the whole heart in the first instance but only the ventricles in the second.

Ordinarily, the A-V node (or a lower point in the bundle of His or his branches) takes over the pacemaking function within a short time (nodal or idioventricular rhythm). If this fails to occur, *ventricular escapes* usually follow. However, the pause may be of such duration as to cause *dizziness* or *syncope*. If the automatic function of the specific tissue of the heart is poor, there may be no automatic contractions of the ventricles (escapes) and death ensues.

The most common cause of cardiac or ventricular standstill is stimulation of the vagus which may be the result of carotid sinus pressure or other reflex disturbances.

The seizures resulting from such a reflex mechanism are usually abolished by *atropine* or *ephedrine*.

TREATMENT

Treatment of the standstill is based on the use of either *epinephrine plus procaine* or *barium chloride* by intracardiac injection. *Resuscitation of the heart* may also be obtained by *manual percussion* of the precordium. If these maneuvers are not successful, artificial respiration, *opening of the chest* (through a transverse incision in the 3rd or 4th left interspace by sectioning the costal cartilages), and *manual massage*, are indicated. A simpler procedure consists of the application of two needle-electrodes to the chest and use of an *artificial pacemaker* (164).

Ventricular Flutter and Fibrillation

An abnormal mechanism of rapid excitation, similar to that more frequently observed in the atria, may develop in the ventricles. The latter occurrence is far more dangerous than the former and frequently results in death.

CAUSE AND MECHANISM

Animal experimentation demonstrates that ventricular flutter and fibrillation may be induced by certain drugs (digitalis in toxic doses, chloroform, cyclopropane, or ether plus epinephrine); ligation of the coronary arteries (116); injection of irritant substances into the myocardium; or electric faradization of the heart. *Oxygen deficiency* seems to be the cause of ventricular fibrillation after coronary ligation (117).

Both clinical and experimental evidence indicate that the coronary circulation is the chief element to be considered in ventricular fibrillation (118). Both coronary lesions and functional disturbances causing coronary insufficiency may be effective, and reflex elements may be involved.

Ventricular flutter or fibrillation may follow coronary occlusion, an attack of rapid heart beat (atrial flutter, atrial or ventricular tachycardia, ventricular anarchy), or ventricular standstill.

Rapid *dilution of the blood*, like that occurring *in drowning in fresh water*, is often followed by ventricular fibrillation. This does not occur in sea water drowning where hemoconcentration occurs (150).

SIGNS

The patient suddenly *faints* and his face shows a *livid color*. The arterial pulse and every other cardiac manifestation, including the apical impulse and the undulations of the jugular veins, disappear. A faint *buzzing murmur* has been described in ventricular flutter while *no sound can be heard* in fibrillation.

ELECTROCARDIOGRAM

Large, regular, monophasic ventricular waves follow each other at a rate of 250 to 300 per minute in ventricular flutter; rapid, irregular, bizarre, small complexes are typical of ventricular fibrillation.

DIAGNOSIS

Absence of any cardiac manifestation is typical of both ventricular standstill and fibrillation. The former is usually of abrupt onset and end; the latter is usually preceded and followed by ventricular premature beats.

Ventricular flutter is not always fatal and some patients may survive repeated attacks; on the other hand, ventricular fibrillation is nearly always fatal; recovery is possible (146) but extremely rare. Respiration may continue for some time after the beginning of an attack of fibrillation.

TREATMENT

Artificial respiration or inhalation with 100 per cent oxygen should be started immediately. *Intracardiac epinephrine with procaine* is sometimes able to reactivate the heart but only if the injection is made *after* the end of any electric manifestation; at an early stage, it might only accentuate the fibrillation.

As already said, cyclopropane or ether anesthesia, and epinephrine, may cause ventricular fibrillation. Various drugs may prevent the occurrence of this lethal disturbance. One single dose of *procaine* (30–70 mg.) or *pronestyl* (**26**) injected intravenously after the onset of anesthesia has a favorable effect (147). *1262* F. has a similar action (148). *Atabrine* (*quinacrine*) and *papaverine* seem to have also similar effects (149). *Procaine*, as well as *1262* F., has a direct action on the myocardium; the other drugs cause coronary vasodilation.

Defibrillation of the ventricles may be obtained in the following way (114):

a) Injection of 2 cc. of 5 per cent procaine into the right ventricle.

b) Manual cardiac massage after opening of the chest.

c) Application of two large electrodes to the heart and sending an alternating current of 1.5 ampères through the organ.

This permits transformation of fibrillation into standstill. Then the procedures indicated for this condition may be used for the *resuscitation of the heart* (page 396).

Cardiac Death and Clinical Death

Four types of cardiac death have been recognized (3).

1) There is a *complete A-V block*, followed by *ventricular standstill*. The atria continue to contract for some time.

2) There is a *total standstill* of the heart.

3) There is *ventricular fibrillation*, followed by *total standstill*.

4) There is a *slow or agonal death*. The ventricular rate gradually becomes slower and is interrupted by premature beats. The ventricular complexes become more and more deformed. The origin of the stimulus may be in the node or in one of the ventricles; S-T is displaced from the basal line; T is inverted. *Total standstill* finally occurs.

Clinical death is not always accompanied by cardiac death. Electrical manifestations of the heart have been recorded for 20 to 30 minutes after the suspension of respiration.

BIBLIOGRAPHY

1. DRY, TH.J. *Manual of Cardiology*. Philadelphia, Saunders, 1943.
2. a) HOFF, H. E., NAHUM, L. H., AND KISCH, B. Am. J. Physiol., 1941, **131**, 687, 693 and 700.
   b) HOFF, H. E. In *Howell's Textbook of Physiology*. Philadelphia, Saunders, 1946.
3. a) PAZZANESE, D. *Modificaçoes de Forma do Electrocardiograma*. São Paulo, Gráfica da Prefeitura, 1942.
   b) STROUD, M. W., AND FEIL, H. S. Am. Heart J., 1948, **35**, 910.
4. WILSON, F. N., AND CO-WORKERS. Am. Heart J., 1934, **9**, 447; and **10**, 46.
5. POTAIN, P. C. E. Ctr. Assoc. Fr. Avanc. Sc., 1885, I, **14**, 201.
6. LUISADA, A. A. *Cardiologia*. Bologna, Cappelli, 1938.
7. LAUBRY AND PEZZI. *Les Rythmes de Galop*. Paris, Doin, 1926.
8. BATTRO, A., BRAUN-MENENDEZ, E., AND ORIAS, O. Rev. Arg. Card., 1934, **1**, 117. Also J. de Phys., Path. Gen., 1935, **33**, 51.
9. a) MOZER, J. J., AND DUCHOSAL, P. Arch. Mal. Coeur, 1930, **23**, 65 and 247.
   b) ROUTIER, D., AND VAN BOGAERT, A. Arch. Mal. Coeur, 1934, **27**, 389, 541 and 588.
10. a) WOLFERTH, C. C., AND MARGOLIES, A. Am. Heart J., 1933, **8**, 41.
    b) CALÒ, A. Cuore e Circ., (Rome), 1937, **21**, 422.
11. CARLYLE, H. F. Canad. M. A. J., 1941, **44**, 260.

12. CHINI, V. L'Alternanza del Cuore. Roma, Ediz. Accad. d'Italia, 1935, **6**, V, 14.

13. VOLHARD, F. Muench. med. Woch., 1905, **52**, 590.

14. WENCKEBACH, K. F., AND WINTERBERG, H. *Die unregelmaessige Herztaetigkeit.* Leipzig, Engelmann, 1927.

15. MACKENZIE, J. Brit. Med. J., 1908, **1**, 23. Also Heart, 1911, **2**, 273.

16. GALLAVARDIN, L., AND GRAVIER, L. Prov. Méd., 1913, **24**, 421.

17. GALLAVARDIN, L., AND GRAVIER, L. Lyon Méd., 1912, **119**, 1144 and 1151.

18. LIAN, C. Presse Méd., 1911, **19** (1), 777.

19. GALLI, L. Muench. med. Woch., 1906, **53**, 1956.

20. SCHERF, D., AND ZDANSKY, E. Fortsch. Geb. Roentgstr., 1929, **40**, 60.

21. BATTRO, A., AND QUIRNO, N. Rev. Arg. Card., 1936, **3**, 267.

22. a) POUMAILLOUX, M. *Le Pouls Alternant.* Paris, Masson, 1930.

    b) GRAVIER, L. *L'Alternance du Coeur.* Paris, Baillière, 1914.

23. CONDORELLI, L. Arch. Pat. Clin. Med., 1929, **8**, 428.

24. MAHAIM, I. *Les Maladies Organiques du Faisceau de His-Tawara.* Paris, Masson, 1931.

25. a) CHINI, V. Atti Acc. d'Italia, 1935, **6**, N. 14.

    b) VAQUEZ, H., AND DONZELOT, E. *Les Troubles du Rythme Cardiaque.* Paris, Baillière, 1926.

26. WILSON, F. N. Form of the Electrocardiogram. In *Stroud's Cardiovascular Disease.* Philadelphia, Davis, 1945.

27. MASTER, A. M., AND CO-WORKERS: Am. Heart J., 1940, **20**, 186.

28. LUISADA, A. A. Rev. Arg. Cardiol., 1942, **9**, 169.

29. GRAYBIEL, A., AND SPRAGUE, H. B. Am. J. M. Sci., 1933, **185**, 395.

30. PARDEE, H. F. B. *Clinical Aspects of the Electrocardiogram.* New York, Hoeber, 1933.

31. BENCHIMOL, A. B. *Bloqueo de Ramo em Clínica.* Rio de Janeiro, Thesis, 1943.

32. a) BAGNARESI, G. Cuore e Circ., 1934. **18**, 65.

    b) KISCH, B., AND GRISHMAN, A. Exper. Med., Surg., 1944, **2**, 277.

    c) GONZALES SABATHIÉ, L., GASPARY, F. V., AND ROJAS, R. A. Rev. Arg. Card., 1944, **11**, 297.

33. COMEAU, W. J., AND HAMILTON, J. G. M. Am. Heart J., 1938, **15**, 276.

34. WILSON, F. N., JOHNSTON, F. D., BARKER, P. S., AND MACLEOD, G. Am. Heart J., 1934, **9**, 447, 459, and 472.

35. WILSON, F. N., HILL, I. G. W., AND JOHNSTON, F. D. Am. Heart J., 1935, **10**, 596 and 903.

36. WILSON, F. N. J. Mt. Sinai Hosp., 1942, **8**, 1110.

37. PERERA, G. H., LEVINE, S. A., AND ERLANGER, H. Brit. Heart J., 1942, **4**, 35.

38. LIAN, C., AND GOLBLIN, V. Arch. Mal. Coeur, 1937, **30**, 787.

39. WOLFERTH, C. C., AND MARGOLIES, A. Am. Heart J., 1935, **10**, 425.

40. BATTRO, A., BRAUN-MENENDEZ, E., AND ORIAS, O. Rev. Arg. Card., 1936, **3**, 325.

41. BATTRO, A., BRAUN-MENENDEZ, E., AND ORIAS, O. Arch. Mal. Coeur, 1938, **31**, 250.

42. BRAUN-MENENDEZ, E., AND SOLARI, L. A. Arch. Int. Med., 1939, **63**, 830.

43. WOLFF, L., PARKINSON, J., AND WHITE, P. D. Am. Heart J., 1930, **5**, 685.

44. LEVINE, S. A., AND BEESON, P. B. Am. Heart J., 1941, **22**, 401.

45. HOLZMANN, M., AND SCHERF, D. Zeit. klin. Med., 1932, **121**, 404.

46. WOLFERTH, C. C., AND WOOD, F. C. Am. Heart J., 1933, **8**, 297.

47. KENT, A. F. S. J. Physiol., 1914, **48**, 22 and 57.

48. PALADINO. Il Movim. Med.-Chir., 1876.

49. ROSENBAUM, F. F., HECHT, H. H., WILSON, F. N., AND JOHNSTON, F. D. Am. Heart J., 1945, **29**, 281.

50. HUNTER, A., PAPP, C., AND PARKINSON, J. Brit. Heart, 1940, **2**, 107.

51. a) WOOD, F. C., WOLFERTH, C. C., AND GECKELER, G. D. Am. Heart J., 1943, **25**, 454.

    b) SEGERS, M., AND CO-WORKERS. Acta Cardiol., 1947, **2**, 21.

    c) LEVINE, H. N. E. Heart Assoc., 1948.

52. WHITE, P. D. *Heart Disease.* New York, Macmillan, 1944.

53. SCHERF, D., AND SHOOKOFF, C. Zeit. exp. Med., 1926, **49**, 302.

54. ROTHBERGER, C. J., AND SCHERF, D. Zeit. exp. Med., 1927, **53**, 792.

55. SCHERF, D., AND BOYD, L. F. *Clinical Electrocardiography.* St. Louis, Mosby, 1940.

56. a) LAUFER, S., AND RUBINO, A. Clin. Med. Ital. (Milan), 1936, **67**, 365.

    b) LUISADA, A. A. J. Lab. & Clin. Med., 1940, **25**, 1146.

57. RUBINO, A. Arch. Sci. Med. (Turin), 1937, **63**, 201. Also Clin. Med. Ital. (Milan), 1936, **67**, 168.

58. Scherf, D., and Siedeck, H. Zeit. klin. Med., 1934, **127**, 77.

59. Géraudel, E. *Le Mécanisme du Coeur et ses Anomalies*. Paris, Masson, 1928. Also Presse Méd., 1935, **43**, 297.

60. Duclós, F. Arch. Card., Hemat., 1935, **17**, 175.

61. Dominguez, C., and Bizzozero, R. C. Arch. Mal. Coeur, 1937, **30**, 820.

62. a) French, A. J., and Weller, C. V. Am. J. Path., 1942, **18**, 109.
   b) Wells, A. H., and Sax, S. G. Am. Heart J., 1945, **30**, 522.

63. Helwig, F. C., and Schmidt, E. C. H. Science, 1945, **102**, 31.

64. a) Klinefelter, H. F. Am. J. M. Sci., 1942, **203**, 34.
   b) Winsor, T., and Burch, G. E. Am. Heart J., 1945, **29**, 685.

65. von Bonsdorff, B. Acta Med. Scand., 1939, **100**, 352.

66. a) Franceschetti, A., and Mach, R. S. Helvet. Med. Acta, 1944, **11**, 887.
   b) Evans, W. Brit. Heart J., 1944, **6**, 41.

67. Pianese. Quoted by Aresu in *Tratt. Ital. Med. Int.*; Milan, S. E. L., 1931.

68. Letulle and Natau-Larrier. *Anatomie Pathologique*. Paris, Masson.

69. Brin, L., and Giroux, L. *Le Syphilis du Coeur et de l'Aorte*. Paris, Doin, 1924.

70. Tedeschi, C. Giorn. Batt., Imm. (Turin), 1929, **4**, 1097.

71. Bettoni, I. Cuore e Circ., 1929, **13**, 210.

72. Kuelbs. The Diseases of the Heart; in *Internal Medicine* by Mohr and Staehelin.

73. Dionisi, A. *Anatomia Patologica della Malaria*. Rome, Ferri, 1927.

74. Segre, R. *Le Malattie del Miocardio*. Bologna, Cappelli, 1932.

75. Chagas, C. Arch. Mal. Coeur, 1928, **10**, 641.

76. Dévé, F. Ctr. Soc. Biol., 1917, **80**, 859.

77. Peters, J. H., Dexter, L., and Weiss, S. Am. Heart J., 1945, **29**, 143.

78. a) Buchbinder, W. C., and Saphir, O. Arch. Int. Med., 1939, **64**, 336.
   b) de Navasquez, S. J. Path. & Bact., 1939, **49**, 33.

79. a) Rich, A. R., and Gregory, J. E. Bull. Johns Hopkins Hosp., 1943, **72**, 65.
   b) Case Record 30 441 of Mass. Gen. Hosp. New England J. Med., 1944, **231**, 628.

80. a) Fiedler. Festschr. d. Stadtkrankenhaus. Dresden, Freidrichstadt, 1899, **2**, quoted from H. Sikl.
   b) Sikl, H. Zeitschr. Path., 1936, **49**, 283.

81. Saphir, O. Arch. Path. 1941, **32**, 1000; and 1942, **33**, 88. Am. Heart J., 1942, **24**, 167.

82. Tedeschi, A. Virchow's Arch., 1892, **128**, 185.

83. Stamer, A. Beitr. path. Anat., 1907, **42**, 310.

84. Wearn, J. T. Bull. New York Acad. Med., 1941, **17**, 754.

85. Myers, V. C. Mo. Conc. Cardiov. Dis., 1944, **13**, N. 6.

86. Wendkos, M. H., and Noll, J. Am. Heart J., 1944, **27**, 414.

87. Freundlich, J. Zeit. klin. Med., 1938, **133**, 768.

88. Gamna, C. Min. Med. (Turin), 1938 (pt. 2), **29**, 5.

89. a) Banti, G. Ziegler's Beitr., 1895, **6**, 5.
   b) Vannucci, O. *Lo Sperim.* (Florence), 1923, 425.

90. Condorelli, L. Verh. Deut. Ges. Kreislauff, 1931, 4th Meeting.

91. Ferrari, E. Cuore e Circ., 1940, **24**, 381.

92. Walser, J. *La Myocardie*. Paris, Doin, 1925.

93. Evans, W., and Wright, G. Brit. Heart J., 1942, **4**, 91.

94. Doumer, E. Soc. Méd. Hôp., 1936, **52**, 819.

95. Langeron, L. Arch. Mal. Coeur, 1937, **30**, 609.

96. Ravid, J. M., and Sachs, J. Am. Heart J., 1943, **26**, 385.

97. a) Schlomka, G., and Schmitz, G. Zeit. Kreislauff, 1928, **30**, 41.
   b) Bright, E. F., and Beck, C. S. Am. Heart J., 1935, **10**, 293.

98. Sternberg, M. *Das chronische, partielle Herzaneurysma*. Leipzig and Vienna, 1924.

99. Wilson, F. N., and co-workers. Am. Heart J., 1944, **27**, 19.

100. Scherf, D., and Erlsbacher, O. Med. Klin., 1934, N. 51.

101. Taran, L. M., and Szilagyi, N. Am. J. Med., 1948, **5**, 379.

102. Le Roy, G. V., and Roberts, R. C. Am. Heart J., 1941, **21**, 114.

103. Nordenfelt, O. Acta Med. Scand., 1939, **102**, 101.

104. Friedman, S., and White, P. D. Ann. Int. Med., 1944, **21**, 778.

105. Jetter, W. W., and White, P. D. Ann. Int. Med., 1944, **21**, 783.

106. Fisher, R. L. Am. Heart J., 1945, **30**, 133.

107. a) Lutembacher, R. Arch. Mal. Coeur, 1917, **10**, 145.
   b) Lutembacher, R., and Mahaim, I. Ann. Méd., 1928, **23**, 79.

108. Taussig, B. L. Am. Heart J., 1937, **14**, 744.

109. Cossio, P. *Aparato Circulatorio*. Buenos Aires, El Ateneo, 1944.

110. Dressler, W. *Clinical Cardiology*. New York, Hoeber, 1942.

111. ROUTIER, D., AND HEIM DE BALSAC, R. Am.
     J. Roentgenol., 1940, **44**, 834.
112. a) ROESLER, H. *Clinical Roentgenology of
        the Cardiovascular System.* Springfield,
        Thomas, 1943.
     b) SCHWEDEL, J. B. *Clinical Roentgenology
        of the Heart.* New York, Hoeber, 1946.
113. a) GOEDEL, A. Wien. klin. Woch., 1929, **42**,
        427.
     b) BLAND, E. F., BALBONI, G. M., AND
        WHITE, P. D. J. A. M. A., 1931, **96**, 840.
114. HOYNE, A., AND WALFORD, N. T. Journ.
     Pediat., 1934, **5**, 642.
115. a) PEZZI, C. Arch. Mal. Coeur, 1925, **18**, 753.
     b) ORSI, A., AND VILLA, L. Arch. Mal.
        Coeur, 1928, **21**, 353.
116. SMITH, F. M. Arch. Int. Med., 1918, **22**, 8;
     and 1923, **32**, 497.
117. RESNIK, W. H. J. Clin. Investigation, 1925,
     2, 93, 117 and 125.
118. HARRISON, T. R. *Failure of the Circulation.*
     Baltimore, The Williams and Wilkins Co.,
     1939.
119. a) DECHERD, G. M., RUSKIN, A., AND
        BRINDLEY, P. Am. Heart J., 1946, **31**,
        352.
     b) BLACKFORD, L. M. Am. Int. Med., 1947,
        27, 1036.
     c) EDELSTEIN, J. M. Am. Heart J., 1946, **31**,
        496.
120. EVANS, W. Brit. Heart J., 1948, **10**, 92.
121. BOUILLAUD. *Traité Clin. Mal. Coeur.* Paris,
     1835.
122. LUISADA, A. A., AND MAGRI, G. Am. Heart J.,
     1952, **44**, 545.
123. LUISADA, A. A., AND ROITMAN, M. Arch. Inst.
     Card. de Mexico, 1948, **17**, 345.
124. FUCHS, G. Wien. med. Woch. 1949, **99**, 535.
125. LUISADA, A. A., ROMANO, F. J., AND TORRE,
     J. M. Proc. Soc. Exper. Biol. & Med., 1948,
     69, 23.
126. WOLFERTH, C. C. Cyclopedia of Medicine.
     Philadelphia, Davis, 1943, vol. III.
127. LUISADA, A. A., MENDOZA, F., AND ALI-
     MURUNG, M. Brit. Heart J., 1949, **11**, 41.
128. WILSON, F. N., AND CO-WORKERS. Am. Heart
     J., 1944, **27**, 19.
129. GOLDBERGER, E. *Unipolar Lead Electro-
     cardiography.* 2nd Edit. Philadelphia,
     Lea and Febiger, 1950.
130. SODI PALLARES, D., AND CO-WORKERS.
     Am. Heart J., 1947, **33**, 819.
131. HELLERSTEIN, H. K., AND SANTIAGO-
     STEVENSON, D. Circ., 1950, **1**, 93.
132. RASMUSSEN, LT., AND MOE, T. Brit. Heart
     J., 1948, **10**, 141.

133. KISS, A. Wien. Zeit. inn. Med., 1947, **28**, 397.
134. BEAUDET, S. C., AND BOERMAN, C. Rev.
     Med. de Liège, 1947, 2/23, 621.
135. a) WEISS, S., AND CO-WORKERS. Arch. Int.
        Med., 1943, **71**, 749.
     b) BANKS, B. M. New England J. Med., 1941,
        225, 443.
136. STEINLIN, J. Schweiz. med. Woch., 1947, **77**,
     72.
137. a) GORE, I., AND SAPHIR, O. Am. Heart J.,
        1947, **34**, 831.
     b) SAPHIR, O., AND AMROMIN, G. D. Am. Int.
        Med., 1948, **28**, 936.
     c) GORE, I., AND SAPHIR, O. Am. Heart J.,
        1948, **36**, 390.
138. a) SAPHIR, O., AND WILE, S. A. Am. J.
        M. Sci., 1942, **203**, 781.
     b) GEFTER, W. I., AND CO-WORKERS. Am.
        Heart J., 1947, **33**, 228.
     c) LUDDEN, T. E., AND EDWARDS, J. E.
        Proc. Staff Meet., Mayo Clin., 1948, **23**,
        379.
139. a) DIAS, E., LARANJA, F. S., AND NOBREGA,
        G. *Doença de Chagas.* Rio de Janeiro,
        Imprensa Nacional, 1946. Also Brasil
        Medico, 1948, **42**, N. 8–9.
     b) AZEVEDO PONDÉ, A. *A Doença de Chagas
        na Bahia.* Bahia, Imprensa Vitoria,
        1947.
140. COSTERO, I., AND DE BUEN, S. Arch. Inst.
     Card. de Mexico, 1947, **17**, 605.
141. a) DEZA, D., AND ROJAS, R. Proc. II
        Interamer. Cong. Cardiol., 1946, **3**,
        1478.
     b) SPRAGUE, H. B. Am. Heart J., 1946, **31**,
        426.
142. ASHWORTH, H., AND JONES, A. M. Brit.
     Heart J., 1946, **8**, 207.
143. OEHNELL, R. F. Acta Med. Scand., 1944,
     Suppl. 152.
144. REED, J. C., AND CO-WORKERS. III Inter-
     american Congress, Chicago, 1948.
145. VAN BOGAERT, A., AND VAN GANABECK, A.
     Cardiol., 1946–47, **2**, 255.
146. ZIMDAHL, W. T., AND FULTON, F. T. Am.
     Heart J., 1946, **32**, 117.
147. BERNSTEIN, C. Anesthesiol., 1946, **7**, 113.
148. BOVET, D., AND CO-WORKERS. Ctr. Soc. Biol.,
     1939, **130**, 29.
149. MELVILLE, K. I. J. Pharmacol. & Exper.
     Therap., 1946, **87**, 350. Also Rev. Canad.
     Biol., 1948, **7**, 236.
150. SWANN, H. G., AND CO-WORKERS. Texas Rep.
     Biol. & Med., 1947, **5**, 423
151. GRAYBIEL, A., AND WHITE, P. D. *Electro-*

cardiography in Practice. 2nd Edit. Philadelphia, W. B. Saunders Co., 1946.

152. LIAN, C., AND WELTI, J. J. Arch. Inst. Card. Mexico, 1949, **19,** 445.

153. CONTRO, S., AND LUISADA, A. A. J. Mt. Sinai Hosp., 1952, **19,** 70.

154. LUISADA, A. A., AND FLEISCHNER, F. G. Proc. Soc. Exper. Biol. & Med., 1947, **66,** 436.

155. SAMET, P., MEDNICK, M., AND SCHWEDEL, J. B. Am. Heart J., 1950, **39,** 841.

156. GOLDBERGER, E., AND SCHWARTZ, S. P. Am. J. Med., 1948, **4,** 243.

157. FORD, R. V., AND LEVINE, H. D. Am. Heart Assoc. Meet., 1949.

158. SCHERF, D., AND BROOKS, A. M. Am. J. M. Sci., 1949, **218,** 389.

159. WUHRMANN, F. Schweiz. med. Woch., 1950, **80,** 715.

160. a) WESSLER, S., AND FREEDBERG, A. S. Arch. Int. Med., 1948, **82,** 1.

  b) DAHLIN, D. C., AND EDWARDS, J. E. Proc. Staff Meet. Mayo Clin., 1949, **24,** 89.

  c) JONES, R. S., AND FRAZIER, D. B. Arch. Path., 1950, **50,** 366.

161. FRANKE, H. Zeit. klin. Med., 1950, **147,** 131.

162. COAKLEY, J. B. Brit. Heart J., 1951, **13,** 148.

163. POTTS, W. J. Proc. Inst. Med. Chicago, 1953, **19,** No. 14.

164. ZOLL, P. M.: New Eng. J, Med., 1952, *247,* 768.

CHAPTER 18

Metabolic, Vitamin, Endocrine, and Traumatic Heart Diseases

Metabolic Disturbances
VON GIERKE'S DISEASE (1)

This is a rare disease, due to faulty glycogen metabolism. Enlargement of the heart is chiefly due to deposition of glycogen in small cavities between the cardiac fibers. A similar involvement of other organs, especially the liver, is present. Death occurs early, usually in the first months of life, but occasionally the age of 4 or 5 is reached.

FATTY HEART

Fatty degeneration of some parts of the heart muscle is present, not only in acute and subacute myocarditis, but also in certain anemias (mainly pernicious anemia). The striped appearance of the myocardium is the cause of the terms "tiger" and "tiger-lily" heart.

Fatty infiltration of the myocardium, chiefly involving the right ventricle, is common in middle-aged or old people. Fatty infiltration is then associated with *deposition of fat around the heart*, mainly around the root of the great vessels, along the coronary arteries, and in the sulcus between the ventricles and the atria (fig. 243). As a rule, there is a close relationship between deposition of fat on the heart and in other parts of the body. It is a sign of general *obesity*.

It is sometimes difficult to know whether the symptoms of these patients are due to the increased weight of the body, the high level of the diaphragm, or the mechanical load carried by the heart. Whenever the patients have hypertension, emphysema of the lungs, or both, additional causes of strain are present.

The most important element in the treatment of obesity is *decrease in food intake*. A daily diet of 1000 to 1500 calories usually results in a steady loss of weight (4 to 8 lbs. per month) without causing hunger, weakness or dizziness (diet III). *Benzedrine sulfate* may depress the appetite if taken 15 minutes before meals. *Thyroid extract* is useful in certain cases.

Vitamin Deficiencies
THIAMINE DEFICIENCY

Thiamine deficiency causes different clinical pictures involving both the cardiovascular and the nervous systems. The pictures are different in the oriental and the occidental countries.

Oriental Thiamine Deficiency (Shôshin or Beri Beri) (3, 4, 5)

This clinical picture occurs in Japanese or Javanese people subsisting on a main diet of polished rice. It appears suddenly with *precordial oppression* and *pain, dyspnea, cyanosis*, and *distention of the veins*. The pulse is rapid and full; the liver is large. The heart is *tremendously dilated and presents several murmurs, both systolic and diastolic*, caused by the enlargement of the chambers and the valvular openings.

There frequently is a *venous murmur* over the right jugular vein (*bruit du diable*). The arterial pulse pressure is high; venous pressure reaches 20 to 40 cm. of water.

The *ECG* shows only atypical changes. *X-ray* reveals *a large heart with tremendous dilatation of the pulmonary artery and its branches*. Death frequently occurs within a few hours.

At autopsy, the heart is flabby and

402

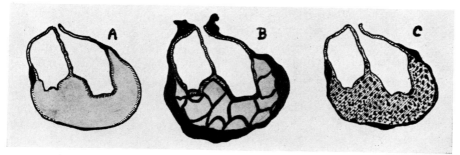

FIG. 243. Distribution of fat within and around the heart (fat indicated by black areas). A, normal; B, heart in obesity; C, fatty degeneration of the heart.

dilated, especially the right chambers, and the liver is very large. Microscopic examination reveals diffuse but not severe lesions of the myocardium.

The clinical picture was interpreted as caused by a primary abnormal dilatation of the small vessels with increased venous return and secondary dilatation of the heart.

Occidental Thiamine Deficiency (6, 7)

This picture was mainly described in the large cities of the United States. The following groups of people are usually affected: alcohol addicts, patients with chronic diseases, poor people with improper diet, and patients with diseases of the gastrointestinal tract. Some of them have neurological signs of thiamine deficiency; some have pellagra. To these should be added many patients with heart failure or hypertension who have been kept for a long time on improper diet.

The syndrome usually starts with *rapid pulse* but this may be followed by a *slow pulse*. There is *cardiac dilatation, triple rhythm, systolic murmur* over the apex or base, *dyspnea*, congestion of the hila and of the pulmonary bases, *venous distention*, and diffuse *peripheral edema*.

The *ECG* may show inverted T, slight aberration and low voltage of the ventricular complexes, and prolongation of Q-T. Premature beats and atrial tachycardia have been described but *the persistence of sinus rhythm is usual* and is important for diagnosis.

On fluoroscopy, an *enlarged cardiac shadow* and decreased amplitude of contraction can be observed. The latter may be caused, at least in part, by pericardial effusion. X-ray reveals severe enlargement of the right heart and often of the pulmonary knob; the left heart remains normal and the pulmonary fields are free from congestion

Low vital capacity, *high venous pressure*, normal arterial pressure, *decreased circulation time*, and increased blood volume and cardiac output, are typical of the syndrome.

At *autopsy*, dilatation and, at times, hypertrophy of the heart are present; the myocardium reveals intracellular and intercellular *edema* and occasional scattered areas of *necrosis;* petechial hemorrhages have been observed. Diffuse *myocardial fibrosis* is frequently present.

The cardiovascular disturbances of occidental thiamine deficiency may cause different clinical pictures with gradual or sudden onset. Fever, vascular collapse, or bronchopneumonia occasionally may be observed.

The exact mechanism of this syndrome is still debated. On the one hand, the components of the vitamin B-complex have a direct influence on the metabolism of carbohydrates (page 32); on the other, the edema is partly the result of *low blood proteins*, favored by malnutrition. Therefore, peripheral edema may be caused both by this mechanism and by heart failure. Whether the edema of the cardiac muscle has the same colloidosmotic mechanism or is a primary factor, is not known; in any case, it may be a contributory factor to heart failure. The possibility of a neurogenic disturbance of the cardiac functions because of sympathetic and vagal lesions has been discussed (7c). Also, it has been pointed out that thiamin-deficient animals have an increased epinephrine level in the blood and excessive amounts of epinephrine or epinephrine-like substances in the myocardium (47). As adrenal cortex is often found hypertrophied, it has been suggested that the adreno-sympathetic system is somehow involved and causes many of the typical signs and lesions (48).

The *increased speed of circulation*, first observed in oriental beri beri (5), is frequently present also in occidental thiamine deficiency, and may be one of the causes of failure by decreasing the peripheral utilization of oxygen. It resembles the phenomena observed in thyrotoxicosis. Cardiac failure may be present with *normal or even increased cardiac output*, though this is reduced in comparison with figures obtained when no failure was present (46).

The diagnosis may not be easy, especially in patients with valvular lesions who also have thiamine deficiency. The diagnosis is based on the following data (7b): insufficient evidence of other etiology; signs of neuritis or pellagra; enlarged heart with sinus rhythm; dependent edema; high venous pressure; recovery with decreased size of the heart; or autopsy consistent with beri beri heart disease.

Thiamine treatment may not cause a prompt improvement because the duration and severity of the deficiency may lead to irreversibility of the process (7c). It may be followed by inversion of the T wave in the electrocardiogram.

Treatment is based on intramuscular or intravenous injections of vitamin B_1 or, better still, of vitamin B-complex (**68**). High protein diet is indicated.

PELLAGRA (8)

The heart is not enlarged in pellagra and may be *small*. *Peripheral edema* is explained by the low protein content of the plasma. The electrocardiogram may show low or inverted T waves and depressed S-T. *The Q-T interval is prolonged.* These changes are probably of metabolic origin, niacin being essential to the metabolism of carbohydrates (page 32), and disappear promptly after administration of *niacin* in daily oral doses of 300 to 500 mg.

SCURVY

Dilatation of the right heart has been described in severe cases of scurvy. It is still to be demonstrated whether it is actually caused by vitamin C deficiency or by associated causes, including deficiency of thiamine.

RICKETS

Dilatation of the heart has been described in children with vitamin D deficiency. It is possible that, in many cases, the thoracic deformity and not the vitamin D deficiency caused the observed changes (page 510). Moreover, associated vitamin deficiencies may be involved.

MALNUTRITION

Malnutrition and starvation may be followed by severe cardiovascular disturbances. Prolonged starvation causes reduction of size and decreased functional capacity of the heart (62). Both systolic and diastolic pressures are lower; cardiac output and stroke volume are reduced; venous pressure is also low (62). The heart rate may be as low as 30 per minute.

The *electrocardiogram* presents a prolonged Q-T interval, large U waves, abnormal T waves, and occasionally a depression of S-T (63). Prolonged protein and carbohydrate starvation and electrolyte imbalance seem to be responsible for these changes even without vitamin deficiency.

Tachycardia and dyspnea may occur between the 12th and the 20th weeks of rehabilitation.

Endocrine Disturbances

HYPERTHYROIDISM

The most typical picture is encountered in thyrotoxicosis.

Signs and Symptoms

The patients have several symptoms caused by the thyroid condition which may simulate organic heart disease. Dizziness and visual disturbances are common. *Palpitation, precordial tightness or pain,* and various sensations caused by irregular heart beat are frequent. Exertion may be followed by *dyspnea* in more advanced cases where a *sensation of fullness in the upper right abdominal quadrant* and *precordial pain* may also exist.

The *radial pulse is rapid,* frequently above 120, and at times it may reach 200 (9). *Irregular pulse* may be found because of *premature beats* or *atrial fibrillation.* The latter is more common in old age and in rheumatic heart disease.

Peripheral signs simulating aortic regurgitation may be present. They include *pistol shot sound, Corrigan's pulse,* and *the double murmur of Duroziez* (10a) (page 240). There may be a loud murmur over the right jugular vein (*bruit du diable*) and over the 2nd right interspace (10b).

The apex impulse is forceful and rapid. There may be the impression of an *apical thrill.* The heart frequently seems enlarged and often presents acute dilatation after exertion.[67] There may be dulness of the manubrium.

Auscultation reveals loud heart sounds and, frequently, *murmurs: a soft apical* and

[67] Hyperthyroidism is not a cause of cardiac enlargement *per se.* It is likely that cases with enlarged heart also have other cardiac diseases. However, the rapid heart action increases cardiac strain in valvular lesions or coronary heart disease.

a *harsher pulmonic systolic murmur.* There may be a *triple rhythm,* or a *diastolic rumble* simulating that of mitral stenosis.

High sensitivity to adrenalin and poor response to vagus stimulation are typical.

Lesions

Serous inflammation of the myocardium, myocardial fibrosis or fibroblastic myocarditis, have been described (49). It is likely that these are concomitant lesions.

Electrocardiogram

The ECG usually reveals *sinus tachycardia* but may show *atrial flutter, tachycardia* or *fibrillation,* or *premature beats.* Prolongation of P-R is rare (12); high T wave in all leads, which was thought common (13), is present only in some cases (14, 15). Intraventricular block is not unusual.

Phonocardiogram

In most cases, the *first heart sound is of large amplitude.* The frequent report of murmurs may not be confirmed by the tracing. The most common finding seems to be a *low-grade systolic murmur* over the mid-precordium (64).

Circulatory Dynamics

Blood pressure is normal or high, with increased pulse pressure. *Cardiac output, blood volume, and speed of circulation are typically increased and are proportional to the basal metabolic rate* (16–19). Outputs of 6 to 12 liters per minute are frequent and are made possible by the severe increase of heart rate while venous pressure is usually normal. Circulation time is usually below 10 seconds.

X-Ray

The heart is less enlarged than clinical data would indicate (19, 20). It has a globular shape and shows enlargement of the pulmonary artery. The aortic arch is high but not large; the left atrium is normal; the superior vena cava may be large.

Mechanism

Hyperthyroidism causes no specific lesion of the myocardium but undoubtedly affects the functions of both the heart and the peripheral vessels. It has been shown that thyroxin deeply affects the chemical equilibrium of the cardiac fibers in experimental animals (21). The glycogen and phosphocreatine metabolisms are so disturbed that the cardiac fibers present an actual loss of creatine, potassium, and phosphates (21). The increased oxidation and circulation speed and the greater excitability of the sympathetic system cause increased cardiac work and favor disturbances of the heart rate and rhythm. Further, it has been shown that the sympathin production of the heart itself is increased under the influence of the thyroid hormone (48).

It has been suggested that the similarity between the clinical picture of the thyroid heart and that of beri beri heart is due to a vitamin deficiency in the former on account of increased requirement in the presence of a normal or inadequate supply (50).

In conclusion, the hearts of these patients perform increased work under abnormal physico-chemical and hemodynamic conditions.

Varieties—Diagnosis

The most common and typical *thyroid heart* is found in thyrotoxicosis or Graves disease. The diagnosis of these cases is easy.

Other cases have no exopthalmos, tremor, nervousness, or enlarged thyroid gland but suffer from *congestive failure with atrial fibrillation* and may be recognized because they have (23): a) sinus tachycardia, not responding to rest and digitalization; b) unexplained loss of weight; c) high BMR, ranging from +30 to +40 and occasionally reaching +60.

Transient atrial fibrillation, transient glycosuria, and transient periods of diarrhea also may be a clue to the diagnosis of hyperthyroid heart (10).

The most difficult diagnosis is that of hyperthyroid heart in patients with valvular defects or coronary heart disease, an association which is often overlooked, and that of thyroid disturbances in elderly people.

Radioactive iodine may be used to estimate the rate at which the drug enters and leaves the thyroid. In thyrotoxicosis, iodine is concentrated in the gland more quickly and in greater quantity than in normal subjects. Geiger counters are used in order to detect the concentration of the tracer in the blood.

Differential diagnosis with the different valvular lesions is necessary when the murmurs and peripheral signs simulate their existence. X-ray and phonocardiographic data, and the existence of a high BMR usually facilitate the diagnosis.

Treatment

Treatment should be medical at first, if necessary, then surgical. *Iodine* (**73**) causes a temporary reduction in the function of the thyroid, which may be of help. *Digitalis* is less effective than in patients without hyperthyroidism because the slowing action of the drug on the heart is less marked. However, the stimulating action of digitalis on the myocardium (page 583) may lead to definite improvement whenever there is heart failure.

Quinidine can be given if atrial fibrillation is present and is usually well tolerated. However, objections have been raised to its use (9).

Sedatives may be of help and are more necessary than in other cardiac patients.

Surgical treatment may be effected as soon as the cardiac condition is improved by the use of iodine, rest, a high caloric diet, and vitamin B. Surgery consists of subtotal or total thyroidectomy. Whenever the general condition of the patient argues against a radical intervention, *ligation of one or more thyroid arteries or x-ray treatment* may be attempted. Surgical intervention frequently restores the sinus rhythm of fibrillating hearts. The choice of anesthesia will be discussed later (page 580).

Radioactive iodine shows promise of good results.

Propylthiouracil can be used in the treatment of the condition (51). Fifty mg. every 8 hours is the optimum dose for routine treatment of the severe cases while 50 mg. every 12 hours is adequate for mild cases. After control of the disease, smaller maintenance doses should be employed. Rare toxic reactions are agranulocytosis, pericarditis, and heart block (52).

HYPOTHYROIDISM AND MYXEDEMA HEART (24)

Hypothyroidism is either a primary disturbance or is secondary to extensive surgery on the thyroid gland.

The hearts of myxedematous patients may be greatly enlarged. The increase of interstitial fluid separates the myofibrils creating *cardiac edema.* This is frequently associated with *pericardial effusion* and edematous infiltration of the pericardium. Destruction of the myofibrils has been described (29). As some cardiac enlargement is also due to dilatation, the tremendous size of these hearts is easily explained. Enlargement of the heart may occur as early as 3 weeks after thyroidectomy (24).

Functional symptoms are: exertional dyspnea and palpitation and weakness.

Physical data are: typical *"edema,"* mild cyanosis, *small and slow pulse* (50 to 70 in most of the cases), and *low blood pressure with reduction of the pulse pressure.* However, cases with normal or high blood pressure are not unusual (26). *The venous pressure is usually high* but not because of heart failure (25).

Examination of the heart reveals that the apex impulse is weak or absent; *cardiac dulness is large while the heart sounds are faint.*

The *electrocardiogram* shows *low voltage*

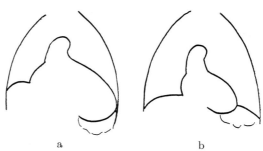

a   b

FIG. 244. *The heart in myxedema.* Cardiac silhouette at x-ray: a, before; b, after treatment with thyroid extract. (Inspired by originals of oesler.)

and frequent inversion of T in all leads (24). The low voltage, thought to be due to increased electric resistance and capacity of the skin (27, 28) may disappear by using subcutaneous needles as electrodes (29).

X-ray frequently reveals a severe increase of the cardiac silhouette (20) with weak pulsations of the margins. A striking reduction in size is obtained by thyroid therapy (fig. 244). When the heart is of normal size, it is further reduced by administration of thyroid extract (26). The vascular peduncle may be enlarged (28) but this finding is not always present.

Cardiac output is usually reduced (14).

Circulation time is prolonged; the blood flow to the skin is extremely reduced as shown by observation of the capillaries. There often is severe *anemia. Blood cholesterol is high* and the abnormal cholesterol metabolism seems to increase the frequency of coronary arteriosclerosis (53).

Angina pectoris is rare in myxedema. When present, it is due to coronary heart disease and is less severe than in cases without myxedema. However, in exceptional cases, the basic coronary lesion is mild and only functional elements due to myxedema cause angina (26).

Treatment

Treatment of myxedema heart is effected by the use of *thyroid extract* or thyroxin. The doses must be small at first and then slowly increased in order to avoid accidents (31). As a rule, 15 mg. (¼ gr.) of desiccated thyroid is well tolerated in most of the cases; at times, a smaller dose is indicated. Maintenance dose varies from 30 to 200 mg. (½ to 3 gr.) (31).

Treatment leads to disappearance of all symptoms and signs and to a tremendous reduction of the heart size.

DIABETES (65)

Diabetes is not known to affect the heart directly in spite of the great importance of changes of the carbohydrate metabolism for the cardiac muscle. However, diabetes seems to predispose to arteriosclerosis. Actually, the number of patients with coronary heart disease or peripheral arterial lesions is far greater among diabetics than among others and their lesions start at an earlier age.

Both insulin deficiency and hypoglycemia are bad for the heart. This is shown by the fact that a low or inverted T wave, S-T depression, and prolonged Q-T, may be found in diabetic acidosis and hypoglycemia (36).

Diabetic acidosis is frequently accompanied by *hypopotassemia.* High insulin doses caused discharge of epinephrine. This results in tachycardia, hypertension, and increased cardiac work with possible coronary insufficiency.

Therefore proper and early compensation of the diabetes by means of insulin, and avoidance of excessive insulin action, are advisable. For these reasons the following rules should be followed: a) administration of a larger dose of carbohydrates, and b) preference given to slow-acting insulin, whenever possible.

It is advisable to allow a moderate hyperglycemia (150–180 mg.) and a slight glycosuria.

The average diabetic with organic heart disease may be given a diet of 60 to 70 gm. proteins, 70 gm. fats, and 250 gm. carbohydrates. If there is obesity, it is important to obtain a reduction in weight, thus reducing the load on the heart. It should be remembered that myocardial infarction may disturb the diabetic control and may cause acidosis and coma (54).

ADRENAL DISEASES

A small heart and a small aorta have been described in *Addison's disease.* Actual diminution of cardiac weight is present in most cases, but the frequent loss of body weight may somewhat invalidate the above findings (30). Low voltage of the electrocardiogram has been noted in advanced cases of Addison's disease (36) but may be absent. The Addisonian crises are usually accompanied by low blood pressure and a further reduction in cardiac size which is secondary to the decrease of circulating blood volume (31).

The *endocrine-cardiac syndrome* (32, 33) with heart failure, liver cirrhosis, pigmentation, and infantilism, is probably due to a multiple endocrine insufficiency. The importance of the adrenal cortex is revealed by the excellent results obtained with the use of adrenal cortical hormone.

Pheochromocytoma is a benign tumor of the adrenal medulla and is accompanied by sudden attacks of extreme hypertension (frequently above 300 mm.) lasting from some minutes to many hours (page 499). Surgical removal of the tumor may result in the complete cure of this condition.

HYPOPARATHYROIDISM

Pulse, blood pressure, and cardiac function may be normal during the course of the disease. However, the electrocardiogram may reveal changes which are similar to those found in animals with experimental low blood calcium: *a prolongation of the Q-T interval* (34), i.e. of electrical systole. Restoration of normal blood calcium by means of *dihydrotachysterol* results in the return to a normal electrocardiogram.

Paget's Disease

Diffuse and severe Paget's disease may be accompanied by increased cardiac output.

Enormous increase of the blood flow through the affected bones has been observed. This causes phenomena similar to those of an arteriovenous fistula including high venous pressure, short circulation time, and finally heart failure (60).

Ovarian Insufficiency

It has been stated that ovarian insufficiency may be accompanied by a depression of S-T, maximal in lead 2, and by low T waves (35). These changes have been found both in young women with poor development of the ovaries and at the time of the menopause. However, these changes are not specific or typical.

The menopausal syndrome is accompanied by slight hypertension, tachycardia, and hot flushes. Vague precordial distress, exertional dyspnea, palpitation, weakness, and sighing respiration, may occur. Treatment with natural or synthetic estrogens improves the clinical syndrome.

Anemia and the Anemic Heart

Acute hemorrhagic anemia may lead to cardiovascular disturbances because of sudden reduction in the blood volume. The great majority of *chronic anemias*, however, have a series of changes which are mainly brought about by the altered composition of the blood.

When the hemoglobin level is below 7 gm. per 100 cc. (around 50 per cent hemoglobin), typical changes occur: *rapid pulse*, low systolic and diastolic pressures, *increased cardiac output at rest, increased blood velocity*, decreased peripheral resistance, and decreased difference in the oxygen contents of the arterial and venous bloods (37 and 46a). These changes are due to the fact that the body requirements for blood are increased so that there may be heart failure while the heart is pumping more blood than normal.

The increased cardiac output of severe anemia seems to be caused by at least two factors, *increased venous filling pressure* and *rapid heart rate* (55). Cardiac enlargement may be considerable. A decrease in cardiac size occurs early in treatment; it does not follow the improvement in hemoglobin level but may be dependent on a drop in venous pressure and cardiac output. As the blood volume in anemia is low (56), there must be diminution of the capacity of the vascular bed, especially marked in the capillary and venous sections of the circulation.

Myocardial changes have been found in hemolytic anemias.

Possible clinical data are: violent pulsation of both the jugular veins and the carotid arteries; typical *machinery murmur* over the veins of the neck (*venous hum, bruit du diable*); forceful apical thrust; slight enlargement of cardiac dulness; loud heart sounds; different murmurs: the most common are a *systolic apical murmur* and a *systolic pulmonic murmur*; less common are a *systolic aortic* and a *diastolic aortic* or *pulmonic*. A *diastolic rumble at the apex* simulating mitral stenosis is possible. These murmurs are due not only to the enlargement of the cardiac chambers and of the large arteries but also to increased speed of the circulation and decreased viscosity of the blood (38, 39). These also explain the venous hum. Increased respiratory minute volume and decreased vital capacity favor exertional dyspnea.

There is a hyperkinetic heart. Resting *cardiac output* may reach 13 liters per minute and *utilization of the available oxygen* may reach as much as 90 per cent (normal 33 per cent). The high cardiac output is maintained both by tachycardia and by increase of venous pressure. The latter must be due to widespread venous constriction because blood volume is reduced and the arterioles are dilated.

Electrocardiogram. In about one-third of the cases, low voltage, flat or inverted T, or depressed S-T, have been noted in V5-V6, especially in patients with anginal pain (57).

X-ray frequently reveals an enlarged heart.

A severe picture of congestive failure has

been described in *pernicious anemia*; autopsy showed hypertrophy of the heart and fatty degeneration of the myofibrils (40). The hypertrophy may be a compensatory phenomenon because cardiac output is increased in these patients.

Differentiation of the picture of congestion (exertional dyspnea, edema, large liver) caused by the anemia itself from that due to *heart failure* may be made on the basis of the lack of orthopnea and venous engorgement in the former and their presence in the latter. Absence of cyanosis, on the other hand, may occur in both if hemoglobin is extremely low (61).

Blood transfusion is frequently beneficial. However, rapid transfusion may lead to severe disturbances, including pulmonary edema, through overloading of the heart and the pulmonary circulation (55). Venous infusion of 2000 cc. at a rate below 15 cc. per minute usually seems to be well tolerated. Small transfusions of concentrated corpuscles may be advantageous but these also should be done slowly. A propped-up position is best in severe cases. Any engorgement of the neck veins is evidence of increased venous pressure (55).

Polycythemia (Vaquez-Osler Disease)

Polycythemia vera is associated with increase in the number of red cells and blood viscosity, and increase in blood volume. Circulation time is longer while cardiac output is normal or lowered (58). Thromboses are common, especially in the cerebral arteries. Coronary occlusion is frequent.

Poisonings—Toxic States

Carbon monoxide poisoning often causes depression of S-T and flattening of T in the electrocardiogram. *Poisonous mushrooms* may produce extreme electrocardiographic changes including bundle branch block (59). *Mercury poisoning* may be followed by changes similar to those of uremia.

Alcohol intoxication may cause sinus tachycardia and paroxysmal atrial fibrilla-

tion, especially in elderly persons. The same is true of acute *diseases of the liver* (59).

Inhalation of *tobacco smoke* causes a transient increase in heart rate and may cause depression or even inversion of T in one or more leads. Severe *sinus tachycardia* reveals sensitivity to nicotine and should advise against its use. The same is true for dizziness, blanching of the fingertips or face, palpitation, or increase of blood pressure.

Trauma and Wounds

Myocardial damage may follow a *penetrating wound or a contusion*. A foreign body can enter the heart through the skin, the esophagus, the venae cavae, or the pulmonary veins (44).

Evaluation of the cardiac damage should take into account: the condition of the heart before the accident; the severity and seat of the lesion; the type of lesion; and the immediate and subsequent signs and symptoms.

A damaged heart is injured more easily than a normal heart, so that underlying mild cardiac changes may lead to severe disturbances in the presence of trauma. While trauma may precipitate *congestive failure* if the heart is not normal, a severe injury of the ventricular wall may cause *acute dilatation and failure*, even without heart disease.

Premature beats, atrial flutter or fibrillation, or paroxysmal tachycardia, may follow *trauma* or *electric shock*. The latter may cause death through subsequent ventricular fibrillation. A-V block is rare except in the *hemorrhage of the septum*.

Rupture of one of the ventricles or a penetrating wound are followed by *hemopericardium* with fatal *tamponade* (page 448). Progressive arterial hypotension and venous hypertension are the usual signs.

The manifestations of *penetrating cardiac injuries* may be due to: a) lesions of the intrinsic structures of the heart (a valve, a coronary artery, the conducting system); b) blood loss caused by hemorrhage; c) compression of the heart. If the patient survives, the signs are usually only those of b and c (44).

Bullets entering the ventricular wall may stop there and become *cardiac* guests for the rest of life without further disturbance. However, premature beats may be caused by them.

The *electrocardiogram* may reveal the injury to the myocardium by giving a picture which resembles that of infarction (43) with the following reservations: a) the lesion is frequently smaller than in infarction; b) it usually occurs in a normal heart; c) it frequently involves the right heart; d) pericarditis is practically constant. On the other hand, *laceration of a coronary artery* may cause extensive infarction (43b).

If the bullet reaches one of the cardiac cavities, there may be a long period during which no disturbance is noted except for occasional murmurs. However, sooner or later, the bullet may cause a severe *embolism*.

Both *cardiac contusion* and *partial rupture of the cardiac wall* are far more common than thought in the past and may heal spontaneously. An ECG recorded soon after the wound or trauma may be of help in the diagnosis and localization of the damage by revealing evolutionary changes of T and S-T (52).

Rupture of the heart may be cured by *suture of the cardiac wall* if an immediate operation can be performed.

Intracardiac foreign bodies should be removed in order: a) to prevent embolism by the foreign body itself or an associated thrombus; b) to reduce the danger of bacterial endocarditis; c) to prevent recurrent pericardial effusions; and d) to diminish myocardial damage (45). Surgery is frequently justified and usually successful.

Air Embolism (41)

Air embolism may be venous or arterial. In *venous embolism*, air bubbles enter a systemic vein and form a foam in the right ventricle through the churning action of the heart. This foam may either stay in the heart or move into the pulmonary artery causing pulmonary air embolism.

In *arterial embolism*, air bubbles penetrate the left heart from the pulmonary veins or through a patent foramen ovale; they form a foam in the left ventricle and may lead to occlusion of a cerebral, splenic, or renal artery.

A *harsh, bubbling rumble (millwheel murmur)* and a *thrill* are noted in systole. There may be vascular collapse. A correct diagnosis may lead to recovery through *aspiration of the air foam from the heart* by means of a syringe.

BIBLIOGRAPHY

1. von Gierke, F. Beitr. path. Anath., Path., 1929, **82,** 497.
2. Pompe, J. C. Ann. Anat. Path., Anat. Norm. Med.-Chir., 1933, **10,** 23.
3. Shimazono, J. *Beriberi.* Berlin, 1927. Also Erg. inn. Med., 1931, **39,** 10.
4. Aalsmer, W. Ch. Wien. Arch. inn. Med., 1931, **21,** 1.
5. Wenckebach, K. F. *Der Beri-Beri Herz.* Berlin, Springer, 1934.
6. a) Weiss, S., and Wilkins, R. W. Ann. Int. Med., 1937, **11,** 104; and J. A. M. A., 1937, **109,** 7861.
   b) Weiss, S. J. A. M. A., 1940, **115,** 832.
7. a) Cossio, P. Rev. Asoc. Med. Arg., 1941, **55,** N. 473, 474.
   b) Blankenhorn, M. A. Ann. Int. Med., 1945, **23,** 398.
   c) Blankenhorn, M. A., and co-workers. J. A. M. A., 1946, **131,** 717.
8. a) Feil, H. Am. Heart J., 1936, **11,** 183.
   b) Rachmilevitz, M., and Braun, K. Brit. Heart J., 1945, **7,** 72.
9. Thomas, H. M. In *Stroud's Cardiovascular Disease.* Philadelphia, Davis, 1945.
10. a) Levine, S. A. *Clinical Heart Disease.* Philadelpha, Saunders, 1937.
    b) Cossio, P. *Aparato Circulatorio.* Buenos Aires, El Ateneo, 1939.
11. Friedberg, C. K., and Sohval, A. R. Am. Heart J., 1937, **13,** 599.
12. Wilson, F. N. In *Stroud's Cardiovascular Disease.* Philadelphia, Davis, 1945.
13. Zonek, H. Deut. Med. Woch., 1920, **46,** 1239.

14. White, P. D. *Heart Disease*. New York, Macmillan, 1944.
15. Gordan, G., Soley, M. H., and Chamberlain, F. L. Arch. Int. Med., 1944, **73**, 148.
16. Thomson, W. O. J. Clin. Investigation, 1926, **2**, 477.
17. Robinson, S. C. J. A. M. A., 1926, **87**, 314.
18. Burwell, E. S., and co-workers. Am. J. M. Sci., 1929, **178**, 159.
19. Blumgart, H. L. Medicine, 1931, **10**, 1.
20. Roesler, H. *Roentgenology of the Cardiovascular System*. Springfield, Thomas, 1945.
21. Herrmann, G. R. *Synopsis of Diseases of the Heart and Arteries*. St. Louis, Mosby, 1941.
22. Peserico, E. Cuore e Circ., 1931, **18**, 33.
23. Hamilton, B. E. J. A. M. A., 1924, **83**, 405.
24. Zondek, H. Muench. med. Woch., 1918, **65**, 1180; and 1919, **68**, 681.
25. Davis, D., Weinstein, A. A., Riseman, J. E. F., and Blumgart, H. L. Am. Heart J., 1934, **10**, 17.
26. Musso-Fournier, J. C., Cerviño, J. M., and Bazzano, J. J. *El Aparato Cardiovascular en las Insuficiencias Tiroideas*. Buenos Aires, Salvat, 1944.
27. Lueg, W. Arch. ges. Phys., 1926, **212**, 649.
28. Pasoli, E. Cuore e Circ., 1932, **16**, 141.
29. Noebel and Rosenbluth. Zeit. exp. Med., 1924, **43**, 332.
30. Barr, D. In *Stroud's Cardiovascular Disease*. Philadelphia, Davis, 1945.
31. a) McGavack, T. H. Am. Heart J., 1941, **21**, 1.
    b) McGavack, T. H., Lange, K., and Schwimmer, D. Am. Heart J., 1945, **29**, 421.
32. Donzelot, E. Arch. Mal. Coeur, 1936, **29**, 1.
33. Oumansky, V., and Longuet, A. Presse Méd., 1938, **46**, 388.
34. Hecht, H., and Korth, C. Zeit. Kreislauff., 1937, **29**, 577.
35. Scherf, D., and Boyd, L. F. *Clinical Electrocardiography*. St. Louis, Mosby, 1940.
36. Roesler, H. Mo. Conc. Cardiov. Dis., 1941, **10**, n. 9.
37. Dautrebande, L. Ctr. Soc. Biol., 1925, **93**, 1029.
38. Luisada, A. A., and Mautner, H. Exper. Med. & Surg., 1943, **1**, 282.
39. Garb, S. Am. Heart J., 1944, **28**, 568.
40. Bouchut, L., and Froment, R. Arch. Mal. Coeur, 1936, **29**, 1.
41. Stallwarth, J. A., *et al.* J. A. M. A., 1950, **143**, 1250.
42. Bland, E. F. Am. Heart J., 1944, **27**, 588.
43. a) Parkinson, J., Bedford, D. E., and Thomson, W. A. Quart. J. Med., 1938. **31**, 455.
    b) Noth, P. H. Am. Heart J., 1944, **27**, 713.
44. a) Beck, C. S. *Surgery of the Heart and Pericardium*. In *Stroud's Cardiovascular Disease*. Philadelphia, Davis, 1945.
    b) Barber, R. F., and Madden, J. L. Am. J. Surg., 1944, **64**, 151.
45. Harken, D. F., and Zoll, P. M. Am. Heart J., 1946, **32**, 1.
46. a) Brannon, E. S., Merrill, A. J., Warren, J. V., and Stead, E. A., Jr. J. Clin. Investigation, 1945, **24**, 332.
    b) Richards, D. W. Bull. New York Acad. Med., 1946, **22**, 630.
47. Raab, W., and Supplee, G. C. Exper. Med. & Surg., 1944, **2**, 152.
48. Raab, W. Ann. Int. Med., 1948, **28**, 1010.
49. Torres, U. L. Hospital (Rio), 1948, **33**, 505.
50. Williams, R. H., and co-workers. Arch. Int. Med., 1943, **72**, 353.
51. a) Astwood, E. B., and Vanderlean, W. P. Ann. Int. Med., 1946, **25**, 813.
    b) Bartels, E. C. New England J. Med., 1948, **218**, 6.
52. Bain, C. Brit. Heart J., 1945, **7**, 1.
53. Higgins. Am. J. M. Sci., 1936, **191**, 80.
54. Brams, W. A. *Treatment of Heart Disease*. Philadelphia, Saunders, 1948.
55. Sharpey-Schafer, E. P. Lancet, 1945, **2**, 296.
56. McMichael, J., and co-workers. Lancet, 1943, **1**, 637.
57. Wintrobe, M. M. Blood, 1946, **1**, 128.
58. a) Altschule, M., and co-workers. Am. J. M. Sci., 1940, **200**, 478.
    b) Stewart, J. J., and co-workers. Am. Heart J., 1941, **21**, 511.
59. Ashman, R., and Hull, E. *Essentials of Electrocardiography*. New York, Macmillan, 1944.
60. Edholm, O. G., Howarth, S., and McMichael, J. Clin. Sci., 1945, **5**, 249.
61. Blumgart, H. L., and Altschule, M. D. Blood, 1948, **3**, 329.
62. Keys, A., Henschel, A., and Taylor, H. L. Am. J. Physiol., 1947, **150**, 153.
63. Ellis, L. B. Brit. Heart J., 1946, **8**, 53.
64. Bassi, G. Med. Internaz., 1948, July–August.
65. Liebow, I. M., and Hellerstein, H. K. Am. J. Med., 1949, **7**, 660.

CHAPTER 19

Diseases of the Coronary System and Myocardial Infarction

Congenital Abnormalities of the Coronary Arteries

Anomalies of the coronary arteries are rare but important. Three types of isolated anomalies have been described:

a) Either the right, or both, coronary arteries arise from the pulmonary artery. If only the right, the difference in pressure between the two coronary arteries and their anastomotic vessels causes diffuse dilatation of both vessels (1, 151).

b) One of the coronary arteries has not developed (1).

c) There is a congenital aneurysm of the right coronary artery (1).

Whenever complex malformations of the heart are present (common trunk, transposition, or tetralogy of Fallot), the coronary arteries are involved from a structural and a functional viewpoint.

In type a, *enlargement of the heart* and fibrosis of the ventricular walls are present. A *triple rhythm* has been noted.

The *electrocardiogram* shows a pattern of ischemia and injury (inverted T wave and displacement of S-T) (page 416).

The patients suffer from attacks of *precordial pain* during which the electrocardiographic changes are further accentuated (3). Death usually occurs within the first months of life.

When the coronary arteries arise from the common arterial trunk, similar disturbances may occur. They are, however, less severe because the blood of the trunk contains a higher amount of oxygen than that of the normal pulmonary artery.

Lesions of the coronary arteries may be responsible, at least in some cases, for endocardial fibroblastosis (149).

A Potts-Gibson fistula at the root of the aorta has been suggested for treatment of these anomalies (150). This would direct oxygenated blood close to the origin of the anomalous coronary, when this vessel arises from the pulmonary artery.

Aneurysm of the Coronary Arteries (122)

CAUSE

a) The most common type is congenital.

b) A certain number of cases are due to septic coronary embolism.

c) A third possible cause is arteriosclerosis.

d) Rare cases are due to lues, rheumatic disease, or panarteritis nodosa.

Described cases range from 5 to 84 years, irrespective of the cause; even congenital types may be found in old patients.

LESIONS

The aneurysm may involve the left coronary twice as often as either the right or both coronary arteries. The aneurysm may be *localized* or *diffuse*, and may reach a large size. The aneurysm may be followed by thrombosis or rupture. If the rupture involves a coronary vein, an *arteriovenous fistula* results.

CLINICAL PICTURE—DIAGNOSIS

The signs and symptoms are atypical in most of the cases and may be confused with those of coronary heart disease and myocardial infarction. Rupture of the coronary artery is followed by *hemopericardium* and *cardiac tamponade* (page

448). Here again, erroneous diagnosis of rupture of the cardiac wall is frequently made.

Coronary arteriovenous fistula is the cause of a *thrill* and a *continuous machinery murmur* which in one case was located at the 4th right interspace (123); there may be a pulsating mass in the same area. As the electrocardiogram is not significant, differential diagnoses should include patent ductus (in cases of transposition) and aortic septal defect.

Coronary Heart Disease

The term "coronary heart disease" is applied, as a pathologic connotation, to lesions of the arterial system of the heart and to the resulting changes of the myocardium. On the other hand, the same term is applied to the clinical pictures caused by these lesions. As the electrocardiogram permits recognition of coronary heart disease in cases without appreciable symptoms or signs, the term cannot be restricted to purely clinical entities.

CAUSE

Acute and subacute infections may cause inflammation of the coronary arteries (coronary arteritis) resulting later in chronic lesions of these vessels. Among them, pneumonia, diphtheria, influenza (5), typhoid fever, and rheumatic fever (7–9) have been cited. Syphilis may damage the proximal portions of the coronary arteries (4).

Panarteritis nodosa (periarteritis nodosa) involves the coronary arteries in 70 per cent of the cases with this disease and is neither rare nor always severe as generally thought (13). It is one of the causes of coronary lesions in young people.

Buerger's disease (thromboangiitis obliterans) is an occasional cause of coronary obstruction (14) and stenosis and is the second most common cause of coronary lesions in youths (15).

Neoplasms involving the heart may compress the coronary arteries, or may invade them causing occlusion.

Arteriosclerosis is the most common cause of coronary lesions and is present in about 90 per cent of cases. The prevalence in the *male sex* has been explained by inherited characteristics of the coronary intima (125) but seems more related to the action of sex hormones on the localization of arteriosclerosis in the coronary arteries (140).

The *familial incidence* seems to be related to either an abnormality in the metabolism of cholesterol or hypertension. Large molecular complexes containing cholesterol and other lipids with variable amounts of protein are normally present in the blood and increase in number in patients with coronary arteriosclerosis (141). Coronary heart disease is more frequent in hypertension, diabetes and gallbladder diseases. While hypertension is also important because of strain, the three conditions seem to be related through the common link of an abnormal metabolism of lipids, including cholesterol.

STRUCTURAL LESIONS

Acute coronaritis may arise by extension or be mycotic in origin; secondary thrombosis may produce arterial blockage. The microscopic aspects of acute and subacute arteritis are similar to those taking place in other arteries.

Severe stress at the ostia of the coronary arteries causes diffuse thickening of the intima which gradually becomes denser with age (12a). Unusual stress and early lesion occur at the right-angle turns of the left coronary and its circumflex branch.

With the lesser degrees of coronary arteriosclerosis, the heart undergoes little or no hypertrophy. With more severe involvement, impaired nutrition is followed by less efficient work and, subsequently, by *cardiac dilatation* and *hypertrophy* (16). In patients who suffer from heart failure, *the weight of the heart is considerably increased* (16).

Coronary sclerosis is almost always due to

atherosclerosis. Unusual stresses occur at the ostia of the coronary arteries and this may explain a diffuse thickening of the intima of these vessels, starting in early life as a cellular fibrous tissue and becoming denser with age (12a). Early arteriosclerosis is frequently limited to the first 2 to 3 per cent of the left coronary artery and its descending branch.

In *youth*, excess cholesterol in the lipoid cells invading the intima excites a mesenchymal cell reaction which stimulates the formation of connective tissue. The growing tissue progressively narrows the lumen; necrosis occurs near the media; new intramural blood channels develop until the inner layers of the thickened intima at times resemble a granulation tissue and extend to the other coats. In cases of thrombosis, *hemorrhages* from ruptured blood channels and associated fibrinoid necrosis extend from the site of the rupture up to the endothelium, causing a *thrombus* and communicating with it. Another possibility in arterial thrombosis is the *breaking through the intima of newly-formed blood channels* (fig. 245).

In *middle age*, more collagen is formed and *scarring* is typical. The development of lesions is slower and more irregular. There are regions of dense scarring, representing the healed lesions of processes which occurred at an earlier age. Narrowing of the coronary lumen and myocardosis (page 384) are frequent.

In *old age*, the reaction of tissues to excess cholesterol is diminished; lipoid cells accumulate in the intima and atheromatous plaques with calcification are typical. Occlusion may be due to the rupture of such a plaque.

THE CONCEPT OF CORONARY INSUFFICIENCY

Coronary insufficiency is a condition in which the need of the myocardium for blood and oxygen is greater than the amount which can be supplied. Coronary insuf-

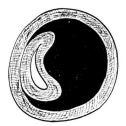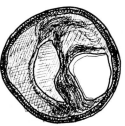

FIG. 245. Two different types of *occlusion of a coronary artery*: a, following an *intramural hemorrhage*; b, by *proliferation of the intima*. (Sketched after Winternitz, Thomas and Le Compte's *The Biology of Arteriosclerosis*. Courtesy of the authors and Charles C Thomas, Publisher.)

ficiency may occur as the result of one of the following mechanisms:

a) A structural lesion causing narrowing of the arteries.

b) A functional constriction due to nerve stimulation or chemical action.

c) Impairment of coronary flow due to low diastolic pressure (aortic valvular defects, patent ductus arteriosus, shock, or extreme bradycardia) or to shortness of diastole (paroxysmal tachycardia).

d) Poor oxygen saturation of the arterial blood (congestive failure, cor pulmonale, congenital heart disease, anemia).

Two or more of these mechanisms are frequently associated. In particular, coronary arteriosclerosis of large branches may be associated with vasomotor narrowing of the smaller ones.

Coronary insufficiency does not occur when both blood supply and blood demand are reduced, as in the senile heart and in certain forms of vascular collapse.

The most common manifestation of coronary insufficiency is cardiac pain, the so-called "angina pectoris."

Coronary heart disease may lead to various clinical-anatomical pictures: a) the senile heart, b) myocardial infarction, c) cardiac pain (angina pectoris), or d) congestive failure.

DEFINITIONS

Coronary occlusion. Occlusion of a coronary artery, whether slow or sudden.

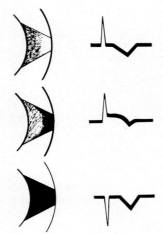

FIG. 246. The three patterns of myocardial damage due to coronary lesions. A, pattern of ischemia; B, pattern of injury; C, pattern of necrosis (transmural).

Clinically, it is applied only to an acute occlusion. Gradual occurrence, excellent collateral circulation, or both, may prevent the establishment of an infarction after an occlusion (18).

Coronary thrombosis. The term has an exact structural meaning. Clinically, it is impossible to know whether the picture is due to thrombosis or another mechanism.

Myocardial infarction. Anatomical-clinical picture which may be caused by coronary thrombosis, prolonged coronary insufficiency, or, more seldom, coronary embolism.

Coronary failure. Prolonged coronary insufficiency (over 20 minutes) not followed by infarction (19). This definition is not widely accepted.

Acute coronary insufficiency. Diminution of coronary flow. If severe or prolonged, it may cause myocardial infarction without occlusion (20).

ELECTROCARDIOGRAPHY

Coronary disease is frequently accompanied by decreased blood supply to the myocardium (ischemia). The latter may be followed by damage (injury) to the heart muscle and, if severe, by its necrosis (death). Consequently, three basic electro-cardiographic patterns have been recognized: ischemia, injury, and death (fig. 246).

Pattern of ischemia. According to widely accepted studies (142), the spreading of the stimulus within the ventricular wall takes place from the subendocardial toward the subepicardial layers. The front of the wave of depolarization is preceded by positive and followed by negative ions. Therefore, an *epicardial electrode* records the wave of depolarization as a *positive deflection* while an electrode introduced into a ventricular cavity records it as a negative deflection. Repolarization of the ventricular wall *in the human heart* has features which are different from those of other species. On account of slow repolarization of the sub-endocardial layers, the front of repolarization starts from the subepicardial layers and moves toward the endocardium (142). As the front of repolarization is preceded by negative ions and is followed by positive ions, an *epicardial electrode* records a *positive T* while a cavity electrode records a negative T.

Ischemia affects the subepicardial layers to a greater extent and slows down their process of repolarization. Following this, the vector of repolarization of the ischemic ventricle proceeds from the cavity toward the surface and *a negative T is recorded by an epicardial electrode* (fig. 249a). The Q-T interval is prolonged because of slower repolarization.

Pattern of injury. Injury of the cardiac tissue leads to formation of an area which is strongly positive during depolarization in relationship to normal tissue. In *sub-epicardial* or *transmural injury of the anterior wall*, an anterior electrode "faces" the positive aspect of the boundary and an *upward displacement of S-T is noted.* In *subendocardial injury of the anterior wall*, an anterior electrode "faces" the negative (normal) aspect of the boundary and a *downward displacement of S-T is noted* (142) (fig. 249b).

Injury to the *posterior wall* would cause

opposite changes in the direction of an S-T displacement, as recorded by an anterior electrode.

Both the chest and the limb unipolar leads of clinical studies use an exploring electrode at some distance from the epicardium; therefore *a mixed pattern of injury plus ischemia (raised S-T and inverted T wave) is usually recorded* unless the area of injury is large.

Pattern of necrosis. The destruction of an area of ventricular muscle results in the disappearance of the electrical forces due to the activity of that area during the process of excitation. As a result, the dead tissue acts like "an electrical window" and the electrode records the negative potentials of the ventricular cavity.[68] Necrosis or death of the tissue is revealed by *a deep QS followed by an inverted T*, if an electrode is placed over the epicardium (fig. 249c).

Unipolar limb or chest leads may register *both the pattern of necrosis and that of the surrounding areas of injury and ischemia*, if the area of necrosis is small. Then a deep Q, an elevated S-T, and a small inverted T are observed. On the other hand, if the infarction is large, the unipolar leads record typical "cavity potentials".

Whenever the necrosis does not involve the entire thickness of the ventricular wall (*intramural infarcts*), potentials from the surrounding healthy tissues reach the electrode. Then, it is impossible to distinguish between prolonged diffuse ischemia plus some degree of injury, and partial necrosis, except by the duration and evolution of the pattern.

Myocardial Infarction

CAUSES

Myocardial infarction is more common in males than in females, having a ratio of 3.4

[68] Put in a different way: the normal vector of electrical forces within the ventricular wall is directed from the endocardium toward the epicardium; whenever necrosis of the wall occurs, the electrode records currents directed away from it, therefore negative.

to 1 in the total series and 5.5 to 1 in patients under the age of 40. Hypertension, diabetes, or both, are present in 88.3 per cent of the females and in 59 per cent of the males (117). Actually, myocardial infarction is very rare in women below 40 unless obesity, hypertension or hyperlipemia are present (118). On the other hand, it is not rare in males between 18 and 40 (119), especially if they have a broad, heavy-set body build. Hypofunction of the thyroid, hypertension, or diabetes, are frequently present in these subjects.

Myocardial infarction may occur in the very young and even in newborn infants (120). In the latter, infectious, traumatic or toxic elements have a predominant importance. Myocardial infarct of the newborn has been observed as a result of treatment of the mother with pitressin during labor.

Myocardial infarction may follow a lesion of the coronary arteries in this order: a) anterior descending branch, 50 per cent; b) right main coronary artery, 23 per cent; c) left circumflex branch, 18 per cent; d) left main coronary artery or right circumflex branch, 4 per cent in each group; e) posterior descending branch, 1 per cent (fig. 247).

Myocardial infarction may be the result of prolonged coronary insufficiency or coronary occlusion. Occlusion due to *embolism* is rare. In about 50 per cent of the cases

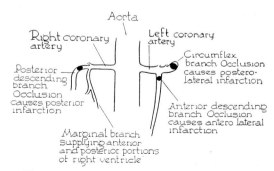

FIG. 247. A diagrammatic representation of the coronary arterial system and the common sites of coronary artery occlusion. Dark discs indicate sites of obstruction. (From Burch and Winsor. Courtesy of the authors and of Lea & Febiger.)

there is the *gradual occlusion* of an arterio-sclerotic vessel by the concentric prolifera-tion of the intima. Prolonged coronary insufficiency usually acts by hastening the occlusion of an already damaged, arterio-sclerotic vessel.

Another possibility, which seems to take place in about 50 per cent of the cases, is that of a *sudden occlusion because of intra-mural hemorrhage* (fig. 245) This may cause obstruction either by pushing an ather-omatous plaque into the lumen or by destroying the endothelium and causing thrombosis of the vessel (28). Sudden increase of blood pressure in the vessels and decreased pressure in the soft, atheromatous tissue, favor the hemorrhage. Rapid clotting of the blood favors and extends the occlusion after the initial stage. *Acute decrease of blood flow due to functional causes* may lead to infarction, especially if there is extensive damage of the vessels.

Effort, emotion, hemorrhage, exposure to cold, visceral reflexes, trauma, and the action of vasoconstricting hormones, drugs or metabolites, may act as *precipitating factors* of an infarct due to coronary insuf-ficiency. The importance of these factors should also be admitted in cases of occlusion due to intramural hemorrhage.

LESIONS

According to the stage reached by the infarction, the following lesions can be observed:

a) *Initial stage.* Necrosis of the myo-cardium is more or less widespread. Blood extravasation and inflammatory reaction are present in the surrounding area. Rupture of the ventricular wall or of the septum may occur.

b) *Advanced stage.* There is proliferation of the connective tissue which is first soft, then fibrous; it later substitutes for the degenerated myofibrils. Hematic pigment, either free, or included in mesenchymal cells, results from the previous hemorrhagic diffusion. The infarcted area gradually becomes a *scar* and may become thinner and distended because of internal pressure and sclerotic involution. The pericardium is first congested, then shows evidence of fibrinous exudate. Later on, the pericardial sac frequently adheres to the heart as a result of *limited fibrous pericarditis* (22).

The infarcted area may vary from 10 to 50 mm. in diameter. The area may be limited by a regular or irregular rim. In some cases, the rim is replaced by a shaded area.

The following types of lesion may be found:

a) *Massive infarction*, involving the entire thickness of the ventricle wall. This is due to blockage of one of the main stems or obstruction of a smaller one when there is diffuse coronary disease.

b) *Small infarction*, limited to a portion of the ventricular wall. This is frequently caused by occlusion of a small branch in the presence of diffuse lesions. Coronary insuf-ficiency may cause it.

c) *Scattered small islands of scar tissue.* These may be caused by occlusion or insufficiency of the coronary system.

Atrial infarction is not very common but has been observed in 17 per cent of a series of cases of ventricular infarction as a concomitant lesion (53). In most of these cases, the infarction was in the right atrium, and frequently in the right ap-pendage. Cases of atrial without ventricular infarction are possible but not frequent (40). *Atrial thrombosis* is common in cases of atrial infarction.

Multiple infarctions are common and autopsy frequently shows that they occurred at different times (fig. 248). The occurrence of coronary thrombosis without infarction is revealed by injection of the coronary system and is by far more frequent when both coronary arteries participate equally in the supply of the left ventricle than other-wise (page 25).

Occlusion of the right coronary artery may give more serious results in that part

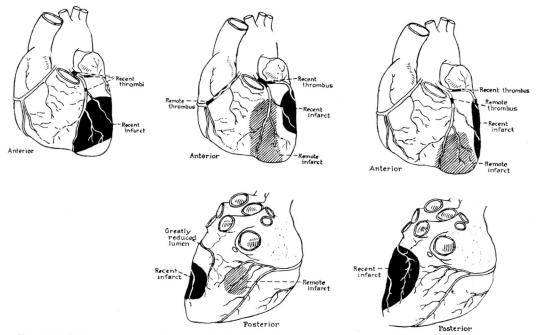

FIG. 248. Different aspects of *myocardial infarctions* due to various occlusions. (From the Am. J. M. Sci. Courtesy of Drs. Feil and Thomson and Lea & Febiger.)

of the left ventricle which is supplied by it than in the right ventricle. This is due to functional causes (page 55).

FUNCTIONAL RESULTS OF ACUTE ISCHEMIA

Acute ischemia is followed by severe functional changes in the myocardium. The ischemic area becomes cyanotic and its contractions weaken rapidly (23). Then the area cannot oppose the sudden rise of ventricular pressure which takes place during each contraction, and dilates in systole, forming a *dynamic ventricular aneurysm* (23). There is a sudden fall of pressure in both the aorta and the pulmonary artery (23, 24) which may be partly compensated within a few minutes. The area surrounding the infarction becomes *hyperexcitable*. Stimuli arising in this area may cause premature beats, ventricular tachycardia, atrial flutter or fibrillation, or ventricular flutter. These disturbances of cardiac rate and rhythm are favored by cardiocardiac reflexes. Stimuli arising in the

same area cause pain, dyspnea, vascular collapse, mental and physical agitation, and gastrointestinal disorders, and contribute to acute pulmonary edema. They may cause a "stress syndrome."

SIGNS AND SYMPTOMS

Premonitory symptoms may precede myocardial infarction by some hours (29). They consist of mild precordial pain or severe pain lasting for only a short time. *Restlessness, sleeplessness,* or *nausea* may precede the attack.

In the severe attack of coronary occlusion, *cardiac pain* is the most striking symptom. It is extremely severe and resistant to treatment. It is frequently located *at the lower part of the sternum or at the epigastrium.* It may be felt as a crushing sensation deep inside the chest, behind the sternum or in the upper right abdominal quadrant. It is described as boring, tearing or constricting, and may be referred to the neck, the throat, the left scapula, the spine, or both arms; it may not be transmitted at all. The pain is usually diffuse.

The pain may persist for several hours or days without remission. It is not influenced by respiration, unless severe complicating pericarditis or pleurisy is present. Pain may be absent but this is unusual except in patients in coma, in alcoholics, or in patients receiving sedation.

Oppression, moderate *dyspnea*, and sensation of impending death are often present. *Nausea*, vomiting and diarrhea are frequent. An attack of *pulmonary edema* may take place at the onset. The patient may be immobile, crushed by the pain. However, psychic and physical *restlessness* may be present, so that the patient sometimes walks, talks, or tosses himself about the bed.

Ashen-gray color, profuse perspiration, *fall in blood pressure*, and a weak pulse are frequently present. The pulse may be *rapid* or *slow*, and is frequently *irregular*. It may *alternate*. The changes of rate and rhythm are due to sinus tachycardia or bradycardia; ventricular premature contractions; atrial tachycardia, flutter, or fibrillation; or atrioventricular block. Several of them may be present.

Examination of the heart reveals a weak apex impulse, moderate cardiac enlargement, and a *remarkable weakening of the heart sounds*, especially the first, which may become inaudible. A *triple rhythm* (gallop rhythm) is frequently noted. It is common to hear a *soft apical systolic murmur*, while a long musical, systolic murmur is occasionally present (96). A *pericardial rub* may be heard between the 2nd and the 4th day in the anterior infarction and is usually of brief duration. It is frequently faint and transient, disappearing after 1 or 2 days. It is a sign which is present only in anterior infarction and found only if sought.

Blood pressure, both systolic and diastolic, usually drops. An extremely low level may be reached so rapidly that the patient goes into *shock*. However, the blood pressure may fall slowly, or may present only an initial drop, to rise again within a few days to one-half or two-thirds of the usual level. Increased blood pressure may be noted in the first few days, probably in connection with the pain.

In the less severe attacks, any of these symptoms and signs may be absent or mild. It is not unusual for precordial pain lasting several hours to be followed by no other symptoms or signs except those revealed by the electrocardiogram.

TEMPERATURE—BLOOD—URINE

A moderate *increase in temperature* is almost always an attending symptom. It usually starts on the 2nd day, reaches its highest level on the 3rd, lasts a few days, then gradually disappears. The temperature may vary between 37.2° and 38.9° (99 to 102°F.) but the lower figures are more common.

Sedimentation rate is constantly increased in myocardial infarction (31). The increase starts between the 2nd and the 4th day, reaching a rate of 60 mm. in an hour and occasionally higher. The maximum is usually reached 2 to 3 days later, then there is a gradual subsiding with a return to normal after 2 or more weeks.

Leucocytosis may start early, from 1 to 2 hours after the attack, reaching 12,000 to 20,000 per mm^3, paralleling the course of the fever. The return to normal may occur within a week or two.

The *urine* frequently contains a trace of albumin, indican, and possibly, urobilin. *Glycosuria* and *hyperglycemia* often occur in the acute stage of myocardial infarction, not preceded by diabetes (59). *Serum cholesterol* is nearly always high in cases of myocardial infarction (113). After the attack, an initial drop and a subsequent rise have been observed (113).

ELECTROCARDIOGRAM

The typical changes of the electrocardiogram are those of the sequence—

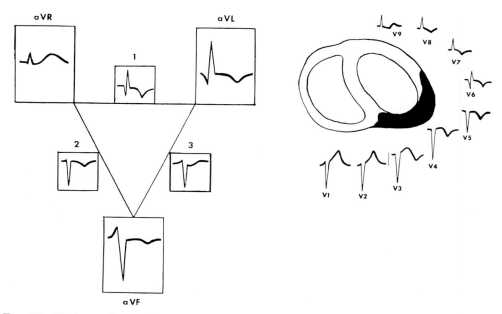

FIG. 249. Electrocardiographic pattern of *old anterolateral infarct*. (From Luisada, Med. Clin. North America. Courtesy of W. B. Saunders Co.).

ischemia, injury and necrosis, as outlined above. Different pictures occur according to the localization of the infarct. The older division of infarcts into *anterior* (Q1-T1) and *posterior* (QT-T3) may be maintained for large infarcts. Otherwise it should be replaced by a more precise description of localization such as anteroseptal, antero-lateral, posterolateral or posterobasal. A high anterolateral or posterolateral infarct may occur (97) (figs. 249, 250).

The typical evolutionary changes of the tracing are well known. They consist of the appearance of a *QS type of initial complex* (or a deep Q followed *by R*), *a convex (or cove-shaped) S-T, and an inverted T wave* (fig. 251). In the process of healing, the negative T wave becomes deeper at first, then decreases, and may become isoelectric. These changes are due to the spreading toward definite areas of the body of negative "cavity potentials" recorded through the necrotic tissue. It could be said that those areas "look inside the ventricle through an electrical window." Table 21 describes the changes of the unipolar chest leads in anterior infarctions.

ELECTROCARDIOGRAPHIC VARIETIES

The *anteroseptal variety* does not affect the limb leads, though it causes important variations in V2 and V3 (or V4), and occasionally in VE. The *anterolateral variety* affects typically the *unipolar lead of the left arm* and partly that of the left leg. This causes the well-known changes in the stand-ard leads 1 and 2. Reciprocal changes take place in the right arm lead. The *chest leads* V4 to V6 reveal the infarction and may permit a gross evaluation of its size (fig. 249).

Both in the *posterolateral* and *posterobasal varieties*, the typical inversion of the initial complex and of the T wave, again due to the "electrical window," is best recorded by the *unipolar lead of the left leg*. A reciprocal change is recorded by the right arm. The resulting balance is revealed chiefly by the standard leads 2 and 3. In the *posterolateral variety*, the posterior chest leads V7 to V9

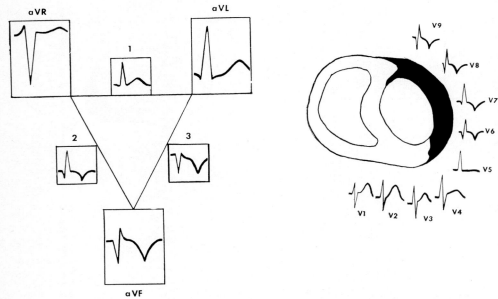

FIG. 250. Electrocardiographic pattern of *old posterolateral* infarct. (From Luisada, Med. Clin. North America. Courtesy of W. B. Saunders Co.).

and the esophageal lead VEs may reveal typical changes (fig. 250). In the *postero-basal variety*, only the unipolar lead of the xiphoid process (VE) reveals the typical picture. On the other hand, the chest leads V1 to V4 present reciprocal changes in both varieties.

Infarcts may occur in any part of the myocardium including *the atria* and *the septum*. They may occur *near the epicardium* or *near the endocardium*; they may be *transmural*, in which case they are like a combination of the above two types; they may be *intramural* because small. In the last instance, the electrical forces around the infarcted area are equal and opposite, so that no pattern of injury or necrosis may be recorded; if, on the other hand, a large area of ischemia surrounds one of these small infarcts, a pattern of ischemia is recorded.

The direction of the S-T displacement may give data on the location of a myocardial lesion because the changes of the S-T segment are different according to the depth and location of the lesion. Elevation

of S-T is found in anterior chest leads when there is an *anterior subepicardial injury*. A *posterior subendocardial injury* (or an *injury of the septum* on the left ventricular side) is also revealed by elevation of S-T in these leads. Opposite ECG changes (S-T depression) reveal *anterior subendocardial* or *posterior subepicardial injury*.

Atrial infarct (40). This rare lesion is revealed by abnormalities of the P wave, premature beats, atrial fibrillation, wandering pacemaker, or nodal rhythm. Later, either *elevation or depression of the P-Q interval with a cone-shaped aspect*, has been observed. There is elevation of P-Q in lead 1 when the left atrium is involved; in lead 3 when the right atrium is damaged. Later, in the stage of inversion of the T-atrial wave, there may be some slurring of QRS because repolarization of the atria (Ta) (page 37) occurs during the QRS complex.

Atypical forms; multiple infarcts. Atypical electrocardiographic patterns are found in about one-third of the cases with infarct. Some are due to preexisting intraventricular

TABLE 21. *Evolution of electrocardiographic changes in anterior infarction*

ECG STAGE	ECG CHANGES RECORDED BY A PRECORDIAL ELECTRODE	MECHANISM	CLINICAL STAGE	EXPLANATION OF CHANGES
1	Primary T wave changes (inverted T).	The area becomes ischemic.	Prodromic stage (brief).	Ischemia.
2	Upward S-T displacement and transient QRS changes. The early primary T wave changes disappear.	The central area is in a state of injury and extends to the epicardium.	The infarction is in the process of establishment but may still be prevented by better coronary flow.	Injury plus ischemia.
3	Severe S-T displacement. QR or QS is present. So-called "cavity potentials" are recorded. T is inverted (new primary change).	The injured area extends and is surrounded by a thin periphery of ischemia. Death of the tissue occurs in the central area (necrosis).	The infarction has occurred (fever, leucocytosis, and increased sedimentation rate).	Necrosis plus injury.
4	The primary T wave changes reappear. The S-T displacement and most of the QRS changes disappear.	The periphery of injured area reverts to the ischemic stage. The injured and necrotic areas are no more in contact with the epicardium.	Early stage of healing of the infarction (2 to 4 weeks).	Ischemia plus necrosis.
5	The primary T wave changes and the Q wave may disappear.	Large part of the ischemic area reverts to normal. There is necrosis in the central area.	Later stages of healing (subsequent months).	Normal tissue (plus necrosis).
6	The permanent QRS changes and the permanent secondary T wave changes persist or disappear according to the extension of the scar.	There is a scar tissue surrounded by normal tissue.	The infarction has healed.	Normal tissue or large scar.

block or older infarcts; some, to gradual production of necrosis with successive involvement of anterolateral and posterolateral parts of the left ventricle. Multiple infarcts are common and may consist of various combinations of recent and old infarcts. In some cases, an inverted T wave in all leads has been observed (*type Tn*) (49). This may be due to: 1) massive infarct involving both the anterior and posterior walls of the left ventricle; 2) anterior infarct in patients already having an inverted T3; 3) posterior infarct in patients already having an inverted T1. Serial electrocardiograms in

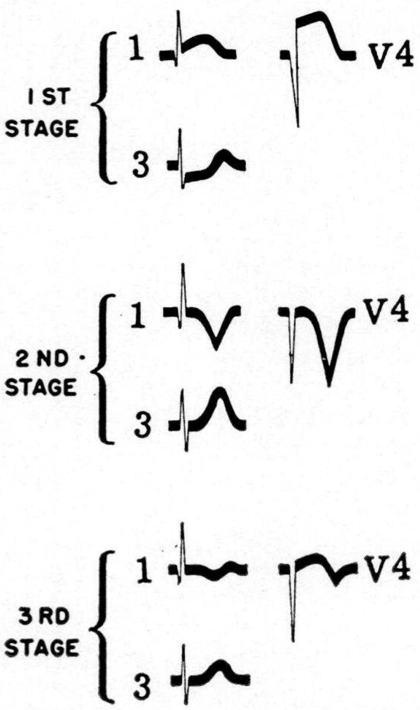

I ST STAGE
1 V4
3

2 ND STAGE
1 V4
3

3 RD STAGE
1 V4
3

FIG. 251. Electrocardiographic changes in the various stages of evolution of an anterolateral infarct.

successive infarcts may reveal either the Tn type of evolution or changes of T; this wave first assumes a frank anterior, then a frank posterior type (or vice versa), in spite of previous abnormalities.

PHONOCARDIOGRAM

The most typical change is the disappearance of the rapid vibrations of the first sound. This presents a prolonged series of *slow vibrations* which are frequently small but may be of normal height. After the acute stage, it is possible to observe *large diastolic sounds* (triple or quadruple rhythm) (page 370). These additional sounds are heard only if they are loud, on account of their low pitch.

LOW FREQUENCY TRACING (CARDIOGRAM)

Cardiographic tracings are obtained with difficulty in the acute stage of myocardial infarction because of the weak cardiac action. When a good tracing is obtained, a slow development of all waves is frequently observed. This is due to the existence of an

area of soft tissue in the left ventricle. By absorbing part of the energy of contraction, this area prevents a rapid rise of pressure and a rapid closure of the mitral valve. Therefore, while the first sound becomes altered the low frequency vibrations of the chest also become slow.

X-RAY

Fluoroscopy may reveal evidence of *calcification of the coronary arteries*. A *diffuse or localized dilatation of the heart* is frequently observed in the early stage after an infarct. Congestion of the lungs, mainly apparent in the hilar vessels, is also frequent (42). Abnormalities of ventricular pulsation may be detected by fluoroscopy (fig. 253) and are better studied by electrokymography. Many months after an infarction, in addition to the functional signs described above, *ventricular aneurysm* (page 391) or *calcification of a section of the ventricular wall* may be observed.

ROENTGENKYMOGRAM

The abnormal movements of the left ventricular wall following myocardial infarction have been repeatedly investigated by means of roentgenkymography.

The most common abnormalities described were: diminution or absence of pulsation in a segment of the left ventricular contour; systolic expansion over the lower left contour; and diastolic splintering (20–23).

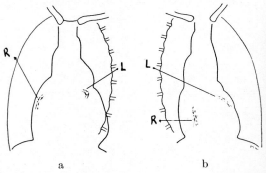

a   b

FIG. 252. Calcification of the coronary arteries at x-ray in the right anterior (a) and in the left anterior oblique (b) positions. R, right; L, left. (From Menendez de Oliveira.)

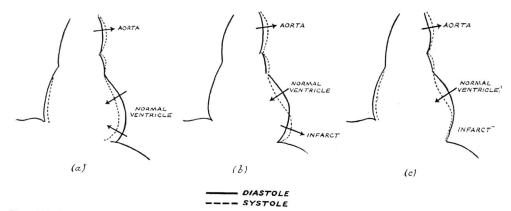

FIG. 253. Fluoroscopic aspect of: a, normal contraction; b, reversal of pulsation (myocardial infarction); c, absence of pulsation (myocardial infarction). (From Ungerleider's *Roentgenology* in Stroud's *Cardiovascular Diseases*. Courtesy of the author and F. A. Davis Co.)

ELECTROKYMOGRAM

Electrokymography permits an accurate study of these movements and gives tracings which may have diagnostic value (143–145).

Several abnormal patterns can be observed in either systole or diastole (143). However, some of the abnormalities can be found in other conditions or can be simulated by improper application of the slit. Therefore, they have no diagnostic significance as to myocardial infarct. Some of the diastolic abnormalities are connected with an abnormality of systole and represent a necessary consequence of the latter (return of the wall after abnormal pulsation). Furthermore, some of these deviations from the normal tracing, and particularly those extending over a large portion of the left ventricular contour, may be favored by positional changes of the heart.

Two definite abnormalities of the sytolic wave should be considered as indicative of localized myocardial damage, in the majority of instances this being identical with myocardial infarct. 1) *Reduced amplitude of the ventricular wave or disappearance of this wave in a circumscribed region of the left ventricle.* Whenever the surrounding areas present large waves, this sign is definitely related to infarction. As that area is functionally (and usually also anatomically) excluded from participating in active contraction, the author suggested the name of *local paralysis* for the phenomenon thus revealed by electrokymography. 2) *Inverted pulsation (paradoxical pulsation) of a circumscribed area of the ventricular myocardium.* In typical cases, this inverted pulsation assumes the aspect of a *plateau*, indicating that the inert wall is passively distended by intraventricular pressure (fig. 254). This type of pulsation may be associated with the existence of a well-defined bulge of the ventricular profile on chest films (*ventricular aneurysm*). In other cases the bulging occurs only in systole while no bulge is present in diastole (*dynamic aneurysm*).

MECHANISM OF THE SIGNS

Cardiac pain is due to stimuli which start from the area of ischemia of the cardiac muscle and reach the nerve centers along sympathetic fibers and through the stellate ganglia. Other stimuli, caused by inflammation of the pericardium and, occasionally, of the pleura, are also frequently present.

Nausea and *sensation of impending death* also are due to stimuli which follow the sympathetic fibers toward the centers.

Dyspnea, restlessness, sweating, diarrhea

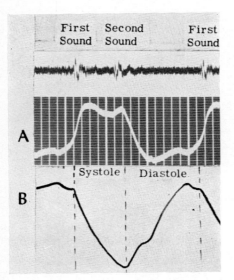

First   Second   First
Sound   Sound   Sound

A

Systole   Diastole

B

FIG. 254. *Old anterolateral infarct*. Expansive systolic pulsation above the apex (dynamic aneurysm) revealed by the electrokymogram. For comparison, a normal ventricular pattern (in black). (From Luisada, Med. Clin. North America. Courtesy of W. B. Saunders Co.).

and *vomiting* should be considered as reflex phenomena. The most likely efferent pathway is the vagus (54). Glycosuria likewise has been attributed to a neurogenic mechanism (59).

The *vascular collapse* is due to multiple causes: a) The exclusion of a group of cardiac fibers from the contraction. b) The fact that the area of infarction becomes softer and forms an *elastic reservoir (dynamic aneurysm)*. On the one hand this decreases the systolic discharge, on the other it increases the residual blood within the left ventricle (106, 107). c) The fact that *reflex elements* cause a series of peripheral phenomena which resemble those of *shock* and may lead to the establishment of this irreversible syndrome (page 520).

The reflex component is maximal at the beginning and may be partly abolished by drugs; the cardiac component is more lasting and not influenced by them. This is shown by the following facts: experimental ligation of one coronary artery causes a sudden drop of pressure in both the lesser and the greater

circulations (47); signs of congestion in the venous system may be missing (48); and autonomic depressants may raise blood pressure. Arterial vasoconstriction, caused in a reflex way by precordial pain, seems to be responsible for the *arterial hypertension (absolute or relative)* which can be observed during the first days in a minority of cases.

The *signs of heart failure* are due to the sudden abolition of one part of the cardiac muscle as an active participant in the contraction and also to the formation of a *dynamic aneurysm* in the area of infarction. They are, therefore, influenced only to a limited extent by drug therapy. Increased work of the rest of the heart may obviate the failure unless prevented by extensive or severe coronary disease.

Acute pulmonary edema has been interpreted as due to acute left ventricular failure. This interpretation is undoubtedly too simple (106). Displacement of a large mass of blood from the greater to the lesser circulation due to cardiovascular reflexes plays an important role in this syndrome.

Leucocytosis, high sedimentation rate, and *fever* are due to necrosis of the cardiac tissue and to the inflammatory reaction which results from it. Inflammation of serous membranes (pericardium, pleura), secondary pulmonary infarctions, and other complications may contribute to these signs.

The *sudden death* of these patients is due to cardiac arrest or ventricular fibrillation. The last is caused by anoxia of the area of partial damage where foci of high excitability are set up. Anoxia may create various degrees of block, favoring filbrillation.

The *musical systolic murmur*, a rare occurrence, can be explained by eddies, formed in the ventricular cavity and favored by the localized area of dilatation (96).

Some of the cardiopulmonary disturbances, such as bradycardia, low blood pressure, and bronchoconstriction seem to be caused by serotonin (5-OH-Tryptamine) liberated from platelets in the process of blood coagulation (155).

COURSE AND COMPLICATIONS

Many patients withstand myocardial infarction without severe embarrassment of the heart and may even discover the existence of a lesion much later. In other cases, there is obvious impairment of cardiac function. Other patients die suddenly or present severe cardiac failure which will be the cause of fatality after weeks or months. Despite the favorable onset, there is always the possibility of extension of the infarct or formation of a new one. The most dangerous phase is in the first 2 weeks, after which scar tissue is usually formed.

Sudden death may be caused by either *cardiac arrest* or *ventricular fibrillation*, the incidence of these being about equal (108).

Rupture of the ventricular wall into the pericardial sac, resulting in *tamponade of the heart* (page 441) or rupture of the *interventricular septum* causing heart failure, may occur within the first 2 weeks. The same can be said for the possible *rupture of a papillary muscle* or a *chorda tendinea*.

Diffuse pericarditis is not rare. If severe, it definitely adds to the dangers of the syndrome. It may be revealed by displacement of R-T in all leads, x-ray data, and prolonged duration of the recovery period.

A condition of *shock* is present in some cases. If prolonged for more than a few hours, it indicates an extensive infarction and, therefore, a serious outlook.

Acute pulmonary edema may be an initial manifestation. Once started, it is more lasting and resistant to treatment than acute pulmonary edema without infarction. The patient may have scanty expectoration and dyspnea but is ashen-gray and is suffocated by the foam present in the trachea and bronchi.

Pulmonary embolism is a frequent complication. It may be caused by mural thrombi *of the right ventricle* (infarction involving the right ventricle or the septum) or the *right atrium* (atrial infarction, congestive failure). In all these cases, the pulmonary occlusions are likely to be *multiple* and *small*. On the contrary, occlusion of the main pulmonary trunk may be due to a larger embolus which usually originates in the large veins of the legs (128) (pages 507 and 539).

Cerebral, renal, or *splenic embolism* are other complications due to detachment of a mural thrombus from the left ventricle (5 to 15 per cent of the cases, in various statistics).

Two-thirds of the patients survive the first attack of myocardial infarction (46a) and one-half of the total survive for many years (46b).

The first 7 days are the most dangerous but sudden death may occur in the second week, even when the course seems favorable. After the 15th day, recovery is probable; after the 21st, it is practically certain in the absence of severe congestive failure.

In some cases of myocardial infarction, persistent pain of the left shoulder, arm, and hand, is due to a reflex (so-called *shoulder-hand syndrome*) (154). Following pain in the left shoulder with painful, stiff, and swollen fingers, deformities of the fingers and atrophy set in, and culminate in *Dupuytren's contracture*.

VARIETIES

In a certain number of cases, *pain is absent.* This may be due to weakness and prostration, or predominance of gastrointestinal, neurological, or pulmonary symptoms. The mortality is higher in these cases on account of the greater incidence of incorrect diagnoses (109).

Cases of coronary occlusion *simulating perforation of a gastric or duodenal ulcer, rupture of a gangrenous appendix, or a gall bladder attack,* are not unusual.

An associated coronary and cerebral syndrome is possible (110). This may be caused by neurological signs of the coronary occlusion. A secondary cerebrovascular accident is also possible as a result of low blood pressure, shock, vascular reflexes, or cerebral edema. This is more severe and more common in cases with combined arteriosclerosis of the coronary and cerebral arteries. Symptomatology may be dominated by restlessness, confusion, syncope, or epilepsy. Hemiplegia may be due to either cerebral embolism, or thrombosis, favored by the sudden circulatory disturbance.

DIAGNOSIS

The diagnosis is not difficult when a typical picture is present and electrocardiography is possible. However, the great number of coronary attacks with atypical symptomatology and the possibility of attacks of a different nature simulating myocardial infarction sometimes present delicate diagnostic problems.

The electrocardiogram is of great help if typical. However, differential diagnosis from tracings of different conditions may be necessary. A typical QS pattern followed by an inverted T is diagnostic. There may be doubt in the *first few days*, during the establishment of the pattern, or if the infarct is *intramural*. In the latter case, a persistent and evolutionary pattern of ischemia may be the only ECG evidence of the infarct. Special diagnostic problems are presented by *multiple infarctions* and by *infarcts in cases of bundle branch block*. It should be kept in mind that bundle branch block may occur suddenly as a result of an infarct. In general, serial electrocardiograms are more informative than one tracing.

Angina pectoris is accompanied by attacks of pain of short duration (10 to 20 minutes); in coronary failure there are longer attacks of pain (20 to 30 minutes) but no persistent ECG changes and no laboratory evidence of infarct.

The possibility of differentiating *myocardial infarction caused by occlusion from that caused by coronary insufficiency* has been discussed. The problem, however, is of little practical importance inasmuch as the immediate prognosis and treatment are the same in both conditions.

Frequent mistakes are made between *myocardial infarct* and *pulmonary infarct*. The latter may or may not give typical ECG signs (page 509). Whenever the ECG is typical, it reveals not only changes in leads AVF and 3 but also evidence of right ventricular "strain" in V1-V2. On the one hand, this would not be present in a posterior infarct; on the other, an anteroseptal infarct would cause changes of V2-V3 and none in aVF and 3.

It should be kept in mind that myocardial infarct may be followed by pulmonary embolism and that pulmonary infarct may be followed by a myocardial infarct, favored by the severe drop in pressure and by the resulting coronary insufficiency.

Differential diagnosis is frequently necessary between *myocardial infarct* and *perforated gastric or duodenal ulcer*. It should be kept in mind that an acute internal hemorrhage may cause S-T and T changes lasting for several days (56) and even precipitate a myocardial infarct through prolonged coronary insufficiency (57).

A *dissecting aneurysm of the aorta* may simulate myocardial infarct (page 485). However, the pain has a different radiation; there may be disappearance of one or both radial pulses; and the ECG changes are atypical, unless the compression of the coronary arteries is of such severity that myocardial infarct actually occurs.

PROGNOSIS

The *prognosis* is much better in initial than in later attacks and becomes worse with each subsequent attack. The prognosis is better in the young, worse in the older age groups. However, the probable shortening of life is greater in the younger group whose life expectancy, if no attack had happened, would have been greater.

Dyspnea, cyanosis, tachycardia, and alternans are serious prognostic signs. Heart failure, embolization, and heart block increase mortality and indicate a grave prognosis.

Myocardial infarction, complicated by acute pulmonary edema, has a mortality of about 50 per cent. Leucocytosis is significant of a severe lesion if above 15,000, while figures above 25,000 are found only in fatal cases. The same is true for fever, if higher than 101 or lasting more than a week.

The duration of fever, leucocytosis, and high sedimentation rate may indicate a persisting inflammatory condition, although this may be caused by complications and not by the infarction itself.

Prognosis is similar in anterior and posterior infarctions.

So far as the blood pressure is concerned, the immediate prognosis is better when blood pressure is high than when it is low because shock may be reached less easily (95). On the other hand, the ultimate prognosis is worse in hypertensive patients (95) and it should be kept in mind that rupture of the ventricular wall is three times more common when blood pressure is high than when it is low (111).

Cases with ruptured ventricular septum seldom live more than 1 month (112).

Ultimate prognosis is difficult because it is based not only on the outcome of the present attack, but on the possibility of complications and on the possible occurrence of other attacks. Among the patients who survive, most have a life span of 4 to 5 years, but certain cases have lived 25 years or more after an attack. Some of the latter led a normal life without restrictions and one had a successful pregnancy (127). Prognosis in centenaries is not different from that in relatively younger patients (156).

TREATMENT

Treatment of acute coronary occlusion has the following program:

a) *To reduce, as far as possible, the work of the heart.* This is obtained by the use of *sedatives* and *bed rest.* If there is danger of shock, sedatives should be used with caution. *Armchair treatment,* advocated by some (153), is frequently unsatisfactory, partly for psychological reasons. However, bedrest should not be unduly prolonged, especially in old individuals, because it may lead to embarrassment of the venous circulation and poor ventilation of the lungs. Whenever there is heart failure, the patient should be propped up in bed. *Morphine sulfate,* 10 to 15 mg. plus *atropine sulfate* 0.5 mg. by hypodermic injection every 4 to 6 hours, or *demerol* (115) 100 mg. at similar intervals, should be given during the first 3 to 6 days. With improvement, the doses can be cut by one-half while *papaverine hydrochloride* (43) 50 mg., *phenobarbital,* or both, are gradually added.

b) *To alleviate pain and anxiety.* This is already obtained by morphine or demerol. *Oxygen* is also helpful.

c) *To prevent autonomic reflexes.* Apart from the action of morphine, phenobarbital, and atropine, the endpoint of reflexes may be depressed by means of 0.2 gm. *quinidine sulfate* per os every 4 hours, or 0.5 gm. *procaine amide* (113) (27) at similar intervals.

d) *To obtain the best level of blood pressure.* While high blood pressure is detrimental because it causes cardiac strain, low blood pressure may increase coronary insufficiency and may lead to shock. Several of the above-mentioned drugs tend to lower blood pressure and should be used wisely. If the systolic pressure drops below 90, supportive measures are justified. They include slow intravenous administration of *glucose solution* containing *nor-l-epinephrine* (116). The average infusion should be about 300 cc. every 6 hours, containing from 4 to 7 mg. of the vasoconstrictor drug (56). A successful treatment of shock is obtained much more easily if it is undertaken within the first 3 hours after its initiation.

e) *To prevent extension of the infarcted area of the heart.* The use of anticoagulants, and that of papaverine favors the establishment of collateral circulation and decreases the chance of an extension of the clot with further occlusion of various branches (see below).

f) *To prevent or treat heart failure.* Heart failure can be combated only to a limited extent because it is due to necrosis of some of the cardiac fibers and is favored by fibrosis of the heart muscle. *Oxygen*, and the combined use of *digitalis* and *quinidine* (or *procaine amide*), is often followed by some degree of improvement. Digitalization should be done slowly so that the full dose is reached in 3 days. It is tolerated best by the use of *gitalin* (119) (**8**) (page 589) which has a wide therapeutic index and causes less increase of ventricular excitability.

g) To prevent paroxysmal or disordered cardiac action. *Oxygen, procaine amide* or *quinidine*, and the various sedatives, are usually helpful. Systematic preventive use of these drugs is advocated by some but does not seem necessary.

h) *To prevent formation of clots adherent to the walls of the heart or to those of peripheral veins* (114, 115). While the former are a frequent cause of secondary occlusion of important arterial vessels (especially in the brain), the latter may cause secondary occlusion of pulmonary vessels. This aim is obtained by the early use of intravenous *heparin* (**63**) in dose of 50 to 200 mg. every 4 hours; by the use of oral *dicumarol* (117) (**64**) or *tromexan* (118) (**65**) subsequently. These drugs are given by mouth with an initial dose of 300 mg. of dicumarol (800 mg. tromexan) and subsequent daily doses of 100 to 200 mg. dicumarol (300 to 600 mg. tromexan). Anticoagulants *need not* be used in younger people or mild attacks and *should not* be used in patients with pulmonary cavities or gastrointestinal ulcers. They are imperative in older people and in severe attacks, and in cases with a history of atrial fibrillation or venous thrombosis. Anticoagulants require proper laboratory control about the ability of the blood to clot. A drop of clotting activity to about 30 per cent of normal is considered the best for preventing thromboembolic phenomena without causing hemorrhages. *Vitamin K* (**66**) should be kept handy and administered in dose of 60 to 75 mg. whenever clotting activity becomes too low. Anticoagulants

should be continued for 4 to 6 weeks in the average cases, for longer periods in cases with complications.

i) *To treat acute pulmonary edema.* The best treatment is *oxygen-alcohol vapor by inhalation* for 1 to 12 hours by mask or nasal catheter (146) (page 560). Infusions or transfusions should be curtailed or stopped; morphine, barbiturates, and mercurials should be limited. The former favor pulmonary edema; the latter favor shock. Digitalis should not be given intravenously during the attack.

In general, *alcohol* in moderate amounts is permitted, especially in hypertensive patients, while *tobacco* is forbidden until after completion of convalescence.

While *severe attacks* require long bed rest, prolonged convalescence, and the most serious measures, *mild attacks* may be treated with 2 weeks in bed, 2 weeks of convalescence, and 1 or 2 months of sharply reduced activity.

Myocardial infarction in diabetic patients often causes increase in blood sugar, glycosuria and, sometimes, ketosis (138). The patients often become more resistant to insulin and this renders their treatment particularly difficult. If no acetone is found in the urine, no change in diabetic therapy is required. If, on the other hand, ketosis develops, a 10 per cent solution of glucose will be given intravenously at the rate of 250 cc. per hour up to a total of 1500 to 2000 cc. At the same time, *crystalline insulin* should be given subcutaneously in doses of 15 to 20 units every 2 hours. Very severe cases may need an initial dose of 40 to 60 units of insulin. Later treatment is the same as in severe diabetes without infarction.

PREVENTION

Prevention of coronary occlusion involves: a) Treatment of hypertension. b) Treatment of diabetes. c) Control of cholesterol metabolism (reduced intake; control of metabolism with hormones, iodides, etc; possible use of estrogens). d) Avoidance of severe exertion or excessive excitement.

Some of these aims cannot be completely attained at present but should be in a foreeable future.

Angina Pectoris (68)

Increasing knowledge in the field of coronary heart disease has changed our understanding and definition of "angina pectoris". Fifty years ago this name was applied to any case of coronary heart disease with cardiac pain; cases of myocardial infarction are now excluded. Therefore, angina pectoris is simply "cardiac pain due to coronary insufficiency not followed by an infarct": the expression "cardiac pain" might be substituted for "angina pectoris".

The mechanism of production and the multiple causes of coronary insufficiency have been already described (page 415). Even if hemodynamic, chemical or vasomotor elements may be involved, there is no doubt that *a structural lesion of the coronary system* is present in the great majority of cases. This lesion is severe and extensive in some patients. In others, it is so limited that it acts only as a "trigger mechanism" favoring reflex coronary ischemia.

Experimental and clinical evidence indicates that cardiac pain is the result of a *disproportion between blood supply to and blood demand by the myocardium*. Both increased blood demand and decreased oxygen saturation in the arterial blood favor cardiac pain. Therefore, patients with hypertension, valvular defects, or congenital malformations of the heart frequently complain of cardiac pain.

In most cases, cardiac pain is precipitated by sudden increase in the blood demand while blood supply cannot be increased because of hardening of the coronary arteries. The increase may be due to physical exertion or increase of venous return caused by either intake of food or recumbency. Therefore, the two

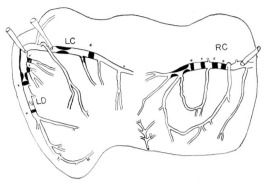

FIG. 255. Diagram of coronary arterial tree in patient with angina pectoris; nine old complete occlusions in all three major coronary arteries. Note large dissectible collateral artery which bridges several occlusions in right coronary artery. (From H. L. Blumgart, Res. Publ. Assoc. Nerv. & Ment. Dis., 1943. Courtesy of the author.)

typical pictures of angina pectoris, *exertional angina* and *decubitus angina* (69), are not too different in the mechanism of their production.

Multiple mechanisms are related to cardiac pain. An occlusion may not be followed by infarction because of well-developed collateral circulation (fig. 255). On the other hand, ischemia may be followed by multiple scars if the collateral circulation is poor. Multiple small occlusions in a wide area have the same result as occlusion of an artery. For these reasons, it is sometimes impossible to say whether, in the individual case, a brief attack of pain is related to structural changes or to a functional mechanism.

The *afferent pathways for cardiac pain* begin in sensory nerve endings which are present in the adventitia of the coronary arteries and possibly of other cardiac structures. The nerve fibers travel by way of *the middle and inferior cardiac nerves* until they reach *the cervical sympathetic ganglia*, and by way of *the thoracic cardiac nerves* until they reach the *upper four or five thoracic sympathetic ganglia* (186). The cervical cardiac fibers descend in the sympathetic chain to the thoracic ganglia;

then, together with thoracic cardiac fibers, proceed through *the white rami communicantes* of the upper four or five thoracic ganglia, and reach their cells in the spinal ganglia.

Anginal pain has been explained in various ways. According to the theory of "poor localization" (72), the brain has a poor localization power and attributes the pain of deep organs to those superficial regions from which it is usually receiving sensory impressions. This is made easy by the fact that sensory fibers from the intercostal nerves have their body cells in the same ganglia as the cardiac fibers. According to the older theory of "irritable focus" (129), painful visceral impulses set up a disturbance in the spinal cord which extends to fibers from the body surface. Pain is referred to the periphery on account of the higher development of skin sensitivity. Disappearance of the pain after local anesthesia (75, 130) seems to confirm this theory and the view has been advocated that *somatic trigger areas* develop within the "reference zone" of the visceral lesion. Chest pain may continue on account of secondary sources of pain in the somatic structures.

Cardiac pain has been attributed to: a) distention of the coronary arteries; b) anoxia of the myocardium; c) accumulation of products of muscular contraction (lactic acid, phosphoric acid, pyruvic acid; histamine, adenosine, or potassium). Either *anoxia* (oxygen deficiency) or *ischemia* (reduction of blood flow) may cause the pain (page 415) and either of the two may be involved though the latter is the more common. Ischemia (as cause of anoxia) and anoxia may cause pain by leading to accumulation of metabolites stimulating the sensory nerve endings, as the cardiac muscle keeps working and is incapable of any important "oxygen debt" (page 33).

It has been pointed out that anginal attacks occur under those conditions which are accompanied by *sympathetic stimulation* and *discharge of epinephrine*, and by *accumulation of sympathin* in the myocardium (physical exertion, exposure to cold, and emotion). It has been shown further that the attacks can be provoked by adrenalin or other drugs stimulating the sympathetic system (nicotine, insulin), and are common in tumors of the adrenal medulla. For these and other reasons, the view was advocated (131) that effort angina is due to an acute anoxia of the myocardium caused by epinephrine and sympathin (page 48), which is particularly severe in patients with sclerotic coronary vessels.

Among the various theories of angina pectoris, one explains the attack as due to a *reflex mechanism*. Beneficial results of carotid sinus compression (136) were interpreted as confirming this theory. However, this maneuver is followed by lowering of blood pressure and decreased work of the heart.

Elements favoring angina pectoris are the following: sudden change from a warm to a cold temperature; severe atmospheric fluctuations (hurricanes); physical effort; emotion; abundant meals; and the copious ingestion of fluid. Nicotine definitely favors angina pectoris; intestinal poisons may do so.

Increased excitability of the vagus nerve, sudden increase of the blood pressure, and distention of the abdominal viscera favor angina pectoris. Hyperthyroidism also favors angina pectoris. In other words, any cause of increased cardiac work, decreased coronary blood supply, or visceral reflexes favors angina pectoris.

SYMPTOMS AND SIGNS

The main symptom of angina pectoris is *cardiac pain*. This is usually referred to the precordial area but may be felt in the left shoulder, in the left side of the neck, and, more rarely, in the left scapular region. The pain is described in various ways: as *an oppressive, crushing, tearing, squeezing, or choking pain*. It may be described as an oppressing, choking, or crushing sensation with complete denial that it is pain. The pain is usually transmitted to the left shoulder, the throat, and the left arm, forearm, or hand. In some cases, it is transmitted to the 4th and 5th fingers of the left hand.

A *sensation of impending death*, once thought typical, is present only in a small number of cases.

In typical cases, the patient, frequently a man in the early fifties, feels the pain when leaving a warm apartment after supper on a cold night. After a few steps, the patient feels a crushing pain in the chest and stops suddenly, afraid to proceed. He often leans against a wall, avoids movements and talking, breathes slowly, and has a pale face with a suffering or fixed expression. After a few minutes, the attack is over and the patient continues his walk.

Attacks occurring early *in the morning* when the patient leaves his home are equally typical. Other attacks may occur *at night*, waking the patient from a bad dream or a nightmare.

Physical examination during the attack fails to reveal much: the pulse is usually full and regular and may present occasional premature beats. Blood pressure is either at the same or at a higher level than before the attack. The face is pale and drawn, occasionally perspiring. Gastric manifestation, like gastric oppression and eructations, are frequent. Salivation, sweating, and an urgent desire to urinate, are present in some cases.

DIAGNOSIS—VARIETIES

The diagnosis of angina pectoris is, in many cases, purely clinical because the ECG fails to show appreciable changes at the moment of the examination. In others, however, the existence of ECG changes lends support to the diagnosis. When the ECG is negative, functional tests should be done or the patient may be studied during a spontaneous attack (cases where the

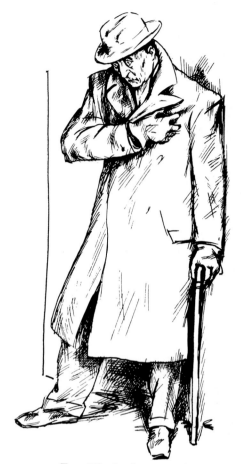

FIG. 256. Angina pectoris

pain coincides with definite events of the daily life). In difficult cases, the beneficial action of nitroglycerine may have diagnostic importance. Once the diagnosis of angina is made, one should try to find how important is the part played by structural lesions, reflex elements, and emotional factors.

In patients with frequent attacks of cardiac pain, the electrocardiogram should be taken between the attacks and also during the attack.

The electrocardiogram, taken during a spontaneous attack of pain, frequently reveals depression of S-T and a diphasic or inverted T wave in one or more leads. The changes are transitory.

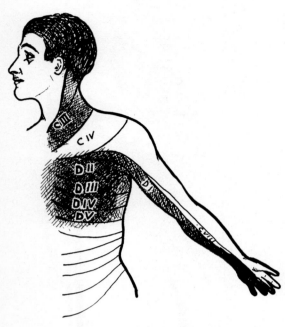

FIG. 257. Distribution of pain in angina pectoris.

Doubtful cases, where history suggests angina pectoris but the electrocardiogram is normal, will be studied by means of *functional tests*. The most used are *Master's two-step exercise test* (147) and *Levy's anoxemia test* (77). The *amyl nitrite test*, described in the author's laboratory (148), is simple and practical. Changes of the ECG, revealed by these tests, are similar to those observed in spontaneous attacks.

Functional tests lead to division of the patients into three groups:

1) The electrocardiogram between attacks reveals severe abnormalities indicative of coronary and myocardial lesions (no functional tests should be performed). A predominant structural component is at the basis of the attacks.

2) The electrocardiogram between attacks reveals slight abnormalities or is normal. Functional tests reveal typical changes of the electrocardiogram. The structural lesion is mild, and functional components contribute to the attack.

3) The electrocardiogram is normal between attacks. Functional tests fail to reveal abnormalities in the tracing. The pain is probably not related to the heart.

Differential diagnosis should exclude a long list of diseases.

Substernal pain may be due to infections, arthritis, mediastinal lesions, gastric and esophageal conditions, aneurysm, and pericarditis.

Precordial pain may be due to mastitis, hematoma, or hypertrophy of the left breast; neurofibromata; abscess or myalgia of the pectoral muscle; neuralgia of the intercostal nerves; radicular pain, occasionally accompanying herpes zoster, periostitis; osteomyelitis; pleurisy; diaphragmatic lesions; and abdominal disorders (aerophagia with pneumatosis, among others).

Pain in the left upper extremity, the shoulder, or the rest of the limb, may be caused by neuritis, arthritis, bursitis, spondylitis, cervical rib, diaphragmatic lesions, and many other conditions.

Pain from noncardiac causes is almost always more diffuse than anginal pain, overlapping the areas of the radial, median, or ulnar nerve. The pain of angina pectoris is never localized to the left of the anterior axillary line.

Differential diagnosis from gastric conditions is frequently necessary because they may simulate angina pectoris and the latter often is accompanied by gastric disturbances.

It should be known that a small percentage of individuals with normal hearts experience pain when taking *coffee*. The pain is not severe, is not increased by exertion, and is of long duration. It is not relieved by nitroglycerin (84).

PROGNOSIS

The prognosis in angina pectoris should be based on the evaluation of all functional and structural elements causing the pain; this means also evaluation and prognosis of the coronary heart disease.

The division of the patients into different

groups (see above) may be used for the prognosis. Extensive and severe myocardial lesions and severe coronary lesions, as revealed by the electrocardiograph and the history, have a severe prognosis. This is based on the knowledge that, sooner or later, myocardial infarction will occur with all the possibilities implied in this event.

Concerning the pain itself, it is difficult to foretell the far distant course. Some patients have angina pectoris for years; then a myocardial infarction occurs. After recovery, the anginal pain is milder or has disappeared. In other cases the opposite is true; an initial infarction starts a series of anginal attacks and these continue throughout life.

In general, angina pectoris in youth has a more severe prognosis unless dynamic or functional elements (tachycardia, valvular defects, anemia, hyperthyroidism), which can be fully or partly relieved, explain the pain.

TREATMENT

The treatment of angina pectoris is often difficult. However, the complete negativism of some authors is not justified.

A proper evaluation of the dynamic, functional, and psychic elements, may permit the exclusion of at least some of them. Removal of a damaged gall bladder; treatment of thyrotoxicosis, paroxysmal tachycardia, or anemia; improvement of gastric conditions; proper diet; better habits; and sometimes a divorce, may avoid the need for further treatment in many cases. Obese patients should reduce; diabetic patients should be treated for diabetes.

Patients with angina should be advised not to take a heavy meal at night and not to go to bed with a full stomach. They should be cautioned against drinking too much fluid *with* their meals and against using tobacco.[69] A diet excluding foods

causing fermentation should be prescribed. *Alcohol* can be allowed but with moderation. Alcohol is a peripheral vasodilator though an extremely poor coronary dilator. Therefore its beneficial effect is based on either reduction of blood pressure or central depression. The latter relieves tension and decreases the severity of possible constrictor reflexes.

Physical exercise may be continued in many cases but open-air exercise, heavy work, and exposure to cold should be forbidden.

Any cause for increased cardiac work, vagal reflexes, or anoxemia should be prevented as far as possible.

Treatment of the attack of angina pectoris is based on vasodilators having a rapid action like sublingual *nitroglycerin* (**53**).

Between the attacks, many drugs can be used; the most effective are:

a) Vasodilators which have a prolonged action like *mannitol hexanitrate* (**51**), *papaverine* (**43**), *aminophylline* (**41, 42**), *khellin* (**48**) (121).

b) *Belladonna* or *atropine* and, in some cases, a total inhibition of the autonomic nervous system (**35**).

c) Hypnotics, like *phenobarbital, nembutal, sodium amytal*, and *chloral hydrate* (**33**).

d) *Quinidine* (**25**).

These drugs have the purpose of reducing cardiac work (and thus blood demand) and of decreasing possible noxious reflexes.

Treatment with small doses of *thyroid extract* may be beneficial in hypothyroid patients. In the others, either *radioactive iodine* (132) or *propylthiouracil* have been advocated for reducing basal metabolism and cardiac work. However, this treatment is destined only for a selected group of cases.

Different *surgical treatments* have been tried.

---

[69] There is considerable variability in the effect of smoking on the circulation. In susceptible persons, smoking is followed by a *rise* in blood pressure (135). Therefore, ultimate decision may be based on a practical test, by taking blood pressure before and after smoking.

a) *Surgical interventions on the cervico-thoracic section of the sympathetic system* (85) attempting the prevention of centripetal, painful stimuli from reaching the higher centers. They consist of removal of the superior cervical ganglia; of these plus the sympathetic chains down to the level of the 1st thoracic ganglion; or of the inferior cervical ganglia plus the 1st thoracic ganglia (stellate ganglia). Alternate interventions are *the section of the rami communicantes T1 to T5 or the paravertebral injection of alcohol* in order to destroy the rami of the upper thoracic nerves (85). The operation was extended later to *the thoracolumbar section of the sympathetics*, attempting to lower the blood pressure and decrease the work of the heart (86).

The fact that pain prevents exertion which may damage the heart, and the possibility of accidents resulting from the lack of innervation of the pulmonary vessels, advise restriction of the first type of operation to a small number of patients, those with unbearable pain, resistant to every other treatment, who are likely to avoid exertion and to follow instructions. The more extensive intervention is indicated mainly in hypertensive patients. Roentgen treatment of the adrenal glands has also been advocated in the latter (87).

b) *Partial or subtotal thyroidectomy* (88). The purpose of this operation is to lower the metabolism and, thereby, the work of the heart. The patients frequently suffer from secondary myxedema and need medical control and treatment. This fact should limit the application of this intervention to a selected group of patients.

c) *Attempts to create a new collateral circulation for the myocardium.* They were done by grafting either the omentum (88) or one bundle of pectoral muscle (89) to the heart or by injecting substances causing adhesive pericarditis (90). These interventions are still in the experimental stage. The same holds true for *pericoronary neurectomy* (93) and *ligation of the coronary*

sinus (85j) which may be combined in the same patient (85k).

Transplantation of the left internal mammary artery into the left ventricular wall has been tried, first in animals (85l) then in man (152). *Graft of a systemic artery into the coronary sinus (arterialization of the coronary sinus)* is also in the experimental stage (134).

Coronary Heart Disease without Cardiac Pain

Coronary heart disease can be followed by severe changes in the myocardium without association with cardiac pain. This is probably due to slow, uniform, and widespread damage of the arteries with subsequent fibrosis of the myocardium. If the fibrosis of the myocardium precedes or accompanies the hardening of the larger vessels, cardiac work and blood demand are decreased without disproportion to the amount of blood supplied by the larger coronary vessels. As a result of myocardial fibrosis, cardiac reserve is decreased.

Whenever the lesion is moderate, the picture of the *senile heart* is observed. On the other hand, if severe lesions occur within a short time, or damage is extensive, *heart failure* may follow. Many cases, which a few decades ago were called "myocarditis," represented advanced coronary heart disease with heart failure. The same picture occurs in patients with a history of previous myocardial infarcts whenever the remaining ventricular wall undergoes a process of fibrosis.

The treatment of heart failure is the same as in other cardiac patients. However, the best results are obtained by *sodium restriction*, a *proper diet* including large doses of vitamin B1, and *mercurial diuretics*, rather than by the use of digitalis glycosides.

Myocardial fibrosis may be widespread in areas of the myocardium outside the ventricular walls. Extensive damage of the atrial wall or of the conducting system may cause atrial fibrillation, nodal rhythm, atrioventricular block, or bundle branch block. Most of these patients have no cardiac pain, and many of them live for several years without myocardial infarct or cardiac failure.

BALLISTOCARDIOGRAM

The ballistocardiogram of patients with coronary heart disease is frequently abnormal. The possible abnormalities are: 1) H wave of amplitude equal or higher than that of the J wave (early M-type); 2) absence of the J wave; 3) J wave M-shaped at its peak (late M type); 4) J wave late in systole and deep K wave (late downstroke type); 5) R-J interval longer than 0.29 second; 6) L wave and after-waves accentuated; and 7) upward bowing of the J-K segment.

It is still open to question which part is played by hypertension or atherosclerosis of the aorta and large vessels in causing these changes. As they are similar to those observed in elderly individuals, they have a definite meaning only if observed in younger subjects. It is also open to question whether the abnormalities of left ventricular contraction causing these changes might not be more clearly detected by the study of the electrokymogram of the left ventricle and the aortic arch, or by recording a carotid tracing.

BIBLIOGRAPHY

1. a) ABBOTT, M. E. In *Nelson Loose-Leaf Medicine*. New York, Nelson, 1944.
   b) DRY, T. J. *Manual of Cardiology*. Philadelphia, Saunders, 1943.
2. a) RICH, A. R., AND GREGORY, J. E. Bull. Hopkins Hosp., 1945, **72**, 65; and **73**, 239.
   b) FOX, R. A., AND JONES, L. R. Proc. Soc. Exper. Biol. & Med., 1944, **55**, 294.
3. BLAND, E. F., WHITE, P. D., AND GARLAND, J. Am. Heart J., 1933, **8**, 787.
4. LAMB, A. R., AND TURNER, K. B. In *Nelson Loose-Leaf Medicine*. Philadelphia, Davis, 1942.
5. SPRAGUE, H. B. In *Nelson Loose-Leaf Medicine*. Philadelphia, Davis, 1942.
6. SMITH, F. M. In *Cyclopedia of Medicine*. Philadelphia, Davis, 1945.
7. VON GLAHN. *The Pathology of the Coronary Arteries*, in "*Diseases of the Coronary Arteries and Cardiac Pain*". Edited by Levy, R. L. New York, Macmillan, 1936.
8. GROSS, L. *The Blood Supply to the Heart in Its Anatomical and Clinical Aspects*. New York, Hoeber, 1921.
9. GROSS, L., KUGEL, M. A., AND EPSTEIN, E. Z. Am. J. Path., 1935, **11**, 253.
10. LEVY, R. *Diseases of the Coronary System*. New York, Macmillan, 1936.
11. ROESSLE. Quoted by von Glahn (7).
12. a) LEARY, T. Arch. Path., 1934, **17**, 453. Also Mo. Conc., Cardiov. Dis., 1942, **11**, N. 11.
    b) SCHLESINGER, M. J., AND ZOLL, P. M. Arch. Path., 1941, **32**, 178.
    c) FRENCH, A. J., AND DOCK, W. J. A. M. A., 1944, **124**, 1233.
13. GRANT, R. T. Clin. Sci., 1940, **4**, 245.
14. SAPHIR, O. Arch. Path., 1942, **33**, 88.
15. VON ALBERTINI, A. Schw. med. Woch., 1943, **73**, 796.
16. DAVIS, D., AND BLUMGART, H. L. Ann. Int. Med., 1937, **11**, 1024.
17. LEVY, R. In *Stroud's Cardiovascular Disease*. Philadelphia, Davis, 1945.
18. SCHLESINGER, M. J. Am. Heart J., 1938, **15**, 528.
19. BLUMGART, H. L., SCHLESINGER, M. J., AND CO-WORKERS. Am. Heart J., 1940, **19**, 1; and 1941, **22**, 1. Am. J. M. Sci., 1937, **194**, 493. J. A. M. A., 1941, **116**, 91. Arch. Int. Med., 1941, **68**, 181.
20. a) OBRASTZOW, W. P., AND STRASCHESCO, N. D. Zeit. klin. Med., 1910, **71**, 116.
    b) HERRICK, J. B. J. A. M. A., 1919, **72**, 387.
21. MASTER, A. M., AND CO-WORKERS. Am. Heart J., 1944, **27**, 803.
22. STERNBERG, M. Wien. med. Woch., 1910, **60**, 14.
23. WIGGERS, C. J. In *Diseases of the Coronary System*. Edited by Levy. New York, Macmillan, 1936.
24. RUBINO, A. Folia Med., 1937, **23**, 1166.
25. MASTER, A. M., DOCK, S., AND JAFFEE, H. L. J. A. M. A., 1937, **109**, 546.
26. BLUMGART, H. L. J. A. M. A., 1945, **128**, 775.
27. LEARY, T. Am. Heart J., 1935, **10**, 328.
28. WINTERNITZ, M. C., THOMAS, R. M., AND LeCOMPTE, P. M. *The Biology of Arteriosclerosis*. Springfield, Thomas, 1938.
29. a) WILLIUS, F. A. Proc. Staff. Meet., Mayo Clin., 1936, **11**, 414.

b) WAITZKIN, L. Ann. Int. Med., 1944, **21,** 421.

c) BOYER, N. H. New England J. Med., 1942, **227,** 628.

30. a) DRESSLER, W. Am. Heart J., 1944, **28,** 81.

b) ROSENBAUM, F. F., WILSON, F. N., AND JOHNSTON, F. D. Am. Heart J., 1945, **30,** 11.

31. a) LIBMAN, E. Am. Heart J., 1925, **1,** 2.

b) BICKEL, G., MOZER, J. J., AND SCICLOUNOFF, F. Arch. Mal Coeur, 1935, **28,** 73.

c) SHOOKHOFF, C., DOUGLAS, A. H., AND RABINOWITZ, M. A. Ann. Int. Med., 1936, **9,** 1101.

32. WILSON, F. N., JOHNSTON, F. C., AND HILL, I. G. W. Am. Heart J., 1935, **10,** 176.

33. PARDEE, H. E. B., AND GOLDENBERG, M. Am. Heart J., 1945, **30,** 367.

34. a) BELLET, S., AND McMILLAN, T. M. In *Stroud's Cardiovascular Disease.* Philadelphia, Davis, 1945.

b) WILSON, F. N. In *Stroud's Cardiovascular Disease.* Philadelphia, Davis, 1945.

35. WOOD, F. C., WOLFERTH, C. C., AND BELLET, S. Am. Heart J., 1938, **16,** 387.

36. a) PARDEE, H. E. B. Arch. Int. Med., 1920, **26,** 244.

b) WILLIUS, F. A. Atlantic M. J., 1925, **29,** 9.

c) PARKINSON, J., AND BEDFORD, D. E. Lancet, 1928, **1,** 4.

d) LEVINE, S. A. Medicine 1929, **8,** 245.

37. BOSCO, G. A. *Sindrome Coronario Lateral.* Buenos Aires, Ferrari, 1943.

38. WILSON, F. N. Rev. Arg. Card., 1944, **11,** 1.

39. THOMPSON, H. W., AND FEIL, H. Am. J. M. Sci., 1944, **207,** 588.

40. YOUNG, E. W., AND KOENIG, B. S. Am. Heart J., 1944, **28,** 287.

41. WEINBERG, H. B., AND KATZ, L. N. Am. Heart J., 1941, **21,** 699.

42. MASSIE, E., AND MILLER, W. C. Am. J. Med. Sci., 1943, **206,** 353.

43. MASTER, A. M., AND CO-WORKERS. Mo. Conc. Cardiov. Dis., 1941, **10,** N. 6.

44. UNGERLEIDER, H. E., AND GUBNER, R. In *Stroud's Cardiovascular Disease.* Philadelphia, Davis, 1945.

45. BLUMER, G. Ann. Int. Med., 1937, **11,** 499.

46. a) ROSENBAUM, F. F., AND LEVINE, S. A. Arch. Int. Med., 1941, **68,** 913.

b) WHITE, P. D. *Heart Disease.* New York, Macmillan, 1944.

47. CATALDI, G. Cuore e Circ. (Rome), 1937, **21,** 2.

48. STEAD, E. A., AND EBERT, R. V. Arch. Int. Med., 1942, **69,** 369.

49. LUISADA, A. A. Atti Congr. Soc. Ital. Cardiol., 1935.

50. HESS, L. Deut. Arch. klin. Med., 1932, **173,** 283.

51. COELHO, E., AND ROCHETA, J. Ann. Med., 1933, **34,** 91.

52. CATALDI, G. M. Policl. (sez. med.) (Rome), 1937, **44,** 170. Arch. Mal. Coeur, 1935, **28,** 604.

53. CUSHING, E. H., FEIL, H. S., STANTON, E. J., AND WARTMENT, W. B. Brit. Heart J., 1942, **4,** 17.

54. a) GILBERT, N. C., FENN, G. K., AND LeROY, G. V. J. A. M. A., 1940, **115,** 1962.

b) McMILLAN, R. L., COWDEN, F. E., AND REINHART, J. B. Am. Heart J., 1945, **29,** 580.

55. a) LEVINE, S. A. Mo. Conc. Cardiov. Dis., 1942, **11,** N. 6.

b) ROSENBAUM, F. F., AND LEVINE, S. A. Arch. Int. Med., 1941, **68,** 913 and 1215.

c) MASTER, A. M. Mo. Conc. Cardiov. Dis., 1936, **5,** N. 12.

56. SCHERF, D., REINSTEIN, H., AND KLOTZ, S. D. Rev. Gastroenterol, 1941, **8,** 343.

57. a) MASTER, A. M., AND JAFFE, H. L. J. Mt. Sinai Hosp. 1940, **7,** 26.

b) KINNEY, T. D., AND MALLORY, K. New England J. Med., 1945, **232,** 215.

58. SCHERF, D., AND SCHOENBRUNNER, E. Klin. Woch., 1937, **16,** 340.

59. RAAB, A. P., AND RABINOWITZ, M. A. J. A. M. A., 1936, **106,** 1705.

60. DONATH, F. Wien. klin. Woch., 1936 (1), **49,** 692.

61. BUCHBINDER, W. C. Proc. Soc. Exper. Biol. & Med., 1944, **56,** 228.

62. BARACH, A. L., AND LEVY, R. L. J. A. M. A., 1934, **103,** 1690.

63. ASKEY, J. M., AND NEURATH, O. J. A. M. A., 1945, **128,** 1016.

64. KISCH, B. Exper. Med. & Surg., 1945, **3,** 1.

65. McGUIRE DOLES, H. South M. J., 1943, **36,** 709.

66. MOKOTOFF, R., AND KATZ, L. N. Am. Heart J., 1945, **30,** 215.

67. a) FRIEDMAN, S., AND WHITE, P. D. Ann. Int. Med., 1944, **21,** 778.

b) JETTER, W. W., AND WHITE, P. D. Ann. Int. Med., 1944, **21,** 783.

68. HEBERDEN, W. *Commentaries on the History and Cure of Diseases.* London, Payne, 1802.

69. VAQUEZ, H. *Maladies du Coeur.* Paris, Bailière, 1928.

70. a) WOOD, F. C., WOLFERTH, C. C., AND BELLET, S. Am. Heart J., 1938, **16,** 387.

b) RISEMAN, E. F., WALLER, J. V., AND BROWN, M. G. Am. Heart J., 1940, **19**, 683.

71. LEVINE, S. A., ERNSTENE, A. C., AND JACOBSON, B. M. Arch. Int. Med., 1930, **45**, 191.

72. LEWIS, T. *Pain*. New York, Macmillan, 1942.

73. DANIELOPOLU, D. *L'Angine de Poitrine*. Paris, Masson, 1927.

74. LUNEDEI, A., AND GIANNONI, A. *Il Dolore Viscerale*. Bologna, Cappelli, 1929.

75. WEISS, S., AND DAVIS, D. Am. J. M. Sci., 1928, **176**, 517.

76. DIETRICH, S., AND SCHWIEGK, H. Klin. Woch., 1933, **12**, 135.

77. LEVY, R. L., BRUENN, H. G., AND RUSSELL, N. G. Am. J. M. Sci., 1939, **197**, 241.

78. RISEMAN, J. E. F., WALLER, J. V., AND BROWN, M. G. Am. Heart J., 1940, **19**, 683.

79. a) ROEMHELD, L. Fortschr. d. Med., 1913, **3**, 936.

b) V. BERGMANN, G. Deut. Med. Woch., 1932, **58**, 605.

80. CHAPMAN, E. M., AND ASMUSSEN, E. J. Clin. Investigation, 1942, **21**, 393.

81. KERR, W. J. Am. Heart J., 1938, **16**, 544.

82. MILLER, H. R. *Angina Pectoris*. Baltimore, The Williams & Wilkins Co., 1939.

83. LEVY, R. L. In *Stroud's Cardiovascular Disease*. Philadelphia, Davis, 1945.

84. LEVY, R. L. Ann. Int. Med., 1937, **11**, 833.

85. a) JONNESCO, T. Bull. Acad. Méd., 1920, **84**, 93. Also Presse Méd., 1922, **30**, 353.

b) DANIELOPOLU, D. *L'Angine de Poitrine*. Paris, Masson, 1927. Also Brit. M. J., 1924, **11**, 553.

c) LERICHE, R., AND FONTAINE, R. Arch. Mal. Coeur, 1927, **20**, 513.

d) FONTAINE, R. Strasb. Méd., 1926, **84**, 85 and 146.

e) COFFEY, W. B., AND BROWN, P. K. Arch. Int. Med., 1923, **31**, 200.

f) CUTTER, E. C. Am. J. M. Sci., 1927, **173**, 613.

g) SWEETLOW, G. I. Am. Heart J., 1925/1926, **1**, 393.

h) WHITE, J. C., AND WHITE, P. D. J. A. M. A., 1928, **90**, 1099.

i) RICHARDSON, E. P., AND WHITE, P. D. Am. J. M. Sci., 1929, **177**, 161.

j) FAUTEUX, M., AND PALMER, J. H. Canad. M. A. J., 1941, **45**, 295.

k) FAUTEUX, M. Am. Heart J., 1946, **31**, 260.

l) VINEBERG, A. M. Canad. M. A. J., 1946, **55**, 117.

86. WHITE, J. C., AND SMITHWICK, R. H. *The Autonomic Nervous System. Anatomy, Physiology and Surgical Application*. New York, Macmillan, 1941.

87. RAAB, W., AND SOULE, A. B. Am. J. Roentgenol., 1944, **51**, 364.

88. a) BLUMGART, H. L., LEVINE, S. A., AND BERLIN, D. D. Arch. Int. Med., 1933, **52**, 866.

b) BLUMGART, H. L., RISEMAN, J. E. F., DAVIS, D., AND BERLIN, D. D. Arch. Int. Med., 1933, **52**, 165. J. A. M. A., 1935, **104**, 17. Ann. Int. Med., 1934, **7**, 1469.

89. O'SHAUGHNESSY, L. Brit. J. Surg., 1936, **23**, 665. Also Lancet, 1937 (1), 185 and 1938 (2), 1.

90. BECK, C. S. In *Disease of the Coronary System*. Edited by Levy. New York, Macmillan, 1936.

91. THOMPSON, S. A., AND RAISBECK, M. G. Ann. Int. Med., 1942, **16**, 495.

92. a) LESSER, M. A. New England J. Med., 1942, **226**, 51; and 1943, **228**, 185.

b) LEVINE, S. A., AND LIKOFF, W. B. New England J. Med., 1943, **229**, 770.

93. FAUTEUX, M., AND SWENSON, O. Un. Méd. Canada, 1945, **74**, 1505.

94. VELA, M. *Valor Pronostico del Electrocardiograma*. Madrid, Libr. Edit. Cient. Med. Esp., 1944.

95. DONALD, T. C. New Orleans Med. & Surg. J., 1945, **98**, 195.

96. a) CASTEX, M. R. Prensa Med. Arg., 1931, **18**, 781.

b) CAPACCI, A., AND MERLI, A. Cuore e Circ., 1943, **27**, 16.

97. ROSENBAUM, F. F., WILSON, F. A., AND JOHNSTON, F. D. Am. Heart J., 1946, **32**, 135.

98. BAYLEY, R. H. Am. Heart J., 1942, **24**, 514; and 1943, **26**, 769.

99. BURCH, G., AND WINSOR, T. *A Primer of Electrocardiography*. Philadelphia, Lea and Febiger, 1945.

100. a) WILSON, F. N., AND CO-WORKERS. Am. Heart J., 1934, **9**, 477; and 1946, **32**, 277.

b) GOLDBERGER, E. *Unipolar Lead Electrocardiography*. Philadelphia, Lea and Febiger, 1947.

101. MYERS, G. B., AND KLEIN, H. A. Am. Heart J., 1948, **35**, 727.

102. HELLERSTEIN, H. K., AND KATZ, L. N. Am. Heart J., 1948, **36**, 184.

103. WILSON, F. N., AND CO-WORKERS. Am. Heart J., 1945, **30**, 11; and 1946, **32**, 277.

104. GUBNER, R., CRAWFORD, J. H., AND UNGERLEIDER, H. E. Am. Heart J., 1939, **18**, 8 and 729.

105. MASTER, A. M., AND CO-WORKERS. Am. Heart J., 1940, **19**, 453 and 464; and 1940, **20**, 475.
106. LUISADA, A. A. J. Am. Geriat. Soc., 1953, **1**, 331.
107. a) TENNANT, R., AND WIGGERS, C. J. Am. J. Physical., 1935, **112**, 351.
 b) MURRAY, G. Ann. Surg., 1947, **126**, 523.
108. STROUD M. W., AND FEIL, H. S. Am. Heart J., 1948, **35**, 910.
109. a) HAYMAN, A. S. Rev. Cub. Card., 1947, **3**, 1.
 b) STROUD, W. D., AND WAGNER, J. A. Ann. Int. Med., 1941, **15**, 25.
110. CHINI, V. Settim. Med. (Milan), 1947, **35**, 443.
111. EDMONSON, H. A., AND HOXIE, H. J. Am. Heart J., 1942, **24**, 719.
112. a) WEBER, M. L. Ann. Int. Med., 1943, **19**, 973.
 b) CARROLL, D., AND CUMMINS, S. D. Am. Heart J., 1947, **34**, 894.
113. WELIN, G. Nordisk Med. (Stockholm), 1948, **37**, 324.
114. WRIGHT, I. S., MARPLE, C. D., AND BECK, D. F. J. A. M. A., 1948, **138**, 1074.
115. a) ALLEN, E. V., AND CO-WORKERS. Ann. Int. Med., 1947, **27**, 371.
 b) PARKER, R. L., AND BARKER, N. W. Proc. Staff Meet., Mayo Clin., 1947, **22**, 185.
116. WOOD, F. C. Med. Clin., North America, 1946, **30**, 1275.
117. MASTER, A. M., DACK, S., AND JAFFE, H. L. Arch. Int. Med. 1939, **64**, 767.
118. UNDERDAHL, L. O., AND SMITH, H. L. Proc. Staff Meet., Mayo Clin., 1947, **22**, 479.
119. YATER, W. M., AND CO-WORKERS. Am. Heart J., 1948, **36**, 372, 481 and 683.
120. RAVICH, R. M., AND ROSENBLATT, P. J. Pediat., 1947, **31**, 251.
121. WILBURNE, M., et al. Am. Heart J., 1947, **34**, 860.
122. SCOTT, D. H. Am. Heart J., 1948, **36**, 403.
123. PAUL, O., SWEET, AND WHITE, P. D. New England Heart Assoc., 1948.
124. ROESLER, H., AND DRESSLER, W. Am. Heart J., 1947, **34**, 817.
125. DOCK, W. J. A. M. A., 1946, **131**, 875.
126. WARTMAN, W. B., AND HELLERSTEIN, H. K. Ann. Int. Med., 1948, **28**, 41.
127. HORWITZ, O., et al. J. A. M. A., 1943, **121**, 1342.
128. FOORD, A. G. J. A. M. A., 1948, **138**, 1009.
129. a) Ross, J. Brain, 1887–88, **10**, 333.
 b) HEAD, H. Brain, 1893, **16**, 1.
 c) MACKENZIE, J. Symptoms and Their Interpretation. London, Shaw and Sons, 1909.
130. a) RINZLER, S. H., AND TRAVELL, J. Am. Heart J., 1948, **35**, 248.
 b) RINZLER, S. H. Am. J. Med., 1948, **5**, 736.
131. RAAB, W. Ann. Int. Med., 1948, **28**, 1010.
132. BLUMGART, H. L., AND CO-WORKERS. Proc. Sox. Exper. Biol. & Med., 1948, **67**, 190.
133. FISHER, R. L., AND ZUCKERMAN, M. Michigan State M. Soc. J., 1947, **46**, 1059.
134. BECK, C. S., AND STANTON, E. J. A. M. A., 1948, **137**, 436.
135. LEVY, R. L., AND CO-WORKERS. III Inter-American Congress of Cardiology, Chicago, 1948.
136. FREEDBERG, A. S. New England Heart Assoc., 1948.
137. RUSKIN, A. Am. Heart J., 1947, **34**, 569.
138. BRAMS, W. A. Treatment of Heart Disease. Philadelphia, Saunders, 1948.
139. BURCH, G. E., AND REASER, P. A Primer of Cardiology. Philadelphia, Lea and Febiger, 1947.
140. PICK, R., STAMLER, J., RODBARD, S., AND KATZ, L. N. Circ., 1952, **6**, 858.
141. GOFMAN, J. W., et al. Circ., 1950, **2**, 161.
142. BARKER, J. M. The Unipolar Electrocardiogram. New York, Appleton-Century, 1952.
143. LUISADA, A. A., AND FLEISCHNER, F. G. Acta Cardiol., 1948, **3**, 308.
144. SAMET, P., SCHWEDEL, J. B., AND MEDNICK, H. Am. Heart J., 1950, **39**, 749.
145. DACK, S., PALEY, D. H., AND SUSSMAN, M. L. Circ., 1950, **1**, 551.
146. a) LUISADA, A. A., WEYL, R., AND GOLDMANN, M. Circ. 1952, **5**, 363.
 b) GOLDMANN, M., AND LUISADA, A. A. Ann. Int. Med., 1952, **37**, 1221.
147. MASTER, A. M. Ann. Int. Med., 1950, **32**, 842.
148. CONTRO, S., AND HARING, O. M. Circ., 1952, **6**, 250.
149. JOHNSON, F. R. A. M. A. Arch. Path., 1952, **54**, 237.
150. GASUL, B. M., AND LOEFFLER, E. Ped., 1949, **4**, 498.
151. DUTRA, F. R. Arch. Int. Med., 1950, **85**, 955.
152. VINEBERG, A. J. Thoracic Surg., 1952, **23**, 42.
153. LEVINE, S. A., AND LOWN, B. J. A. M. A., 1952, **148**, 1365.
154. STEINBROCKER, O., et al. Ann. Int. Med., 1949, **19**, 433.
155. COMROE, J. H., et al. Am. J. Physiol., 1953, **173**, 379.
156. MEDALIA, L. A., AND WHITE, P. D. J. A. M. A., 1952, **149**, 1433.

Diseases of the Pericardium

Congenital Anomalies of the Pericardium (1)

These may vary from the *complete absence of the pericardial sac* to a more or less extensive *defect of its left portion.* In the latter case, the pericardial cavity communicates freely with the left pleural cavity. A displacement of the left phrenic nerve toward the right is usually present.

Associated anomalies of the heart, lungs, kidneys, and peritoneum are common. The heart is enlarged in 50 per cent of the cases, but this has no influence on life expectancy.

Mild precordial pain has been observed in some cases; *herniation* of the heart followed by *strangulation* occurred in others.

When there is a *common pleuropericardial cavity,* the anomaly may be suspected because of unexplained cardiac displacement to the left, abnormal cardiac mobility, and cardiac enlargement.

Traumatic Rupture of the Pericardium (2)

Traumatic rupture is usually the result of penetrating wounds or thoracic compression, with or without fracture of the ribs, sternum, or vertebrae. It is found most frequently in persons who have been struck or run over by automobiles but may occur after falling from a height or as the result of crushing or burying. *Contusion* and even *strangulation of the heart* may complicate *pericardial tears* produced by compression.

The most common lesion is a tear on the left side with the heart protruding through the opening. *Intense precordial pain* is present in some cases. A *friction rub* sometimes develops.

A *curious systolic murmur,* with alter-nating loud and soft sounds sharply interrupted by a pause (*millwheel murmur*), was audible in one case; in another, there was a murmur, occurring once every so many pulsations and similar to the sound produced by blowing into an empty bottle (3).

The condition may result in pneumo-pleuropericarditis, simple pericarditis, or *retraction* of the torn margin with *herniation* and, possibly, *strangulation of the heart,* followed by death.

Herniation of the Heart

As seen above, herniation of the heart may follow congenital anomalies or traumatic rupture of the pericardium. *Surgical removal of part of the parietal pericardium* may also be followed by herniation and strangulation of the heart followed by vascular collapse (58).

Hemopericardium (25)

Hemorrhage into the pericardial cavity occurs under the following conditions: penetrating wound of the heart and large vessels; contusion of the heart, with or without rupture; rupture of the ventricular wall soon after myocardial infarction or after formation of an aneurysm; rupture of an intrapericardial aortic aneurysm; scurvy; hemorrhagic diseases; and cardiac tumors. Hemopericardium occurred, in some instances, following intracardiac injection of epinephrine.

The hemorrhage may occur *rapidly* or *slowly;* it may be constant or recurrent. If the bleeding is slow or intermittent, a large amount of blood collects in the pericardial cavity and gives the symptoms and signs of effusion. If the bleeding is rapid, *shock* and *acute tamponade* result.

While rapid and multiple blood transfusions are carried out, one or more *pericardial aspirations* should be performed. If bleeding persists, surgical intervention is resorted to. It consists of suture of the ruptured ventricular wall (only in cases of trauma).

Coagulation and organization of the extravasated blood may result in *chronic tamponade* or *constriction* (page 448). *Decortication of the heart* is then necessary.

Pneumopericardium

This condition may be caused by putrid pericarditis, rupture of a pulmonary cavity into the pericardium, or by an esophageal or gastric tumor (70). It may follow paracentesis of the pericardium. When the amount of fluid is small, the gas which distends the pericardium *causes* the *disappearance of cardiac dulness.* X-ray easily reveals the existence and amount of gas because the pericardial sac is visible as a thin line, separated from the cardiac silhouette (fig. 263).

Tumors

Tumors of the pericardium are most frequently *sarcomata*, usually metastatic. Sometimes they invade the pericardial sac as a result of extension from nearby organs (lungs, mediastinal lymph nodes, etc.); at other times they lie beneath the epicardium after hematogenous implantation. *Metastatic carcinomata*, rare *primary sarcomata*, and benign tumors (such as *fibromata, lipomata,* or *angiomata*) have been described. These may give purely local disturbances or, if diffuse, the picture of constrictive mediastinopericarditis.

Hydatid Cysts

Hydatid cysts may occur in the pericardium. They may rupture into one of the ventricles if they invade the heart muscle and may cause pericardial adhesions (page 450).

Pericarditis

CAUSES

There are three main routes along which infection can be carried into the pericardial serosa: a) through the blood stream in cases of sepsis; b) from the heart and vessels in cases of myocarditis or aortitis; c) from the surrounding organs in cases of pleurisy, hepatitis, peritonitis, pulmonary abscess, lymphadenitis, esophageal foreign body, or penetrating wound of the chest.

Numerous diseases and agents may cause pericarditis. a) Rheumatic disease. b) Tuberculosis. c) Bacterial infections caused by the Pneumococcus, Streptococcus, Staphylococcus, Meningococcus, Gonococcus, *Escherichia coli, Brucella melitensis, Bacillus tularense,* or *Hemophilus influenzae.* d) Myocardial infarction. e) Chronic glomerulonephritis and malignant hypertension. f) Syphilis. g) Amebiasis or actinomycosis. h) Tumors. i) Scurvy. j) A recently described form is part of a polyserositis and is associated with either *scleroderma* or *Libman-Sacks' endocarditis* (86). k) Acute benign forms. The last group probably includes various types, some caused by a *virus* while others seem to follow an upper respiratory infection.

Tuberculous pericarditis is frequently part of a more diffuse lesion involving many serous membranes (*polyserositis*). *Rheumatic pericarditis* is usually associated with myocardial and endocardial lesions (*pancarditis*). An *allergic reaction* has been advocated for both, in the former case to tubercular and, in the latter, to streptococcal antigens. An allergic reaction to bacterial proteins has also been postulated in some cases of "benign, nonspecific pericarditis" (71, 72).

The possibility that a slight change of either the pH or the permeability of the serous membrane, due to mild infection, may cause local fixation of toxins, has been considered.

Pneumococcic pericarditis may occur during pneumonia but most frequently is the result of an empyema of the left side.

Streptococcic pericarditis is the result of sepsis, pulmonary abscess, or esophageal ulcer.

While most forms of pericarditis may result in the production of *adhesions*, the occurrence of constrictive pericarditis is relatively rare. *Most of the cases of constrictive pericarditis are caused by tuberculosis* (73, 63). However, other causes are definitely possible, including collagen diseases (86).

Acute and Subacute Pericarditis

LESIONS

Two different stages or phases can be recognized: dry pericarditis and pericarditis with effusion. The former is always present, the latter may follow. Either stage may be followed by a chronic stage and may result in the formation of adhesions.

Dry pericarditis. This may be limited to the vascular pedicle, the apex, the region of the inferior cava, or may be diffuse. The epicardium is red, opaque, and covered by loose, yellowish, fibrinous exudate. The pericardial fluid, normally limited to a very small amount, becomes more abundant and thicker because of fibrin and leucocytes. More strata of fibrinous exudate may be added until an irregular mass, which may attain even 10 mm. in thickness, forms between the heart and pericardial sac (*cor villosum*). A connective tissue reaction gradually leads to organization of the exudate which is partly reabsorbed and partly transformed into fibrous tissue.

Pericarditis with effusion. After an initial "dry" phase, the pericardial fluid rapidly increases and distends the serous cavity. The exudate may attain a volume of 600 to 800 cc. and varies in composition.

a) *Serofibrinous effusion.* The fluid is yellow or rose-colored and contains fibrin, leucocytes, a few red cells, and droplets of fat. It is typical of rheumatic and tubercular pericarditis.

b) *Purulent effusion.* The fluid is yellowish or grayish and thick. It contains a large percentage of pus cells and drops of fat. It is typical of pneumococcic or streptococcic infections but may be found in tubercular infection (*caseous pericarditis*).

c) *Hemorrhagic effusion.* The fluid is pink or reddish and contains a large percentage of red cells. It may be found in tubercular, streptococcic, neoplastic, or uremic pericarditis.

Pericarditis with effusion should not be confused with *transudation* of the pericardial cavity, a common event in congestive failure, nephrosis, myxedema, thiamine deficiency, and prolonged agony. The fluid then contains a smaller percentage of albumin, fibrin, and cellular elements (page 453).

Involvement of the superficial layers of the myocardium is present in all cases of pericarditis.

SYMPTOMS AND SIGNS

When pericarditis is a complication of an acute infection, its onset is marked by increase in temperature, restlessness, and slight dyspnea. Both in these cases and when pericarditis is the only lesion, the following symptoms and signs may be present: *sticking or dull precordial pain, palpitation, obstinate nonproductive cough,* and, occasionally, *dysphagia.* The pulse is small and rapid.

DRY PERICARDITIS

The area of cardiac dulness may be enlarged (4). Auscultation reveals the existence of *friction rubs* which may be of fine, coarse, or creaking type. They are poorly transmitted, seem superficial and are louder with the patient in the sitting position. They are usually present in two different phases of the cardiac cycle ("to-and-fro" rubs) and are similar. When the rubs are short and occur both in systole and diastole, they cause a typical sequence, called *locomotive rhythm.* This is different from a quadruple rhythm of a more common type (page 370) because in the latter the extra-

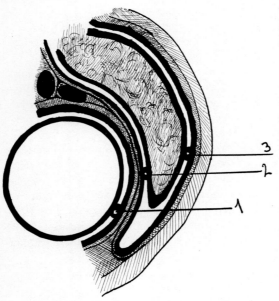

3
2
1

FIG. 258. *Sites of friction rubs.* 1, pericardial; 2, pleuro-pericardial; 3, pleural.

sounds are dull and of poor intensity, while in the former they are loud and snapping; moreover, in locomotive rhythm, the two additional sounds are *in systole and diastole* while, in a quadruple rhythm, they are both in diastole.

Graphic Tracings

Electrocardiogram. The *ECG* may be completely normal in the phase of dry pericarditis, except for *sinus tachycardia.* However, electrocardiographic changes consisting of *low voltage of the QRS complex* and *changes of S-T and T* may be observed.

Phonocardiogram. The *friction rubs* are transcribed as vibrations of various pitches, with those of higher pitch prevailing. These are grouped in either two or three phases of the cardiac cycle. The most common are those which occur during *presystole* and *systole* (to-and-fro rubs); a third group may take place in *early diastole* (5).

Course

Three possibilities should be considered: a) The pericarditis has a favorable evolu-

tion and heals without appreciable effusion, leaving no trace. b) Effusion takes place. c) Multiple adhesions develop.

Diagnosis

The diagnosis is based upon auscultation of friction rubs. These are seldom mistaken for anything else, but, on the other hand, other sounds may be mistaken for them. The systolic rub, which is usually louder and longer than the presystolic, lags after the first sound and is well separated from it.

The rapid succession of *two or three systolic clicks* (page 455) may simulate a systolic rub (6). However, in such cases, no abnormal extra-sound occurs during diastole, a fact which is unusual in pericarditis.

Harsh or grating systolic murmurs may be mistaken for rubs. Their blowing type and the absence of diastolic murmurs help to rule out friction rubs. The differentiation of *pleuropericardial* from *pericardial friction rubs* (fig. 258) is sometimes difficult. The former are due to inflammation of the pericardial pleura and may have a cardiac rhythm. They are usually heard along the left margin of the pericardium and are far more influenced by respiration than pericardial rubs.

In certain normal individuals with flat chests, either heart sound or both may be associated with a superficial *crunching sound* when the stethoscope is placed at the lower left border of the sternum (19). This has been attributed to rubbing of the heart against the superficial structures.

PERICARDITIS WITH EFFUSION

The patient may present *pallor, ashen-gray color,* or *cyanosis. Dyspnea* is common and may be so severe that the patient *bends forward* (9b) and occasionally stoops in the *Mohammedan prayer position* (34) in order to relieve the compression of the fluid on the large veins. *Nausea, dysphagia, hiccup,* and *dysphonia,* are possible.

Peripheral edema is present in cases of large effusion. It may predominate in the district of the superior cava in the morning and in that of the inferior cava in the late afternoon, as the result of different decubitus of the patient (7).

The *jugular veins are engorged* and fail to show appreciable pulsations (34b). The pulse is small, weak, and regular (except in rheumatic cases). Forced inspiration may cause the *double inspiratory phenomenon* of *Kussmaul* (8): increased swelling of the jugular veins and decreased radial pulse during inspiration (so-called *paradoxical pulse*) (fig. 269).

The precordial area may present a certain bulging due to flattening of the intercostal spaces. In purulent pericarditis, there may be *edema of the chest wall*.

The apical thrust is seldom visible, a fact which is important only in children or when it was previously present. When the apical thrust is *visible within the area of dulness*, this may be significant.

The area of *cardiac dulness* becomes roughly *triangular* due to extension near the apex and *obtuseness of the cardiohepatic angle* (9) (fig. 259). A coincidence between relative and absolute dulness and the abrupt transition from dulness to normal resonance are typical.

Percussion of the heart in supine, lateral, and sitting positions, reveals *changes of*

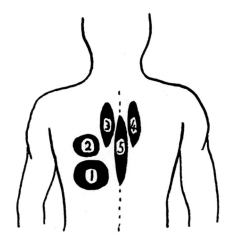

FIG. 260. Different areas of dulness on the posterior surface of the thorax in pericarditis with effusion. 1, Pins' sign (left base); 2, Ewart's sign (angle of scapula); 3, Germe's sign (left paravertebral area); 4, Ewart-Teissier's sign (right paravertebral area); 5, Ewart's sign (spine).

the area of dulness due to shifting of the fluid. When the effusion is large, there is an increase of the area of dulness in the 2nd and 3rd spaces (10). The *area of Traube may become dull*, owing to descent of the left hepatic lobe (11).

An area of dulness, situated *in various points of the back* (fig. 260) and accompanied by bronchial breathing, has been described by different authors (12).

Auscultation reveals *dull, muffled*, and *distant cardiac sounds*. *Friction rubs* may still be heard and there may be a *triple rhythm*.

The liver is frequently enlarged but its enlargement may be simulated by lowering of the diaphragm. *Ascites* is possible. When present, it is usually caused by peritonitis of the same etiology as the pericarditis.

Arterial pressure is normal or low; *venous pressure* is elevated.

Graphic Tracings

Electrocardiogram. Three different electrocardiographic stages are recognized (13, 68, 69).

1) *Acute stage.* The pattern consists of

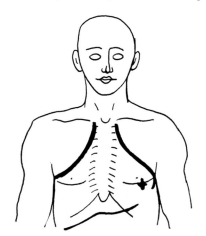

FIG. 259. Area of dulness in *pericarditis with effusion.* + marks the seat of the apical thrust.

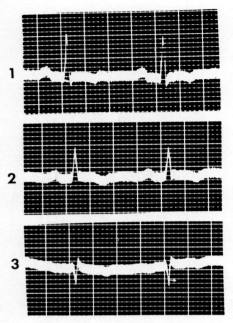

FIG. 261. Electrocardiogram in a case of *pericarditis with effusion*. Subacute stage.

elevation of S-T in the limb and chest leads. This elevation is maximal if the exploring electrode is placed over the area where a friction rub is audible.

2) *Subacute stage.* The S-T elevation gradually decreases and a moderate inversion of T in the limb and the chest leads becomes apparent. The T waves are *not* cove-shaped (fig. 261).

3) *Chronic stage.* The inverted T wave may last for a long time, but it usually returns to normal within a few weeks.

In general, the maximum inversion of T occurs between the 16th and the 43rd day of disease; it may involve only one or two leads while the others present low T.

No deep Q wave is ever present. Low voltage may be observed in large effusions.

Electrokymogram. The electrokymogram of both cardiac borders reveals small (and even absent) pulsations in pericarditis with effusion. Theoretically, the pulsations of the aortic arch should be normal but, in some cases, the aortic pulsations also are small.

Jugular tracings. It is typical to obtain tracings with poor amplitude of all waves. This is in contrast with the engorgement of the veins.

X-Ray

The unexplained finding of an enlarged cardiac silhouette is important. A small effusion is revealed by a bulging of the posterior-inferior part of the silhouette (15a). Later on, the grooves around the heart and vessels fill out, the pedicle shortens, and the waist of the heart is straightened. If the patient changes from the erect to the supine position, the basal shadow widens.

A large effusion frequently gives *a water-bottle shape* in the erect, and *a globular or rectangular shape*, in the recumbent position. However, two different profiles have been described: *the effusion with tense*, and *the effusion with flaccid pericardium* (14). The former may fail to reveal the effusion because the main landmarks of the cardiac silhouette are preserved and only the functional data are changed (fig. 262) (15).

Roentgenkymography may show contrast between strong pulsations of the aorta and weak pulsations of the ventricular margin (16). This contrast, however, is absent if the ventricular contractions are small by effect of compression on the veins, or failure.

Circulation Time

Arm-to-tongue time is usually *normal* (76). This is in contrast with the prolonged circulation time of the enlarged hearts.

Mechanism of the Signs

Experimental studies on pericardial effusion have shown that the fluid collects first over that portion of the heart which lies between the diaphragm and the anterior chest wall. As the amount increases, the effusion extends around the right margin and over the apex. The easily expanding lung tissue allows the fluid to follow gravity

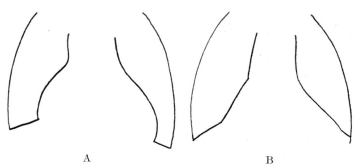

FIG. 262. Cardiac silhouette in two types of *pericarditis with effusion*. A, tense pericardium; B, flaccid pericardium. (Inspired by originals of Heckmann.)

except when the effusion is very abundant, the pericardial sac is very tense, or the elasticity of the lung is altered.

The compression developed by the fluid is exerted mainly on organs which have low pressure and small contractions, i.e. *the large veins and the atria*. This compression is usually felt to a greater extent by the inferior cava and the hepatic veins (which sometimes enter the cava within or near the pericardium). On the contrary, the superior cava is mainly compressed if the patient lies supine, as sometimes during a deep sleep.

A rapidly accumulating massive effusion may compress *the whole heart* with maximum effect over the right atrium. In such a case, both the superior and the inferior cava are dilated and congested (62).

Animal experimentation has proven that *the rise of venous pressure takes place both in the systemic and in the pulmonary circulation* (77). This is the cause of the "inflow stasis" (43). *High venous pressure has a compensatory action because it increases the filling gradient of the heart* (venous pressure minus intrapericardial pressure).

The *enlargement of the heart* is more marked than previously thought (4) and may be explained by superficial myocarditis and myocardial edema. These are more severe in rheumatic and bacterial forms than in tubercular cases. *Superficial myocarditis is the cause of the electrocardiographic changes.*

As previously discussed (page 416), a subepicardial lesion is followed by: a) a *pattern of ischemia* (inversion of the T wave) due to slower repolarization in the superficial layers and inversion of the vector of repolarization; and b) a *pattern of injury* (upward displacement of S-T) due to the fact that the electrode faces the damaged zone which is *positive* in relationship to the normal layers during depolarization. *Low voltage*, if present, is caused by the effusion which short-circuits some of the changes of potential.

The heart moves freely within the effusion, as proven by the frequent persistence of rubs.

It is generally admitted that the pericardium is insensitive to ordinary stimuli. However, distention of the pericardial cavity and irritation of the anterior surface of the parietal pericardium cause severe *substernal pain* (21a).

Varieties—Complications

Different types of pericarditis are due to different causes.

Rheumatic pericarditis. Pericarditis has usually a favorable evolution and disappears within 3 to 20 days. If effusion develops, there is a longer course but the fluid may be readsorbed spontaneously within 1 to 2 months. Adhesions may develop but no constriction takes place, except in rare cases.

Tubercular pericarditis. In general, the inflammation starts insidiously and may cause large effusions before the patient complains. Readsorption is limited or absent and the course is long. The fluid is frequently hemorrhagic; it often tends to become thicker and may be transformed into a caseous mass which is later organized by fibrous tissue. If pleural and peritoneal effusions are present, the pericardial inflammation is part of a *polyserositis (Concato's disease)*. Tubercular pericarditis frequently causes pericardial adhesions and may lead to constriction. In some cases, the course is progressive and fatal.

Pyogenic pericarditis. It is accompanied by a purulent exudate and causes a severe clinical picture. Abscesses of the myocardium, the diaphragm, or the liver, or left-sided empyema, may be associated.

Uremic pericarditis causes only limited signs and may be a post-mortem finding. The fluid may be abundant and is frequently hemorrhagic. The electrocardiographic changes are variable and often minimal (60). The altered blood chemistry may contribute to this type of effusion.

One of the possible complications of pericarditis is *cardiac tamponade*, due to rapid and progressive rise of intrapericardial pressure. When the venous pressure cannot rise further and its level is reached by the pressure of the effusion, venous return is blocked and cardiac output fails.

Purulent pericarditis at times may cause the formation of a *hydropneumopericardium* through formation of gas (*putrid peri-*

carditis) or perforation of a lung. In such cases, auscultation reveals a splashing noise, called *millwheel murmur (bruit de moulin)* and the x-ray shows that the fluid is limited by an horizontal level. The same picture may be observed after paracentesis of the pericardium followed by the introduction of air (fig. 263).

Diagnosis

The diagnosis of pericarditis offers no difficulty when rubs are heard as confusion with a valvular murmur is unlikely (page 85). Recognition of the effusion is easy when large; otherwise it may be confused with cardiac enlargement. Changes of the area of dulness in different positions, abrupt change from a clear to a dull percussion sound, apical thrust within the area of dulness, x-ray and electrocardiographic data, are of help.

If there are severe changes of the electrocardiogram and prolonged pain, *confusion with myocardial infarction* is possible. The differential diagnosis is based on the fact that, in pericarditis, fever and friction rubs start at the time of the pain, while in myocardial infarction pain is the first manifestation, and fever and rubs occur from 12 to 36 hours later. The ECG of myocardial infarction shows a gradual and rapid evolution culminating with the pattern of necrosis (deep Q or QS complex); this is never observed in pericarditis. However, anterior subepicardial infarction may give the same

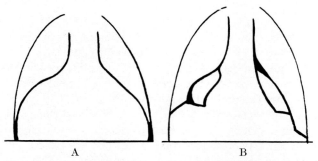

A   B

FIG. 263. Cardiac silhouette of *pericarditis* before (A) and after *paracentesis* (B). The latter reveals the thickness of the pericardial sac because of the pneumopericardium, and the heart within the sac. (Inspired by originals of P. D. White.)

ECG changes as pericarditis. A slower evolution, less striking changes, and the absence of a clear-cut localization may frequently allow the ECG diagnosis of pericarditis.

Differentiation between *rheumatic* and *benign pericarditis* is usually possible. The former has a more severe myocardial involvement revealed by murmurs and changes of P-R and Q-T; murmurs, leucocytosis, and joint involvement are not present in benign pericarditis.

Differential diagnosis between the effusion due to *transudation* and that caused by inflammatory *exudation* is made by examining the physico-chemical properties of the fluid (page 453).

Differential diagnosis between pericarditis with effusion and *dilatation of the heart* can be made with the help of x-ray (78). The cardiac silhouette decreases during *the Valsalva* and increases during *the Mueller test*, in cases with dilatation; it fails to show any marked change in cases with effusion. When pulsations are present, they become more prominent with the Valsalva test, in cardiac dilatation. Widening of the angle of the main bronchi is in favor of dilatation while an obscured angle of bifurcation is in favor of effusion. Absence of lateral and posterior displacement of the esophagus is likewise in favor of effusion.

Treatment

Whenever possible, causal treatment should be undertaken. Therefore, infections due to pyogenic bacteria, amebae, or syphilis should be treated with specific drugs or antibiotics as early as possible. *Cortisone, ACTH,* or *aspirin* in adequate doses (page 198) favorably influence rheumatic pericarditis (page 447).

A specific and prophylactic therapy is possible in many acute forms. *Penicillin* treatment of pneumonia and of streptococcic sore throat has already decreased the occurrence of secondary pericarditis due to the Pneumococcus or Streptococcus. The same therapy should be used if the pericarditis is present. Whenever possible, culture of the agent and testing of its resistance to antibiotics should be done. *Aureomycin* (1 gm. orally every 6 hours for 4 days; then one-half that dose for 3 days) has proved useful in cases of benign pericarditis (74). Early use of *streptomycin* in tubercular pericarditis is helpful and may prevent development of constriction (61, 75). It should be given both by intramuscular injection and intrapericardial instillation.

Morphine is necessary in cases with severe pain or dyspnea. A *light ice-bag*, placed over the precordial region, is useful in the acute stage and gives comfort to the patient.

Digitalis is usually not helpful because the signs of congestion are not due to cardiac failure. On the other hand, it is not contraindicated because the fall of venous pressure, caused by digitalis in congestive failure, is not observed in pericarditis. *Metrazol* or *coramin* (61) may be given in cases with low blood pressure, and *quinidine* if premature beats or paroxysmal tachycardia occur.

Venesection in general is harmful because it decreases the venous pressure, a useful compensatory phenomenon.

Paracentesis of the pericardium. Aspiration of the pericardial fluid is indicated in the acute stage only if severe compression occurs. Otherwise, it is advisable to wait until the subacute stage is reached when there is a less rapid production of exudate. The procedure should be done under local anesthesia. The needle may be introduced either outside the apex or at the junction of the xiphoid process with the left costal arch (21b) (figs. 264 and 265). Posterior paracentesis has been accomplished in cases with posterior dulness without causing discomfort. If this does not control the effusion, a valvular surgical drainage is necessary (85).

Aspiration of the fluid should be accompanied by introduction of air which is

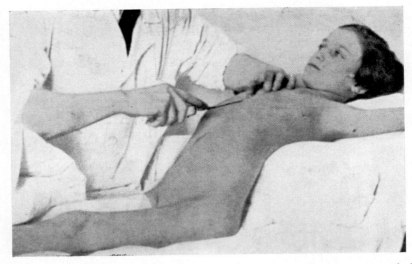

FIG. 264. Position of the patient for *pericardial paracentesis* using Marfan's technique

later gradually absorbed. This procedure limits the production of new fluid and the formation of adhesions (22, 23).

In cases or purulent or putrid pericarditis,

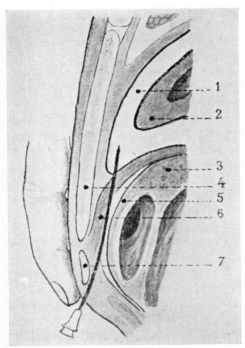

FIG. 265. Course followed by the needle in *pericardial paracentesis*. 1, pericardial fluid; 2, heart; 3, liver; 4, sternum; 5, peritoneum; 6, diaphragm; 7, xiphoid process.

the pericardial cavity may be irrigated with physiologic solution but *open surgical drainage* is often necessary. *Intrapericardial injection of penicillin* has proved helpful in such cases (24) and may accompany parenteral treatment. Surgical intervention may be needed if medical treatment is unsuccessful.

Chronic, Adhesive, and Constrictive Pericarditis

While most types of acute pericarditis may result in chronic inflammation, the fibrous bands resulting from this process cause "constriction" only in a minority of cases. The majority of cases with constrictive pericarditis are due to tuberculosis (73) while a few may be due to other bacterial infections, rheumatic fever, collagen diseases (86), or other causes.

LESIONS

Diffuse constrictive pericarditis (8, 27). The chronic inflammation results in the formation of fibrous tissue which connects the heart with the pericardial sac and this with the surrounding organs. There is a complete obliteration of the pericardial cavity and partial obliteration of the pleural cavities. A solid fibrous mass may enclose the heart.

the large vessels, and the diaphragm, and is connected with the lungs and the sternum (fig. 266). The subdiaphragmatic organs may also be involved. There may be *calcification or ossification of the pericardium*. Cardiac function is still possible, either because only loose adhesions are present within the pericardial sac or because incomplete adhesions are present outside.

Partial adhesive (possibly constrictive) pericarditis. This may present different aspects:

a) *Complete internal without external adhesions (concretio cordis)*. The pericardial sac adheres to the heart but is free from the surrounding organs: "the pericardium moves with the heart like a glove on the hand" (22).

b) *Extensive external without internal adhesion (accretio cordis)*. The heart is free within the pericardial sac but the latter is extensively connected to the sternum, the lungs, and the diaphragm.

c) *Periaortic adhesions*. This is frequently of luetic etiology and is usually associated with aortitis or aortic aneurysm; the upper part of the pericardial sac may be obliterated.

d) *Peri-superior cava*. This is frequently due to tuberculosis, syphilis, or tumors, and presents a typical compression picture (superior caval syndrome) (page 463).

e) *Peri-inferior cava*. This is usually tubercular and also presents a typical picture. (inferior caval syndrome) (page 464).

f) *String-like adhesions of different types* (fig. 267). Among them, a ring-like calcification of the A-V groove is particularly important and may be constrictive. Another important lesion is that which may develop in the interventricular groove because it may cause compression of the anterior descending branch of the left coronary artery.

A *peritonitis with perihepatitis* may be present and is one of the causes of *frosted liver*.

Different opinions have been expressed about the *volume of the heart* in adhesive pericarditis. A moderate increase is possible (28) but normal or decreased volume can be observed. *In general, the heart of rheumatic pericarditis is increased while that of tubercular pericarditis is normal or slightly decreased.* Different elements may contribute to these variations: existence of valvular defects *before* the compression started; prolonged compression by abundant exudate; initial constriction in the region of the venae cavae decreasing venous return; age of the patient; and condition of the myocardium. Impairment of the venous return due to constriction may cause decreased work followed by *atrophy and reduction in size of the myofibrils* (29).

Calcification of the pericardium is due to deposition of calcium salts. In general, either calcification is not complete, leaving an opening in the region of the apex, or there are many *plaques*, connected by fibrous tissue and permitting the same degree of mobility which is enjoyed by a lobster. *Ossification of the pericardium* is rare but possible.

Both the fibrous and the calcific processes may involve the myocardium and penetrate as deeply as the A-V valves. Valvular insufficiency and even stenosis may result, but the latter is rare. Stenosis of the venae cavae by diffuse or localized fibrosis is more

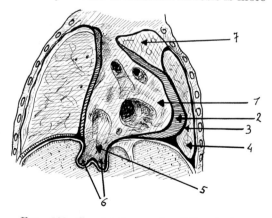

Fig. 266. *Constrictive pericarditis*. 1, heart; 2, adherent, thickened pericardial tissue; 3, adhesion with left pleura; 4, left lung; 5, dilated inferior cava; 6, dilated hepatic veins. (Sketched after Elias and Feller.)

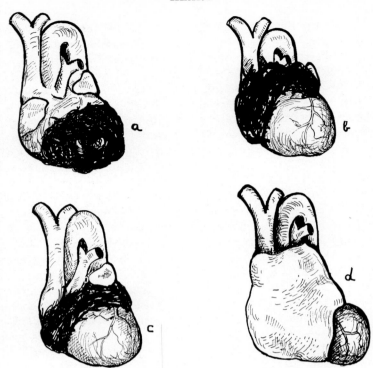

FIG. 267. Different types of *partial adhesive pericarditis*. a, peri-apical type; b, peri-basal type; c, string-like type; d, calcified pericardium with opening at apex.

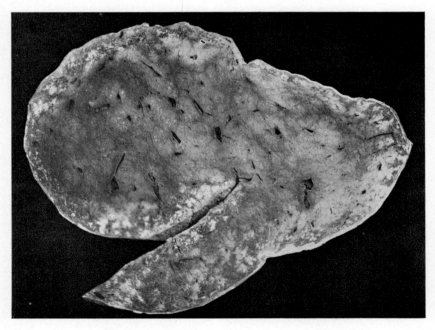

FIG. 268. Frosted liver

common. Stenosis of the hepatic veins is possible and may be due to either *compression* (30) or *thrombosis* with recanalization (63). The most common *hepatic lesion* is *sclerosis of the hepatic and portal veins* (86). This is frequently associated with liver cirrhosis. The *spleen* presents fibrosis of the pulp, hyperplasia of the sinuses, and fibroadenia.

A *systemic and pulmonary phlebosclerosis* is common and is accompanied by capillary fibrosis of the lungs (86).

The *frosted liver* is a special, less common, lesion. The organ is covered by a whitish coat of fibrous tissue and is adherent to the diaphragm (31, 32) (fig. 268); strong spokes of fibrous tissue penetrate into the liver and form a network within which the dilated veins are visible. This lesion is due to *simultaneous action of chronic engorgement of the hepatic veins plus chronic inflammation of the peritoneum*. It is, therefore, typical of *Pick's syndrome*[70] where constrictive pericarditis is associated with a mild peritonitis, mainly acting on the upper part of the abdomen. The abundant ascitis is due to both exudation (peritonitis) and transudation (liver cirrhosis). Pick's syndrome is, therefore, a special type of polyserositis (*Concato's disease*) and is usually, though not always, tubercular (32).

SIGNS AND SYMPTOMS

The signs of constricive mediastinopericarditis vary according to the extension and localization of the lesions.

The patients are usually semiinvalids because of *weakness*, possible malnutrition, and inability to perform any effort. They suffer no pain. *Exertional dyspnea* is practically constant while *orthopnea* is slight and may be absent. There is no jaundice. *Cyanosis* is frequent; it may be limited to

[70] The name of *Pick's syndrome* has been applied to all varieties of constrictive pericarditis with ascitis. According to the original description, this extension is not justified.

the face, to the upper parts, or extend over the entire body. It is not necessarily severe.

Venous engorgement is usually apparent. It may predominate in the area of the superior or inferior cava, or may be diffuse. The veins of the neck, though distended, *fail to present active pulsations*.

Simultaneous tracings of the jugular veins and of the radial pulse reveal the frequent existence of *Kussmaul's phenomenon:* inspiration causes swelling of the jugular veins and simultaneous weakening (8) (or even disappearance (42)) of the radial pulse (fig. 269). This represents accentuation of a normal phenomenon.

There may be *edema* of the upper half of the body, presenting special consistence and appearance.

An interesting modification of respiratory dynamics is often present. Under normal conditions, the sternum is thrust anteriorly during inspiration; in these patients, the upper part of the sternum is thrust forward while the lower part is pulled back during inspiration (*crossed respiration*) (7, 22).

Pleural effusion is possible. The abdomen is distended because of *ascites*. The fluid is either a transudate or is of mixed character.[71] The *liver is large*, occasionally very large, but not pulsating. *Dependent edema* may be absent or slight but is usually present in the terminal stages of the disease.

Observation of the thorax may elicit a certain number of signs. Their importance

[71] Summary of the differences between transudates and exudates is given here:

	TRANSUDATES	EXUDATES
Aspect	Clear	Opaque
Clotting	Absent	Possible
Specific gravity	From 1.008 to 1.015	From 1.018 to 1.030
Albumin	From 0.2 to 3 per cent	From 3 to 6 per cent
Rivalta test	− or +−	From ++ to +++

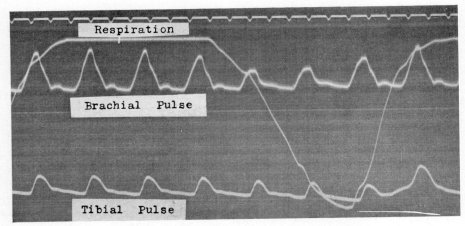

Respiration

Brachial   Pulse

Tibial   Pulse

Fig. 269. "Paradoxical" pulse

is limited because they are not always present. They are:

a) *Absence of the apical thrust.*

b) *Systolic retraction* of either the apical region (33) or a wide anterior or posterior region (33–35); apical retraction followed by diastolic thrust (36).

c) *See-saw movement* between the left and right sides of the chest (37).

Percussion of the precordial area reveals the following data. The area of cardiac dulness is frequently *smaller* than in normal persons or, at least, is not enlarged. However, a large heart is present in about one-third of the cases (63). There is coincidence between the relative and absolute areas of dulness; no inspiratory expansion of the pulmonary margins can be detected; and there is the same area of dulness in different positions, because the heart has lost its mobility.

Auscultation usually reveals *regular heart sounds*, occasionally *weak or distant. Cardiac murmurs* may be present because of valvular defects (rheumatic or bacterial pericarditis, fibrous or calcified processes reaching the valves) or because of disturbance of the cardiac function due to traction or compression (relative insufficiency or relative stenosis). *Increased loudness or splitting of the 2nd pulmonic sound is evi-*

dence of constriction of the left cardiac chambers (64).

Extra-sounds are frequently present. There may be a *triple rhythm* of either the atrial or the ventricular type (page 370). The latter may reveal a snapping quality of the additional sound (*protodiastolic click* (38)). There may be a *systolic snap* or *click*. When located at the apex, it is due to partial, external, pericardial adhesions. In rare cases, there is a *quadruple rhythm*, due to addition of a systolic and a diastolic click to the normal heart sounds.

ARTERIAL AND VENOUS PRESSURE—
CARDIAC OUTPUT

Circulation Time

Arterial pressure is normal or low with decreased pulse pressure. *Cardiac output is usually low*, in some cases only 50 per cent of normal (44). *Venous pressure is elevated* (45). A difference in the venous pressure of the two arms or between arm and leg has diagnostic importance showing different severity of compression (46). Cases with isolated or predominant compression of the hepatic veins, a rare occurrence, may present a low venous pressure, similar to that of patients with liver cirrhosis.

Both arm-to-tongue and arm-to-lung times

are increased. However, there may be important individual variations.

Blood—Urine—Ascites

Blood count is usually normal. Leucocytosis indicates the continued existence of an inflammatory process.

Serum proteins are reduced in cases having peripheral edema. The *urine* usually does not contain bile.

Examination of the abdominal (or thoracic) fluid reveals either a pure transudate or a borderline fluid (page 453).

GRAPHIC TRACINGS—CATHETERIZATION

Electrocardiogram

Disturbances of cardiac rate and rhythm are sometimes present because of myocardial or coronary lesions or because the traction of adhesions favors premature beats, paroxysmal tachycardia, or atrial flutter; atrial fibrillation may occur. However, the most usual findings are: *regular sinus rhythm; low voltage* in the limb leads; low, flat, or inverted T waves in one or more limb leads; occasional splintering of the ventricular complex (45b). Right axis deviation has been observed when there is predominant compression of the left ventricle (47). S-T may be depressed. Changes of the P wave consisting of broadening, notching, and increased voltage, have been noted.

The study of the *deviation of the electric axis in different positions* may reveal that the heart is fixed and is not displaced by gravity, a fact which may be used in the differential diagnosis with congestive failure (49). This sign is observed when extensive internal and external adhesions are present and not in cases having only internal adhesions.

Phonocardiogram

It is possible to note increased *loudness of the second pulmonic sound*, which is evidence of constriction of the left cardiac

chambers with higher pulmonic pressure (47). The second sound may be *split.*

A *triple rhythm* of either the atrial or ventricular type is frequently recorded; a high-pitched *diastolic click* is frequently recorded in calcification of the pericardium. This occurs at the time of rapid filling and is the equivalent of a third sound.

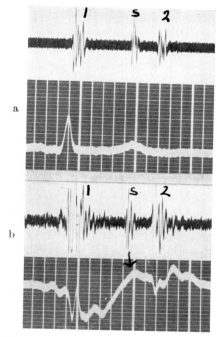

FIG. 270. Systolic snap (S) in the sound tracing of a case of *adhesive pericarditis.* a, compared with the ECG; b, compared with the pulsation of the area of best auscultation.

A typical finding is that of a *systolic click* or *snap.* This is a high-pitched vibration at, or after, the middle of systole, frequently followed by a few smaller vibrations (fig. 270). Cases where two or three small extra-sounds are present in systole may occur.

Electrokymogram

A typical sign of constrictive pericarditis is the following (80). The border tracing of the left ventricle presents a sharp and deep

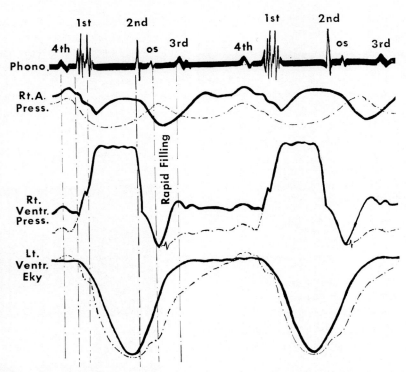

Fig. 271. Scheme of the V type of electrokymogram and of the typical pattern of intracardiac tracing in constrictive pericarditis. Dotted lines, normal patterns.

drop followed by a rapid rise. There is a flat line during most of diastole and no evidence of the normal rebound which marked the end of isometric relaxation period. However, this pattern, called the *V type of ventricular contraction* (fig. 271), can be found in other conditions impairing ventricular diastole (amyloid, fibroelastosis).

Catheterization

Catheterization of the heart reveals high venous pressure and normal or low right atrial pressure in cases with predominant constriction around the venae cavae. *High venous and right atrial pressures with low right ventricular pressure* indicate compression of the right atrium (66). *High right ventricular and pulmonary blood pressures indicate constriction of the left heart* (64).

The ventricular pressure curve shows a very rapid phase of passive filling in early diastole followed by *a diastolic plateau* (81) (fig. 271).

Jugular Vein Tracing—Liver Tracing

In general, the jugular and hepatic waves are small and difficult to record. *Kussmaul's sign* may be recorded (page 445). The adhesive and constrictive process tends to limit the transmission of the waves caused by cardiac dynamics; therefore, possible abnormal waves are *not* due to the adhesive process and are decreased in amplitude by it.

X-RAY

In many cases, roentgen-ray study gives only scarce data; in others, however, the following data can be observed (50).

a) *Abnormality in the profile of the cardiac silhouette* due to adhesions with the lungs; the angles or irregularities may be increased by deep respiration.

b) *Disappearance of the known landmarks* of the cardiac silhouette with *straightening of the borders.*

c) *Thick, diffused shadows around the heart* obscuring the anterior and posterior

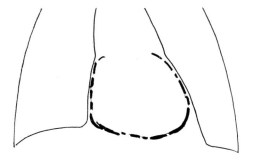

Fig. 272. Cardiac silhouette in a case of *calcified pericardium.*

spaces (lateral views). Observation of an opaque ring or scattered spots, due to *calcification of the pericardium,* is possible (fig. 272).

d) *Decreased amplitude of pulsation of the cardiac margins.* This is important when accentuated in some areas.

e) Transmission of cardiac pulsations to the left diaphragm.

f) Poor visibility of the hilar shadows and of the pulmonary network. This is important in cases with congestion of the systemic venous circulation.

Interesting data may be obtained with the *pneumo-mediastinum* (51) (page 152) and *pneumo-peritoneum* (page 152). The former may reveal anterior extrapericardial adhesions; the latter, subdiaphragmatic adhesions (fig. 273).

Roentgenkymography may confirm the above described data and reveal that the motion of some part of the heart is due to traction or is otherwise abnormal.

MECHANISM OF ORIGIN OF THE SIGNS

The clinical picture of adhesive and constrictive pericarditis includes three groups of signs and symptoms:

a) Those caused by disturbed function of nerves, lymph-vessels, bronchi, trachea, and esophagus.

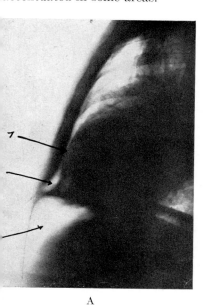

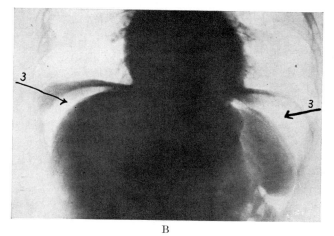

A   B

Fig. 273. A. *Pneumo-mediastinum* in a case of adhesive mediastino-pericarditis (lateral view). 1, anterior adhesion; 2, air below adhesion (pneumo-mediastinum); 3, air below the diaphragm (pneumo-peritoneum). B. Same case, frontal view showing the *pneumo-peritoneum.* The air has detached the diaphragm from the liver and spleen (3, 3).

b) Those connected with venous and hepatic engorgement.

c) The effusion in the abdominal cavity and, possibly, in one or both pleural cavities.

The signs of the first group are apparently caused by compression. The second group has been attributed to heart failure, decreased forces contributing to venous return, or compression of the large veins.

Limited mobility of the diaphragm and more intimate connections between sternum, diaphragm, and mediastinum, may favor enlargement of the liver, partly through lack of the rhythmic compression by the diaphragm (page 60) (22, 52).

Ventricular contraction may be hindered by adhesions which add to the normal effort, because of traction exerted on resistant structures (ribs, sternum, diaphragm, and subdiaphragmatic organs) (53) and because of angulation and rotation of the heart (25). This obstacle, mainly present during inspiration, can be admitted only in cases with extensive systolic retraction of the chest wall.

Ventricular dilatation is hindered by the formation of constrictive masses or by calcification (25, 54). This is proven by the data of the electrokymogram (80) and by right heart catheterization (81). This obstacle is particularly important in preventing further dilatation, one of the physiological means for increasing cardiac output. Actually, these patients are often incapable of even limited efforts.

Myocardial and valvular lesions, connected with and due to the same process causing adhesions, may be present (52). However, their importance is secondary.

Of special importance is *the localization of the adhesions.* It is apparent that when they develop around the venae cavae or the hepatic veins (30), they cause venous congestion, decreased venous inflow, and decreased cardiac output. *Compression of the atria or pulmonary veins* has been demonstrated in certain cases; *predominant compression of the left ventricle,* in others (64).

The *effusion of various serosae* has been explained as the result of heart failure (37), venous compression (52), or inflammation (32). It is the author's view (26, 55) that heart failure is present only in a small number of cases, usually toward the end of the clinical course; that the main factor is compression of the large veins (venae cavae, hepatic veins, vena azygos); and that, in some cases, an inflammatory component is also present, as revealed by the fluid and by autopsy.

Increased venous pressure is a direct result of the compression exerted on the large veins. This increase is less useful than in pericardial effusion because it is unable to overcome the compression (57). However, it may accelerate the flow through the constricted areas.

The chief mechanism by which these patients can increase their cardiac output is *tachycardia.* This should be considered as a useful phenomenon, within limits (57).

VARIETIES

Different etiology, severity, and extension, cause different clinical pictures.

High mediastinal syndrome with superior vena cava compression. This picture is often described under the name of *mediastinitis* but pericardial lesions are seldom absent. It will be described later (page 463).

Diffuse constrictive pericarditis with predominant compression of the right heart. It is usually due to tuberculosis. The patients have frequently a typical triad (25): high venous pressure; quiet, small heart; and transudative ascites. The jugular veins are distended and immobile. The liver is large, the spleen is normal. There is no edema of the legs. The urine is normal. There may be transudation in the right pleural cavity.

Diffuse constrictive pericarditis with predominant compression of the left heart. It is usually due to tuberculosis. There is dyspnea. The 2nd pulmonic sound is loud. Catheterization reveals increased systolic pressure in the right ventricle and pulmonary artery. The liver is normal or only slightly enlarged.

Constrictive pericarditis with peritonitis (Pick's syndrome). The clinical picture is due to a *polyserositis.* The inflammation usually starts in the right pleura or the pericardium and then diffuses to the upper part of the peritoneum. The process predominates either in the right pleural cavity and involves the pericaval part of the pericardium (31) or in the pericardial cavity (32). The liver is *frosted*; there are adhesions between diaphragm, liver, stomach, and spleen. *The ascitic fluid is borderline between exudate and transudate* and may be a frank exudate. The spleen may be enlarged. In a special variety, only observed in children (56), the liver shows both *stasis* and *active tuberculosis.*

Partial pericardial adhesions may be entirely asymptomatic and harmless. One type is revealed by a *systolic click or snap.* Patients with this sign may complain of *precordial pain*, especially when stretching their arms or after exertion; of *palpitation*; and of *anxiety.* Therefore, they are often mistaken for patients with more serious cardiac lesions (67).

Cases of adhesive pericarditis with valvular lesions are usually due to rheumatic disease. The heart is enlarged and any clinical evidence of the chronic process of the pericardium may be absent. The process seldom develops serious constriction but may be responsible for increased severity of venous or hepatic engorgement through compression developed by bands of connective tissue.

DIAGNOSIS

In spite of recent contributions, diagnosis of constrictive pericarditis may be difficult. The clinical pictures of superior or inferior cava compression are usually easily recognized and the difficulty lies mainly in the evaluation of the lesions.

Diffuse constrictive pericarditis should be differentiated from *rheumatic heart disease with mitral and tricuspid stenosis.* The data of the electro- and phonocardiogram, and of the electrokymogram; the size of the heart (smaller in pericarditis); if necessary, the data of catheterization allow a correct diagnosis.

Differential diagnosis between *constrictive pericarditis* and *an amyloid heart* is extremely difficult (83).

The differential diagnosis between *constrictive pericarditis* and *cardiac failure* is based on the fact that, in the latter, there usually is a rapid and irregular pulse, congestion of the lungs, dyspnea, active venous pulsations, and a much slower circulation time. Digitalis is more effective in cardiac failure.

PROGNOSIS

Prognosis of these syndromes should be based on nature and extension of the lesions, age of the patient, existence of associated lesions and seat of the compression, cardiac function, and the possibility of surgery. In general, these cases last many years because the engorgement due to compression has a different significance from that due to cardiac failure.

TREATMENT

Medical treatment is based on the use of *mercurial diuretics* by injection (11, 12) and *ammonium chloride* by mouth (13). *Digitalis* is not contraindicated but is seldom helpful unless cardiac failure also sets in.

Paracentesis of the abdominal cavity is necessary whenever abundant ascites is present and no surgical intervention is possible; it should be repeated at regular intervals.

Surgery should be performed in the great majority of the cases. According to a recently advocated viewpoint, surgery of tubercular cases should be undertaken at the time of the effusion and before organization of the exudate (82).

Various interventions are possible. The simplest procedure consists of the *mobilization of an anterior chest plastron* (*sternum plus ribs*); this is beneficial in cases with predominant external adhesions and in cases with extensive calcification (54). The best procedure, however, consists of the *complete decompression and decortication of the heart* (25, 54, 55). In a large majority of cases, the operation is successful and is followed by abundant diuresis and increased cardiac output. This operation allows the heart to assume a more physiological position and removes the scars constricting the various chambers and organs.

While various approaches, from the left or right side, have been advocated, the entire surgical field may be exposed by *median sternotomy* (84). This approach permits excision of the pericardium beyond both cardiac borders and around the venae cavae.

Quinidine or *pronestyl* is given in the last two days before surgery in order to reduce the excitability of the heart. *Atropine* and *morphine* are employed as preanesthetic drugs, then light anesthesia, with *nitrous oxide, oxygen,* and *ether,* is used (25). If the heart reacts to superficial stimulation, 2 per cent *procaine,* directly applied, is of help.

BIBLIOGRAPHY

1. a) Ash, R. In *Stroud's Cardiovascular Disease.* Philadelphia, Davis, 1945.
   b) Sunderland, S., and Wright-Smith, R. J. Brit. Heart J., 1944, **6,** 167.
2. Hunter, W. C., and Crynes, S. F. Mo. Conc. Cardiov. Dis., 1940, **9,** N. 2.
3. Lavallée. Quoted by Hunter and Crynes (2).
4. Wolff, L. New England J. Med., 1943, **229,** 423.
5. Cossio, P., Berconsky, I., and Dambrosi, R. G. Am. Heart J., 1942, **24,** 223.
6. Wolferth, C. C., and Margolies, A. Int. Clin., 1940, **1,** Suppl. 3.
7. Wenckebach, K. F. Zeit. klin. Med., 1910, **71,** 402.

8. Kussmaul, A. Berl. klin. Woch., 1873, **10,** 433.
9. a) Ebstein, W. Virchow's Arch., 1892, **130,** 148.
   b) Blechmann. Thèse, Paris, 1913.
10. a) Banti, G. Deut. med. Woch., 1888, **12,** 897.
    b) Sibson. In *Reynolds System of Medicine,* 1877, v. 4.
11. Auenbrugger. *Inventum Novum.* Vienna, Trattner, 1761.
12. a) Pins, E. Wien. med. Woch., 1889, **39,** 209 and 248.
    b) Ewart, W. Brit. M. J., 1896, **1,** 717.
    c) Levine, S. A., and Gevalt, F. Trans. Assoc. Am. Physicians, 1940, **55,** 106.
13. a) Porte, D., and Pardee, H. E. B. Am. Heart J., 1929, **4,** 586.
    b) Scott, R. W., Feil, H. S., and Katz L. N. Am. Heart J., 1929, **5,** 68 and 77.
    c) Picchini, G. Cuore e Circ., 1932, **16,** 300.
    d) Hermann, G., and Schwab, E. H. Trans. Assoc. Am. Physicians, 1934, **49,** 229. Also Arch. Int. Med., 1935, **55,** 917.
    e) Bellet, S., and McMillan, T. M. Arch. Int. Med., 1938, **61,** 381.
    f) Van der Veer, J. B., and Norris, R. F. J. A. M. A., 1939, **113,** 1483.
    g) Groedel, F. M., and Reichert, P. Cardiol., 1941, **5,** 4.
    h) Urschel, D. L., Bondy, P. D., and Salley, S. M. New England J. Med., 1945, **233,** 399.
14. Heckmann, K. Muench. med. Woch., 1937, **84,** 60.
15. a) Roesler, H. *Cardiovascular Roentgenology.* Springfield, Thomas, 1945.
    b) Schwedel, J. B. *Clinical Roentgenology of the Heart.* New York, Hoeber, 1946.
16. Bordet, E., and Fischgold, H. *La Radiokymographie du Coeur et des Vaisseaux.* Paris, Masson, 1937.
17. Fletcher, C. M. Brit. Heart J., 1945, **7,** 143.
18. Wolff, L. New England J. Med., 1944, **230,** 422.
19. Blumer, G. Arch. Int. Med., 1914, **14,** 605.
20. Cohnheim, J. *Lectures on General Pathology.* London, 1889.
21. a) Porter, W. B. In *Cyclopedia of Medicine.* Philadelphia, Davis, 1944.
    b) Marfan, A. B. Sem. Méd., 1913, **33,** 469.
22. Wenckebach, K. F.
    a) Zeit. klin. Med., 1910, **71,** 402.
    b) *Ueber pathologische Beziehungen zwischen Atmung und Kreislauf*; Volkmanns Samml. klin. Vortr., 1937, N. 465-466.
    c) *Herz und Kreislaufinsuffizienz.* Dresden, Steinkopff, 1931.
23. Lucherini, T. Cuore e Circ., 1936, **10,** 3.

24. WISE, A. W., AND SHAFER, L. E. J. A. M. A. 1945, **127, 583.**

25. BECK, C. S. In *Stroud's Cardiovascular Disease.* Philadelphia, Davis, 1945. Also in *Medical Physics.* Year Book Publishers, 1947.

26. LUISADA, A. A. *Le Mediastino-Pericarditi Adesive.* Roma, Pozzi, 1936.

27. GRIESINGER, W. Dissertation, Tuebingen, 1856.

28. a) SMITH, H. L., AND WILLIUS, F. A. Arch. Int. Med., 1932, **50, 171** and 410.

    b) MUSSER, J. H., AND HERMANN, G. R. J. A. M. A., 1926, **87, 459.**

29. ROBERTS, J., AND BECK, C. S. Am. Heart J., 1941, **22, 314.**

30. ELIAS, H., AND FELLER, A. *Stauungstypen bei Kreislaufstoerungen.* Vienna, Springer, 1926.

31. CURSCHMANN, H. Deut. med. Woch., 1884, **10, 564.**

32. PICK, F. Zeit. klin. Med., 1896, **29, 385.**

33. WILLIAMS, C. J. B. London J. Med., 1850, vol. 2. Also in *System of Treatment.* New York, Latham and English, 1915.

34. a) HIRTZ, E. Rév. gen. clin. Thér., 1898, **12, 689.**

    b) OGLE, C. Proc. Roy. Soc., London, Feb.-March, 1910.

35. BROADBENT, J. F. H. Lancet, 1895, July 27.

36. SKODA, J. Allg. Wien. med. Zeit., 1863, N. 10, 11, 36, 37.

37. VOLHARD, F., AND SCHMIEDEN, V. Klin. Woch., 1923, **2, 5.**

38. FRIEDREICH, N.

    a) Virchow's Handb. Pathol. und Ther., 1868, vol. 5.

    b) Deut. Arch. klin. Med., 1865, **1, 241.**

39. LIAN, C., MARCHAL, M., AND PAUTRAT, J. Bull. Mém. Soc. Hôp., 1933, **49, 20.**

40. WOLFERTH, C., AND MARGOLIES, A. In *Stroud's Cardiovascular Disease.* Philadelphia, Davis, 1945.

41. GALLAVARDIN, L. Lyon Méd., 1913, **121, 409.**

42. RIEGEL, F. Berl. Klin. Woch., 1877, **14, 657.**

43. a) CHURCHILL, E. D. Arch. Surg., 1929, **19, 1451.**

    b) CUTLER, E. C. In *Nelson's Loose-Leaf Surgery.* New York, Nelson, 1927.

44. a) BURWELL, C. S., AND STRAYHORN, W. D. Arch. Surg., 1932, **24, 106.**

    b) BURWELL, C. S., AND FLICKINGER, D. Arch. Int. Med., 1935, **56, 250.**

45. BECK, C. S. Arch. Surg., 1929, **18, 1659.** Ann. Surg., 1935, **102, 801.** J. A. M. A., 1935, **104, 714.** Am. Heart J., 1937, **14, 515.**

46. a) CONTI, A. Giorn. Clin. Med., 1933, **14, 902.**

    b) SERRA, V. Cuore e Circ., 1929, **13, 381.**

47. WHITE, P. D. In *Stroud's Cardiovascular Disease.* Philadelphia, Davis, 1945.

48. a) HOCHREIN, M., AND WEISS, S. Arch. Int. Med., 1929, **44, 290.**

    b) HOCHREIN, M., AND LAPLACE, L. Deut. Arch. Klin. Med., 1936, **176, 113.**

49. a) CARTER, E. P., AND DIEUAIDE, F. R. Bull. Johns Hopkins Hosp., 1921, **32, 219.**

    b) DIEUAIDE, F. R. Arch. Int. Med., 1925, **35, 362.**

50. ZDANSKY, E. Med. klin., 1931, **27, 156.** Also Wien, klin. Woch., 1933, **46, 993.**

51. CONDORELLI, L. Min. Med., 1936, (P. 1), 27, 81. Presse Méd., 1937, **45, 1831.** Cardiol., 1937, **1, 26.**

52. SCHUR, M. Erg. inn. Med., 1934, **47, 348.**

53. a) GALVAGNI, E. Clin. Med. Ital., 1898, **37, 756.**

    b) SACCONAGHI, G. L. *La Clinica della Adesione Pericardica.* Roma, Pozzi, 1924.

54. a) BRAUER, L. *Erkrankungen des Perikards.* In *Atlas und Grundriss der Roentgendiagnostik* by F. M. Groedel. Muenchen, Lehmann, 1921.

    b) BRAUER, L., AND FISCHER, H. *Herzbeutelfunktion und Herbeutelerkrankungen.* In *Textbook of Path. Physiology* by Béthe and Bergmann. Berlin, Springer, 1927.

    c) BRAUER, L. *Die Herzchirurgie.* Same textbook as b above.

55. DELORME, E. Gaz. Hôp. Paris, 1913, **86, 2269;** and 1914, **87, 341.**

56. HUTINEL, V. Rév. Mens. Mal. Enf., 1893, p. 529; and 1894, p. 15.

57. LYONS, R. H. AND BURWELL, C. S. Brit. Heart J., 1946, **8, 33.**

58. BETTMAN, R. B., AND TANNENBAUM, W. J. Ann. Surg. 1948, **128, 1012.**

59. BARNES, A. R., AND BURCHELL, H. B. Am. Heart J. 1942, **23, 247.**

60. KEITH, N. M., PRUITT, R. D., AND BAGGENSTOSS, A. N. Am. Heart J. **31, 527.**

61. MEREDITH, H. C. Am. Heart J. 1949, **37, 129.**

62. GREISMAN, H., BROWN, C. R., AND SMETANA, H. Am. Heart J. 1947, **34, 447.**

63. PAUL, O., CASTLEMAN, B., AND WHITE, P. D. Am. J. M. Sci. 1948, **216, 361.**

64. WHITE, P. D., ALEXANDER, F., CHURCHILL, E. D., AND SWEET, R. H. Am. J. M. Sci., 1948, **216, 378.**

65. GILLICK, F. G., AND REYNOLDS, W. F. California Med. 1949, **70, N. 5.**

66. BLOOMFIELD, R. A., LAUSON, H. D., AND CO-WORKERS. J. Clin. Investigation, 1946, **25, 639.**

67. LUISADA, A. A., AND ALIMURUNG, M. Acta Cardiol. (Bruxelles): 1949, **4, 309.**

68. BARNES, A. R. *Electrocardiographic Patterns*. Springfield, Thomas, 1940.

69. BELLET, S., AND McMILLAN, T. M. Arch. Int. Med., 1938, **61,** 381.

70. HARP, V. C., AND PEEKE, E. S. Am. Heart J., 1949, **37,** 134.

71. LEVY, R. L., AND PATTERSON, M. C. Am. J. Med., 1950, **8,** 34.

72. PORTER, W. B., CLARK, O., AND PORTER, R. R. J. A. M. A., 1950, **144,** 749.

73. ANDREWS, G. W. S., PICKERING, G. W., AND SELLORS, T. Quart. J. Med., 1948, **17,** 291.

74. TAUBENHAUS, M., AND BRAMS, W. A. J. A. M. A., 1950, **142,** 973.

75. FALK, A., AND EBERT, R. V. J. A. M. A., 1951, **145,** 310.

76. BELLET, S., *et al.* Ann. Int. Med., 1951, **34,** 856.

77. METCALFE, J., AND WOODBURY, J. W. J. Clin. Investigation, 1951, **30,** 661.

78. ARENDT, J., AND CARDON, L. Radiol., 1949, **53,** 371.

79. ENSELBERG, C. D., LESSE, S., AND SCHWEDEL, J. B. Meet. of A. H. A., 1951.

80. McKUSICK, V. A. Public Health Serv. Publ. No. 59; 1951, 125.

81. HANSEN, T., *et al.* Circ., 1951, **3,** 881.

82. HOLMAN, E., AND WILLETT, F. J. A. M. A., 1951, **146,** 1.

83. FINDLEY, J. W., AND ADAMS, W. Arch. Int. Med., 1948, **81,** 342.

84. HOLMAN, E. Lancet, 1951, **71,** 420.

85. DONALDSON, J. K. *Surgical Disorders of the Chest.* 2nd Ed. Philadelphia, Lea and Febiger, 1947.

86. MOSCHCOWITZ, E. J. A. M. A., 1953, **153,** 194.

CHAPTER 21

Diseases of the Large Vessels

Congenital Anomalies of the Veins (80)

Anomalies of the superior cava. This trunk may be *hypoplasic* or *very large* (*megacava superior*). There may be *two superior cavae,* the right and the left; the left superior cava usually terminates into the left atrium but it may join the ending of the coronary sinus. It is due to persistence of the *left duct of Cuvier.*

Anomalies of the inferior cava. There may be *two inferior cavae,* one terminating into the right atrium; the other, into the left. There may be a single inferior cava terminating into the left atrium.

Septal defects or stenosis or atresia of the pulmonary artery are frequently associated.

Congenital Anomalies of the Pulmonary Veins (79)

Anomalous drainage of the pulmonary vessels is possible. There may be either *complete* or *incomplete* drainage of the pulmonary veins into the right atrium or its tributaries. Incomplete drainage is compatible with life and has been reported even in adults. The best chances for survival are when less than 50 per cent of the vessels have anomalous drainage or when there is association with an atrial septal defect. The clinical picture may be similar to that of uncomplicated atrial septal defect (page 278) and even catheterization may not reveal the lesion. Only angiocardiography gave diagnostic data in certain cases.

When anomalous venous drainage from the lungs is *partial,* the most common sites of entry are the superior cava, the right atrium, and the left innominate vein. In the *complete* anomalous drainage, the sites of entrance may be the above mentioned, and also the coronary sinus, the inferior cava, or the portal vein. Complete anomalous drainage may be found in newborn infants and is due to anomaly of development in the system of the *ductus venosus* (page 11).

If the anomalous veins increase to a great extent the flow of the right atrium and there is an atrial shunt, *cyanosis* is constant and is increased by feeding. In such cases, survival is possible. When the drainage occurs into the superior cava or the innominate veins, catheterization reveals a high oxygen content before reaching the right atrium.

The *physical data* may simulate atrial septal defect including a systolic pulmonic murmur and a loud P_2 (page 279).

The *x-ray* shows the same data of an atrial septal defect (page 280) while this shunt is not present. *The superior cava may be broad* (drainage into this vessel). The left atrium is small.

The *arterial blood* may present a slightly low saturation.

Anomalous pulmonary drainage should be corrected *before* surgical correction of an atrial septal defect.

The Superior Caval Syndrome (83)

The superior caval syndrome is a clinical picture characterized by venous engorgement, cyanosis, and edema in the district of the superior vena cava. It may be caused by either *occlusion* or *compression of the cava* or by an *aortic-caval fistula.* Occlusion or compression may be due to bronchogenic carcinoma, mediastinal tumors, aneurysm of the aorta (page 478), mediastinopericarditis (page 450), or thrombophlebitis of the superior cava. The aortic-caval fistula is usually due to rupture of an aneurysm of the ascending aorta (page 481) into the cava.

When the obstruction is *above* the entrance of the azygos vein, blood from the upper half of the body may still reach the lower part of the cava through collateral venous channels which finally drain into the azygos. When the obstruction is *below* the entrance of the azygos vein, blood from the upper part of the body reaches the right atrium only through collateral channels which drain into the inferior cava.

SIGNS AND SYMPTOMS

The face is flushed and cyanotic. Cough, hemoptysis, hoarseness and dysphagia are frequent. Fullness in the head, *headache*, *drowsiness, stupor*, and paroxysmal dyspnea may occur. These symptoms may be alleviated by the erect position. *Edema, cyanosis, and venous engorgement of the head, neck, arms, and upper part of the body are typical*. The superficial veins of the trunk are dilated and tortuous.

If there is an aortic-caval fistula, a loud, continuous, *machinery murmur* is audible over the right side of the chest and back.

X-RAY

The heart is normal in size. The shadow of the superior cava may be widened. The data of an aneurysm, a mediastinal tumor, or a mediastinopericarditis, may be found. *Venograms* with diodrast may reveal the site of obstruction.

VENOUS PRESSURE—CIRCULATION TIME

Venous pressure in the arm veins is from 30 to 40 cm. of water. A significant difference between the two arms may be found. The femoral venous pressure is frequently normal; when elevated, it is still lower than the venous pressure of the arm.

The *circulation time* is found to be normal in arm-to-tongue tests, revealing a striking difference from cases of heart failure.

When *thrombosis of the cava* occurs, the severity of the symptoms depends, to some

extent, upon the rapidity with which the collateral circulation develops and upon the level of the occlusion. The anastomosis of deep collateral veins frequently causes passive congestion of the kidneys, as revealed by albuminuria.

Diagnosis is possible from the study of the physical signs and by means of venograms, venous pressure measurements, and circulation time tests.

Therapy. Venous obstruction due to occlusion of the superior cava in experimental animals has been relieved by the creation of shunts. The most satisfactory was found to be that between superior cava above the obstruction and right atrium. Clinical applications are possible.

The Inferior Caval Syndrome

The inferior cava can be ligated in man without producing edema of the lower extremities. This procedure has actually been performed in cases of thrombophlebitis (81) or for relief of chronic congestion (82). Occlusion of the inferior cava may be due to thrombosis (84) and its obstruction may be caused by ascites, neoplasm, or fibrous constriction (page 458). The results are less favorable than in surgical ligation.

The typical picture consists of *edema and venous engorgement of the lower extremities*. *Collateral veins* develop on the surface of the abdomen and chest and discharge some of the blood of the lower part of the body into the superior cava. The lymphatic vessels of the legs increase their flow.

The venous pressure is high in the legs, normal in the arms.

Right Aortic Arch and Vascular Rings

LESIONS

There are three major types (fig. 274).

a) There is a *right aortic arch* (3). The aorta arises from the left ventricle, then rises higher than it does normally, *turns right*, and follows the right side of the vertebral column. Before reaching the dia-

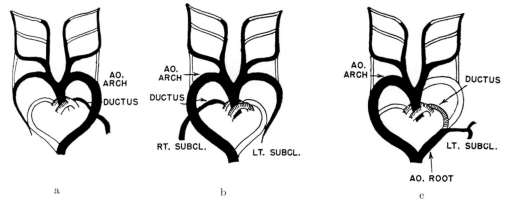

FIG. 274. a, Development of the normal aortic arch. b, Right aortic arch with symmetrical inversion of the large vessels. c, Right aortic arch with persistent *aortic root*.

phragm, the descending aorta may cross the spine to the left and follow a normal course (figs. 275 and 276). *The aortic arch, which passes over the right bronchus, lies to the right of the trachea and esophagus and pushes the esophagus toward the left.* The fibrosed remnants of the ductus arteriosus may form a vascular ring encircling the trachea and esophagus together with the pulmonary artery and the aortic arch.

b) The ascending aorta has a course similar to that in section (a) but *the arch passes behind the esophagus* (1). A *diverticulum (aortic root)* branches off the ascending aorta and gives off the left subclavian artery; the obliterated ductus arteriosus connects it with the pulmonary artery. In these cases, esophagus and trachea are again encircled (fig. 277).

c) There is a *double aortic arch* (1, 4). The right (or posterior) arch is usually larger; the left (or anterior) arch, is smaller. The right is retroesophageal; the left passes anteriorly to the trachea, enclosing the trachea and esophagus in a vascular ring (fig. 277). The ascending aorta may consist of either a single or a double trunk.

Possible associated abnormalities are tetralogy of Fallot or Eisenmenger complex (pages 310 and 318), coarctation or atresia of the left aorta (page 467), abnormalities in origin of the left subclavian artery, per-

sistent common arterial trunk, and dextrocardia.

These congenital lesions are due to the obliteration of the 4th left branchial artery (fig. 5) or to persistence of both the right and left 4th arteries. They may reproduce conditions which are normal in amphibia and reptilia. Persistence of the 4th right arch leads to a condition similar to that seen in birds.

Several varieties of *vascular rings* surrounding the esophagus and the trachea are possible and may be caused by anomalies of origin of the carotid and subclavian arteries, in addition to the above described lesions (54).

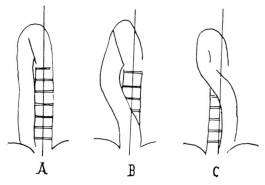

FIG. 275. Different courses of the descending aorta in cases with *persistent right aortic arch*. (From G. Canali.)

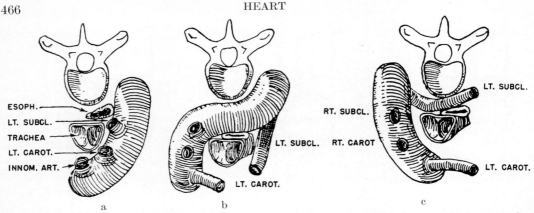

ESOPH.
LT. SUBCL.
TRACHEA
LT. CAROT.
INNOM. ART.

RT. SUBCL.
LT. SUBCL.
LT. CAROT.

RT. SUBCL.
RT. CAROT.
LT. SUBCL.
LT. CAROT.

a   b   c

FIG. 276. Transverse section of the thorax seen from above. a, normal aorta; b, right aorta turning to left; c, right aorta which stays at the right of the spine. (From G. Canali.)

SIGNS AND SYMPTOMS

The first type of anomaly is probably more frequent than generally thought and may be discovered in mature or elderly people. On the contrary, type (c) is rarer and seldom found in adults. The general signs described in some cases, particularly cyanosis and clubbed fingers, are due to associated lesions and not to the aortic malformation.

Double aortic arch may cause *cyanosis* and *stridor* and favor pulmonary infections in children (5). *Difficulty in swallowing*

(dysphagia lusoria) is not uncommon in the anomalies of types (b) and (c), especially when arteriosclerosis causes dilatation of the aorta.

Certain physical signs may be present: *dulness* along the upper right sternal border extending to the right sternoclavicular junction; *visible and palpable systolic pulsation* in the 2nd and 3rd right interspaces near the sternum and at the supraclavicular fossa; loud cardiac sounds to the right and above their normal site; and possibly a systolic murmur in the 2nd right interspace, in the 2nd left, or in both.

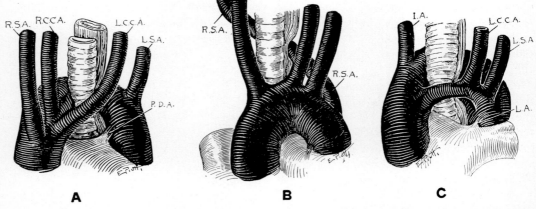

R.S.A. R.C.C.A.   L.C.C.A.
                    L.S.A.
                              P.D.A.

R.S.A.
            R.S.A.

I.A.   L.C.C.A.
                    L.S.A.
            R.S.A.
                              L.A.

A   B   C

FIG. 277. Various types of vascular rings. A, *Right aortic arch.* Left common carotid artery compressing front of trachea. Pulmonary artery drawn against the trachea by the ductus arteriosus. B, *Anomalous right subclavian artery* which arises from the left side of the aortic arch and presses on the posterior wall of the esophagus. C, *Double aortic arch.* The ascending aorta divides into two limbs which subsequently join and form the descending aorta. (From Gross and Ware, Surg., Gyn., and Abst. Courtesy of Dr. R. E. Gross).

X-RAY (3, 4)

In the *frontal position*, the aortic knob is absent on the left side and either a knob or a band-like shadow is present on the right, extending up to the clavicle (type a). In the absence of the aortic knob, the pulmonic knob appears larger. Either the diverticulum or the left aortic arch may show on the left in types (b) and (c). A barium swallow reveals that the esophagus is indented and displaced to the left.

In the *right anterior oblique*, the esophagus and the trachea are either normal or pushed forward and the esophagus shows a posterior indentation. In the *left anterior oblique*, the esophagus shows an indentation which is toward the left instead of the right; the descending aorta is visible between the esophagus and spine.

A *right aortic arch* passing posterior to the esophagus deviates the latter to the left and causes a rounded defect on its posterior aspect. A *constrictive double aortic arch* causes narrowing of the trachea and esophagus from both sides. A *right subclavian artery* arising from the left side of the arch of the normal aorta may pass to the right either in front of the trachea or behind the esophagus causing a typical indentation (55).

DIAGNOSIS

Diagnosis of the right aortic arch is based on x-ray observation but the pulsation at the right supraclavicular region, the typical dulness, and the dysphagia may indicate the presence of the lesion. Differential diagnosis from aortitis and aortic aneurysm is necessary, and the x-ray data are decisive. Diagnosis of double aortic arch or anomalous vessels constricting the trachea and esophagus is very important, especially in infants.

COURSE

Many cases with anomaly type (a) reach old age with few or no symptoms. On the other hand, anomaly type (b) is a frequent cause of symptoms and anomaly type (c) often gives disturbances in children; it is seldom observed in adults because of the high mortality.

TREATMENT

Surgery of the double aortic arch and of other anomalies of the arteries of the neck has been accomplished with excellent results (15d). *Division* of the thinner of the two arches, or of an anomalous subclavian artery, relieves the pressure and permits reestablishment of normal conditions. Early surgery insures survival and normal development of an infant.

Coarctation of the Aorta

Coarctation of the aorta is a lesion which usually develops at the junction of the arch with the descending aorta but which in rare cases may develop in other points of the aorta. The clinical picture is four times more common in males than in females. *Early onset of puberty* and precocious physical development are typical (49).

CAUSE AND LESIONS

Most of the reported lesions are *congenital* even if they become manifest at various ages of infancy, childhood, or maturity. Narrowing of the descending aorta by sclerodermic retraction of the diaphragm, an exceptional lesion, is *acquired* (47).

The lesion consists of a narrowing of the aorta which is either slightly above the ductus (*preductal coarctation*) or is opposite to or slightly below it (*postductal coarctation*) (fig. 278). Both types are *congenital* and are caused by faulty development of the IVth arterial arch, its junction with the dorsal aorta, and the VIth arterial arch, during the second month of fetal life (7, 68). The cases with preductal coarctation (so-called *infantile type*) usually succumb within the first months of life unless there is a patent ductus arteriosus which has a compensatory function. The cases with postductal coarctation (so-called *adult type*) soon develop an adequate *collateral circulation* and frequently survive until maturity.

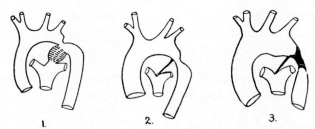

FIG. 278. Different types of coarctation. 1, *preductal type*; patent ductus; 2, *postductal type*; 3, *atresia* of the aorta. (From W. Evans, Quart. J. Med. Courtesy of the author.)

This collateral circulation is developed over the surface of the thorax and abdomen, connecting the aortic arch with the organs which receive their blood supply from the descending aorta. It is made: a) between branches of the superior intercostal arteries (subclavian) and the other intercostal arteries (descending aorta); b) between branches of the subscapular arteries (subclavian) and the intercostal arteries (descending aorta); c) between internal mammary (sub-

clavian) and the epigastric branches of the external iliac arteries (descending aorta) (fig. 279).

These collateral vessels reach a tremendous size and may form *tortuous loops* under the skin of the thorax and abdomen. The intercostal arteries, extremely sinuous, cause *indentations of the ribs* by their pulsation.

In rare cases, coarctation causes only a slight narrowing of the aorta and *a marked*

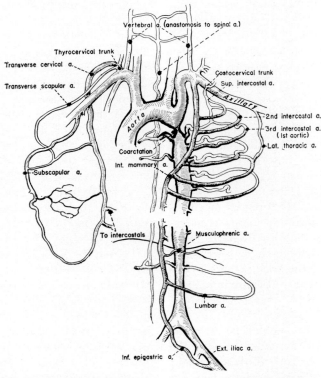

FIG. 279. The major channels in coarctation of the aorta. (From Edwards and coworkers. Proc. Staff Meet., Mayo Clin., 1948, courtesy of the authors).

narrowing of the left subclavian artery (9). In other exceptional cases, there is *a narrowing of the descending or the abdominal aorta* (10, 72).

The ascending aorta, the aortic arch, and the great vessels of the arch are dilated in all three types; exceptionally, the left carotid and subclavian are small. The descending aorta and its branches are thin and poorly developed in all types.

Associated lesions, such as interventricular septal defect, aortic stenosis, bicuspid aortic valve, mitral stenosis, aneurysm of the sinus of Valsalva, common trunk giving both carotid arteries, or bicuspid aortic valve (7), are possible in the preductal type.

SIGNS AND SYMPTOMS

Infants with a *preductal* coarctation usually develop the first symptoms within 2 weeks of life and about three-fourths die within the first 8 weeks. A small number may survive and even reach senility (68). Patients with a *postductal* type of coarctation, on the contrary, may experience only minor disturbances during infancy and adolescence while the most important signs and symptoms become apparent between 20 and 45 years of life.

One of the first symptoms is *exertional or precordial pain. Chest or back pain* may be caused by erosion of ribs or root compression by enlarged arterial channels (including spinal anastomoses) (52). There is a frequent association with *thyrotoxicosis*, probably because of increased blood supply to the thyroid gland (52). *Headache, nausea, vomiting, vertigo, diplopia,* and *hemoptysis,* may occur. *Dry, nonproductive cough, weakness,* and *sensation of cold in the legs* are frequent.

The carotid and subclavian arteries show a visible pulsation with rhythmic expansion of the suprasternal notch and the supraclavicular regions. The apical thrust is displaced to the left and downwards, evidence of left ventricular enlargement. Both a *thrill* and a *late systolic murmur* may be present over the 2nd left interspace, and

the latter also *at the back,* but they are not constant. A *systolic murmur* can be heard over the aortic area, the suprasternal notch, and at the first left interspace. An *aortic diastolic murmur* is not uncommon (16).

One of the more obvious signs is the *pulsation of multiple arterial vessels* over the surface of the thorax and abdomen. These may reach the caliber of a normal radial artery and are easily palpable in the intercostal spaces. When these are not apparent, they become more obvious *if the patient stoops forward with his arms hanging down* (53).

The *radial pulse is full on both sides* (often, more on the right); *the femoral pulse and that of the arteria dorsalis pedis are small or absent* (fig. 280). When the pulse is palpable, a *marked delay* between apical thrust and femoral pulse can be appreciated.

The *blood pressure is elevated* in both arms and forearms. It is *lowered,* or impossible to estimate, in both thighs and legs.

The *temperature* of the legs is low; *circulation time* is prolonged in the lower extremity (11). The *basal metabolic rate* is frequently increased (21).

GRAPHIC TRACINGS

Electrocardiogram. This tracing may reveal the existence of *left axis deviation.* There may be evidence of *left ventricular hypertrophy, left intraventricular block,* or *both.* On the other hand, coarctation plus patency of the ductus is usually followed by *right ventricular hypertrophy* and *strain.*

Phonocardiogram. A *systolic murmur,* caused by the narrowing of the aorta, is frequently recorded. The vibrations of this murmur have usually a *diamond-shaped aspect* but may be nondescript in type. This murmur is well recorded over the base, especially at the left of the sternum. It may be recorded even better at the back, between left scapula and spine (69). When the murmur is louder at the back, an important differential datum with any valvular defect is obtained. An *early-diastolic murmur,*

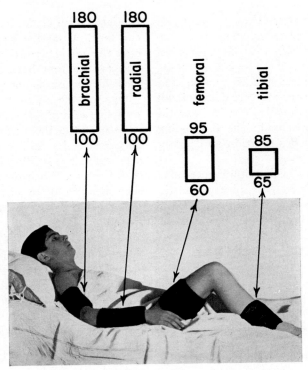

Fig. 280. Blood pressure difference in *coarctation of the aorta*.

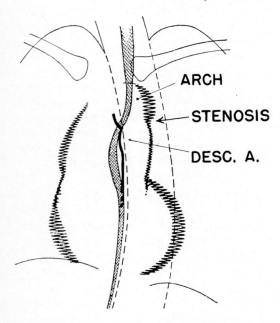

Fig. 281. Roentgenkymogram in a case of *coarctation of the aorta*. Left anterior oblique. Sudden reduction of pulsation beyond the coarctation. (From Laubry and Heim de Balzac.)

similar to that of aortic insufficiency, is recorded in most cases at the back, even though it may not be heard with a stethoscope (69). It is caused by the blood flowing through the narrow section of aorta during diastole (fig. 283).

Roentgenkymogram, electrokymogram. Roentgenkymography shows a sharp contrast between the pulsations of the aortic arch and those of the descending aorta (fig. 281).

Electrokymography also shows that the densogram of the aortic arch has large pulsations while that of the descending aorta has small pulsations or none at all (70).

Ballistocardiogram. The ballistocardiogram presents typically the absence of the K wave (71) (fig. 283). This pattern, which has diagnostic value, becomes normal after surgery.

X-RAY

There may be *reduction in size of the descending aorta.* On the other hand, *the*

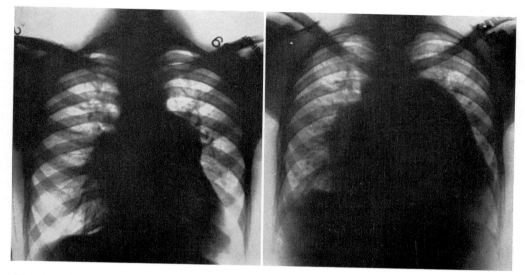

FIG. 282. Cardiac silhouette in a case of coarctation plus ductus arteriosus (p.m. control). The two roentgenograms were taken 5 years apart.

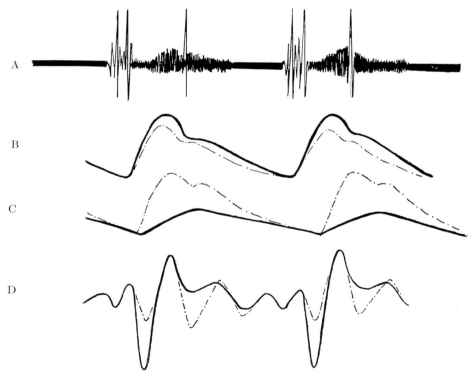

FIG. 283. Scheme of graphic tracings in coarctation of the aorta. A, phonocardiogram recorded over the back. B, pulse tracing of the brachial artery. C, tracing of the femoral artery. D, ballistocardiogram. Dotted lines, normal patterns. Deep I and lack of K in the BCG.

ascending aorta and aortic arch are dilated and show active pulsations; therefore, a sharp contrast is present between them and the descending aorta which shows weak pulsations or none at all.

A *bulbous* or *spindle-shaped dilatation of the descending aorta* beyond the constriction may be observed. It can be recognized by typical displacement of the esophagus. *Calcifications* can be observed in the wall of the descending aorta.

A leftward convexity may be present in the upper mediastinum. This is due to a *dilated left subclavian artery* and may be mistaken for the aortic knob.

The cardiac silhouette is often typical of left ventricular enlargement.

The ribs show marked *notching* because of irregular erosion of their inferior borders by the dilated and tortuous intercostal arteries. In doubtful cases, intravenous injection of diodrast may outline the narrowed section of the aorta and some of the collateral arterial vessels.

VARIETIES—COURSE

The two types, preductal (infantile) and postductal (adult) cause two somewhat different pictures.

a) The *preductal type* is most often observed in infants, even though occasional patients develop an adequate collateral circulation and reach adolescence or even maturity or old age. These patients, on account of the usual persistence of the ductus have the following peculiarities: *possible cyanosis, more marked in, or exclusive of the lower extremities* (49); right axis deviation; loud machinery murmur over the 2nd left interspace; poorly developed collateral circulation; large pulmonary knob (fig. 282).

b) The *postductal type* is usually observed in young people or adults. Its presence *at birth* is proven by occasional autopsies in infants and by increasing reports of correct diagnoses in children. These patients present typical clinical signs described above (page 469) and may complain only in their late

thirties of disturbances of the cerebral circulation or of the circulation of the lower extremities.

Coarctation between innominate artery and left subclavian, as well as coarctation of the abdominal aorta, are rare possibilities (72). The former causes a *reduced pulsation of the left radial and carotid arteries;* the latter has a less well developed collateral circulation and less difference in pressures between the upper and lower extremities. Notching of the ribs is not visible; pulsation of the abdominal aorta above the umbilicus may be present.

Coarctation of the aorta and atypical origin of the right subclavian artery, arising from the aorta below the constriction, may cause *hypertension in the left arm only* (50).

MECHANISM

The mechanism of production of the hypertension is still under debate. Both the mechanical effect of the constriction and the secondary renal ischemia have been advocated. So far, conflicting evidence has been presented for both theories.

Left ventricular hypertrophy is responsible for left axis deviation in the postductal type. In the preductal, on the contrary, the right ventricle supplies the lower half of the body, thus preventing some of the overload for the left; in these cases, the hypertrophied right ventricle causes right axis deviation. In the former group, the murmur is due to passing of the blood through the narrow section of the aorta in late systole (and even early diastole). In the latter, the murmur is chiefly due to patency of the ductus.

DIAGNOSIS

Diagnosis is simple in the "adult" type because the clinical picture is typical and associated lesions are rare. It is based on the finding of arterial hypertension in the upper extremity with hypotension in the lower, in young patients. However, the possibility of a similar difference of pressure caused by an atheromatous plaque, should not be forgotten. *Cases where the blood pressure of the arm is normal and that of the legs is very low, are possible* (13). In these, even more than in the others, observation of the collateral circulation and x-ray data are of great importance.

The diagnosis is more difficult in children and infants. However, *palpation of the femoral arteries* usually reveals weak or absent pulsation, even in cases with patency of the ductus.

The diagnosis of an abnormally located coarctation is always difficult and an aortic aneurysm must be excluded first.

The most common confusion in adults is between coarctation and essential hypertension.

PROGNOSIS—COMPLICATIONS

The prognosis is better in the postductal type than in the other. Initial heart failure may be revealed by *intermittent claudication* and *night cramps*, the already poor circulation being made more defective by the failure. Death may be caused by *cerebral hemorrhage*[72] or *thrombosis; coronary occlusion; paroxysmal pulmonary edema;* or *rupture of the aorta. Congestive failure* often terminates the clinical course in the other cases. Poor circulation of the lower extremities favors *thromboarteritis of the leg.* A possible complication is represented by a *subacute bacterial infection* with localization on the constricted site (and possibly on an associated bicuspid aortic valve).

TREATMENT

Surgical treatment of this condition has been accomplished successfully. At first anastomosis between the left subclavian and descending aorta was attempted (14). Later, *resection of the narrow aortic section with anastomosis of the aortic ends* became the procedure of choice (15).

In infants with preductal coarctation,

[72] The hemorrhage is usually due to rupture of a congenital cerebral aneurysm.

surgery should be attempted as early as possible. In them, resection of the aorta is successful only if simultaneous ligation of the ductus is performed; this is a dangerous operation which, however, has succeeded in isolated cases (73). Anastomosis of the subclavian artery to the descending aorta has also been tried (51).

In the postductal type, the optimal age for surgery is between 6 and 20 years of age because, later on, *arteriosclerosis* of the descending aorta frequently makes this vessel unsuitable for manipulation and suture (48). However, successful correction has been reported even at the age of 40. Pregnancy is a definite indication for surgery. Stenosis of either the mitral or the aortic valve is a contraindication (74).

When resection of the constricted area is impossible, *thoracolumbar sympathectomy* for relief of the hypertension may be attempted.

Congenital or Dynamic Changes of the Aorta and Pulmonary Artery

a) *Congenital dilatation of the ascending aorta* has been described in rare cases in association with arachnodactyly (17). The patients died between the ages of 14 and 25. The aorta presented malformation of the media, involving both the muscular and the elastic elements. Either a systolic or a double murmur was heard over the aortic area.

b) *Congenital, or idiopathic dilatation of the pulmonary artery* can be found as an isolated abnormality. Dulness, and systolic or double murmur, can be found at the left of the sternum. The right ventricle is not dilated; *the aorta is usually small.* This process is usually asymptomatic. *Catheterization* shows either a normal or a slightly increased gradient of pressure between right ventricle and pulmonary artery. The x-ray aspects of this lesion may simulate an atrial septal defect. The lesion has been attributed to abnormal division of the fetal *truncus* (63); it is often associated with an intrinsic weakness of the arterial wall (7, 18) and the dilatation often extends to the main stems. Atherosclerosis of the pulmonary artery is a frequent complication, even in children. In these cases, *wrapping of the pulmonary artery in cellophane* can be tried, though the experience is not favorable, so far (64).

c) *Dynamic dilatation.* Both the aorta and the pulmonary artery may present a dilatation which is due to increased pressure or flow, not sufficient to cause permanent stretching. Physical examination and x-ray observation reveal a dilatation which, however, is not confirmed by autopsy.

Dynamic dilatation of the aorta is frequently present in aortic insufficiency, aortic stenosis, coarctation of the aorta, patent ductus arteriosus, hypertension, and tetralogy of Fallot.

Dynamic dilatation of the pulmonary artery is frequently found in pulmonic insufficiency, patent ductus arteriosus, atrial septal defect, Eisenmenger complex, and chronic cor pulmonale.

Thyroid, anemic, and thiamine-deficient hearts are frequently associated with dynamic dilatation of both the pulmonary artery and the aorta.

d) *Hypoplasia of the aorta (aorta angusta).* The aorta of these patients is poorly developed but is uniform in its course (19). However, in exceptional cases (75), only the thoracic descending aorta is narrow. Early arteriosclerosis of the vessel may be present. Older descriptions associated a status thymico-lymphaticus with this rare condition. The hypoplasia associated with atrial septal defect is said to be present at birth, whereas other types may be due to faulty development.

X-ray frequently allows recognition of the small caliber of the aorta (fig. 284).

Poor development of the entire body or abnormality of the genitalia may be present. The blood pressure may be normal or low. Cases with high blood pressure probably have some degree of coarctation, even if diffuse hypoplasia is present. Unexplained heart failure or rupture of the aorta may be the result of this condition.

A *secondary or dynamic hypoplasia* is found in patients with low blood pressure or

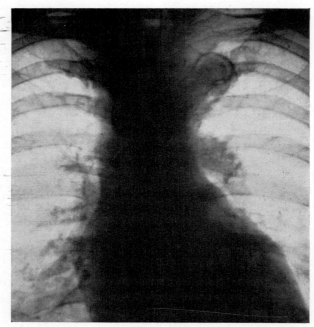

FIG. 284. Cardiac silhouette in a case of aortic hypoplasia with calcified aortic arch.

low cardiac output (mitral stenosis, aortic stenosis, chronic consumptive diseases, etc.).

Aortitis—Atherosclerosis of the Aorta

These two processes have been classified in the past under the same name of "aortitis." It is preferable to keep them apart because of different etiologies and manifestations. However, inasmuch as the two forms can be associated, a clinical differentiation is not always possible.

Aortitis is due to an inflammatory lesion. It may be caused by *rheumatic disease, typhoid, influenza,* or *streptococcic infections* (22a). However, the most frequent cause of aortitis is *syphilis* (page 201).

Atherosclerosis of the aorta, with exceptions, does not occur in young people but, as a rule, is found after 50 and is frequent in old age. It is favored by diabetes, obesity, and hypertension.

LESIONS

The lesions of *acute aortitis* are similar to those of acute arteritis in general (page 529). One type, revealed by extensive areas of inflammation in the intima, seems due to mycotic emboli and may result in multiple aneurysms (20). In some cases, acute aortitis may simulate the aspects of syphilitic aortitis.

Syphilitic aortitis is usually located in a limited portion of the vessel and in one or few of its branches. The ascending aorta and the aortic arch are preferred sites. The descending aorta is usually normal but may be damaged.

The gross changes of the aorta are characteristic. Elevated gray or bluish-gray, translucent *plaques* are present on the surface of the intima. Multiple foci of infiltration, formed by lymphocytes, plasma cells, and, rarely, giant multinuclear cells, are present in the media. The elastic and muscular structures are destroyed or present evidence of degeneration. Miliary gummata may be found in the adventitia. In some areas, the foci are replaced by scar tissue

which may penetrate through the entire thickness of the aorta. The small nourishing vessels are frequently narrowed or occluded. Proliferation of the connective tissue of the intima is typical. The inflammatory foci are *miliary gummata* and may contain *Treponemata.* The aortic lesion is frequently associated with lesions of the aortic valve, and coronary mouths, and also with myocardial, pericardial, and mediastinal lesions.

The *atherosclerotic aorta* is longer and larger than a normal vessel. The typical lesions, which may be present in any section, are frequently located in the abdominal aorta: they are the *atheromatous plaque,* the *atheromatous ulcer,* and the *fibrous plaque.*

Newly-formed blood channels in the aortic wall may favor subintimal hemorrhages. Thrombotic precipitates frequently form on the damaged intima, mainly in the abdominal aorta. A fibrotic process is frequently present in the aortic or the mitral valve, in the coronary arteries, and in the initial parts of the large arteries.

SIGNS AND SYMPTOMS

Mild disturbances may be present for many years. However, the symptoms may start suddenly: *substernal oppression* or *pain, dyspnea, palpitation,* and *obstinate nonproductive cough.* Substernal oppression and pain are often connected with coronary lesions; dyspnea (especially paroxysmal nocturnal dyspnea) may be related to aortic insufficiency. Only cough is related to the aortic lesions and is interpreted as a reflex phenomenon. However, sometimes pain is transmitted *to both arms and is increased by changes in position,* a fact which is typical of the aortic lesion.

Dysphonia and, occasionally, a *bitonal voice* are caused by lesion of the left recurrent nerve. *Dizziness* is frequent and due to cerebral arteriosclerosis or to the dynamic changes of aortic insufficiency. *Weakness* is frequent. *Luetic aortitis* is often accompanied by rigidity of the pupils to light (*Argyll-Robertson's sign*).

The carotid arteries and the suprasternal notch show active pulsations. In particular, *a kinking of the right common carotid artery* due to dilatation of the aortic arch is revealed by intensive pulsations *at the right side of the suprasternal notch.* The aortic arch may be palpated at the suprasternal notch, and a *systolic thrill* is felt in that area. Percussion reveals *a cap of dulness* at the sternal manubrium, encroaching on the 2nd and 3rd right interspaces.

The 2nd aortic sound is ringing and is much louder than normal. This is important in the absence of high blood pressure (23). There frequently is prolongation of the 1st aortic sound or a definite *systolic murmur* over the 2nd right interspace. The murmur may become *musical or similar to the cry of a sea gull.*

The radial pulse is usually *celer;* the abdominal aorta is easily palpable and pulsates strongly. Other signs vary with different localizations (see below).

VARIETIES

Aortitis or atherosclerosis of the ascending aorta and aortic arch.

This localization is frequently accompanied by coronary sclerosis (atherosclerosis) or aortic insufficiency (lues). The right radial pulse is frequently smaller because of narrowing of the mouth of the subclavian artery (atherosclerosis). *Friction rubs* may be heard near the sternum (lues).

GRAPHIC TRACINGS

Electrocardiogram. This tracing may present different patterns caused by associated lesions. Thus, changes due to aortic insufficiency (page 242), hypertension (page 497), bundle branch or intraventricular block (pages 376 and 379), and coronary heart disease (page 434), are frequently encountered. There is no relative bradycardia as in aortic stenosis.

Phonocardiogram. The phonocardiogram may reveal the following data:

1) An *opening click (or snap) of the aortic valve;* this is a high and loud vibration which precedes the rise of the carotid pulse and is due to lesion of the semilunar valves (24).

2) A *triple rhythm* due to addition of a *loud systolic vibration* (so-called *systolic gallop*).

3) The second sound consists of three to four large vibrations and is prolonged by two or three smaller vibrations equivalent to a *short diastolic murmur.*

4) A *systolic murmur* is also frequently present; its vibrations have the aspect of a short, early-systolic murmur, or that of a diamond-shaped murmur. It is recorded best over the second or third right interspaces, but may be loudest at the left of the sternum.

Pulse and pressure tracings. The pulse tracings reveal a steep rise, a sharp peak, and a quick descent. These changes may be due to either aortic insufficiency (syphilis) or increased rigidity of the aortic wall (atherosclerosis) (fig. 285). There is no anacrotic depression as in aortic stenosis. The pulse and pressure tracings of the lower extremities frequently reveal an increased pressure. Atherosclerosis of the aortic arch may cause smaller pulse and lower blood pressure in the arms (narrowing of the subclavian arteries).

There is an *increased pulse pressure* (decreased elasticity of the aorta, chiefly in atherosclerosis) *and a relative increase in pressure of 30 to 50 mm. at the tibial arteries.* Diastolic pressure is low.

X-ray. The ascending aorta is of increased opacity. It is dilated and shows an increased amplitude of pulsations, particularly in the left anterior oblique position. The aortic arch is frequently dilated, as shown both by the profile of the aortic silhouette and by the section of the aortic knob. *Calcification of the ascending aorta and the aortic arch* can be observed in a large percentage of cases

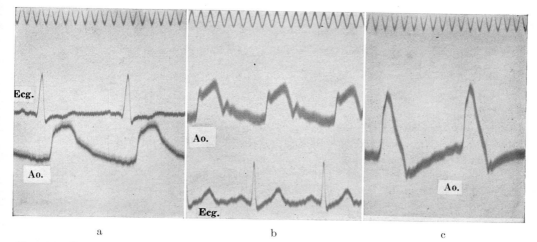

a   b   c

FIG. 285. Tracing of the abdominal aorta in three patients. a, aneurysm of the abdominal aorta; b, atherosclerosis of the aorta; c, abdominal aortitis.

with atherosclerosis of the aorta or aortitis (57).

The so-called *aortic arch syndrome* or *reversed coarctation* consists of weak pulsations of all the vessels of the aortic arch with hypertension of the lower extremities. It may be caused by atherosclerosis, lues, trauma, Buerger's disease, polyarteritis nodosa, or a congenital lesion (76).

Aortitis of the descending aorta (posterior aortitis) (25). This syndrome is usually due to lues. The patient complains of pain which is girdle-like or is fixed in the left interscapular region. The x-ray reveals dilatation and increased density of the descending aorta, mainly apparent in the oblique positions. Areas of calcification are frequently visible.

Abdominal atherosclerosis. The patients complain of *paroxysmal epigastric pain* with posterior radiation. The pain is accompanied by *nausea, pallor*, and occasionally, *anguish* (26). These attacks are usually caused by exertion but may follow meals. When hyperacidity, belching, vomiting, or mucous diarrhea occur, the attacks are easily mistaken for gastrointestinal disorders. Weakness and unpleasant pulsations in the abdomen are present between the attacks.

The abdominal aorta is easily palpated above the umbilicus. It is a sinuous and large vessel with a *strong, expansive pulsation* and is *very tender*. The femoral arteries have strong pulsations and present a *pistol-shot sound* and a *thrill*.

Sectional measurements of blood pressure reveal that *the blood pressure of the femoral and tibial arteries is from 50 to 80 mm. higher than the brachial pressure* (27).

Pulse tracing. The pulse tracing of the femoral arteries has a great amplitude. Its pattern consists of a sharp rise and a rapid drop (fig. 285). Simultaneous pulse tracings of the suprasternal notch and the femoral arteries reveal an *increased speed of the pulse in the descending aorta.*

COURSE AND COMPLICATIONS

The syndromes caused by atherosclerosis have a longer and milder course than those caused by lues. Very often the lesions of the coronary arteries or of the aortic valves dominate the clinical picture. Formation of an *aneurysm* is possible. Hypertension is frequent (29). *Rupture of the aorta* and *formation of a dissecting aneurysm* are dreaded possibilities. Sudden death may occur in the early stages of luetic aortitis (30). Acute pulmonary edema or heart failure are other possibilities.

DIAGNOSIS

The general diagnosis of an aortic lesion is made on the basis of obstinate dry cough, precordial pain influenced by position and transmitted posteriorly, changes of the voice and of pupils, sternal dulness, and suprasternal or epigastric pulsation. The x-ray data are frequently helpful. Different signs are present according to the predominant localization.

Recognition that the aortic lesion is due to syphilis can be made following these criteria (56): age below 40; history or evidence of lues plus positive serology; or, in the absence of unequivocal clinical data, repeatedly positive serology; conditions of the vascular system insufficient to explain dilatation of the aorta.

Differential diagnosis is always more difficult when there is aortic regurgitation.

In elderly people, the diagnosis of atherosclerosis is made only after exclusion of syphilis. Differential diagnosis from aortic aneurysms is not always possible, especially in lesions of the descending or abdominal aorta. In the latter case it has been observed that *compression of the abdominal aorta* decreases the femoral pulse in cases of aortitis but increases it in some cases of aneurysm.

PROGNOSIS

Prognosis is better in the atherosclerotic than in the syphilitic lesions. However, if there is no aneurysm, treatment may limit the extension of the vascular damage in the latter.

TREATMENT

In the case of *atherosclerosis*, the treatment is based on rest, diet, avoidance of strain, hypotensive and vasodilator drugs, and sedatives. *Potassium iodide* (**73**) may be helpful.

General dietary measures *restricting fat and especially cholesterol intake*, and *use of* *estrogens* are under study (page 528). They may not only check the progress of atherosclerosis, but also cause its regression.

In the case of *luetic aortitis*, antisyphilitic treatment gives symptomatic relief and may arrest the progress of the disease. This treatment may be effective if started early; much less so if the lesions are far advanced; it is often impossible to treat the patient if there is heart failure. The most commonly accepted plans of treatment have been already sketched (page 201).

The treatment of patients with cardiac failure is that common to the condition.

Atherosclerosis or Arteritis of the Pulmonary Artery

Atherosclerosis of the pulmonary artery is much rarer than that of the aorta. It is encountered in cases with hypertension of the lesser circulation, secondary to congenital, pulmonary or mitral diseases; it will be discussed below (page 510). The possibility of a *primary atherosclerosis* has been advocated but proof of this is lacking.

Pulmonary arteritis may be caused by rheumatic disease, or by gonococcic or pneumococcic infections. Luetic arteritis is possible; in most of the cases it is transmitted from the aorta through a patent ductus or by way of mediastinal inflammation. There are, however, cases of isolated luetic arteritis.

Because of the thin wall of the pulmonary artery, both atherosclerosis and arteritis frequently determine the formation of an aneurysm of this vessel.

Aortic Aneurysms

Aneurysm is the partial or diffuse dilatation of an artery.

CAUSE

The great majority of aneurysms are due to *syphilis*. Diffuse arteritis is followed by weakening of the wall and by a more severe, localized lesion. A few aneurysms are caused by *rheumatic disease*. *Atherosclerosis* may cause aneurysms, especially in the abdominal aorta. *Arterial hypertension* and *trauma* favor the formation of aneurysms. Rare congenital aneurysms of the aorta, in association with various other congenital lesions, have been described.

LESIONS

The aneurysm may be *elongated (fusiform)* or *pouch-like (saccular)*. When the aortic wall ruptures and the blood is contained by the surrounding structures and by a limiting membrane of connective tissue, there is a *periaortic hematoma (aneurysma spurius)*. Penetration of blood between the aortic walls creates a *dissecting aneurysm* (page 485).

Thirty-two per cent of the aneurysms are in the ascending aorta, 40 per cent in the aortic arch, 12 per cent in the descending aorta, and 7.2 in the abdominal aorta. The others are either multiple or in the aortic bulbus (31) (fig. 286). Therefore, the ascending aorta and the arch are the most common seats of aneurysms.

The wall of the aneurysm consists of connective tissue and is supported by the surrounding layers; these are thickened by an inflammatory reaction, partly due to mechanical irritation and partly to the specific cause of the aortitis. The process contributes to containment of pressure but also favors extension by slowly invading the surrounding structures.

The *size* of the aneurysm is extremely variable, from that of a green pea to that of a child's head.

The blood contained in the pouch may remain fluid; in such a case the aneurysm acts like a *reservoir* which dilates during systole and shrinks with diastole. In many cases, however, stratified, whitish thrombi fill the pouch, which behaves like a *solid mass*. The thrombi usually do not organize because the wall is unable to produce newly formed blood channels.

The aneurysm may penetrate all surrounding structures and break through the

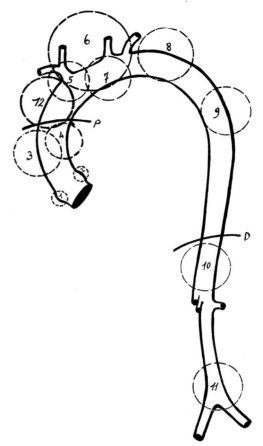

Fig. 286. Possible location of aneurysms. 1, 2, sinus of Valsalva; 3, 4, intrapericardial; 5, right aortic angle; 6, convexity of arch; 7, concavity of arch; 8, left aortic angle; 9, descending aorta; 10, 11, abdominal aorta; 12, ascending aorta; P, pericardium; D, diaphragm.

chest wall or rupture into the pericardial or pleural cavities, the esophagus, the trachea, a bronchus, or one of the venae cavae. Sometimes the rupture occurs through a minute hole which closes later, permitting survival of the patient.

SYMPTOMS AND SIGNS

The main signs and symptoms can be grouped under three different headings: compression phenomena, physical signs directly due to the mass, and changes of circulatory dynamics.

COMPRESSION PHENOMENA

The *sensitive nerves* react to compression and irritation with a sensation of *pain*, radiating to the neck, back, and arms; this may be elicited by changes in position, effort, or deep respiration. Lesion of one of the *recurrent nerves* causes hoarse or bitonal voice through paralysis of the respective vocal cord. Lesion of the *vagus* may cause dysphagia, vomiting, or bradycardia. Lesion of the *phrenic nerve* causes hiccup and, possibly, a unilateral paralysis of the diaphragm. Lesion of the *sympathetic chain* of one side causes vasomotor, thermal, and perspiration disturbances; among them, *ipsilateral dilatation of the pupil* is typical.

Compression of the *trachea* or one of the *main bronchi* produces obstinate *cough* and *stridor*; there may be *atelectasis* of one of the pulmonary lobes. Pressure on the lung parenchyma or on a bronchus may cause *hemoptysis*.

Compression of the *esophagus* may cause *dysphagia*.

Compression of the *large venous collectors* (innominate trunks, superior cava, azygos) causes severe venous congestion.

Compression of the *thoracic duct* may cause edema, or abdominal effusion (pseudo-chylous effusion).

Compression of one or more *arteries* is possible and may lead to unilateral or bilateral disappearance of the radial pulse.

PHYSICAL SIGNS DUE TO THE MASS

When the aneurysm expands outward, it may create a round *mass* which has an *expansive pulsation*. The apex impulse may be in an abnormal site because of displacement of the heart. There may be a *double pulsation*; the systolic impulse is then followed by *a diastolic thrust*, caused by the recoil of the retrocardiac aneurysm (32a).

Percussion may reveal an aneurysm before it has reached the chest wall.

Auscultation of the mass reveals the heart sounds and, frequently, a *double murmur*, caused by the blood entering and leaving the pouch through a narrow entrance. Distinction between this and the murmurs of an aortic valvular lesion is not always possible.

Auscultation at the mouth may reveal a *rhythmic oral whiff* (32b). The trachea presents rhythmic pulsations when the cricoid cartilage is raised (*tracheal tug*) (33a) and when it is pushed toward the left (33b); it transmits the cardiac sounds clearly (33c). The head of the patient may present rhythmic nodding movements (34).

CHANGES OF CIRCULATORY DYNAMICS

These take place when the sac is large, elastic, and contains fluid blood. The sac behaves like *a reservoir* because it distends in systole, decreasing the systolic pressure below it by virtue of its capacity, and retracts in diastole, increasing the diastolic pressure below it. Therefore, a comparison between an artery above and one below the sac reveals that the pulse is smaller and has a slower rise (*pulsus tardus*) in the arteries placed below. The *slow rise gives the impression of a delayed pulse because the palpating finger feels the peak and not the onset of the wave* (35). Actual delay does not occur (78). Certain aneurysms increase the amplitude of the pulse, distal to the sac, if they have a rigid wall (35).

VARIETIES

Aneurysms of the Valsalva Sinuses (36, 61)

These aneurysms are rare. They may be favored by congenital dilatation and may be caused by syphilis or bacterial infection (more frequently in cases of bacterial endocarditis). Aneurysm of the right sinus is relatively more common and compresses the right ventricle. It may rupture into the right atrium or ventricle or into the left ventricle creating a *cardio-aortic fistula*. The fistula is revealed by a *continuous machinery murmur* behind the sternum having greater variations of intensity in the case of the ventricles. Aortic insufficiency, bundle branch block and even A-V block are not infrequently caused by this type of aneurysm. It may rupture into the pericardial sac causing *hemopericardium* and *tamponade*.

Aneurysm of the left sinus compresses the pulmonary artery causing right ventricular enlargement and cyanosis. It may rupture into that artery giving physical signs which simulate a patent ductus (page 291); the murmur, however, is of maximal intensity in the 3rd and not in the 2nd left interspace.

Aneurysm of the posterior sinus may rupture into the left atrium or ventricle again creating a *cardio-aortic fistula* and a *rough machinery murmur.*

Intrapericardial Aneurysm of the Ascending Aorta (37)

It may develop toward the right or toward the left. That developing *toward the right* causes the following signs: *attacks of paroxysmal dyspnea and precordial pain*, often transmitted to the right arm; *severe cyanosis and edema* in the upper part of the body and head (compression of the superior cava); *diffuse venous engorgement* with peripheral edema and hepatic enlargement (compression of the right atrium); *or a bulge in the 3rd or 4th right interspace having a nonexpansive pulsation.* The *electrocardiogram* presents *left axis deviation* and, possibly, a *small or flat P wave.* The *x-ray* shows a shadow which displaces the angle between right atrium and vascular pedicle downward.

The aneurysm developing *toward the left* causes a greater increase of the transverse diameter of the heart. There frequently are signs of congestion simulating congestive failure. *There is a nonexpansive pulsating bulge in the 3rd and 4th left interspaces.* The *electrocardiogram* presents *no axis deviation* and a *high P wave.* The *x-ray* reveals a deformity of the left border of the cardiac silhouette.

Death is caused by rupture into the pericardial cavity, the pulmonary artery, one of the atria, the superior cava, the esophagus, the right ventricle, or one of the lungs.

When there is rupture into another vessel, death is delayed. Auscultatory signs, caused by the *fistula*, become apparent.

Aneurysm of the Ascending Aorta in the Extrapericardial Section

This is one of the most common sites for aortic aneurysm. The sac develops anteriorly and toward the right, creating an expansive *pulsating bulge in the 2nd and 3rd (occasionally 4th) right interspaces.* There is dulness at the right of the sternum, a systolic thrill, and a systolic or double murmur. There often is *tracheal tug.* The radial pulses are equal. The cardiac apex may have a *double impulse* or a *diastolic thrust.* The aneurysm may cause compression of the superior cava, the right innominate vein, or the innominate artery. Therefore, diffuse edema of the upper part of the body, edema of the right side of the chest and right arm, and a small radial and carotid pulse on the right, may occur. The aneurysm may enlarge toward the right supraclavicular region causing displacement of the trachea to the left, and paralysis of the right recurrent nerve. In rare cases, the sac may cause a symmetrical pulsation on both sides of the sternum.

The *x-ray* reveals a large shadow at the right of the sternum, especially apparent in the left anterior oblique position (fig. 287A). The *electrocardiogram* frequently reveals atrial tachycardia, premature beats, or fibrillation.

Rupture may take place into the pericardium, the pulmonary artery, the right pleura, one of the atria, or outwards.

Aneurysm of the Aortic Arch

This is one of the most common aortic aneurysms. When not too large, the signs of compression are moderate and only changes of the pulse are typical; *the left radial pulse is smaller and may be delayed when compared with the right.* There is *tracheal tug*, nonproductive cough, bitonal voice, dysphagia, attacks of paroxysmal dyspnea, and precordial pain. If the sac

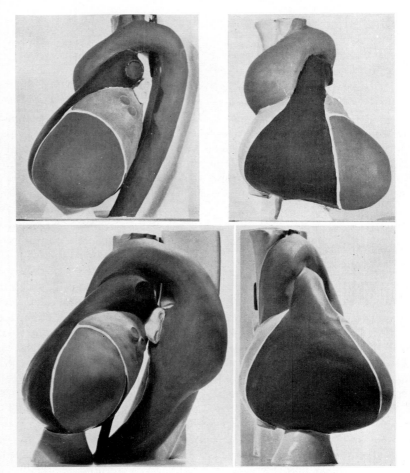

FIG. 287. Cardiovascular lues. a, aneurysm of ascending aorta and aortic regurgitation; b, aneurysm of descending aorta (from originals of the American Heart Association).

becomes large, there may be compression of the trachea and of the innominate veins. The aneurysm usually bulges at the suprasternal notch and in both supraclavicular regions; it may lift and later perforate the manubrium.

The *x-ray* chiefly reveals a round shadow in the oblique positions.

Rupture may occur into the left bronchus, the trachea, the esophagus, the pleural cavities, the pulmonary artery, or outwards.

Aneurysm of the Descending Aorta

This often develops insidiously for a long time, then suddenly causes compression of essential organs. Thoracic or lumbar pain

have been observed for as long as 10 or 15 years. Then, boring pain develops in the back, left shoulder, or left side; stiffness of the back may occur. The aneurysm may cause dysphagia and, by destroying the spine, paraplegia. It may cause left pleural effusion. It may push the heart forward. There may be a pulsating mass at the left of the spine (22b). *Hematemesis* and *hemop- tysis* are frequent. *The pulse of the femoral arteries may be small and seem delayed* over that of the upper extremities.

X-ray in the lateral and in the left anterior oblique positions may reveal the aneurysm (fig. 287B). There may be dense shadows due to *calcified plaques*. A barium swallow may show deviation of the esophagus and a clear indentation caused by the aneurysm.

Rupture may occur backwards, through the chest wall, into the esophagus, or into one of the pleural cavities.

Aneurysm of the Abdominal Aorta

Aneurysms of the upper part are usually luetic; those of the lower, arteriosclerotic. Luetic aneurysms cause *dull, aching, sharp, or throbbing pain* in the abdomen or back; arteriosclerotic aneurysms cause pain only if large. There may be episodes simulating ileus paralyticus, caused by mechanical compression of the intestines or lesions of the mesenteric arteries.

The aneurysm is usually palpable as a pulsating mass in the supraumbilical region. *The pulsation is expansive.* A rough systolic murmur, rarely a double murmur, is audible over the mass. *The pulse of the femoral and tibial arteries is small and delayed.* Compression of the mass causes normalization of the pulse.

The *graphic tracings* of the mass reveal a rounded and slow pulsation which is different from that of abdominal aortitis (fig. 285).

The *x-ray* may reveal the aneurysm if the wall is calcified. Insufflation of the colon and distention of the stomach with gas may permit visualization of the mass. The *aortogram* permits visualization of the mass in difficult cases; *exploratory laparotomy* has been occasionally resorted to (38).

GENERAL DIAGNOSIS

The diagnosis of aortic aneurysms is easy when they are of average size. It may be difficult when the aneurysm is either very small or very large, and when the blood is clotted within the aneurysm so that the sac behaves like a tumor. The most difficult diagnoses are those of aneurysms of the Valsalva sinuses and those of the abdominal aorta. *X-ray data* are always of great value while roentgenkymography, and especially electrokymography, are helpful for the differential diagnosis between aneurysms and mediastinal tumors (60). Mediastinal tumors may reveal a transmitted pulsation (border tracing), not an expansion (densogram). Aneurysms, on the contrary, present both a transmitted and an expansive pulsation (border tracing similar to densogram).

Angiocardiography has proven useful in the diagnosis of aneurysms of the sinus of Valsalva before perforation (59). *Catheterization* reveals the shunt if there has been perforation.

Differential diagnosis should exclude: mediastinal tumors, cardiac tumors, cardiac cysts, goiter, abscesses, localized pericarditis, and many other more rare conditions.

PROGNOSIS

Prognosis is always guarded. The earlier the diagnosis, the longer the course. Early antiluetic treatment, symptomatic treatment, and rest may improve the outlook.

TREATMENT

The medical treatment of the aneurysm is that of the underlying aortitis or atherosclerosis (pages 201 and 528). Rest is very important and frequently causes a remarkable improvement.

Pain may be controlled by the use of analgesics and sedatives or by the *paravertebral injection of alcohol* into the ganglia in order to destroy the pathways of pain. The latter may be preceded by *injection of novocain* which, by giving temporary relief of pain, shows the effectiveness of the more radical procedure.

Surgery of the aneurysms becomes more and more effective. Small aneurysms and the large ones where the vessels are not diseased (those following wounds) respond best to *end-to-end suture of the vessel.* In general, those of the abdominal aorta are the easiest to approach. Aneurysms of the lower thoracic aorta have been resected in a few cases. Ligation of the thoracic aorta, however, is not possible unless there is coarctation of the aorta with an extensive collateral circulation.

In the case of large thoracic aneurysms, the best technique seems to be the *wrapping of the pouch in polythene cellophane* (58). This causes an intense fibrotic reaction preventing further expansion with eventual rupture, and reducing the existing dilatation. When venous engorgement is present, *venesection* may increase the patient's comfort.

Aneurysm of the Pulmonary Artery and Its Branches (62)

CAUSE—LESIONS

Because of weaker structure, the pulmonary artery is easily distensible. The principal dilatation occurs in the anterior and lateral parts of the trunk where the elastic and muscular components are particularly thin. The dilatation often involves part or all of the left stem which is like a prolongation of the trunk. However, both branches may be involved. Congenital anomalies, atherosclerosis of the pulmonary artery, and hypertension of the lesser circulation are the most frequent causes. Syphilis is present in nearly one-third of the cases. Other infections may initiate the changes in mitral or congenital cases which already have high pressure in the pulmonary artery. Among the most common congenital lesions, patent ductus arteriosus, high atrial septal defect, and Eisenmenger complex are associated most frequently with this type of aneurysm. Lutembacher's syndrome follows.

SIGNS AND SYMPTOMS

Cyanosis, orthopnea, and *precordial pain,* mainly localized in the 2nd and 3rd left interspaces, are common. Tracheal tug is usually absent while *paralysis of the left vocal cord is possible.* There may be bloody sputum.

The heart becomes broader on percussion. There is a *cap of dulness* in the 2nd and 3rd left interspaces, usually with *no bulge* and *no pulsation.* There may be a systolic thrill.

In most cases, auscultation reveals a *systolic murmur* over the 2nd left interspace; occasionally a *diastolic murmur* is also heard if the pulmonic valve is involved or the ostium is dilated.

The *electrocardiogram* reveals *right axis deviation.* There may be abnormalities of S-T and T if the left coronary artery is compressed.

The *x-ray* reveals a rounded shadow, actively pulsating, to the left of the heart which is particularly evident in the right anterior oblique. *The whole cardiac shadow becomes more triangular* because of cardiac rotation and burying of the apex into the diaphragm. The Valsalva test (page 85) shows a dilatation of the aneurysm on fluoroscopy. There may be unilateral or bilateral *hilar dance.*

Angiocardiography and *catheterization of the heart* give definite data in difficult cases. Abnormally high pressure in the pulmonary artery should be considered evidence against a congenital aneurysm of this artery.

COMPLICATIONS

Thrombosis of the pulmonary artery may be the cause of death. Congestive failure is otherwise inevitable. Rupture of the aneurysm is not common and never takes place externally.

DIAGNOSIS

Diagnosis is possible after exclusion of aortic aneurysms, paracardiac tumors, and cysts. It should be kept in mind that the aneurysm may complicate a congenital lesion.

Rupture of the Aorta and Dissecting Aneurysm

Complete Rupture of the Aorta (42, 44)

Traumatic rupture of the aorta is rare; it may occur when a terrific blow is given the thorax and sudden torsion of the head and trunk takes place. The rupture usually occurs at the junction of the arch and the descending aorta, probably because the latter is the most mobile portion.

Spontaneous rupture of the aorta may occur at any age. It may be caused by rupture of a luetic, atherosclerotic, or mycotic aneurysm; it may be connected with coarctation or hypoplasia of the aorta; or it may be due to secondary rupture of a dissecting aneurysm. In some cases, no apparent aortic lesion, or only abnormal thinness of the wall, is present.

Arterial hypertension is a favoring cause in about one-half of the cases. In older patients, arteriosclerotic changes are frequent. In the young, the most common causes are toxic or infectious, but degenerative changes may be present. Alteration of blood lipids, which occurs in pregnancy, may be another cause. Medial necrosis is usually present (page 526).

Death is usually sudden. It may be delayed if the rupture occurs in stages or if the blood flow is temporarily dammed by mediastinal structures or serous membranes.

Incomplete Rupture of the Aorta (43)

This condition takes place after tearing of the wall but before dissection. The tear usually occurs in the ascending aorta, often near one of the leaflets. It may be oblique or longitudinal but is usually transverse. It varies from 5 to 20 mm. in length. The condition is not rare; it is favored by a local predisposition (aortic hypoplasia, aortic coarctation, etc.) and by arterial hypertension. Trauma or effort may precipitate it.

The most common symptom is a *choking sensation* followed by *stabbing or tearing pain.* Occasionally, *cough, bloody sputum,* and *fever* are present.

A *systolic or diastolic aortic murmur or both* are frequently heard after the rupture. The systolic murmur is harsh and seems due to vibrations caused by the abrupt edge of the tear. The diastolic murmur is soft and caused by *aortic insufficiency.* This is due to dilatation of the initial part of the aorta,

lack of support of one or more cusps, and loosening of the commissures.

Incomplete rupture may heal. On the other hand, it may be followed by a dissecting aneurysm, either within a short time or after a new tear.

Dissecting Aneurysm

CAUSE AND LESIONS

Dissecting aneurysm has the same causes and is favored by the same conditions as aortic rupture because it is the most common outcome of the latter. Atherosclerosis, aortitis, or hypertension, are commonly found in the old-age groups. In younger patients, coarctation, hypoplasia, or congenital thinness of the aorta, or pregnancy, may favor dissection. Pregnancy causes changes of the blood lipids, and dissection usually occurs before labor (44c).

The most frequent seats of the tear are the ascending aorta, shortly above the valves, and the aortic arch at the isthmus; the descending or abdominal aorta may be involved.

It is thought that *dissection starts in the media* with a transverse or oblique tear. Rupture of the intima follows immediately, and the blood penetrates between media and adventitia, either in one direction or in both (fig. 288). The cause of the necrosis of the media (page 526) is still somewhat obscure.

Sometimes the dissection of the aortic wall proceeds along the entire vessel reaching the semilunar valves on one end and the bifurcation at the other.

After a period of from a few minutes to some days after the initial tear, *the adventitia also ruptures.* This causes a *hemorrhage* into the pericardium, the pleura, or the peritoneum, and is followed by death. If the hemorrhage is intrapericardial, there is compression of the atria and *tamponade.* If it is in the other serous cavities, there is *vascular collapse* and death.

In rare cases, a new endothelial coating of the newly-formed cavity takes place and the

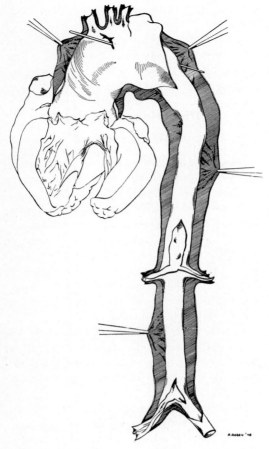

FIG. 288. Dissecting aneurysm of the aorta. (From the New England J. Med. Courtesy of Dr. T. B. Mallory and the Massachusetts Med. Soc.)

aorta becomes *like a double-barrel gun* until a new rupture takes place.

It is common for the dissecting aneurysm to cause compression of one or more of the large arteries. The coronaries, the carotid, the subclavian, or the iliac arteries, are usually involved.

SIGNS AND SYMPTOMS

Pain is the most important sign. It starts suddenly and is *boring* and *tearing* in nature. It is deeply located and is transmitted *toward the back and both arms*. Transmission *toward the groin and both legs* may occur later but is initial when the tear is in the abdominal aorta. Thus the distribution of pain gives a clue to the progressive dissection of the aorta. The pain may become similar to that of angina pectoris if there is compression of the coronary arteries. Rare cases present a *silent dissection* (66).

Pulsation of a sternoclavicular joint has been reported.

Vascular collapse and *fainting* may occur initially or may be delayed, occurring as a terminal episode. Compression of different arteries may cause the *disappearance of the radial and carotid pulses on one or both sides;* numbness and paresthesias are usually associated. Later, *disappearance of the femoral pulse,* paraplegia, numbness of the legs, and urinary disturbances may occur.

Sudden onset of a *diastolic murmur,* strange splashing noises, or *friction rubs* may appear over the aortic area.

The *blood pressure* may be normal or elevated but *drops suddenly in most cases.* It should be measured in different arteries in order to exclude a local drop, caused by compression of an artery by the aneurysm.

Hematuria, anuria, or *ileus paralyticus may be present.* Slight fever, leucocytosis, and increased sedimentation rate are frequently observed.

The *x-ray* may reveal a diffuse increase of the aortic caliber.

The *electrocardiogram* does not show typical changes. Decreased voltage, inverted T and raised S-T, have been encountered and are probably caused by compression of the coronary arteries. The ECG may reveal the occurrence of a myocardial infarction due to the same mechanism (44b, d).

COURSE AND COMPLICATIONS

The course may vary from a few minutes to many days. In rare cases, *clinical healing* takes place through canalization of the channel and formation of a new endothelium (65). Autopsy reveals in such cases the so-called *double-barrel aorta.* Sometimes a progressive increase or extension of the symptoms and signs takes place. Cerebral ischemia may cause monoplegia, hemiplegia, or disturbance of speech. The signs of effusion in one of the pleural cavities, usually the left, are due to rupture of the aneurysm and precede death only by a short time. *Friction rubs* may be caused by rupture into the pericardial cavity. *Slight jaundice* may be caused by absorption of blood pigment from a periaortic hematoma.

DIAGNOSIS

The diagnosis of dissecting aneurysm is now frequently made during life. Differential diagnosis between incomplete rupture and dissecting aneurysm is based on the compression phenomena and the more diffuse pain of the latter. *Angiocardiography* may be used, after the acute state is over, and may permit demonstration of the size and extent of the aneurysm (67). Differential diagnosis from pulmonary embolism and myocardial infarction is necessary and may be difficult. The most difficult cases are those having a secondary myocardial infarct (page 417).

TREATMENT

There is no treatment for the rupture. *Bed rest* and *morphine* may prevent the extension of an incomplete rupture and the formation of a dissecting aneurysm. Once the latter is formed, rest may further delay rupture of the aneurysm. Once the acute stage is over, *wrapping of the aorta in cellophane* may be tried (67). This procedure, if successful, may alleviate the symptoms and permit a normal activity.

Embolism and Thrombosis of the Abdominal Aorta (45)

These conditions are unusual, but very serious, and are relatively more frequent in maturity.

Aortic embolism is usually due to detachment of small mitral or aortic vegetations or larger mural thrombi of the left atrial appendage or the left ventricle. Therefore, the occurrence of aortic embolism may take place in bacterial endocarditis, in mitral stenosis, or after myocardial infarction.

The symptoms and signs vary according to the size of the embolus, the site at which it has lodged, the degree of secondary thrombosis, and the extension of the collateral circulation.

A large embolus, lodging at the bifurcation of the aorta, gives *sudden, excruciating pain in the abdomen or back with nausea and vomiting;* it is followed by severe pain in one or both legs, then by numbness and complete loss of sensation. The lower extremities are pallid and cold and no pulsation can be felt in their arteries.

Death usually occurs within a few days through gangrene of one or both legs. In rare cases, the collateral circulation is so adequate that only *intermittent claudication* results (page 534).

Surgical intervention consists of *embolectomy* and must be performed early (at least in the first 24 hours), in order to be successful. Usual therapy for shock, early application of alternating suction and pressure on the extremities, and *papaverine* by injection (52) are part of the medical treatment.

Slow, progressive thrombosis of the abdominal aorta is possible (46); it results in occlusion of the vessel and ischemia of the lower extremities. This condition may be caused by: a) severe ulcerative arteriosclerosis of the aortic wall, b) embolism to the bifurcation, or c) thrombosis of the pelvic arteries after irradiation. It has a slow, protracted course and may not cause gangrene of the lower extremities. Its occurrence is revealed by weakness in the legs after exercise (*bilateral intermittent claudication*) and *absence of the pulse* in both femoral arteries.

The condition may be followed by signs of visceral infarction and, much later, by arterial hypertension if the thrombus slowly extends upwards.

BIBLIOGRAPHY

1. ARKIN, A. Am. Heart J., 1936, **11**, 444.
2. BEDFORD, D. E., AND PARKINSON, J. Brit. J. Radiol., 1936, **9**, 776.
3. a) ASSMAN, H. *Die klinische Roentgendiagnostik der inneren Erkrankungen.* Leipzig, Vogel, 1924.
   b) NEUHAUSER, E. B. D. Am. J. Roentgenol. 1946, **56**, 1.
4. a) LIAN, C., AND MARCHAL, M. Arch. Mal. Coeur, 1937, **30**, 649.
   b) ROUTIER, D., AND HEIM DE BALZAC, R. Arch. Mal. Coeur, 1937, **30**, 504.
   c) ROUTIER, D., JOLY, F., AND HEIM DE BALZAC, R. Ann. Méd., 1937, **41**, 210.
5. BROWN, J. W. *Congenital Heart Disease.* London, J. Bale Publ., 1939.
6. FRANKE, H. Deut. Arch. klin. Med., 1940, **186**, 304.
7. ABBOTT, M. E. In *Nelson Loose Leaf Medicine.* New York, Nelson, 1944.
8. PEZZI, C., AND AGOSTONI, G. Cuore e Circ., 1928, **12**, 525. Also Cardiol., 1937, **1**, 125.
9. GRISHMAN, A., SUSSMAN, M. L. AND STEINBERG, M. F. Am. Heart J., 1944, **27**, 217.
10. MAYCOCK, W. H. Am. Heart J., 1937, **13**, 633.
11. BLUMGART, H. L., LAWRENCE, J. S., AND ERNSTENE, A. C. Arch. Int. Med., 1931, **47**, 806.
12. STEELE, J. M., AND COHN, A. E. J. Clin. Investigation, 1938, **17**, 514.
13. WHITE, P. D., *Heart Disease.* New York, Macmillan, 1944.
14. BLALOCK, A., AND PARK, E. A. Ann. Surg. 1944, **119**, 445.
15. a) GROSS, R. E., AND HUFNAGEL, C. A. New England. J. Med., 1945, **233**, 287.
    b) GROSS, R. E. New England Heart Assoc., 1945, **233**, 586.
    c) CRAFOORD, C., AND NYLIN, G. J. Thoracic Surg., 1945, **14**, 339.
    d) GROSS, R. E., AND WARE, P. F. Surg., Gynec. & Obst., 1946, **83**, 435.
16. PERLMAN, L. Am. Heart J., 1944, **28**, 24.
17. BAER, W., TAUSSIG, H. B., AND OPPENHEIMER, E. Bull. Johns Hopkins Hosp., 1943, **72**, 309.
18. a) WAETJEN, J. Deut. med.Woch., 1924, **50**, 713.
    b) COSTA, A. Arch. Pat., Clin. Med., 1928, **7**, 329; and 1930, **9**, 305.
19. a) MORGAGNI, G. B. *De Sedibus et Causis Morborum.* English trans.; reprinted in *Cardiac Classics* by Willius and Keys. St. Louis, Mosby, 1941.
    b) ROKITANSKY, C. *Handb. der path. Anat.,* 1842.
    c) VIRCHOW, R. *Ueber die Chlorose und die damit zusammenhaengende Anomalien im Gefaessapparate.* Berlin, 1872.

d) IKEDA, K. Minn. Med., 1932, **16**, 172.
e) VALENTINE, W. N., AND RUSSELL, J. N. Am. Heart J., 1945, **30**, 514.
20. a) EPPINGER. Quoted by COSTA (b).
    b) COSTA, A. Clin. Med. Ital., 1930, **61**, 443.
21. MUSSAFIA, A. Cuore e Circ., 1941, **25**, 257.
22. a) PAPPENHEIM, A. M., AND VON GLAHN, W. C. Am. J. Path., 1926, **2**, 15.
    b) VON GLAHN, W. C. In *Nelson Loose Leaf Medicine.* New York, Nelson, 1944.
23. a) ALLBUTT, C. *Diseases of the Arteries.* London, Macmillan, 1915.
    b) HERMANN, G. R. *Synopsis of Diseases of the Heart and Arteries.* Mosby, St. Louis, 1941.
24. WOLFERTH, C., AND MARGOLIES, A. In *Stroud's Cardiovascular Disease.* Philadelphia, Davis, 1945.
25. LAUBRY, C. *Les Sindromes d'Aortite Postérieure.* Paris, Masson.
26. BACCELLI, G. *Patologia del Cuore e dell' Aorta.* Roma, 1867. Also Rif. Med., 1898, **2**, 152.
27. a) TEISSIER, L. J. Semaine Méd., 1902, 389.
    b) MOUGEOT, A. Paris Med., 1919, **9**, 374.
28. LUISADA, A. A. *Cardiologia.* Bologna, Cappelli, 1938.
29. BOYD, L. J., AND SCHERF, D. Urol. and Cut. Rev., 1942, **46**, N. 3.
30. LEARY, T. New England J. Med., 1940, **223**, 789.
31. COSTA, A. Cuore e Circ., 1930, **14**, 481.
32. a) HOPE, J. *A Treatise on the Diseases of the Heart and Great Vessels.* Philadelphia, Haswell and Johnson, 1842.
    b) DRUMMOND, D. Proc. Northumb. a. Durham Med. Soc., 1888–9, 158.
33. a) OLIVER, T. Lancet, 1878, **2**, 406.
    b) CARDARELLI, A. *Gli Aneurismi dell'Aorta.* Naples, Pasquale, 1868. Also Giorn. Intern. Sci. Med. (Naples), 1894, **16**, 361 and 481.
    c) GROCCO, P. Lavori Congr. Med. Int., Roma, 1903, **12**, 191.
34. a) FELETTI, R. Atti. Congr. Ital. Med. Int., Roma, 1895; and Gazz. Osp. (Milan), 1895.
    b) FRENKEL, H. Rev. Med., 1902, **22**, 604.
    c) BOCCIARDO, C. Policl. (sez. med.), 1906, **13**, 56.
35. a) MAREY, E. J. *La Méthode Graphique dans les Sciences Expérimentales.* Paris, Masson, 1885.
    b) FRANÇOIS-FRANCK. Ctr. Soc. Biol., 1880, 6s, **5**, 387; 1880, 7s, **1**, 276; and 1886, 8s, **3**, 1.
36. a) PISTOCCHI, G. Mal. Cuore, Vasi; 1921, **5**, 125.
    b) MACLEOD, A. Brit. Heart. J., 1944, **6**, 194.

c) WARTHEN, R. O. Am. Heart J. 1949, **37**, 975.

37. MARTINI, T., AND JOSELEVICH, M. *Les Anévrismes Intrapéricardiques de l'Aorte.* Buenos Aires, Mercatali, 1931.

38. a) SCOTT, V. Am. J. Syph., Gon., Ven. Dis., 1944, **28**, 682.

b) PRATT-THOMAS, H. R. So. Car. Med. Assoc. J., 1944, **40**, 251.

39. a) HENSCHEN, S. E. *Das Aneurysma Arteriae Pulmonalis.* Leipzig, Breitkopf and Hartel, 1906 (Samm. klin. Beitr., **15**, 2/3, N. 422–423).

b) COSTA, A. Arch. Pat. Clin. Med., 1929, **8**, 257.

40. a) LUISADA, A. A. Min. Med., 1934 (2), **25**, 421.

b) GROEDEL, F. M. Radiol., 1939, **33**, 219.

c) BOYD, L. J., AND MCGAVACK, T. H. Mo. Conc. Cardiov. Dis., 1941, **10**, n. 2.

41. ALEXANDER, J., AND BYRON, F. X. J. A. M. A., 1944, **126**, 1139.

42. a) TAYLOR, F. R., AND MOREHEAD, R. P. Ann. Int. Med., 1944, **21**, 81.

b) MCDONALD, J. B., AND CAMPBELL, W. A. Am. Heart. J., 1945, **30**, 321.

43. a) GALLAVARDIN, L. AND GRAVIER, L. Paris Méd., 1922, **45**, 29.

b) MARESCH, R. Wien klin. Woch., 1929, **42**, 417.

c) PEERY, T. M. Arch. Int. Med., 1942, **70**, 689.

44. a) GLENDY, R. E., CASTLEMAN, B., AND WHITE, P. D. Am. Heart J., 1937, **13**, 129.

b) WEISS, S. New England J. Med., 1938, **218**, p. 512.

c) SCHNITKER, M. A., AND BAYER, C. A. Ann. Int. Med., 1944, **20**, 486.

d) WAINWRIGHT, C. W. Bull. Johns Hopkins Hosp., 1944, **75**, 89.

45. a) FRY, F. W. Mo. Conc. Cardiov. Dis., 1940, **9**, N. 5.

b) MOREST, F. S., AND RUBIN, S. Am. Heart J., 1948, **36**, 227.

46. STRAUS, R., DOMINGUEZ, R., AND MERLISS, R. Am. J. M. Sci., 1946, **211**, 421.

47. GROSSI, L., AND SEITUN, F. Cuore e Circ. (Rome), 1948, **32**, 271.

48. GROSS, R. E. Mo. Conc. Cardiov. Dis., 1947, **139**, 285.

49. TAUSSIG, H. B. *Congenital Malformations of the Heart.* New York, Commonwealth Fund, 1948.

50. ESPINOSA, O. H.: Rev. Arg. Card., 1948, **15**, 68.

51. JOHNSON, J., AND KIRBY, C. K. Am. Surg., 1948, **127**, 1119.

52. BRAMWELL, C. Brit. Heart J., 1947, **9**, 100.

53. CAMPBELL, M., AND SUZMAN, S.: Brit. Heart J., 1947, **9**, 185.

54. EDWARDS, J. E. Med. Clin. North America, 1948, 925.

55. NEUHAUSER, E. B. D. Am. J. Roentgenol., 1946, **56**, 1.

56. DE LA CHAPELLE, C. E. New York Med., 1947, **3**, 17.

57. LENÈGRE, J., KILAIDONIS, P., AND DE BRUX, J.: Arch. Mal. Coeur., 1948, **41**, 193.

58. a) ABBOTT, O. A. J. Med. Assoc. of Georgia, 1947, **9**, 355.

b) DE TAKATS, G., AND REYNOLDS, J. T. Surg., 1947, **21**, 443.

c) POPPE, J. K. Am. Heart J., 1948, **36**, 252.

59. CHAVEZ, I., DORBECKER, N., AND CELIS, A. Arch. Inst. Card. de Mexico, 1947, **17**, 121.

60. LUISADA, A. A., AND FLEISCHNER, F. G. Am. J. Med., 1949, **6**, 756.

61. HERRMANN, G. R., AND SCHOFIELD, N. D. Am. Heart J., 1947, **34**, 87.

62. DETERLING, R. A., AND CLAGETT, O. T. Am. Heart J., 1947, **34**, 471.

63. LAUBRY, C., AND ROUTIER, D. Acad. de Med. de Paris, 1941, **124**, 126.

64. OPPENHEIMER, B. S. Trans. Assoc. Am. Physicians, 1938, **63**, 61.

65. CASSIDY, M., AND PINNIGER, J. Brit. Heart J., 1946, **8**, 130.

66. HOSKINS, J., AND GARDNER, F. Brit. Heart J., 1946, **8**, 141.

67. a) GOLDEN, A., AND WEENS, H. Am. Heart J., 1949, **37**, 114.

b) ABBOTT, O. A. J. Thoracic Surg. In press.

68. CALODNEY, M. M., AND CARSON, M. J. J. Pediat., 1950, **37**, 46.

69. WELLS, B. G., RAPPAPORT, M. B., AND SPRAGUE, H. B. Am. Heart J., 1949, **38**, 69.

70. PANNIER, R., et al. J. Belge Radiol., 1950, **33**, 1.

71. NICKERSON, J. L., et al. Circ., 1950, **1**, 1032.

72. a) BAHNSON, H. T., et al. Am. Heart J., 1949, **38**, 905.

b) KONDO, B., et al. Am. Heart J., 1950, **39**, 306.

c) LARSEN, K. Acta. Med. Scand., 1952, Suppl. 266, 661.

d) OLIM, C. B. Ann. Surg., 1949, **130**, 1091.

73. HAXTON, H. A., AND THOMSON, M. L. Brit. M. J., 1948, **2**, 1062.

74. JACOBSON, G., et al. Am. Heart J., 1953, **45**, 889.

75. FERRIN, A. L., BRIGGS, J. F., AND BARONOFSKY, I. D. Minn. Med., 1950, **33**, 1193.

76. a) LAMPEN, V. H., AND WADULLA, H. Deut. med. Wchnschr., 1950, **75**, 144.

b) ROSS, R. S., AND MCKUSICK, V. A. Meet. Am. Heart Assoc., 1952.

77. LOGUE, R. B., AND SIKES, C. J. A. M. A., 1952, **148**, 1209.

78. WHITTLESEY, R. H. Am. J. Physiol., 1952, **168**, 192.

79. SPECHT, H. D., AND BROWN, A. F. Arch. Int. Med., 1953, **92**, 148.

80. CASTELLANOS, A. *Cardiopatias Congenitas de la Infancia*. La Habana, Fresnada, 1948.

81. GASTON, E. A., AND FOLSOM, H. New England J. Med., 1945, **233**, 229.

82. COSSIO, P., AND PERIANES, J. J. A. M. A., 1949, **140**, 772.

83. a) EHRLICH, W., *et al.* J. Thoracic Surg., 1934, **3**, 352.

   b) OCHSNER, A., AND DIXON, J. L. J. Thoracic Surg., 1936, **5**, 641.

   c) ALTSCHULE, M. D., *et al.* Arch. Int. Med., 1945, **75**, 24.

   d) HUSSEY, H. H., *et al.* Am. Heart J., 1946, **31**, 1.

84. DEROW, H. A., *et al.* Arch. Int. Med., 1939 **63**, 626.

85. GERBODE, F., *et al.* Surg., 1949, **25**, 556.

Chapter 22

Hypertension of the Greater Circulation and Hypertensive Heart Disease

The syndrome of arterial hypertension is one of the most commonly found and is, therefore, of great clinical interest.

Arterial hypertension is frequently a secondary occurrence in diseases of the kidneys or the arteries. It may be present as a solitary occurrence, and, in such cases, the mechanism of origin of the elevation of pressure is still under discussion.

Hypertension is an elevation of blood pressure above normal. *Normal* blood pressure should not be confused with *average* blood pressure. While average blood pressure is 120/80, normal blood pressure varies between various individuals even in basal conditions (page 65). Blood pressure may be considered normal whenever it is below 140/90 in basal conditions unless previous readings proved a lower level. Above 40 years of age, systolic pressure tends to rise slightly and slowly. This increase, which does not represent "disease," is the expression of a common benign arteriosclerotic lesion of the arteries and is present in about two-thirds of the cases. It can be called *senile hypertension*.

Hypertensive heart disease is not the same as *hypertension*. The former term should be used only when there is evidence of ventricular enlargement or "strain." The latter term applies to any case having persistently high blood pressure.

CAUSE

Not less than 58 different morbid states associated with hypertension have been described (1). The following classification simplifies current, more complex, listing of the causes.

Arterial Hypertension

a) Renal
   Vascular
   Parenchymal
   Perinephral
   Pyelourethral
b) Neurogenic
   Lesion of CNS
   Lesion of pressoreceptors
   Hypertensive diencephalic syndrome
c) Vascular
   Coarctation of aorta
   Atherosclerosis of aorta
d) Endocrine
   Cushing's syndrome
   Pheochromocytoma
e) Essential

Renal hypertension may be found first of all in *diseases of the peripheral vessels* involving the kidneys. Among them, arteriosclerosis, panarteritis nodosa, arteritis, congenital abnormalities, obstructions (aneurysm, thrombosis, embolism), and Buerger's disease are the most important. *Affections of the renal parenchyma* occur in acute and chronic nephritis, pyelonephritis, hydronephrosis, renal stones, tumors, infarction and amyloidosis of the kidney, and the toxemia of pregnancy; *a unilateral lesion may be sufficient to cause hypertension.* *Perinephric lesions* may be caused by perinephritis, tumors, or any other cause of external pressure on the kidney; here again *a unilateral lesion may be involved.* The *affections of the urinary passages* include obstruction of the pelvis, ureter, or urethra; prostatitis; and pyelitis.

Neurogenic hypertension is found in cases with increased intracranial pressure because of tumor, trauma, or inflammation. Concussion of the brain and spinal cord injuries

491

are accompanied by hypertension (53). Decreased sensitivity of the *pressoreceptors of the aortic and carotid walls* due to arteriosclerosis may result in hypertension. The hypertensive diencephalic syndrome (29) is another example of neurogenic hypertension.

Cardiovascular hypertension is found in coarctation of the aorta (page 467). The moderate hypertension due to *arteriosclerosis of the aorta* may be a common effect of aging in contrast with other types of arteriosclerosis (65). Cardiovascular hypertension is also found in cases with functional vasoconstriction (anoxemia, heart failure, central stimulation), and in patients with polycythemia.

Endocrine hypertension occurs in certain diseases of the adrenal glands (including pheochromocytoma), and the pituitary gland (acromegaly, Cushing's syndrome).

Hypertension of certain cases of *Graves' disease* has an entirely different mechanism (page 405) and should not be considered here.

Essential hypertension is still an obscure condition. It has been considered as a "disease of adaptation" (66) while psychogenic factors leading to increased activity of the hypothalamus and of the sympathoadrenal system have been considered responsible for its occurrence (67).

Heredity has importance in essential hypertension, as shown by hypertensive families. However, we do not know which psychological, functional, or anatomical abnormality is inherited.

Mental strain and *excitement* are among the factors which cause wide fluctuations of pressure. They probably favor the establishment of a persistently high blood pressure.

Essential hypertension may occur *at any age* but is most frequent between 40 and 50. It is not significantly more common *in either sex*. It has been said that it is rare among Chinese living in China and Africans of Kenya, the environment and diet being more important than race or climate. However, proof has been given that there are racial groups of Negroes with no competitive tension and a high percentage of hypertension.

Obesity is frequently but not necessarily associated with essential hypertension.

MECHANISM OF ORIGIN

The main characteristics of human hypertension are the following: increased pulse pressure, frequently with increased mean pressure, and changes in the form of the central pulse (rapid diastolic collapse) (5).

Three possible factors can be discussed: increased cardiac output (through changes of heart rate or systolic discharge); reduced blood volume due to decrease of capacity and elasticity of the large arteries; and increased arteriolar resistance (6). Experimental studies as well as clinical observations indicate that blood volume and cardiac output are within normal ranges. It is apparent, therefore, that *peripheral resistance is increased*, and since blood viscosity is normal, arteriolar constriction is of paramount importance. Functional or anatomical changes of the aorta (5, 7) and of the large arteries in general have also been demonstrated. Therefore, *a general narrowing of the arterial tree should be admitted*.

It is now widely admitted that *arteriosclerosis and hypertension are frequently independent phenomena*. Therefore, *functional changes* of the arterial system, of either neurogenic or humoral nature, have been postulated. Experimental studies reported below may clarify this point.

In hypertension, the contraction of the left ventricle becomes stronger in order to expel a normal amount of blood against a higher peripheral resistance. This leads to dilatation and hypertrophy of this chamber. If this is within moderate limits, it may not be apparent during life.

Arterial hypertension is accompanied by an increased coronary flow (8). However, the myocardial capillaries fail to increase proportionately with muscle hypertrophy; therefore coronary insufficiency and, later, cardiac failure, are the distant but inevitable results of hypertension (page 367).

In experiments with heart-lung preparations, systemic hypertension is constantly accompanied by pulmonary hypertension (9). This observation cannot be applied to an intact circulation because different factors contribute to compensate for the changes in the latter (10). Actual measurements have demonstrated *normal pressure in the right ventricle* with the exception of malignant hypertension and heart failure (68). *Even if pulmonic pressure does not increase, the blood content of the lungs is increased* (6). Slight failure of the left ventricle or increased venous return cause an immediate rise of pulmonic pressure, a fact which is favored by the already existing distention of the pulmonary vessels. This explains the frequent finding of an enlarged right ventricle in arterial hypertension (11) and the possible episodes of pulmonary edema.

The cause of narrowing of the vascular system has been studied in detail through animal experimentation.

EXPERIMENTAL HYPERTENSION

Different interventions produce permanent hypertension in experimental animals.

a) *Increased intracranial pressure* or *intracisternal injection of kaolin* (12), *veratrin* (69), or *fibrin* (70).

b) *Overdosage with calciferol* (13).

c) *Section of both depressor and both carotid sinus nerves* causes a permanent hypertension in dogs while results in rabbits are less permanent (14). This form of hypertension is accompanied by tachycardia and is prevented or abolished by total sympathectomy. As a result of these studies, the possibility of human hypertension due to carotid sinus dysfunction was advocated.

d) *Administration of desoxycorticosterone in large doses* is followed by hypertension. This is due to the fact that this substance *reduces urinary excretion of sodium* and increases the concentration of sodium in the body fluids. As a logical deduction, *excessive secretion of the adrenal cortex* has been considered as a cause of hypertension. It is self evident that *the adrenal medulla*, source of epinephrine, can be responsible, at least partly, for paroxysmal or sustained hypertension.

e) *Renal lesions*, such as reduction of the renal circulation by means of clamps, wrapping the kidney in cellophane, or unilateral injury after removal of the other kidney, cause hypertension (15). This type of experimental hypertension has the greatest resemblance to clinical types with respect to pulse pressure, heart rate, and cardiac output (16).

The fact that the flow through the glomerulus is regulated by *two* arterioles (the afferent and the efferent arteriole) and the particular efficiency of the renal vasomotor system account for the fact that wide changes of the systemic pressure do not affect glomerular filtration. *Therefore, arterial hypertension is not a compensatory process for decreased kidney function.* Retention of nonprotein nitrogenous substances fails to elevate blood pressure so that even bilateral nephrectomy is seldom accompanied by hypertension (17).

The constriction of both renal arteries is followed by persistent hypertension through a humoral mechanism. During ischemia,[73] a proteolytic enzyme (*renin*) is liberated from the cells of the renal tubules. This enzyme acts upon an α^2 formed in the liver (*renin-substrate*) and leads to formation of a pressor substance called *angiotonin* or *hypertensine*. An inhibitor substance (enzyme?) called

[73] Ischemia of the kidneys is commonly used as the easiest way to produce effects. However, hypertension can be produced without local ischemia either by lowering the systemic pressure or by reducing the intrarenal pulse pressure. It has been proven that *anoxia is not the cause of secretion of renin.* Decrease of pressure below 60 mm. Hg, *acting on pressoreceptors of the kidney itself*, seems to be responsible for the *Goldblatt phenomenon* (71).

angiotoninase later destroys this hypertensive agent.

Angiotonin (hypertensine) affects directly the smooth muscles of the arteries. Small doses act like pitressin and decrease the coronary flow. Large doses elicit vascular reflexes and cause slower heart rate and decreased cardiac output.

Persistent hypertension may be produced by the renal pressor system through *excessive production of angiotonin (hypertensine), absence of angiotoninase (hypertensinase), or lack of balance between the two*. Angiotonin is one of the few substances which cause arterial vasoconstriction without changing capillary flow (18).

A different series of studies has shown that the initial stage of experimental renal hypertension in dogs is associated with the appearance in the blood of a *renal vasoexcitor substance* (VEM) (45). During the chronic hypertensive stage, the blood gives a neutral reaction, because the excitor substance is neutralized by a depressor substance (VDM) while, in malignant hypertension, the depressor substance gradually disappears. It is possible that VEM is identical with *pherentasin*, a prolonged pressor substance which has been isolated from the blood of hypertensive patients (72).

Humoral hypertension may be caused either by a structural lesion of the renal vessels, or by a functional mechanism (narrowing of the renal vessels due to nerve impulses). This seems confirmed by the following observations:

a) Many cases of essential hypertension fail to show appreciable vascular lesions at renal biopsy (19) and present a definite improvement after thoracolumbar splanchnic section (20).

b) Experimental hypertension caused by intracisternal injections and that caused by carotid sinus denervation are prevented by either sympathectomy or denervation of the kidney and are cured by the same surgical procedures (21).

Arteriovenous capillaries, able to by-pass the ordinary glomerular circulation, have been demonstrated in the kidney (49). Nervous stimuli might impede circulation in the glomerulus, cause shunting of blood through the more direct route, and determine ischemia of the cortex. This would

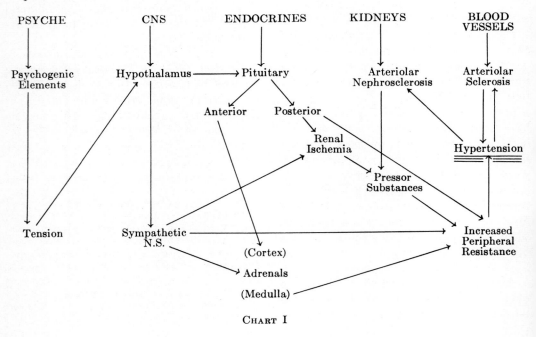

CHART I

start the already known mechanism of humoral hypertension.

Studies on the role of the anterior pituitary and of the adrenal cortex deserve special emphasis. Nephrosclerosis and hypertension have been produced by administration of *anterior pituitary extract, desoxycorticosterone acetate* (46) *plus large doses of sodium chloride, or the latter alone.* On the other hand, pressor substances have been found in the cerebrospinal fluid (47) and seem to be liberated by the arterial walls themselves when submitted to prolonged nervous stimulation (48).

In conclusion, it is impossible to decide whether essential hypertension is due to a neurogenic mechanism acting largely through hormonal and humoral mechanisms or vice versa. It is likely that both are involved in human hypertension even though certain types of hypertension, connected with structural changes, can be explained in a simpler way.

LESIONS

Primary lesions of the kidneys and urinary tract may be present in cases of hypertension due to renal pathology. However, the only typical changes of hypertension are the *secondary lesions* of the heart, kidneys, brain, and arterial system.

Hypertrophy of the left ventricle may be present within 4 weeks from the onset of hypertension. The heart of acute nephritis is actually among the heaviest. In essential hypertension it is frequently twice (600 gm.) and even three times (900 gm.) heavier than a normal heart but may be normal in weight (fig. 289).

Fibrosis of the aortic and mitral valves is frequent. *Coronary sclerosis* and *myocardial fibrosis* are nearly always present, as proven by the fact that 68 per cent of the deaths due to coronary disease are associated with hypertension (22).

Arteriosclerosis is often present as a secondary lesion, favored by the strain of high blood pressure. The change may take place

rapidly, even within a year. The structural changes of the peripheral arteries are similar to those of other types of arteriosclerosis, except for greater hypertrophy of the muscular tissue. While the arteriosclerotic changes are irregular in distribution, hypertrophy is usually diffuse (23).

Renal arteriosclerosis is but an example of diffuse arteriosclerosis and is, therefore, a secondary lesion. It may be minimal or even absent. On the other hand, atherosclerosis of the large renal arteris may be *the cause* of hypertension.

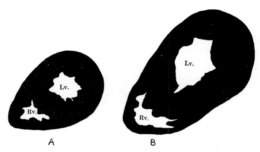

FIG. 289. Transverse section of the heart in chronic hypertension. A, normal heart; B, heart of hypertensive patient. (Inspired by originals of P. D. White.)

SIGNS AND SYMPTOMS

Permanent hypertension may exist for many years without symptoms. This is particularly true in essential hypertension which is frequently an unexpected finding on routine physical examinations. However, emotional instability is frequently present.

The early symptoms vary. *Headache, dizziness, weakness, irritability, and sleeplessness,* are frequent in the early stages. On the other hand, *perspiration, flushing,* and *palpitation* may be present in other patients and may be connected with disturbed thyroid or pituitary function.

Shortness of breath upon exertion is a rather early symptom together with palpitation and, at times, *precordial oppression. Paroxysmal nocturnal dyspnea and paroxysmal pulmonary edema* may occur early in the course of the disease. Their connection with ventricular strain and with diffuse stimulation of the sympathetic system will be discussed later (page 558).

Premature beats and, at times, *paroxysmal tachycardia*, may be connected with stretching of left ventricular walls.

Heart. Examination of the heart in the early stages reveals *increased loudness of the 2nd aortic sound* and, at times, its *prolongation*. At this stage, no heart disease is present. In later stages, a *triple rhythm* is heard (page 370) and an *apical systolic murmur* is often present. These signs indicate ventricular strain and dilatation and justify the diagnosis of hypertensive heart disease. An *aortic systolic murmur* is not unusual. It is caused by dilatation of the vessel or atherosclerosis. The *2nd aortic sound may be prolonged* because of sclerosis of the aortic valve. If it is followed by a *diastolic murmur*, aortic insufficiency is present, being caused by aortitis, atherosclerosis, or incomplete rupture of the aorta. Alternation of the pulse reveals the existence of a severe myocardial lesion.

Changes of the ascending aorta are common. Dynamic dilatation of the aorta (page 473) occurs first but atherosclerosis of the aorta (page 525) is common when the hypertension has lasted for several years. Dulness of the manubrium, pulsation of the suprasternal notch, and prolongation of the first sound (loud and audible vascular component of the 1st sound), are its manifestations.

Renal signs and *symptoms* may be due to a renal lesion causing the rise of blood pressure. In essential hypertension, renal signs may be absent for most of the clinical course or may be limited to a few hyaline casts and slightly low specific gravity. *Cerebral signs*, due to arteriosclerosis and including convulsions, may simulate uremia.

Nervous symptoms may be absent but usually are present. Transient paralysis or aphasia is not exceptional and may be due to a vascular spasm (24), a small hemorrhage, or discrete arterial thrombosis (25). *Headache* is frequent; it may be limited to a

sensation of fullness or pressure. It may be present only during the morning. More severe pain may be connected with severe change in pressure of the spinal fluid (renal hypertension) or structural lesions. Toxic phenomena may contribute to headache in renal diseases. *Dizziness, tinnitus, drowsiness, nausea, dyspepsia,* and *vomiting,* may occur. These are partly connected with the high pressure of the spinal fluid and partly with functional or structural disturbances of the cerebral vessels.

Hemorrhages from the nose, gastrointestinal tract, bronchi or lungs, uterus, kidneys, and urinary tract are common.

A *progressive loss of weight*, which may be rapid, occurs in many patients.

Retinal changes are common and may be grouped into two main classes (26): a) *arteriosclerosis* of the retinal vessels, and b) *papilledema.* The former has a less serious meaning than the latter unless it is accompanied by extensive and multiple hemorrhages. The prognosis of cases with papilledema is always serious.

BLOOD PRESSURE

Different behaviors of the systolic and diastolic pressures may be found.

High systolic pressure with low diastolic pressure is found in bradycardia, aortic insufficiency, patent ductus arteriosus, arteriovenous fistula, hyperthyroidism. The actual burden of the arteries is less because the highest level is maintained only for a short time.

Normal (or slightly raised) systolic pressure with high diastolic pressure is usually found in congestive failure.[74] As the mean pressure is high, the actual burden for the arteries is greater than in the previous group. In many cases there is a "decapitated hypertension," shown by the higher readings of systolic pressure when the patient improves.

[74] Cases having a high diastolic pressure with a normal or low systolic pressure should not be included here. They will be described in chapter 24 (syndrome of hyposphygmia).

Increased systolic and diastolic pressure, with a high level of diastolic, is a very serious condition which is found typically in nephritis and in malignant hypertension.

High systolic and moderately high diastolic pressures are found in many cases of essential hypertension. The lower level of mean pressure accounts for better tolerance of the condition.

Different readings in the two arms, with a high blood pressure in either the right or the left arm (more often the left), are common. *The systolic pressure of the lower extremities* is usually from 30 to 40 mm. higher, while the diastolic pressure is from 10 to 20 mm. higher than that of the arm. A greater difference points to either aortic insufficiency or abdominal atherosclerosis (p. 477). The opposite behavior, namely lower pressure in the legs, is a sign of coarctation of the aorta (page 467). High pressure in the legs with low pressure in the arms may be caused by hypertension plus atherosclerosis of the aortic arch.

It has been said that an isolated hypertension of the lower extremities may precede by years the establishment of hypertension in the higher limbs. This fact, however, needs confirmation.

VENOUS PRESSURE

Venous pressure may be normal or low. However, cases of essential hypertension where venous pressure reached 14 and even 16 cm. of water without any evidence of heart failure have been described. This elevation has been attributed to partial transmission of the high arterial pressure (36).

SPINAL FLUID

High pressure of the spinal fluid is frequent. It may reach from 40 to 60 cm. of water. Its connection with the headache and the beneficial results of lumbar puncture both on headache and arterial pressure have been emphasized (37).

GRAPHIC TRACINGS

Electrocardiogram

The early stages of hypertension may not be accompanied by electrocardiographic changes. However, a short P-R interval (about 0.14 second) with normal QRS has been described (38).

The electrocardiographic evidence of *left ventricular hypertrophy* is considered one of the most important signs of hypertensive

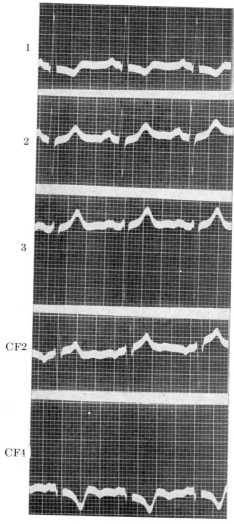

FIG. 290. Electrocardiogram in a case of essential hypertension with left ventricular hypertrophy and "strain".

heart disease (fig. 230). The unipolar limb leads may show an *inverted T wave* either in aVL (left arm) or in aVF (left leg) according to the position of the heart. For this reason, while such a pattern is seen most commonly in lead 1, it may be present occasionally also in lead 3 (fig. 290).

Patients with renal hypertension may also present *low voltage of P and QRS*, and *prolongation of Q-T*. This electrocardiographic picture has been called *cor renale* (73).

Phonocardiogram

This tracing may show high and prolonged vibrations caused by a *loud, booming second aortic sound*; the vibrations of the first aortic sound are often prolonged. A *systolic murmur* is frequently recorded at the apex, over the aortic area, or both. The former is due to left ventricular enlargement causing slight regurgitation, and may be favored by fibrosis of the mitral valve. The latter is caused by enlargement of the left ventricle and the ascending aorta resulting in a "relative aortic stenosis" (page 255).

It is common to record *a triple rhythm*. The meaning and mechanism of this have been already discussed (page 370).

Pulse and Pressure Tracings

The pulse curve may present an *anacrotic depression* indicating left ventricular strain. There may be *pulsus alternans*, evidence of a severe functional abnormality of the left ventricle (page 373).

The pressure tracing, recorded with both the oscillatory and auscultatory methods, frequently reveals an *auscultatory gap*. This consists of the lack of arterial sounds while the pulses are unchanged; the phenomenon seems connected with the anacrotism of the pulse (pages 252 and 254).

X-RAY

In the early stages of the disease the dimensions of the cardiac shadow may not be perceptibly increased even though left ventricular hypertrophy may be suggested by *increased convexity of the left ventricular border*. Later on, progressive enlargement of the left ventricle outwards, downwards, and backwards, is observed, indicating hypertensive heart disease (fig. 291). Arteriosclerotic changes of the aorta may be present in the absence of cardiac enlargement. They are revealed by elongation and tortuosity of the aortic arch, greater density of the shadow, and, occasionally, by signs of *calcification*.

Heart failure is revealed by total enlargement of the heart and by signs of pulmonary congestion.

VARIETIES

The most common type of hypertension is the so-called *essential hypertension*. From

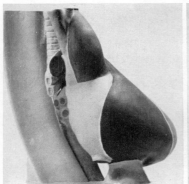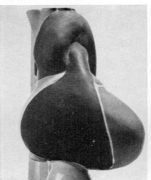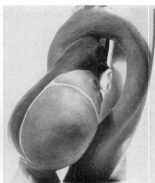

Fig. 291. Cardiac silhouette of hypertensive heart disease. (From models of the American Heart Association.)

the clinical point of view, cases with this type of hypertension can be placed in one of the following three groups (64).

a) *Benign form:* moderate increase of blood pressure; arteriosclerotic changes of the retinal vessels; normal urine; long clinical course.

b) *Intermediate form:* higher and more stable level of blood pressure; early appearance of headache, dizziness or exertional dyspnea; diffuse contraction of the retinal vessels; early appearance of albumine, casts, and red cells in the urine; evidence of left ventricular strain appears early; death occurs within 6 to 10 years.

c) *Malignant form:* early impairment of vision, early occurrence of exertional dyspnea and anginal pain; early and severe renal changes are revealed by the urine; retinal angiospasm and neuroretinopathy are present; cardiac and renal insufficiency cause death, usually in uremia, within 2 years.

A few well-established varieties deserve a separate description.

Hypertensive diencephalic syndrome. This syndrome occurs mostly in young and middle-aged women, but may occur in men (29). The periodic appearance of a blotchy blush, extending over the face and upper trunk, is typical. Tachycardia, hyperperistalsis of the bowels and lachrymation, not associated with emotion, are other signs. The basal metabolic rate may be elevated (from +10 to +30) but thyroidectomy is not beneficial. The name of the variety is due to recognition that similar signs are brought on by diffuse diencephalic stimulation in human beings (30).

Neurogenic hypertension. This variety is still incompletely understood. The patients have a practically normal renal function. High spinal anesthesia produces a marked increase in renal blood flow with decreased renal resistance and lower blood pressure (31). These patients show the greatest improvement after sympathectomy.

Pyelonephritis. The clinical signs and symptoms may resemble those of essential hypertension (32) and diagnosis may be difficult. Intravenous pyelography, separate catheterization of the ureters, and study of the sediment of the collected urine of a 24-hour period are of help. Unilateral pyelonephritis may be the cause of hypertension in some of the patients. If this is the case and the other kidney is normal or only slightly damaged, unilateral nephrectomy may lead to normalization of the blood pressure and cure the clinical syndrome.

Pheochromocytoma, a chromaffin tumor of the adrenal medulla, may cause hypertension. It first causes *paroxysmal attacks of high blood pressure* during which the extreme level of 300 mm. or more may be reached. Later, a *sustained hypertension,* which is difficult to distinguish from essential hypertension, is created. When death occurs during one of the paroxysms, it is frequently preceded by an attack of pulmonary edema (page 555). Histamine gives a paradoxical effect and increases blood pressure in these cases (44). Benzodioxane, an adrenolytic drug, reduces blood pressure in cases of pheochromocytoma, not in cases of renal hypertension (74).

Carcinoma of the adrenal glands is usually a cortical tumor and may simulate Cushing's syndrome. Differentiation between this syndrome and one of the pituitary origin may be made because the excretion of male sex hormone is increased in patients with cortical tumor.

The possibility that *the loss of ovarian function* was responsible for the common hypertension of menopausal syndrome has been advanced. However, this fact has not been demonstrated (1).

Cushing's syndrome is considered as a state of pituitary imbalance connected with tumors of the adrenal cortex or atrophy of hypothalamic nuclei. Increased activity of the pituitary (ACTH), stimulates the adrenal cortex and secondary adrenocortical and renal pressor hyperactivity causes hypertension (75).

Hypertension of pregnancy. Eclampsia, preeclampsia, and toxemia of pregnancy are considered to be related to renal abnormalities. Hydronephrosis and pyelitis are often the precursors of toxemia syndromes (39). Nephritis, pyelitis, and hypertension are frequently interrelated in pregnant women. The cardiorenal strain caused by pregnancy, and the improvement caused by delivery, have masked for a long time the fact that these women often develop typical cardiovascular symptoms in a later stage. In many cases, the vascular and renal disturbances become latent after delivery and recur at a later date whenever a new strain is imposed on the heart and kidneys (40).

Malignant hypertension. Malignant hypertension may appear during several apparently dissimilar diseases, all having high blood pressure (3, 33). The great majority of patients have had hypertension for many years but the malignant syndrome may be present from the onset (1). It is frequently difficult to decide whether the hypertension is primary, or secondary to some unrecognized process. Among the typical signs are papilledema and multiple hemorrhages of the eyegrounds, possibly accompanied by detachment of the retina. The pulse pressure usually tends to be reduced; enlargement of the heart occurs within a short time; hematuria and poor renal efficiency are typical; hemorrhagic arteriolitis and arteriosclerotic changes cause a rapid deterioration of the patient. If the syndrome occurs during pregnancy, delivery may be accompanied by remission of the signs and a much longer clinical course.

Transient hypertension. Transitory elevations of the blood pressure often represent an early stage of essential hypertension (34).

Orthostatic hypertension. Hypertension occurring only in the erect posture has been described in cases of nephroptosis (41). It is a rare occurrence, caused by diminution of renal blood flow and its repercussions on the renal pressor system. The rarity is connected with the fact that, in the majority of cases, a greater blood flow occurs in the standing position.

COMPLICATIONS

The most common complications are due to lesions of the heart, kidneys, or cerebral vessels. Congestive failure, myocardial infarction, angina pectoris, and attacks of paroxysmal dyspnea or pulmonary edema are frequent. Uremia and cardiovascular accidents are possible. Acute infections or pulmonary embolism from phlebothrombosis of the leg may terminate the clinical course.

Thyroid heart, syphilitic aortitis and aortic regurgitation, atherosclerosis of the aorta, and rheumatic valvular lesions may be associated with hypertension, causing a more serious outlook and a shorter clinical course. Neurocirculatory asthenia is a frequent complication of hypertension.

Renal arteriosclerosis or arteriolosclerosis is a possible complication of hypertension.

Attacks of headache, vomiting, convulsions, and coma may be caused by *cerebral edema*. On the other hand, attacks of localized sensory or motor paralysis of brief duration are due to *sudden occlusion of cerebral arterioles* followed by *infarcts*. The extension of the latter is determined by the greater or lesser collateral circulation (51).

DIAGNOSIS

The diagnosis is based on the recognition that a *persistent and significant increase of blood pressure is present.*

Palpation of the superficial arteries, ophthalmoscopic examination of the retinal vessels, urinalysis, and kidney function tests help to determine the degree of vascular change in the respective regions.

Intravenous urography, urine cultures, cystoscopy, and retrograde pyelography, are often necessary in order to detect abnormalities of the urinary tract.

Electrocardiography, phonocardiography, and roentgen-ray examination of the chest complete the cardiac study and reveal the existence and grade of hypertensive heart disease.

Functional tests, including the cold pressor test and measurements during normal or induced sleep, ascertain the degree of reactivity of the vasomotor system.

Ruling out coarctation of the aorta, pheochromocytoma, polycystic kidney, congenital anomalies, glomerulonephritis, and pyelonephritis, is necessary as a first step. Histamine and benzodioxane tests should be undertaken. Exclusion of a unilateral renal lesion is particularly important because of the therapeutic success which is obtained in such cases, especially if the patient is young.

When the diagnosis of essential hypertension is established, an evaluation of neurogenic, endocrine, and renal factors should be made.

High spinal anesthesia may be done in order to demonstrate the value of a possible intervention on the sympathetic system.

Glomerulonephritis and malignant hypertension (35). Differentiation between glomerulonephritis and malignant hypertension (before uremia sets in) is difficult but possible (35). Patients with terminal glomerulonephritis have a lower rate of glomerular filtration (plasma inulin clearance) and of tubular secretory capacity (diodrast clearance) and also a higher proteinuria than patients with malignant hypertension and renal failure. The former develop signs of cardiac failure five times less often, and live four times longer, than those with glomerulonephritis. Blood pressure is higher, cardiac output is lower, and peripheral resistance is greater, in malignant hypertension than in glomerulonephritis. Electrocardiographic signs of hypertensive heart disease are far more common in the former than in the latter.

Neurogenic and endocrine factors may cause hypertension. An extreme example of the neurogenic type is represented by the diencephalic syndrome while the pheochromocytoma is a typical example of

endocrine hypertension. Differential diagnosis between these and the high blood pressure of hyperthyroidism is necessary (1).

PROGNOSIS

Prognosis can be based only upon the general clinical consideration of the case.

Systolic pressure in itself has a definite bearing on prognosis because the highest figures usually imply a shorter life expectancy, but diastolic pressure is even more important in this respect. A diastolic pressure maintained above 150 mm. has a bad prognostic significance.

Signs of malignant hypertension always imply a bad prognosis as do signs of heart failure. The same is true of patients having hypertensive heart disease, vascular disease, albuminuria or encephalopathy. Evidence of myocardial or coronary damage implies a more guarded prognosis. The same is true of obesity and diabetes.

Clear renal involvement is a serious sign; however, it has been shown that terminal glomerulonephritis in a hypertensive patient has a much better outlook than malignant hypertension with renal failure (35).

TREATMENT

Patients with *benign hypertension* connected with senility (a level of 170/100 should be considered within this group in a person of 60) do not require treatment. Therapy should be limited to patients with evidence of hypertensive heart disease, renal disease, or cerebral disease, or having severe symptoms.

DIET THERAPY

Salt restriction (X) (55, 76) or the rice, fruit, sugar *diet of Kempner* (XIV) (54, 77) with its *low sodium, low cholesterol*, and *low protein* contents, benefits about two-thirds of the patients. Following 10 weeks of such treatment, considerable loss of weight, improved symptomatology, and objective improvement take place. However, the results are far greater in obese patients than in others; severe psychological problems often arise; low sodium syndrome may develop; and the results disappear within a few weeks from resumption of a normal diet. Therefore, a more moderate restriction of salt may be indicated (IX). Good results have been obtained also with a *low cholesterol diet* (XII) (56).

Dietary treatment has given good results in certain patients, no results in others. This indicates various mechanisms of action and, therefore, the necessity of selection before indicating a diet. The first two diets are often successful for a certain time but cannot be continued because they are too monotonous. Moreover, excessive deprivation of certain constituents may cause severe debilitation and should be avoided because it may be dangerous (78).

Cation exchange resins have been tried but their success is questionable. Moreover, salt restriction to 1-1.5 gm. daily is still necessary.

HYPOTENSIVE DRUGS

Sedatives. Phenobarbital and other *barbiturates* may be helpful at times. It is the writer's view that they should be given only at night in ambulatory patients. Fractional administration should be reserved for patients with severe hypertension who are assigned to bed rest and should not be unduly prolonged. *Bromides* may be useful in some cases.

Hypotensive drugs. These drugs have been employed at first for pharmacological tests. Later, their continued use seemed justified as it caused appreciable improvement in a number of patients. They are: a) *Tetraethyl-ammonium chloride or bromide* (61); b) *dibenamine* (62) (**37**); c) *hydergine* (63) (**36**); and d) *hexamethonium* (79) (**39, 40**). The first and the last paralyze the ganglia; the second acts on sympathetic endings; the third inhibits sympathetic activity within the CNS. These drugs have powerful hypotensive action. The need of a delicate adjustment of dose in order to prevent a too-sudden drop of pressure, and the various side effects which are more marked in the erect position, limit their use to severe cases and bedridden patients. A girdle and leg bandages may prevent postural hypotension.

Protoveratrine (80) (**47**) lowers blood pressure in a reflex way by stimulating sensitive fibers of the left ventricle, carotid sinuses, aortic arch, and pulmonary arteries. It is very effective and may be given to ambulatory patients. Subcutaneous dose is 4 to 6 micrograms per kilogram every 8 to 12 hours. The oral dose is 0.5 to 0.75 mg. t.i.d. after meals and at bedtime. Side effects, mainly consisting of nausea, are more common by this route. A significant blood pressure drop is obtained in about one-third of the patients.

Rauwolfia (81) (**45**) has a moderate but nearly constant hypotensive action, and no side effects.

Nitrites are frequently disappointing. However, they may lessen the danger of complications. Among them, *mannitol hexanitrate* (**51**) and *peritrate* (**50**) are slow-acting drugs which can be used together with *papaverine* (**43, 44**) in order to obtain additional effects.

Potassium iodide (**73**), alone or with added *bromides*, is frequently helpful though its mechanism of action is incompletely known. It should be employed with caution.

Potassium sulphocyanate (thiocyanate) often causes a definite lowering of blood pressure. However, the toxicity of this drug calls for great caution in its use. Its hypotensive action is nitrite-like while its less severe toxic manifestations are similar to those of the iodides.

Pyrogens have been tried in malignant hypertension (82). However, their administration is difficult.

Psychotherapy has been tried with moderate success. An attempt at removing the strain of professional and social activities, as well as the worries of family tangles, should always be made.

At times *rest* is very important and a few days of bed rest may lower the blood pressure remarkably. However, care shall be taken in order not to transform a person, having many years of possible activity, into a bedridden patient.

Physiotherapy and *roentgen irradiation* of the thyroid, the pituitary, or the adrenal glands have been tried with limited results.

Subtotal thyroidectomy, propylthiouracil, and *radioactive iodine* have been advocated and may give results in selected cases.

Extreme hypertension responds well to *spinal* or *caudal anesthesia.* This procedure has been used in hypertension associated with acute nephritis, cardiac failure, or encephalopathy, and lowers blood pressure by causing peripheral vasodilation.

SURGICAL TREATMENT (19, 20, 42, 43)

Apart from surgical treatment of renal or adrenal conditions and from thyroidectomy, many surgical interventions have been advocated. They include decortication or denervation of the kidneys, bilateral thoracolumbar rhizotomy, splanchnic resection, adrenal denervation, and subtotal adrenalectomy.

Bilateral lumbodorsal splanchnic resection is the most successful. It is performed in two stages. In a fair percentage of patients it is followed by marked reduction of blood pressure. Symptomatic relief, improvement of eyegrounds, decrease of cardiac enlargement, and increase of kidney concentrating ability take place. In some cases, triple rhythm, left axis deviation, inverted T1, pulsus alternans, and ventricular hypertrophy disappear, causing an amazing clinical change. In some cases, the maximum effect is reached from 3 to 5 months after the intervention. It is, sometimes, temporary but may be permanent. It may be out of proportion with the lowering of blood pressure. Sympathectomy requires special precautions (girdle, bandaged legs) for preventing sudden drop of pressure in the erect position.

The effect of the operation does not seem to be dependent upon the condition of the renal arterioles and may be due, at least partly, to decreased peripheral resistance.

The main indications for surgery are hypertensive neuropathy, or a rapidly progressive hypertension in a young person. The main contraindications are heart failure, severe coronary heart disease, and renal insufficiency. However, these may be exceptionally waved aside, with the understanding that surgery will bring only a limited or temporary relief. Pregnant women with hypertension and toxemia may respond favorably to sympathectomy.

The results of sympathectomy have led to the following conclusions.

Cases with humoral or endocrine hypertension may benefit from surgery (57). Hypertensive patients with heart failure who do not respond to digitalis or other remedies may benefit from surgery and attain a cardiovascular equilibrium (58). Hypertensive patients submitted to surgery may experience a remarkable subjective and objective improvement and are better influenced by drugs (59), even though their blood pressure is unchanged or only slightly lower. This has been tentatively explained as due to decreased amount of sympathin and epinephrine in their tissues, including the heart muscle (60).

GENERAL THERAPEUTIC EVALUATION

Different types of hypertension require different methods of treatment.

1) Cases with pheochromocytoma, unilateral renal disease, or coarctation of the aorta require surgery.

2) Cases with benign and stationary hypertension should be treated with mild sedation and mild dietary restrictions.

3) Cases with obesity, high blood cholesterol or both, should be placed on a reducing or rice diet for some weeks. Later, they should follow a moderate diet, poor in cholesterol.

4) If there is cardiac enlargement or

other evidence of left ventricular strain, a
low sodium diet should be prescribed. and
hypotensive drugs should be used.

5) Patients with malignant hypertension
or rapid evolution of the vascular lesions
should be submitted to sympathectomy. If
this is not possible, bed rest, strict diet,
therapy with protoveratrine or sympatholytics, should be prescribed.

BIBLIOGRAPHY

1. PAGE, I. H. In *Stroud's Cardiovascular Disease*. Philadelphia, Davis, 1945.
2. MOSENTHAL, H. O. In *Nelson Loose Leaf
   of Medicine*. New York, Nelson, 1946.
3. DEROW, H. A., AND ALTSCHULE, M. D. New
   England J. Med., 1935, **213**, 951. Also Ann.
   Int. Med., 1941, **14**, 1768.
4. HOUSTON, W. B. In *Stroud's Cardiovascular
   Disease*. Philadelphia, Davis, 1945.
5. WIGGERS, C. J. Ann. Int. Med., 1932, **6**, 12.
   Also Am. Heart J., 1938, **16**, 515.
6. WIGGERS, C. J. *Physiology in Health and Disease*. Philadelphia, Lea and Febiger, 1944.
7. WIGGERS, C. J., AND WÉGRIA, R. Am. J.
   Physiol., 1938, **124**, 603.
8. GREGG, D. E. Am. J. Physiol., 1936, **114**, 609.
9. a) FUEHNER, H., AND STARLING, E. H. J.
      Physiol., 1913, **47**, 286.
   b) ANREP, G. V., AND BULATAO, E. J. Physiol.,
      1925, **60**, 175.
10. KATZ, L. N., AND WIGGERS, C. J. Am. J.
    Physiol., 1927, **82**, 91.
11. THOMPSON, W. P., AND WHITE, P. D. Am.
    Heart J., 1936, **12**, 641.
12. a) CUSHING, H. Mitt. Grenz. Med. Chir.,
       1902. **4**, 773. Also Am. J. M. Sci., 1903,
       125, 1017.
    b) FORSTER, F. M. Am. J. Physiol., 1943,
       139, 347.
    c) HELLER, H. Klin. Woch., 1934, **13**, 241.
    d) PICK, E. P. Wien. klin. Woch., 1935, **48**,
       634.
13. a) APPLEROT, S. Am. J. Physiol., 1933, **105**,
       294.
    b) HANDOWSKY, H. S. J. Physiol., 1937,
       90, 62 P.
14. a) HERING, H. E. *Die Karotissinusreflexe*.
       Dresden, Steinkopff, 1927. Also Zeit.
       Kreislauff., 1927, **19**, 410.
    b) HEYMANS, C., BOUCKAERT, J. J., AND
       REGNIERS, P. *Le Sinus Carotidien*. Paris,
       Doin, 1933. Also Surgery, 1938, **4**, 487.
    c) KOCH, E., AND CO-WORKERS. Krankheits-
       forsch., 1929, **7**, 241. Also Zeitschr. exp.
       Med., 1934, **94**, 105.

d) NOWAK, S. J. G. Ann. Surg., 1940, **3**, 102.
e) BLALOCK, A. Physiol. Rev., 1940, **20**, 159.
f) THOMAS, C. B., AND CO-WORKERS. Am.
   Heart J., 1940, **19**, 316. Also Proc. Soc.
   Exper. Biol., 1941, **48**, 24.
15. a) GOLDBLATT, H., AND CO-WORKERS. Bull.
       Acad. Med. Cleveland, 1932, **16**, 6. Ann.
       Int. Med., 1937, **11**, 69. J. Exper. Med.,
       1934, **59**, 347; 1937, **65**, 671; and 1938,
       67, 809. *Experimental Hypertension In-
       duced by Renal Ischemia*. Harvey Lecture,
       Series 33, Baltimore, The Williams &
       Wilkins Co., 1938; Physiol. Rev., 1947, **27**,
       120.
    b) PAGE, I. H. J. Mt. Sinai Hosp., 1941, **8**, 3.
    c) HOUSSAY, B. A., AND BRAUN-MENENDEZ,
       E. Brit. M. J., 1942, **2**, 179.
    d) BRAUN-MENENDEZ, E., FASCIOLO, J. C.,
       LELOIR, L. F., MUÑOZ, J. M., AND TA-
       QUINI, A. C. *Hipertension Arterial
       Nefrógena*. Buenos Aires, El Ateneo,
       1943.
16. HOLMAN, D. V., AND PAGE, I. H. Am. Heart
    J., 1938, **16**, 321.
17. HARRISON, T. R., AND CO-WORKERS. Tr. Assoc.
    Am. Physicians, 1936, **51**, 281.
18. a) LANDIS, E., AND CO-WORKERS. J. Clin.
       Investigation, 1938, **17**, 189.
    b) ABELL, R. G., AND PAGE, I. H. J. Exper.
       Med., 1942, **75**, 305.
19. SMITHWICK, R. H. Surg., 1940, **7**, 1.
20. CASTLEMAN, B., AND SMITHWICK, R. H. J. A.
    M. A., 1943, **121**, 1256.
21. a) BRAUN, L., AND SAMET, B. Wien. klin.
       Woch., 1933, **46**, 225; 1934, **47**, 65; and
       1935, **48**, 940. Also Arch. exp. Path.
       Pharm., 1935, **177**, 662.
    b) GERBI, C., AND MARTINETTI, R. Arch.
       Scienze. Med., 1936, **61**, 397.
    c) GRIMSON, K. S., BOUCKAERT, J. J., AND
       HEYMANS, C. Proc. Soc. Exper. Biol. &
       Med., 1939, **42**, 225.
22. BELL, E. T., AND CLAWSON, B. J. Arch. Path.,
    1928, **5**, 939.
23. FAHR, T. In Handb. d. Spez. path. Anath. u.
    Hist., 1934, **6**, 807.
24. PAL, J. *Die Gefaesskrisen*. Leipzig, Hirzel,
    1905.
25. ALLBUTT, C. *Arteriosclerosis*. London, Mac-
    millan, 1925.
26. FISHBERG, A. M., AND OPPENHEIMER, B. S.
    Arch. Int. Med., 1930, **46**, 901.
27. BALLANTYNE, A. H. Arch. Ophtalim., 1945,
    33, 97.
28. WHITE, P. D. Am. Heart J., 1945, **30**, 140. Also
    Bull. New England Med. Center, 1945,
    7, 205.
29. PAGE, I. H. Am. J. M. Sci., 1935, **190**, 9.

30. Cushing H. Proc. Nat. Acad. Sci., 1931, **17,** 163.
31. Page, I. H., Taylor, R. D., Corcoran, A. C., and Mueller, L. Proc. Centr. Soc. Clin. Research, 1943, **16,** 13.
32. a) Weiss, S., and Parker, F. Medicine, 1939, **18,** 221.

    b) Abeshouse, B. S. Surg., 1941, **9,** 942; and **10,** 147.
33. a) Volhard, F. and Fahr, T. *Die Brightsche Nierenkrankheit.* Berlin, Springer, 1914.

    b) Fahr, T.: Virch. Arch., 1919, **226,** 119.

    c) Fishberg, A. M.: *Hypertension and Nephritis.* Phila., Lea and Febiger, 1939.
34. Levy, R. L., White, P. D., Stroud, W. D., and Hillman, C. C. J. A. M. A., 1945, **128,** 1059.
35. a) Corcoran, A. C., and Page, I. H. Ann. Int. Med., 1944, **21,** 747.

    b) Taylor, R. D., Kohlstaedt, K. G., Richter, A. B., and Page, I. H. Ann. Int. Med., 1944, **21,** 765.
36. a) Villaret, M., and co-workers. Presse Méd., 1923, **31,** 318.

    b) Schott, E. Deut. Arch. klin. Med., 1912, **108,** 537.

    c) Rotky, H., and Klein, O. Med. Klin., 1923, **19,** 1574.

    d) Schleiter, H. G., and Thomas, A. B. Tr. Am. Clim. & Clin. A., 1931, **47,** 86.
37. Greppi, E. Riv. Neurol., 1933, **6,** 201.
38. Scherf, D. Bull. New York Med. Coll., Flower and Fifth Ave. Hosp., 1941, **4,** 116.
39. Peters, J. P. J. A. M. A., 1938, **219,** 793.
40. Herrick, W. W., and Tillman, A. J. B. Arch. Int. Med., 1935, **55,** 643. Also Am. J. Obst., 1936, **31,** 832.
41. McCann, W. S., and Romansky, M. J. J. A. M. A., 1940, **115,** 573.
42. a) Adson, A. W., and Brown, G. E. J. A. M. A., 1934, **102,** 1115.

    b) Craig, W. M. West J. Surg., 1934, **42,** 146.

    c) Crile, G. Pennsylvania M. J., 1937, **40,** 1017.

    d) Grimson, K. S. Ann. Surg., 1941, **114,** 753.

    e) Grimson, K. S., Kernodle, C. E., and Hill, H. C. J. A. M. A., 1944, **126,** 218.
43. a) Talbott, J. H., Castleman, B., Smithwick, R. H., and co-workers. J. Clin. Investigation, 1943, **22,** 387.

    b) Rojas, F., Smithwick, R. H., and White, P. D. J. A. M. A., 1944, **126,** 15.

    c) Smithwick, R. H. Arch. Surg., 1944, **49,** 180. Also New York State J. Med., 1944, **44,** 2693.

    d) Peet, M. M., and Iseberg, E. M., J. A. M. A. 1946, **130,** 467.
44. a) Hyman, A. and Menscher, W. H. J. Urol., 1943, **49,** 755.

    b) Roth, G. M. and Kvale, W. F. Am. J. M. Sci., 1945, **210,** 653.
45. a) Shorr, E., and Zweifach, B. W. Federation Proc., 1949, **8,** 146.

    b) Shorr, E. Am. J. Med., 1948, **4,** 120.
46. Page, I. H. J. A. M. A., 1949, **140,** 451.
47. a) Page, I. H. Science, 1935, **82,** 550.

    b) Raab, W. Ann. Int. Med., 1948, **28,** 1010. Also Am. J. Physiol., 1948, **152,** 324.
48. Jimenez, Diaz C., and co-workers. Rev. Clin. Españ., 1947, **24,** 417. Also Rev. Españ. Card., 1947, **1,** 1.
49. Trueta, J., and co-workers. *Studies of the Renal Circulation.* Thomas, Springfield, Ill., 1947.
50. Goldberger, E. *Unipolar Lead Electrocardiography.* Philadelphia, Lea and Febiger, 1947.
51. Pickering, G. W. J. A. M. A., 1948, **137,** 423.
52. a) Bloomfield, B. A., and co-workers. J. Clin. Investigation, 1946, **25,** 639.

    b) Lenègre, J., and Maurice, P. Arch. Mal. Coeur, 1947, **40,** 173.

    c) McMichael, J. Ann. Rev. Physiol., 1948, **10,** 201.
53. a) Raab, W. Am. Heart J., 1949, **37,** 237.

    b) Thomson, C. E., and Calhoun, Witham, A. New England J. Med., 1948, **239,** 291.
54. Kempner, W. North Carolina M. J., 1944, **5,** 125; and 1945, **6,** 61 and 117. Am. J. Med., 1948, **4,** 545. Ann. Int. Med., 1949, **31,** 821.
55. a) Grollman, A., and co-workers. J. A. M. A., 1945, **129,** 533.

    b) Bryant, J. M., and Blecha, E. Proc. Soc. Exper. Biol. & Med., 1947, **65,** 227.
56. Dock, W. J. A. M. A., 1947, **134,** 1197.
57. De Takats, G., and Fowler, E. F. Surg., 1947, **21,** 773.
58. Chavez, I., and Méndez, L. Arch. Inst. Card. de Mexico, 1948, **18,** 680.
59. a) Davis, C., and co-workers. Ann. Surg., 1948, **128,** 1770.

    b) Peet, M. M. New England J. Med., 1947, **236,** 270.

    c) Fishberg, A. N. J. A. M. A., 1948, **137,** 670.
60. Raab, W. Discussion, Meeting New England Heart Assoc., 1948.
61. a) Brown, H. S., and Craig, W. McK. Proc. Staff Meet., Mayo Clin., 1948, **23,** 94.

    b) Lian, C., and Bergamo, G. Semaine des Hôp. (Paris), 1948, **24,** 2237.
62. Haimovici, H., and Medinets, H. E. Proc. Soc. Exper. Biol. & Med., 1948, **67,** 163.
63. a) Freis, E. D., Stanton, J. R., and Wilkins, R. W. Am. J. M. Sci., 1948, **216,** 163.

b) BLUNTSCHLI, H. J., AND GOETZ, R. H. Am. Heart J., 1948, **35,** 873.

64. PAGE, I. H. In *Myers, J. A., and McKinlay, C. A. The Chest and the Heart.* Springfield, Thomas, 1948, vol. II.

65. a) MOSCHOWITZ, E. J. A. M. A., 1950, **143,** 861.
    b) DOCK, W. Bull. New York Acad. Med., 1950, **26,** 182.

66. SELYE, H. *Stress.* Montreal, Acta. Inc., Med. Publ., 1950.

67. SCHROEDER, H. A. Am. J. Med., 1951, **10,** 189.

68. LENÈGRE, J., AND MAURICE, P. Arch. Med. Coeur, 1947, **40,** 173.

69. JARISCH, A., *et al.* Klin. Wochn., 1940, **18,** 1440.

70. CAMERON, G. R., AND KUO, S. N. J. Path. & Bact., 1949, **61,** 375.

71. DIVRY, A. Arch. Intern. Phys., 1951, **59,** 211.

72. SCHROEDER, H. A., AND OLSEN, N. S. Meet. Am. Heart Assoc., 1952.

73. ZUCKERMANN, R., *et al.* Arch. Cardiol. Mexico, 1951, **21,** 155.

74. a) SNYDER, C. H. AND VICK, E. H. Am. J. Dis. Child., 1947, **73,** 581.
    b) GOLDENBERG, M., *et al.* J. A. M. A., 1947, **135,** 971.

75. HEIMBECKER, P., AND PFEIFFENBERGER, M. Am. J. Med., 1950, **9,** 3.

76. a) ALLEN, F. M., AND SHERRILL, J. W. J. Metab. Res., 1922, **2,** 429.
    b) PINES, K. L., AND PERERA, G. A. Med. Clin. North America, 1949, 713.
    c) CHAPMAN, C. B., AND GIBBON, T. B. Medicine, 1950, **29,** 29.

77. WATKINS, D. M., *et al.* Am. J. Med., 1950, **9,** 441.

78. CHAPMAN, C. B., *et al.* New England J. Med., 1950, **243,** 899.

79. FINNERTY, F. A., AND FREIS, E. D. Circ. 1950, **2,** 828.

80. a) MEILMAN, E., AND KRAYER, O. Circ., 1950, **1,** 204; and 1952, **6,** 212.
    b) STEARNS, N. S., AND ELLIS, L. B. New England J. Med., 1952, **246,** 397.
    c) WILKINS, R. W. Mo. Conc. Cardiov. Dis., 1951, **20,** 89. Also New England J. Med. 1950, **242,** 535.

81. WILKINS, R. W., AND JUDSON, W. E. New England J. Med., 1953, **248,** 48.

82. PAGE, I. H. J. A. M. A., 1951, **147,** 1311.

CHAPTER 23

Hypertension of the Lesser Circulation and Pulmonary Heart Disease (Cor Pulmonale)

The syndromes caused by hypertension of the lesser circulation have been described more recently than those caused by systemic hypertension. A secondary lesion of the right heart is a frequent, though not inevitable, result.

Acute Cor Pulmonale Caused by Pulmonary Embolism and Infarction

CAUSE

Pulmonary embolism causes sudden obstruction of the pulmonary artery, one of the stems, or one or more secondary branches of the pulmonary artery. The emboli arise either in the right heart or in any part of the systemic venous circulation. The most common sites of origin are the *veins of the pelvis* (obstetrical and surgical cases) and *those of the lower extremities*. Mural thrombi, dislodged *from the endocardium of the right atrium* (congestive failure, atrial fibrillation) *or the right ventricle* (myocardial infarction) (1), are also a possible cause of pulmonary embolism.

Embolism from the pelvic veins may take place in postoperative patients, usually from 8 to 14 days after operation; that from the right heart may occur in cardiac patients. Embolism from the leg veins may occur in patients with a known *phlebitis* or in ambulatory patients having *quiet venous thrombosis* (2, 3) without symptoms. In the latter, the embolism is a sudden, unforeseen occurrence and may be mistaken for a coronary occlusion. While *thrombophlebitis of varicose veins* and *phlegmasia alba dolens*

(*milk leg*) rarely give rise to fatal complications, phlebitis of the deep veins of the lower extremities (*phlebothrombosis*) is more dangerous and carries a higher mortality (page 539).

A *rapidly developing thrombosis* of a branch of the pulmonary artery may, in exceptional cases, give a clinical picture which is similar to that of pulmonary embolism.

Certain *predisposing factors* favor the occurrence of thrombosis and embolism.

a) *Causes affecting the composition of the blood* (*the rapidity of clotting is increased*). Toxemia, infection, dehydration, anemia, leucemia, pregnancy, the puerperal state, and trauma should be included in this group.

b) *Causes affecting the integrity of the endothelium* (*thrombosis is favored*). Typhoid fever, grippe, syphilis, rheumatic disease, bacterial endocarditis, arteriosclerosis, and phlebosclerosis are the most important.

c) *Causes affecting the blood flow* (*circulation is slowed down*). Conditions causing low metabolism, low blood pressure, and slow circulation (either general or in certain areas) are important factors. Cardiac failure is the most frequent cause of *general changes of flow*; varicose veins are the most frequent cause of *local changes of flow*.

The importance of a *sudden increase of venous pressure* in patients with heart disease, phlebothrombosis, or both, in the detachment of a loose mural thrombus should be emphasized (3). This increase may be due to cough, defecation, parturition, coitus, or lifting or straining; any of them, by causing a sudden change in vascular dynamics, may cause sudden death.

FUNCTIONAL AND STRUCTURAL EFFECTS

Complete occlusion of the pulmonary artery causes death within a short time unless the occluding factor is rapidly removed. Occlusion of one of the main stems, or obstruction of the main artery, which is equivalent to from 50 to 66 per cent of the caliber, may be compensated in experimental animals (4). Compensation is based upon increased effort of the right ventricle and dilatation of this chamber and the pulmonary artery (or its proximal section). Dilatation of the pulmonary vessels of the intact lung is also important when one stem is occluded (5). One important factor of compensation is the initial tension of the right ventricle which is dependent upon venous return. A too severe obstruction causes diminished return to the left ventricle with *decreased output and coronary ischemia.* Both cause decreased efficiency of the right ventricle.

Pulmonary embolism is followed by *pulmonary infarction* which is followed in turn by consolidation, often resulting in pneumonia (*infarct pneumonia* (8b)).

Multiple reflexes, arising in the occluded pulmonary artery and causing a diffuse vasoconstriction in both the pulmonary and the coronary arteries, have been demonstrated (5). Reflex bradycardia, hypotension, as well as bronchoconstriction and pulmonary vasoconstriction, seem to be caused, at least partly, by *serotonin* (5-OH-tryptamine) liberated from platelets in the process of coagulation (37). *It is possible that the effect of reflexes on the coronary vessels is less important than that of hypotension in causing coronary ischemia and insufficiency* (38).

Embolic block at the bifurcation of a pulmonary branch is frequent. Pressure in the area supplied by the branches then falls nearly to zero. Stagnation in the affected area and leakage of blood through the vascular walls follow, causing a *hemorrhagic infarct.* It is customary to admit a wedge-shaped infarction with the greater breadth toward the surface of the lung and associ-ated with a certain degree of associated pleurisy. However, rounded or indefinite formations are often revealed by x-ray.

Multiple infarctions are frequent. A recent infarct resembles a blood clot while an older one shows organization, fibrosis, and superficial retraction. *Septic emboli* may be followed by abscesses. *Large occlusions* may affect an entire lobe or even one lung, causing diffuse edema without consolidation. This, however, is usually incompatible with recovery.

SIGNS AND SYMPTOMS

In typical cases, *the patient suddenly becomes cyanotic and dyspneic* and complains of *precordial oppression* and *suffocation.* Ashen-gray color and diffuse perspiration may appear. *The pulse is weak and extremely rapid,* blood pressure falls, and *shock* may occur. *Nausea* and *vomiting* may appear.

If death is avoided, the vascular collapse subsides after 1 to 2 hours, and strain of the right heart becomes apparent (*acute cor pulmonale*). Dilatation of the right ventricle, which is apparent on percussion and fluoroscopy, then occurs. The dilated pulmonary artery may cause violent pulsation of the 2nd left interspace. *Accentuation of the 2nd sound over the pulmonic area,* and *a triple rhythm* over the center of the precordium, are heard (1b, 6).

A *pericardial friction rub* in the 2nd, 3rd, and 4th interspaces, near the left sternal border, has been described and attributed to impingement of the pulmonary conus on the anterior wall (1b, 7).

The *neck veins* are distended revealing a *rise of systemic venous pressure* (8a). Marked systolic pulsations of the jugular veins and the liver may be due to relative tricuspid insufficiency.

One or two days after the onset, the *signs of infarction* appear. They consist of: *cough,* which is frequently followed by *bloody sputum; pain,* limited expansion, and dulness of the corresponding area of the chest; decreased breath sounds or bronchial breathing; and, occasionally, *friction rub.* The latter is evidence of *reactive pleuritis.*

Within 12 to 24 hours from the onset, *fever, leucocytosis,* and *increased sedimentation rate* appear. After the first 2 or 3 days, moderate *jaundice* may be observed (1d). It is caused by hemolysis and readsorption of pigment from the infarcted area but may be favored by liver engorgement.

ELECTROCARDIOGRAM

Tracings taken soon after the attack may present significant changes (1, 6b, 10). They consist of *right axis deviation* (S$_1$-high R$_3$) and evidence of *ischemia (or "strain")* of the right ventricle (depressed S-T and inverted T in leads 2, 3, and VF, as well as in V$_1$-V$_2$). These changes do not appear in cases where the obstruction is not followed by cardiac "strain".

X-RAY

Roentgen-ray evidence of pulmonary infarction is lacking in the early stages but *elevation of the diaphragm on the affected side* may be observed. Later, *a rounded shadow* in one of the pulmonary fields is the most common finding while triangular opacity is infrequently seen. The appearance of the affected area may be that of a bronchopneumonic type of infiltration.

COMPLICATIONS

If the patient survives, possible complications are pneumonia, pleurisy, and pericarditis. If an atrial septal defect has been present, sudden increase of right heart pressure may cause inversion of the blood stream through the shunt, followed by severe cyanosis. New emboli may, furthermore, pass through the defect causing cerebral or renal embolism (*paradoxical embolism*—pages 279 and 316). Myocardial infarction may be precipitated by shock, by anoxemia, and by the reflexes which follow pulmonary embolism (12).

DIAGNOSIS

The diagnosis of pulmonary embolism is not difficult when this condition occurs in congestive failure, after surgery, or in patients with known phlebitis. Otherwise, differential diagnosis from myocardial infarction is necessary. In *anteroseptal infarction,* there is an inverted complex (QS or QR) in V$_3$-V$_4$ while in *pulmonary infarction* there is an inverted T *and no deep Q* in V$_1$-V$_2$. If secondary coronary ischemia is followed by infarction, this is seldom anteroseptal and may be recognized by the usual signs (page 421).

In rare cases, differential diagnosis between acute cor pulmonale and *diaphragmatic hernia* is necessary (18).

TREATMENT

Prevention of the embolism in postoperative patients is done by using *heparin* (13) (**63**) or *dicumarol* (**64**) (page 594), and by *early exercise* of the legs (9) with the intent to accelerate venous circulation.

Surgical exploration of the femoral veins may demonstrate the existence of thrombosis and may be followed by bilateral vein ligation. This has the purpose of preventing the mobilization of a large clot but cannot prevent the formation of small emboli through the collateral circulation.

Preventive ligation in patients with varicose veins and in elderly patients requiring perineal surgery or operations on the legs has been done but may be substituted by anticoagulant therapy. *Ligation of the iliac veins* is necessary in some cases (15).

Embolectomy (Trendelenburg operation (16)) has been performed in cases with occlusion of the main artery or one of the stems. It is successful only when the attack occurs in a hospital so that immediate intervention is possible.

Oxygen is helpful and will be given by mask or tent. *Venesection is contraindicated.* *Anticoagulants* (heparin, followed by dicumarol) should be started at once and continued for several weeks. *Morphine, atropine*, and *papaverine* are given in order to prevent vascular spasm and reflex changes in the pulmonary and coronary circulations (17). However, *care should be taken not to lower blood pressure to a shock level.* A too severe drop of pressure may also favor myocardial ischemia and thus lead to heart failure or myocardial infarct.

If *shock* develops, *infusion of plasma containing nor-epinephrine* should be started at once.

Intravenous digitalis is given if heart failure develops.

Subacute and Chronic Pulmonary Heart Disease (Subacute and Chronic Cor Pulmonale)

CAUSE AND MECHANISM

There are three main types: cases with pulmonary hypertension without obstruction; cases with pulmonary hypertension secondary to obstruction; and cases of pulmonary shunt.

1) *Pulmonary hypertension without obstruction.* These cases have no limitation to oxygen intake; oxygen saturation of the arterial blood is normal; if there is cyanosis, this is a *"peripheral cyanosis"* (large a-v oxygen difference).

a) *Primary hypertension.* This is a group which can be accepted only temporarily. It includes a so-called *idiopathic* or *essential hypertension* (28) found in young persons, and *hypertension due to congenital hypoplasia of the pulmonary vessels with secondary thickening of their walls.*

b) *Secondary hypertension.* This may be due to either increased resistance *beyond* the lung (mitral stenosis) or to increased flow (septal defects, patent ductus, Lutembacher, Eisenmenger, transposition, common trunk). The last conditions have a "central cyanosis" due to mixture of bloods from the greater and lesser circulation. All may have a *late cyanosis* due to secondary lesions of the pulmonary vessels with decreased oxygen intake.

2) *Pulmonary hypertension secondary to*

obstruction (33). In all these cases there is a deficient oxygen intake and a decreased oxygen saturation of the arterial blood while the a-v difference in oxygen is normal (*central cyanosis*).

a) *Cancer of the lung* (miliary carcinomatosis).

b) *Tuberculosis* (fibrotic type).

c) *Pulmonary emphysema* (due to bronchitis, peribronchitis, bronchial asthma, senile emphysema).

d) *Bacterial* (chronic multiple abscesses; bronchiectasis; chronic pneumonia).

e) *Thromboembolic* (multiple embolisms, multiple thromboses) (41).

f) *Arteriosclerotic* (luetic, idiopathic).

g) *Parasitic* (bilharzia).

h) *Exposure to dusts* (pneumoconiosis, anthracosis, berylliosis, silicosis, siderosis, exposure to radioactive dust).

i) *Deformity of the chest.*

j) Lesions of the pulmonary vessels which are part of a "collagen disease" (scleroderma, panarteritis nodosa, reaction to sulfonamides or to serum).

3) *Arteriovenous fistula of the lungs.* These patients have a rapid circulation; part of the blood flow bypasses the pulmonary capillaries, so that the oxygen intake is deficient and there is a "central cyanosis".

In many of the cases with obstruction, inadequate ventilation, reduced vital capacity, and increased CO_2 content of the arterial blood are present. *Whenever anoxia is present, a vasomotor constriction of the pulmonary arterioles may increase the obstruction.*

LESIONS

The main structural changes consist of either of the two following possibilities:

a) *A lesion of the lungs* (fibrosis, silicosis, anthracosis, pneumoconiosis, atelectasis, bronchiectasis, bronchitis and peribronchitis, emphysema) *or of their small vessels* (arteriosclerosis, endarteritis obliterans, periarteritis).

b) *A primary lesion of the heart* (valvular defects, shunts, malformations).

Secondary lesions are:

a) *A secondary lesion of the pulmonary artery and stems* (dilatation, atherosclerosis).

b) *A secondary lesion of the heart* (dilatation and hypertrophy of the right ventricle; possible dilatation of the right atrium) (fig. 292).

c) *Distention of the venous system and liver* (late stages).

SIGNS AND SYMPTOMS

Some of the signs and symptoms are due to the primary disease and may, therefore, precede the establishment of pulmonary heart disease. Attacks of bronchial asthma, chronic obstinate cough, dyspnea, and weakness are common episodes which may precede the cardiac changes by years or decades. They may mask the actual symptoms caused by the heart and make the diagnosis difficult.

General signs are: *severe cyanosis*, which may reach an extreme degree[75]; *clubbing* of the fingers and toes; *polycythemia; low oxygen saturation* of the arterial blood; frequent signs of pulmonary emphysema and chronic bronchitis; and prolonged and forceful expiration.

The heart rhythm is usually regular. *The rate is frequently increased.* Enlargement of the right heart is revealed by a *forceful epigastric pulsation* and by an extension of cardiac dulness to the right.[76] There frequently is *a pulmonic systolic murmur; the 2nd pulmonic sound is loud and occasionally split.* It may be followed by a soft, early-diastolic pulmonic murmur. A soft systolic murmur over the tricuspid area may be

[75] On account of the extremely dark color of the faces of some of these patients, they have been called "black cardiacs." The syndrome of arteriosclerosis of the pulmonary artery with chronic pulmonary heart disease is also called the *syndrome of Ayerza and Arrillaga.*

[76] Right ventricular enlargement may be difficult to detect because of pulmonary emphysema and low level of the diaphragm. For the same reason, sometimes the only sites where the heart sounds can be detected are the suprasternal and xiphoid areas.

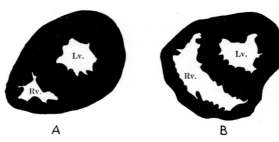

A   B

FIG. 292. Transverse section of the heart in *cor pulmonale*. A, normal heart; B, heart of chronic cor pulmonale. (Inspired by originals of P. D. White.)

heard in a more advanced stage. Arterial blood pressure is usually somewhat low; *venous pressure is high.* The jugular veins and the liver may be engorged.

GRAPHIC TRACINGS

Electrocardiogram

Right axis deviation is frequent. *Right ventricular hypertrophy* is usually noted (page 368) and there may be evidence of *ischemia of the right ventricular wall* (so-called "right ventricular strain"): depressed S-T and inverted T wave in leads 2, 3, and aVF, as well as in the chest leads V_1-V_2 (fig. 293). There may be a *P-pulmonale*, which is evidence of *right atrial enlargement* (page 369). This consists of *high voltage and longer duration of P in leads 2, 3, and aVF.* There is a positive phase of P, followed by a brief and peaked negative phase in V_1-V_2; the duration of P is greater than 0.10 second.

Phonocardiogram

A *diamond-shaped systolic murmur* is often recorded over the second left interspace. The *second pulmonic sound* is loud and occasionally split. It may be followed by a few vibrations "in decrescendo" caused by slight incompetence of the pulmonic valve.

A *triple rhythm* is frequently recorded (page 370) over the epigastrium and the tricuspid area (so-called right ventricular gallop).

The murmurs of the *a-v fistula of the lung*

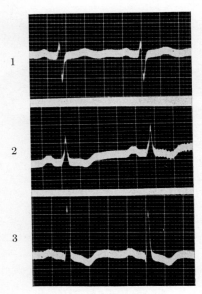

Fig. 293. Electrocardiogram of *chronic cor pulmonale.*

are the following: a *late-systolic murmur* frequently overshadowing the second sound; or an *early-diastolic* murmur.

Low Frequency Vibrations of the Chest and Epigastrium

An apex cardiogram may reveal a systolic depression of the apex. On the contrary, the epigastric tracing usually reveals a high, early, and forceful positive thrust due to the hypertrophy of the right ventricle (page 370). The atrial wave is high in the epigastric tracing (29).

Electrokymogram

The most notable findings are the following (30). High and rapidly expanding pulse of the pulmonary arch. High and rapidly expanding pulse over the hilar shadows. Small or absent pulsation over the lung fields. In cases with unilateral or lobar fibrosis, lack of pulse is limited to the affected side or to the fibrotic lobes.

CARDIOMANOMETRY

Right ventricular systolic pressure is between 35 and 90 mm. mercury (normal

22–23); *right ventricular diastolic pressure* is frequently 3 to 5 mm. mercury (normal 0). If the right ventricle is in failure, its diastolic pressure becomes higher. *The systolic pressure of the pulmonary artery* is about the same as that of the right ventricle, e.g. 35 to 90 (normal 22–23) while the *diastolic* is frequently 10 to 30 (normal 7–9) (31).

The *gradient of pressure* between pulmonary artery and pulmonary capillaries is frequently increased, indicating pulmonary arteriolar vasoconstriction. Oxygen inhalation or intravenous digitalis frequently reduce this gradient, indicating its functional nature.

In cases with a-v fistula of the lungs, the pulmonary artery has a high systolic and a low diastolic pressure.

CARDIAC OUTPUT—PERIPHERAL RESISTANCE

Cardiac output is often increased. This is a compensatory phenomenon due to the poor oxygenation of the blood (39). However, the output may be normal if there is no anoxia, pulmonary resistance is high, or there is heart failure (39, 40).

The data of catheterization correlated with cardiac output reveal the frequent existence of *peripheral vasodilation* which contrasts with pulmonary vasoconstriction. However, this vasodilation is present only in a low percentage of cases.

X-RAY

Both the right atrium and the right ventricle are enlarged, the conus of the right ventricle, the pulmonary artery, and its stems, are *dilated* and show strong pulsations. The hilar shadows are thick and may pulsate (fig. 294).

Lesions of the lungs are revealed by x-ray and, even better, by *angiopneumography*.

COURSE AND COMPLICATIONS

The course of this syndrome is usually long, lasting for many years.

In the most common forms, those second-

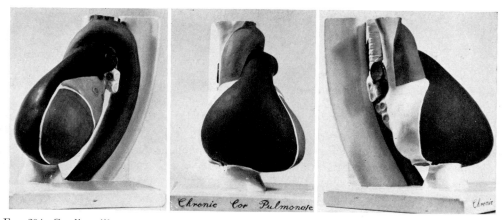

FIG. 294. Cardiac silhouette of chronic cor pulmonale. (From models of the American Heart Associa tion.)

ary to bronchopulmonary lesions, three main periods can be considered:

a) *Phase of bronchial and pulmonary lesions.* The lesion starts in the bronchi, then causes bronchiectasis, peribronchitis, and emphysema. The sputum is often bloody. Periods of improvement alternate with periods of more severe symptoms.

b) *Phase of compensated cor pulmonale.* The pulmonary fibrosis acts as an obstacle to the lesser circulation. Hypertension in the pulmonary artery, enlargement of the right ventricle, hemoptysis, and attacks of paroxysmal dyspnea (largely due to the heart) are frequent. The oxygen saturation of the arterial blood may be lower. Clubbing and cyanosis begin. Electrocardiographic, x-ray, and physical signs of right heart enlargement are apparent. The venous pressure is normal.

c) *Phase of decompensated cor pulmonale.* Cyanosis is very severe; polycythemia is constant. *Chronic dyspnea, headache,* and *somnolence* are typical. The *venous pressure is high; the liver is large;* there may be *peripheral edema.* Congestion of the brain, kidneys, and spleen may be present. There is evidence of *chronic right ventricular failure.* These patients may have superimposed episodes of acute cardiac failure.

VARIETIES

Bronchial asthma (22). Bronchial asthma with pulmonary emphysema is a common cause of cor pulmonale. The strain represented by the severe attacks of dyspnea is a contributory element. The diagnosis of the cardiac complication is often difficult because of the previous existence of dyspnea and distention of the lungs. Peripheral edema is not common and may be present for only a few days before death. A bronchospastic element is often present and should be relieved before evaluating the severity of the cardiac damage.

Chest deformities (23, 36). Severe deformity of the chest, especially kyphoscoliosis, is a frequent and not widely known cause of cor pulmonale. Absolute and relative reduction of lung volume and vital capacity is present. The distortion and rigidity of the thoracic cage causes difficulty in breathing, resulting in a *purely diaphragmatic type of respiration.* This leads to *habitual dyspnea* which gradually increases after the arrest of growth. *Dyspnea is relieved at times by hyperextension in the recumbent position.* Exertion may cause attacks of dyspnea with weakness and fainting. *Dyspnea* and persistent *tachycardia* may be the only early signs of heart failure. The combined cardiac and pulmonic insufficiency may lead to rapid development of symptoms and death within a short time. Mild or latent heart failure in cases with slight deformity has been described.

Multiple and silent pulmonary embolism followed by organization may cause chronic and intractable cor pulmonale (41).

Arteriovenous fistula of the lungs (24, 34). This congenital lesion consists of the formation of vascular pockets connecting branches of the pulmonary artery with pulmonary veins. The resulting shunts cause increased cardiac output and decreased oxygen intake because part of the blood bypasses the pulmonary capillaries. Cardiac enlargement, polycythemia, and clubbing are the result. Weakness, faintness, dyspnea, chest pain, and hemoptysis are common. A *continuous machinery murmur* may be present on the surface of the chest above the fistula.

The diagnosis is simplified by using *angiopneumography* with the same technique which is employed for angiocardiography. This should be performed with caution because of the shunts.

DIAGNOSIS

The diagnosis may be difficult because of the possible confusion with congenital heart disease or mitral stenosis. As both of them can be the cause of *a secondary cor pulmonale*, exclusion of pulmonary components is not always easy. Moreover, a-v fistula of the lung has several points in common with congenital malformations of the heart.

Differential diagnosis from *mitral stenosis* may be necessary. A phonocardiogram may help by showing that no diastolic murmur is present in cor pulmonale. The ECG has a high, notched and prolonged P wave in 1 and 2, in mitral stenosis; in leads 2 and 3, in cor pulmonale (27). No prolongation of P-R is present in cor pulmonale.

Once mitral stenosis and congenital shunts of the heart are excluded, three elements should be evaluated:

a) The part played by the basic lesion (pulmonary disease, deformity, arteriovenous aneurysms), its cause and severity.

b) The part played by right ventricular strain.

c) The possible signs of heart failure.

As no valvular stenosis is present in these patients, the level of the venous pressure is inversely proportional to the efficiency of the right ventricle. On the contrary, cyanosis, polycythemia, oxygen saturation, and dyspnea are largely dependent upon the pulmonary conditions. Severe right ventricular enlargement is evidence of some degree of heart failure.

In most cases, *pulmonary function tests* may give evidence of the degree of impairment of the pulmonary respiratory function. Frequent determinations of the oxygen content of the arterial blood and blood counts are also necessary.

In certain cases, catheterization of the right heart reveals the degree of heart failure and may show the degree of increased resistance of the pulmonary vessels and whether or not there is a functional component.

TREATMENT

In many cases, a careful study of the patient before cor pulmonale has set in may allow a causal treatment so that the cardiac condition is prevented. This prevention includes the entire medical and surgical possibilities of the chest physicians.

Surgical correction of the chest deformity, *lobectomy* in cases of a-v aneurysms, may correct the condition if undertaken before it is too late.

Digitalis is helpful whenever there is right heart failure (32). It may be followed by increased pressure of the pulmonary artery. However, this is temporary and disappears with the improvement of the cardiac condition. Digitalis lowers right atrial and venous pressure, increases peripheral resistance, and decreases pulmonary arterial resistance.

Oxygen is useful. However, care should be taken not to depress the respiratory center. Therefore, 95 per cent oxygen with 5 per cent CO_2 is recommended. In emphysema and pulmonary fibrosis, several *mechanical procedures* are helpful. They include an elastic girdle, raising the foot of the bed, and pneumoperitoneum, in order to favor expiration.

Morphine may be dangerous in many of these conditions, and particularly in those associated with chest deformity. Sudden death may result from respiratory insufficiency following depression of the respiratory center by morphine or oxygen.

ACTH or *cortisone* may be helpful in "collagen diseases". *Surgery* should be resorted to in some of the congenital malformations of the heart.

Ephedrine (57) *and isupral* are useful in cases with bronchoconstriction. Even though there is no known specific vasodilator of the pulmonary vessels (except oxygen), *aminophyllin* (42), *priscoline* (54), or *papaverine* (43, 44) can be tried.

Penicillin aerosol may be helpful in chronic pulmonary infection. *Heparin* should be used in repeated pulmonary embolization.

Venesection is indicated only if there is heart failure while *pulmonary failure alone contraindicates this procedure.*

BIBLIOGRAPHY

1. a) White, P. D., and Brenner, O. New England J. Med., 1933, **209**, 1261.
   b) McGinn, S., and White, P. D. J. A. M. A., 1935, **104**, 1473.
   c) White, P. D., and co-workers. Arch. Int. Med., 1937, **60**, 39; and 1940, **65**, 163.
   d) White, P. D. Am. J. M. Sci., 1940, **200**, 577.
2. Homans, J. New England J. Med., 1934, **211**, 993; and 1943, **229**, 309.
3. Chapman, E. M., and Linton, R. R. J. A. M. A., 1945, **129**, 196.
4. a) Cohnheim, J. F. *Lectures on General Pathology.* London, New Sydenham Soc., 1889, **1**, 54.
   b) Haggart, G. E., and Walker, A. M. Arch. Surg., 1923, **6**, 764.
   c) Fineberg, M. H., and Wiggers, C. J. Am. Heart J., 1936, **11**, 255.
5. a) Hochrein, M., and Schneyer, K. Arch. exp. Path., 1937, **187**, 265.
   b) Hochrein, M. Akt. Kreislauff., 1938, **14**, 24.
   c) Scherf, D., and Schoenbrunner, E. Klin. Woch., 1937, **16**, 340.
6. a) Evans, W. Brit. Heart J., 1943, **5**, 73.
   b) Lewes, D. Brit. Heart J., 1944, **6**, 161.
7. Durant, T. M. In *Stroud's Cardiovascular Diseases.* Philadelphia, Davis, 1945.
8. a) Wood, P. Brit. Heart J., 1941, **3**, 21.
   b) Konschegg, T. Virch. Arch., 1930, **278**, 638.
9. Robinson, C. A. New England J. Med., 1944, **231**, 821.
10. White, P. D. *Heart Disease.* New York, Macmillan, 1944.
11. Smith, K. S. Quart. J. Med., 1938, **7**, 85.
12. Currens, J. Proc. Staff Meet., Mayo Clin., 1942, **17**, 502.
13. Murray, D. W. G., and Best, C. H. J. A. M. A., 1938, **110**, 118.
14. Barker, N. W., Allen, E. V., and Waugh, J. M. Proc. Staff Meet., Mayo Clin., 1943, **18**, 102.
15. a) Tillet, W. S., Cambier, M. H., and McCormack, J. E. J. Clin. Investigation, 1945, **24**, 595.
    b) Fine, J. Bull. New England Med. Center, 1946, **8**, 6.
16. a) Trendelenburg, F. Arch. klin. Chir., 1908, **86**, 686.
    b) Sauerbruch, F. *Die Chirurgie der Brustorgane.* Berlin, Springer, 1920/25.
17. Beckwith, J. R. Virginia Med. Monthly, 1944, **71**, 279.
18. McGinn, S., and Spear, L. M. New England J. Med., 1941, **224**, 1014.
19. Willius, F. A. Canad. M. A. J., 1946, **54**, 42.
20. a) Ayerza, L. Unpublished lecture, 1901. Also Semana Medica, 1925, **1**, 43.
    b) Arrillaga, F. C. *Esclerosis Secundaria de la Arteria Pulmonar y su Quadro Clinico.* Thesis no. 2536, Buenos Aires, 1912. Arch. Mal. Coeur, 1913, **5**, 518. *La Arteritis Pulmonar.* Buenos Aires, Garcia, 1925.
21. Castex, M. R., and co-workers. Prensa Med. Arg., 1932, **19**, 1; and 1936, **23**, 481.
22. a) Kountz, W. B., Alexander, H. L., and Prinzmetal, M. Am. Heart J., 1936, **11**, 163.

b) Schiller, I. W., Colmes, A., and Davis, D. New England J. Med., 1943, **228,** 113.

23. Schaefer, G. Zeit. Kreislauff., 1934, **26,** 689.

24. Sisson, J. H., Murphy, G. E., and Newman, E. V. Bull. Johns Hopkins Hosp., 1945, **76,** 93.

25. Sussman, M. L., Grishman, A., and Steinberg, M. F. New England J. Med., 1943, **228,** 777.

26. Evans, W., and Hunter, A. Brit. Heart J., 1943, **5,** 73.

27. Shleser, I. H., and Langendorf, R. Am. J. M. Sci., 1942, **204,** 725.

28. a) Dresdale, D. T., *et al.* Am. J. Med., 1951, **11,** 686.

    b) Griswold, H. E. Meet. Am. Heart Assoc., 1951.

29. Luisada, A. A., and Magri, G. Am. Heart J., 1952, **44,** 545.

30. Luisada, A. A., and Fleischner, F. G. Am. J. Med., 1949, **6,** 756.

31. a) Bloomfield, R. A., *et al.* J. Clin. Investigation, 1946, **25,** 639.

    b) Richards, D. W. Am. J. Med., 1947, **3,** 434.

32. Ferrer, I., *et al.* Circ., 1950, **1,** 161.

33. Austrian, R., *et al.* Am. J. Med., 1951, **11,** 667.

34. Baer, S., *et al.* Circ., 1950, **1,** 602.

35. Crane, P., *et al.* Am. J. Roentgenol., 1949, **62,** 418.

36. Evans, W. Brit. Heart J., 1946, **8,** 162.

37. Comroe, J. H., *et al.* Am. J. Physiol., 1953, **173,** 379.

    Alinow, M. R., *et al.* Am. Heart J., 1946, **31,**

38. M702.

39. Cournand, A. Circ., 1950, **2,** 641.

40. Fowler, N. O., *et al.* Circ., 1952, **6,** 888.

41. Owen, W. R., *et al.* New Eng. J. Med., 1953, **249,** 919.

CHAPTER 24

Hypotension—Shock—Hyposphygmia

The clinical syndromes caused by or connected with a lowering of the blood pressure deserve greater attention than usually thought. One of the reasons for their neglect is the erroneous belief that "hypotension is good for the patient" (1). This belief is based on the arbitrary fixation of *one level* as a normal level of blood pressure or, even worse, on accepting as "normal" an increasing figure with the progression of years (page 65). This led to inclusion of a large number of normal people in the group of so-called hypotensive patients. On the other hand, studies made by insurance companies deal only with mortality and are usually not interested in symptoms or working efficiency.

The normal level of blood pressure has as its lower limit figures of about 100 systolic and 65 diastolic. This somewhat arbitrary level may be further lowered if the patient is of the African or Mongolian races. Any condition associated with a blood pressure which is lower than the above figures and presents both a low systolic and a low diastolic pressure should be called *hypotension* (2). On the contrary, a different syndrome is that of patients having a slightly lower systolic but a normal or even a high diastolic pressure. As the main characteristic of these patients is the small radial pulse, the author proposed the name of *hyposphygmia* for this syndrome (2).

Hypotension

CAUSE

The causes are different in the acute and chronic types of hypotension.

Acute hypotension may be caused by:

a) Hemorrhagic collapse, due to severe and sudden loss of blood (bleeding wounds, hemoptysis, gastrointestinal hemorrhage, metrorragia).

b) *Direct central effect of emotion or fear* in vasolabile individuals; *invasion of cerebral vessels or vasomotor centers by tumors; sudden distention of cerebral veins* caused by straining in patients with superior caval syndrome (24).

c) *Reflex collapse*, caused by severe and prolonged reflex stimulation, which may or may not be felt as pain. Sensitive nerve stimulation (sciatic, ulnar nerve, testicles); distention of a hollow viscus (gall bladder, stomach); stimulation of a serosa (pleura, peritoneum); stimulation of the myocardium (coronary occlusion), the aorta (dissecting aneurysm), or the pulmonary artery (pulmonary embolism); or distention of the pressoreceptors (carotid sinus in arteriosclerotic persons; pulmonary artery in patients with chronic cor pulmonale) are the most common causes.

d) *Allergic collapse.* Trauma, burns, serum injections, hay fever, intestinal occlusion, favism, and bronchial asthma may be accompanied by a sudden vascular collapse.

e) *Cardiogenic collapse.* Temporary arrest of cardiac activity, extreme slowing of heart rate, or, on the contrary, extremely rapid cardiac action, may cause low blood pressure.[77]

f) *Anoxia* may cause a sudden hypotension through active vasodilation. It is more frequent in infants (but may take

[77] The *cardiogenic collapse* which follows coronary occlusion has not been included in this group because of its partly reflex mechanism. However, cases with extremely severe myocardial damage and cases with severe disturbance of the cardiac rate and rhythm should be included.

place also in older patients) with tetralogy of Fallot following exertion or crying (24).

All these conditions may lead to a state of "shock" which is usually irreversible. Shock will be discussed below.

Subacute or chronic hypotension is present in many clinical syndromes.

a) *Infectious and parasitic diseases*; it is connected with fever and the action of bacterial toxins.

b) Starvation, cachexia, vitamin deficiency, anemia, physical exhaustion, poisoning, and anesthesia, are accompanied by low blood pressure. Low blood pressure is also found in lipoid nephrosis.

c) *A mechanical obstacle to venous return* (liver cirrhosis, extensive varicose veins), *cardiac action* (pericarditis with effusion or constrictive pericarditis, amyloid heart, fibroelastosis) or *systolic discharge* (valvular stenosis) is a further cause of low blood pressure. It is apparent that a decrease of cardiac output due to *cardiac failure* may also cause hypotension.

d) *Endocrine disturbances* may determine hypotension; the most common causes are hypothyroidism and Addison's disease.

MECHANISM

Maintenance of blood pressure is based on a good cardiac output and an optimal peripheral resistance. Therefore, any sudden decrease of either of them causes a drop in blood pressure. Deficiency in cardiac output can be due to heart failure or decreased venous return. The latter may be due to extreme venous dilatation.

Hemorrhagic collapse is easily explained because the sudden decrease of blood volume leads to decreased venous return and, therefore, to decreased cardiac output.

A *reflex collapse* is usually based on a double mechanism:

a) Efferent stimuli along the pathway of the vagus slow down the heart, at times causing asystole.

b) Efferent stimuli along the sympathetic pathways dilate the peripheral vessels.

This double mechanism has been proven for the carotid sinus and aortic reflexes (page 53), and is probably true for other reflexes.

Both arterial and venous dilatation seem to occur (3, 4, 5) resulting in a sudden decrease of peripheral resistance and a decrease of venous return.

Different reactions have been demonstrated in man: at times, reflex vagal slowing of the heart is the main factor of the blood pressure drop (*vasovagal collapse*); at other times, on the contrary, peripheral dilatation is of paramount importance (*vasosympathetic collapse*). It is apparent that atropine is useful in the first case but not in the second, and that both types may be combined.

Allergic or *anaphylactic collapse* is attributed to a sudden drop in venous return. This is caused by *severe dilatation of the peripheral capillaries* (6, 12) and probably by *constriction of the hepatic veins* (7).

Subacute and chronic hypotensions are caused by *arteriolar and venous dilatation* (fever, toxemia), *poor venous return*, or *mechanical hindrance to cardiac action*. Vascular dilatation may be favored by depression of the vasomotor center (bacterial toxins, poisoning) and may be connected with endocrine disturbances (Addison's disease).

The possibility that an abnormal function of the renal pressor system may be the cause of low blood pressure has been advocated but, so far, not proven.

SIGNS AND SYMPTOMS

When a *vascular collapse* occurs, poor cerebral circulation causes different phenomena: *dizziness, fainting, syncope,* or *convulsive attacks.* The severity and duration of the collapse is responsible for the severity of the cerebral symptoms.

Subacute hypotension may cause *disturbances of vision* and *hearing* and strange sensations in the throat, stomach, or chest.

Chronic hypotension is often accompanied

by *exertional dyspnea and palpitation* and also, at times, by precordial pain during exertion. Weakness, lowered resistance to fatigue, and headache are also common.

Physical examination may reveal that the *heart is small* (typical after hemorrhage or in Addison's disease). The apex thrust may be strong and the 1st sound, loud. However, in vascular collapse and toxic states, all manifestations of cardiac activity are weak. *Tachycardia, triple rhythm, and various murmurs* are common. *Venous pressure* is frequently low.

The *electrocardiogram* may reveal a marked respiratory arrhythmia, high T waves, and occasional inversion of T_3 with slight raising of S-T (8).

Orthostatic hypotension. This interesting clinical picture may vary considerably. In some cases, *dizziness* is felt when the patient rises from the recumbent to the erect position. In other patients, on the contrary, the mere fact of raising the head above a certain level causes *syncope*, so that some of these unfortunates even learn to walk in a crouching position (9)!

During the fainting attack, different possibilities exist (5).

a) The heart *slows down* considerably and may even stop (*cardiac type*).

b) The blood pressure drops without bradycardia and usually with *tachycardia* (*vascular type*).

c) Fainting occurs without cardiac or vascular changes because carotid stimuli reach the brain causing syncope (*cerebral type*). An association of these types is possible.

In most of these cases an *abnormal sensitivity of the carotid sinuses is present.* In some patients, these areas have a *low sensitivity* and fail to compensate with adequate reflexes for the pooling of blood in the arterioles of the viscera and in the veins of the lower extremities (5, 10). In others, these areas are *extremely irritable* on external compression and cause severe brady-cardia or cardiac arrest when stimulated

by *internal* (sudden change of position) or *external* (tight collar, sudden turning of head) pressure. Extreme bradycardia may occur in patients with faulty coronary flow. Extreme irritability of the carotid sinus may be favored by atheroma of the carotid arteries and is common in pheochromocytoma. The cerebral type of attacks is common in cases of tabes, encephalitis, or other neuropathy, including that of diabetes.

Either myocardial infarction (11) or cerebral infarction may be determined by a sudden drop in pressure if the vessels of that organ had been previously damaged (coronary or cerebral arteriosclerosis).

Orthostatic hypotension may be the result of surgical splanchnicectomy. It is more marked during the first months following surgery and may occasionally last a few years. It is due to inability of compensatory, reflex vasoconstriction to offset the pooling of blood in the splanchnic area and the lower extremities. Eventually arterial tonus is regained and this type of hypotension is attenuated.

Permanent or orthostatic hypotension may be caused by drugs, especially those inhibiting the sympathetic system (hydergine, dibenamine, benzodioxane) or blocking the ganglia (hexamethonium).

Left lateral hypotension. This unusual phenomenon has been attributed to obstruction of the pulmonary veins with decreased return to the left heart, or to reflexes of unexplained origin (21).

Diagnosis is based on several tests of alternated recumbency and erect position with blood pressure readings, pulse counts, and electrocardiograms.

Compression of either carotid sinus should test the sensitivity of those areas and should be performed before and after an injection of *atropine.*

TREATMENT

In *acute hypotension,* treatment varies according to the cause. When allergy is involved, *adrenalin* (**55**) and *ephedrine* (**57**) shall be used. When hemorrhage is the cause of the collapse, either *rectal or venous infusion* with physiologic salt solution or plasma or *blood transfusion* are the best remedies. When reflexes are involved, *morphine, atropine,* and *phenobarbital* should be used.

In some patients, total inhibition of the autonomic system is indicated (**35**). In others, *atropine* or *phenobarbital* alone should be preferred. The use of a *tight girdle* and of *an elastic bandage* over the lower extremities is useful in certain cases. Avoidance of tight collars is always necessary. In some cases, if the carotid sinus fails to react promptly, a prolonged sojourn in the tilted "head-up" bed (**10**) may be tried in order to "train" the carotid pressoreceptors.

If the myocardium is responsible for the abnormal reaction, *quinidine* (**24**) or *pronestyl* (**26, 27**) are indicated.

Extreme reactivity of the carotid sinus may require *denervation of the sensitive area of one side*. This should be preceded by local infiltration with novocaine which would temporarily benefit the patient.

Chronic hypotension should be treated with *ephedrine* (**57**), *benzedrine* (**58**), *coramine* (**61**), and *strychnine* (**69**).

In patients with a tendency to venous dilatation, *paredrinol* (**59**) should be used. *Ligation of the femoral veins* may be necessary in patients with varicose veins.

Shock

Any condition causing severe hypotension may degenerate into a spontaneously irreversible state called "shock".

CAUSE

Primary shock may be caused by numerous conditions such as hemorrhage, allergy, injuries, burns, surgery, toxemia, gastrointestinal perforation or obstruction, exposure, freezing, or dehydration. Pain and fear may be contributory factors. Sudden cardiac failure or acute disturbances of

cardiac rate and rhythm may be followed by *secondary shock (cardiogenic shock)*.

SYMPTOMS AND SIGNS

The patient is pale or ashen-gray but may be cyanotic and frequently has a cold, clammy skin. Anxious, drawn appearance is common. Restlessness, tremor, muscular twitchings, and weakness may be observed. Sensitivity and reflexes are depressed. The tongue is dry and parched. Nausea, vomiting, diarrhea and oliguria may be present.

The superficial veins are small or invisible and fail to fill on compression. The heart sounds are weak. The heart rate is rapid and regular. The arterial pulse is small and thready. The respiration is superficial and rapid but not belabored. *The arterial pressure is very low*, with reduced pulse pressure. Figures of 80/60 are considered bordering the shock level; lower figures indicate shock. When systolic blood pressure reaches the critical level of from 75 to 60 mm. Hg, a relative slowing of the heart occurs. *The venous pressure is low; the temperature is subnormal; the metabolic rate is reduced.*

COURSE

Three main stages have been recognized: *initial, compensatory,* and *irreversible* (**16**). The initial stage is actually a stage of hypotension which is by no means typical. The development of the irreversible stage may occur with varying speed and may, therefore, cause either *delayed* or *acute forms of shock.*

VARIETIES—MECHANISM

Shock is a circulatory insufficiency due to disproportion between blood volume (decreased) and vascular capacity. It is caused by loss of fluid either outside or within the body.

Primary shock is due to a cardiac or vascular mechanism leading to extremely low blood pressure. *Secondary shock* is caused by a sudden loss of blood, or a sudden increase of capillary permeability with escape of plasma into the interstitial spaces

(12). In both cases, a decrease of blood volume takes place.

Primary shock may also be followed by increased capillary permeability following anoxia. Increased blood concentration and refractoriness to fluid replacement are typical.

Recognition that *noxious principles arise* during hemorrhagic, traumatic, and allergic shock and that they are the direct cause of the vascular disturbance represents an important step in understanding the syndrome (13).

It was shown later that different humoral phenomena occur during the two main stages of shock (14).

a) *Compensatory stage:* this is characterized by an increase of constrictor activity of the metarterioles and the precapillary sphincters.

b) *Irreversible stage:* the precapillary control is lost and blood flows into the capillary bed; this causes a progressive stagnation in the small veins with eventual decrease and failure of the venous return to the heart.

It was further recognized that these changes are due to humoral principles because they can be transferred from one animal to another (14).

It is known that the two stages represent the alternate phase of predominance of two substances: one is a stimulant and vasoconstrictor substance, either *angiotonin* (hypertensine), or the VEM principle, or both; the other is a depressant substance which paralyzes the arterioles and prevents their reaction to epinephrine (VDM or ferritine). This substance is manufactured in the liver (14), as further shown by the greater resistance of animals whose liver had an artificially maintained, adequate blood supply (15). In the last stage, a deficiency of the pressor substance is apparent.

In conclusion, shock is a syndrome caused by disturbance of many functions but based on progressive impairment of the circulation and leading to irreversible failure and death (16). Circulatory impairment, due to de-creased venous return, causes a secondary decrease of cardiac output and arterial pressure. The predominant action of a noxious substance causing arteriolar paralysis is apparent in the later stages. This leads to a vicious circle and an irreversible trend.

TREATMENT

The well-known formula that shock should be treated by means of "reassurance, oxygen, rest, warmth, morphine, fluids, and transfusion" (17) is valid for most of the cases, even if often inadequate.

Transfusions and infusions (whole blood, plasma, plasma derivates or substitutes) are definitely useful. *Arterial transfusion* (500 cc. in 10 minutes into the radial artery, then continued at a slower rate) is not more effective than venous transfusion.

The use of *epinephrine* has been discussed and its utility questioned. Experimental proof that lack of response to epinephrine and dilatation of the small vessels occurs in the last stage of shock, shows that its use in this stage is not contraindicated. Moreover, epinephrine is always useful in allergic shock where several peculiar vascular reactions initiate the vascular disturbance. *Nor-epinephrine* (**56**) is widely used with fair results.

Metrazol, coramine, and *pitressin* (18) have little value. *Paredrine* increases both the arterial and venous pressure but not cardiac output (18).

It is likely that *angiotonin (hypertensine)* would be the most effective remedy, as experiments seem to indicate (19).

Hyposphygmia (2)

Hyposphygmia is the circulatory syndrome of patients with a low systolic pressure and a normal or high diastolic pressure. As a result, *mean pressure is normal or slightly low while pulse pressure is small* (2, 20).

CAUSE

The most typical form is congenital or, at least, is favored by a congenital tendency.

Hyposphygmia is found most frequently in adolescents and young people but can be observed at any age. The patients frequently have evidence of poor function of either the thyroid or the adrenal glands.

Tuberculosis, malaria, lues, vitamin deficiency, or chronic alcohol intoxication, may be present in these subjects. The question may be raised whether these conditions, which frequently exert their influence during childhood and adolescence, favored the circulatory syndrome.

Heart failure and extreme tachycardia may be the cause of a secondary hyposphygmia.

SIGNS AND SYMPTOMS

The patients complain of *weakness, lack of will power,* and sometimes, *somnolence.* They often dislike any kind of physical activity, have a *poor appetite,* and an *extreme fear of cold.* Fatigability, lack of interest in the surroundings, and poor memory are often present. In some cases, there is a definite similarity with neuro-circulatory asthenia (page 547).

Headache is common and is located mainly in the occipital region; it may be influenced by the position.

Vertigo may be present. *Exertional dyspnea* and *palpitation* are common but slight.

Cyanosis of the hands and feet is common and is increased by cold. The extremities are cold and clammy. The heart is frequently in a median position (*vertical* or *"drop" heart*). The apical thrust is often visible and forceful. The 1st sound is loud; the 2nd sound is loud over the pulmonic but weak over the aortic area.

Blood pressure at the arm gives figures of 100/90 or 95/85. *Blood pressure* at the forearm presents *an extreme reduction of the pulse pressure,* with figures of 100/95, 95/90, or 85/80; it may be impossible to measure it because of extreme reduction of pulsations. The difference in pulse pressure is far more marked at the forearm than at the arm and may be present only in the former (2) (fig. 295).

Orthostatic tachycardia and hypotension are constantly present. Orthostatic decrease of pulse pressure is frequent.

The *static blood pressure tests* (page 162) give a paradoxical response: when the arm is raised, pulse pressure increases; when the arm is lowered, pulse pressure decreases.

The study of blood pressure in different

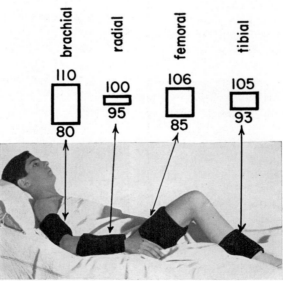

Fɪɢ. 295. Blood pressure in hyposphygmia

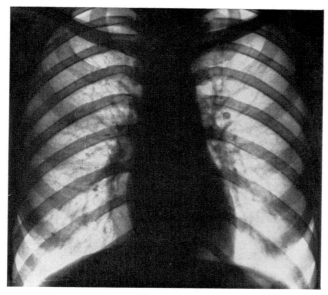

Fig. 296. Small, vertical heart in a case of hyposphygmia

arteries reveals the already mentioned change between arm and forearm. The tibial systolic pressure is frequently equal to that of the arm (fig. 295) but may be higher. The x-ray reveals frequently a small, vertical heart (fig. 296).

Venous pressure is frequently high and may reach even 20 cm. of saline.

MECHANISM

While hyposphygmia caused by tachycardia or heart failure is due to reduced systolic discharge, the most typical form has a peripheral mechanism.

Peripheral dilatation alone would not explain the observed changes. A tentative explanation has been advanced by the writer (2): the arterial wall of these patients has a poorly developed muscular tissue; secondary changes due to toxic, infectious, allergic, or deficiency factors further impair the contractility of the arteries. These behave like elastic tubes, as witness the reduction in pulse pressure at the periphery and upon lowering the arm. The relative increase of blood pressure in the leg of some patients may be explained by the larger caliber of those arteries and by reflected

waves. Secondary disturbances of the capillaries and veins are associated symptoms.

COURSE AND COMPLICATIONS

Patients with hyposphygmia have poor resistance to effort or infections; this may be the cause of a somewhat higher mortality. In general, these patients have a poor efficiency and a reduced capacity for work. Therefore, even if their span of life is normal, they may be a burden to their family and are not an asset to society.

DIAGNOSIS

The diagnosis of hyposphygmia is based on the figures of blood pressure; this should be recorded not only at the arm but also at the lower part of the forearm by means of an oscillometer.

TREATMENT

Secondary hyposphygmia of heart failure or tachycardia requires treatment of the cardiac disturbance.

Secondary hyposphygmia of infectious and consumptive diseases may be treated with drugs stimulating the peripheral vessels, including *ephedrine* (**57**), *benzedrine*

(58), *paredrinol* (59), *and coramine* (61). *Physiotherapy* may be useful in certain cases.

Congenital hyposphygmia, especially of children and adolescents, requires: a) full diet containing the necessary amount of calories; b) large doses of vitamin B-complex; c) *caffeine* (60), *strychnine* (69), *coramine* (61), *or paredrinol* (59); d) *physiotherapy* and *massage*; e) gradual, open air *physical exercise* with sun therapy.

BIBLIOGRAPHY

1. ROBINSON, S. C. New England J. Med., 1946, **223**, 407.

2. a) LUISADA, A. A. Giorn. Med. Prat., March, 1924.
   b) LUISADA, A. A. *Ipotensione e Iposfigmia.* Roma, Pozzi, 1929.

3. HEYMANS, C., BOUCKAERT, J. J., AND REGNIERS, P. *Le Sinus Carotidien.* Paris, Doin, 1933.

4. GOLLWITZER-MEIER, K., AND SCHULTE, H. Pfluegers Arch., 1931, **229**, 251. Also Arch. exp. Path., Pharm., 1932, **165**, 685.

5. WEISS, S. J. Clin. Investigation, 1937, **16**, 73. Also Proc. Assoc. Research Ment. & Nerv. Dis., 1938, **18**, 571.

6. DALE, H. H., AND CO-WORKERS. J. Physiol., 1910, **41**, 318; 1911, **43**, 182; 1918, **52**, 110; 1919, **52**, 355.

7. MAUTNER, H., AND PICK, E. P. Muench. med. Woch., 1915, **62**, 1141. Also Bioch. Zeitschr., 1922, **127**, 72.

8. BATTRO, A., AND LAVALLE COBO. Rev. Arg. Cardiol., 1936, **3**, 215.

9. a) LAUBRY, C. *Semeiologie Cardio-Vasculaire.* Paris, Doin, 1924.
   b) AGOSTONI, G. Arch. Mal. Coeur, 1937, **30**, 101.
   c) TRIPODI, M. Policlin. (sez. prat.), 1932, **39**, 797.

10. MCLEAN, A. R., AND ALLEN, E. V. J. A. M. A., 1940, **115**, 2162.

11. PRIEST, W. S. Mo. Conc. Cardiovasc. Dis., 1942, **11**, N.2.

12. a) MOON, V. H. *Shock and Related Capillary Phenomena.* Oxford Univ. Press, 1938.
    b) BLALOCK, A. Physiol. Rev., 1940, **20**, 159.

13. a) CANNON, W. B. *Traumatic Shock.* New York, Appleton Century Co., 1923.
    b) BAYLISS, W. M. Great Britain Nat. Health Ins. Com., Med. Res. Com., Spec. Rep., series No. 26, 1919.
    d) RAPPORT, D., GUILD, R., AND CANZANELLI, A. Am. J. Physiol., 1945, **143**, 440.

14. a) CHAMBERS, R., ZWEIFACH, B. W., AND LOWENSTEIN, B. E. Am. J. Physiol., 1943, **139**, 123.
    b) ZWEIFACH, B. W., LEE, R. E., HEYMAN, C., AND CHAMBERS, R. Ann. Surg., 1944, **120**, 232.
    c) SHORR, E., ZWEIFACH, B. W., AND FURCHGOTT, R. F. Science, 1945, **102**, 489.
    d) SHORR, E., *et al.* Trans. Assoc. Am. Physicians, 1947, **59**, 28.

15. a) FRANK, H. A., SELIGMAN, A. M., AND FINE, J. J. Clin. Investigation, 1946, **25**, 22.
    b) DEXTER, L., FRANK, H. A., HAYNES, F. W., AND ALTSCHULE, M. D. J. Clin. Investigation, 1943, **22**, 847.

16. WIGGERS, C. J. *Physiology in Health and Disease.* Philadelphia, Lea and Febiger, 1945.

17. FREEMAN, N. E. In *Stroud's Cardiovascular Disease.* Philadelphia, Davis, 1945.

18. a) FRANK, H. A., ALTSCHULE, M. D., AND ZAMCHECK, N. J. Clin. Investigation, 1944, **24**, 54.
    b) FRANK, H. A., SELIGMAN, A. M., AND FINE, J. J. Clin. Investigation, 1945, **24**, 435.

19. FINE, J., FRANK, H. A., AND SELIGMAN, A. M. Ann. Surg., 1945, **122**, 652.

20. FERRANNINI, A. Med. Ital. (Naples), 1903, **1**, 374, 410, 441, 463; 1905, **3**, 82. Also Giorn. Int. Sci. Med., (Naples), 1904, **26**, 529.

21. STEIN, P. Arch. Int. Med., 1952, **90**, 234.

22. a) VEAL, J. R., *et al.* South M. J., 1951, **44**, 1096.
    b) FRENCH, W. E. Memphis M. J., 1951, **26**, 5.
    c) SILBER, E. N. J. A. M. A., 1951, **147**, 1626.

23. ARMSTRONG, T., AND JIMENEZ, R. P. Arch. Med. de Cuba, 1952, **3**, 168.

24. JUDSON, W. E. Med. Clin. North America, 1953, Sept., 1337.

CHAPTER 25

Diseases of the Peripheral Arteries

Arteriosclerosis

CAUSE

Numerous factors have been mentioned in the past as causes of arteriosclerosis but there was insufficient evidence for them in spite of a great deal of speculation.

Arteriosclerosis seemed to be a natural effect of aging, and *senescence* was considered an important cause. However, arteriosclerosis is not always associated with old age and may be found in middle-aged and even young individuals. Moreover, a definite difference between senile and arteriosclerotic changes has been described.

A connection between arteriosclerosis and *arterial pressure and flow* also was described. Arteriosclerosis of the brachial arteries in manual workers and of the cerebral arteries in professional people is common. A greater degree of sclerosis at the branching point of the vessels was further noted.

Once a connection between pressure and sclerosis was admitted, the high incidence of arteriosclerosis in *hypertensive patients* was easily explained. As a consequence, it was admitted that *strain and stress*, as well as *abnormal tonus of the vascular wall*, were responsible for the arteriosclerotic changes. Evidence has been found that either general or local *hypertonus*, if sufficiently severe and lasting, causes arteriosclerotic changes. Ischemic anoxemia of the arterial wall was thought to be the result of *hypertonus* by compression of the vasa vasorum. However, hypotonus also may be associated with arteriosclerosis and, therefore, attention was paid to the reduction in mean and pulse pressures possibly causing ischemic anoxia of the vasa vasorum. Attention was further paid to the lymphatic circulation of the

wall and it was claimed that this may be disturbed by either hypo- or hypertonus (2).

A *toxin theory* also has been advanced, explaining arteriosclerosis as the result of a lesion of the intima, caused by acute infections and other toxic states. The lesion would increase the permeability of the wall to cholesterol and fats.

Once the concept of anoxia of the arterial wall was accepted, it was thought possible that *changes of the normal colloidal state of the blood* might cause the same result by impairing the oxygen and nutritive exchange and reducing the permeability of the wall. Various colloidal plasmatic disturbances have been considered: one type might be due to carbohydrates, one to lipoids, and one to proteins.

Experimental arteriosclerosis was successfully induced in rabbits, dogs, and chicks but much of the older work is vitiated by the fact that these animals are subject to spontaneous arteriosclerosis (3). Two methods, however, can stand the most critical tests:

a) *Adrenalin arteriosclerosis* (4) which causes lesions of the media of a type identical to Moenckeberg's arteriosclerosis.

b) *Cholesterol arteriosclerosis* (5, 28, 31) which reproduces most of the aspects of human arteriosclerosis.

It is likely that, given a high and prolonged intravascular pressure, the normal cholesterol of the blood is injected mechanically into the normal structure of the vessel; an excess of cholesterol would cause earlier and more severe lesions (3). Arteriosclerosis was produced in rabbits (5), chickens (28), and dogs (29) by feeding high cholesterol diets. It was proven that the *height of cholesterol level is not as important as the ratio of total cholesterol to serum phospholipids.* The latter seem to have a stabilizing effect upon the colloidal state of cholesterol in the blood. It was further proven that animals which develop arteriosclerosis have a high concentration of "giant molecules" of lipoproteins,[78] a fact which is similar to that occurring in arteriosclerotic patients (26). The concentration of these molecules is not related to high cholesterol level even though these giant molecules are more numerous in high cholesterolemia.

A significant decrease of plasma cholesterol was found in hyperthyroid animals, and vice versa (27), a fact which coincides with clinical observation. Choline and other lipotropic agents seem to cause regression of experimental arteriosclerosis (32).

STRUCTURAL LESIONS

The arteriosclerotic process may be of three different types:

a) *Atherosclerosis (nodular sclerosis).* In the aorta and larger vessels, the earliest gross evidence of atheroma occurs in the form of yellowish streaks in the intima. These are due to cholesterol, neutral fat, and fat-laden wandering cells. When these lesions increase in size, they lead to the formation of excrescences which project into the lumen and undergo hyaline changes or necrosis. A rich network of blood vessels exists around these lesions (6). The *atheromatous plaque,* so-called because of the soft material contained within the lesion, exhibits various degrees of calcium deposition and, occasionally, of bone formation. The main lesion is intimal but less conspicuous lesions of the media are also present. Ulceration of the surface of the plaque causes the formation of the *atheromatous ulcer* which favors thrombosis, especially in smaller vessels.

b) *Moenckeberg's sclerosis (medial arteriosclerosis).* This type is characterized by the

deposition of calcium in ring-like formations *within the media* of the arteries (*trachea-like radial artery*). The bulging of these formations causes narrowing of the lumen while depressions are present in the intima between them. The calcareous deposits may undergo ossification. Atrophy of the muscular and elastic strata, fibrosis of the media, and moderate thickening of the intima are present.

c) *Arterionecrosis.* There may be: i) *cystic medionecrosis* of unknown etiology with degeneration of the medial coat of the aorta; it frequently leads to rupture and dissecting aneurysm; or ii) *toxic arterionecrosis* with degenerative and necrotic lesions in various parts of all the arterial coats; it is due to exogenous or renal toxins, or adrenal substances.

d) *Hyperplastic arteriosclerosis.* It involves the small arteries and arterioles; there is hyperplasia of the media and, partly, of the intima. It is associated with high blood pressure; it may be found in the pulmonary vessels of congenital heart patients.

Fibrosis of the aortic valves and *sclerosis of the peripheral veins* are usually present in patients having sclerosis of the arteries.

It should be noted that, while arteriosclerosis is a diffuse process, no relationship exists between lesions of the large and small arteries. Moreover, the small arteries of one organ (heart, brain, kidney) may be attacked severely while those of the others are relatively, or even absolutely, untouched.

A lesion of the small arteries goes hand in hand with impairment of the blood supply of the respective organ, causing an increase of connective tissue, called *fibrosis,* which may cause clinical manifestations. It may be asked whether *capillary alterations* are not an important part of this process.

SYMPTOMS AND SIGNS

The clinical picture of arteriosclerosis is extremely variable and depends upon the severity and distribution of the lesion.

When arteriosclerosis is *diffuse,* the entire

---

[78] Utilizing the ultracentrifuge and a special flotation technique, several *lipoprotein complexes containing cholesterol* were separated. Those of the Sf 10–20 class seem to be related to human atherosclerosis (26).

body acquires a *senile aspect*. This may occur with a certain rapidity, even within a few months. The patient is usually pale and his movements are slow and rather stiff. There often is a rapid *loss of weight*, and *cachexia* may be evident.

The skin is either finely wrinkled or flabby; the face may present rapid changes of color, from pale to red, because of vasomotor disturbances. Weakness, loss of appetite, extreme emotional reactions, headache, dizziness, amnesia, dysarthria, and disturbances of hearing and vision are common. Sensory disturbances of the hands and feet may occur.

The *blood pressure* usually presents increased pulse pressure and low diastolic because of increased rigidity of the large arteries. While hypertension is more common, hypotension may occur, the variation being due chiefly to the fact that participation of the renal arteries to the process is not always present.

Patients with Moenckeberg's sclerosis may have a blood pressure of difficult evaluation because of the resistance of the arterial wall to compression. Either increase or decrease of pressure in certain vascular areas is common. The latter is usually due to narrowing of the arterial mouths in the aortic wall, the former to rigidity and dilatation of the larger vessels.

Thrombosis and hemorrhage are possible in any organ.

The visible arteries are tortuous and present a forceful pulsation which increases their curvatures. They are hard and resistant or give the impression of being fleshy. The pulse is frequently *celer* but may be "thready".

There is dulness of the manubrium and there may be evidence of left ventricular enlargement. *The 2nd aortic sound is loud and ringing.* There may be a triple rhythm.

The x-ray may reveal the signs of atherosclerosis of the aorta and *beads of calcification* along the aorta and the peripheral arteries. It frequently shows an enlarged heart.

Serious disturbances are due to arteriosclerosis of the heart and the kidney. The former is a cause of *coronary heart disease* (page 414); the latter, of either benign or malignant *renal sclerosis* and, possibly, of *essential hypertension* (page 491).

GRAPHIC TRACINGS

Pulse and Pressure Tracings

The most varied findings can be obtained. In certain cases, no pulse tracing (and no indirect pressure tracing) can be obtained over certain arteries. This is usually due to occlusion of the vessels. However, extreme narrowing of an artery may still allow a thin, continuous flow of blood which cannot be recognized by the tracing on account of the lack of pulsation.

Senile arteriosclerosis is accompanied by changes in the configuration of both the radial and the digital pulse. In patients with this disease, *crest time* is markedly increased in both the radial and the digital tracings. Younger persons with initial arteriosclerosis may present increased crest time of the digital pulse.

Ballistocardiogram

The ballistocardiogram of arteriosclerotic patients frequently presents abnormal patterns. These are extremely variable and are similar to those described in coronary heart disease. They may have importance if found in relatively young persons.

VARIETIES

Cerebral arteriosclerosis may cause thrombosis or hemorrhage of the brain. When the hemorrhages are small, limited clinical pictures may occur.

Gastric or intestinal arteriosclerosis may cause dyspeptic, hemorrhagic, and enteralgic episodes. Acute diarrhea may be caused by *intestinal edema*, connected with the vascular disturbance.

Arteriosclerosis of the extremities (arterio-

TYPES OF DISTURBANCES OF THE
PERIPHERAL ARTERIAL CIRCULATION

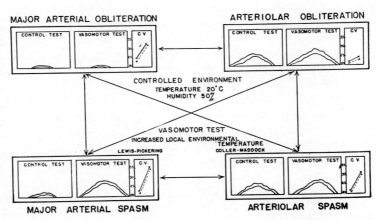

Fig. 297. Changes in the oscillometric and calorimetric readings which characterize the four main types of *arterial disturbances* responsible for deficiencies of the peripheral distribution of arterial blood. Any combination of these types may be met within clinical practice. (From Herrmann, J.A.M.A.)

sclerosis obliterans) may cause intermittent claudication (page 535), vascular occlusion, and gangrene.

Coronary arteriosclerosis has been described previously and is the most common cause of coronary heart disease (page 414).

Renal arteriosclerosis is also common and is a frequent cause of arterial hypertension (page 491).

DIAGNOSIS

The diagnosis of arteriosclerosis is essentially clinical. The general picture may be absent and rigidity of the peripheral arteries may be a late sign. Therefore, only the signs of functional deficiency of an organ may require explanation. Differentiation between the signs and symptoms of hypertension and those of arteriosclerosis is often necessary. Oscillometry and calorimetry are of help in the differential diagnosis of arterial disturbances (fig. 297).

TREATMENT

Contrary to previous belief, it has been proven that arteriosclerotic lesions of the aorta, large arteries, and coronary arteries,

may regress. Several trends are explored; they include a) the use of *estrogens* in the male and in the older female; b) the *restriction of caloric and fat intake* (diets XII and XIII) for obese patients or those having more than 220 mg. per cent of cholesterol in their blood; c) the substitution of vegetable for animal fats; d) the stimulation of oxidations by diet, vitamin B-complex, or small amounts of thyroid extract; e) the decholesterolization of tissues by lipotropic factors (choline, etc.) and the stabilization of cholesterol by lecithin.

The patient should be reassured and it should be pointed out that arteriosclerosis is compatible with long survival. If the main organs do not show signs of deficiency, presence of arteriosclerosis should not be mentioned. If a severe lesion of an essential organ is not present, retirement from work should not be advised because it might cause loss of interest in the surroundings and rapid mental and physical decadence.

When arteriosclerosis of either the heart or the lower extremities is not present, *exercise* is useful.

Obese patients should try to reduce by an

adequate diet (high protein, low fat and carbohydrate diet—III). If azotemia has developed, a *low protein diet* is indicated (IV).

Alcohol, coffee, and *tobacco* may be restricted according to the clinical picture but they seem to have no effect on the arteriosclerosis.

Potassium iodide (**73**) has a mild, beneficial action; it should be used with caution in order not to overstimulate the thyroid.

Theophylline (**78**) and *aminophylline* (**41, 42**) are useful as are the *nitrites* (from the rapid-acting *nitroglycerine* (**53**) to the slow-acting *mannitol hexanitrate* (**51**) and *peritrate* (**50**).

Bromides (**32**) and *chloral* (**33, 34**) are useful in some cases. The barbiturates are useful in most patients, from the rapid *nembutal* to *amytal* (**31**) and to the slow *barbital*.

Toxic and Infectious Polyarteritis

Severe arterial lesions may occur during a toxic process (lead poisoning) or a general infection (7). In the earliest stage, the arteries present focal edema of the media; later, degeneration of the elastic and muscular structures occurs; in the third stage, atypical regeneration, fibrosis, and calcification may be observed. The entire process, which may be more or less diffuse, is limited to the media and seems to be caused by a lesion of the vasa vasorum or the lymphatic vessels of the wall.

Acute Arteritis

CAUSE

Acute arteritis may occur at any age when bacteria (or their toxins) damage the arterial wall. The existence of toxic arteritis also has been proven. Arteritis may be caused by the *Pneumococcus, Eberthella typhi,* and the *Streptococcus hemolyticus* or *viridans*. Arteritis may also be caused by rheumatic disease, typhus, and malaria. Among the different localizations, that of the arteries of the lower extremities is most common.

LESIONS

a) *Disseminated arteritis.* This type is localized mainly on middle-sized arteries like the iliac, carotid, and subclavian arteries, and chiefly at their bifurcations. The subendothelial layers present infiltration and dissociation of the elastic fibers.

b) *Thromboarteritis.* This is the most common type. The artery is either completely (*obliterant thrombo arteritis*) or partially occluded (*parietal thromboarteritis*). The thrombus is a whitish, adherent formation of secondary formation. The thrombus consists of fibrin, platelets, and granular residua of both red and white cells. Where the thrombus adheres to the arterial wall, it is attached closely to the intima which is swollen and infiltrated, having lost its endothelium. Degenerative lesions and inflammatory reaction are present in the other arterial layers. Subsequent organization and fibrosis of the thrombus is customary. *Slowing of the circulation due to the arterial thrombosis is usually followed by venous thrombosis.*

c) *Embolic, septic arteritis.* This type is caused by arterial embolism. The embolus may reach and damage the artery either through the lumen or through the blood channels of the wall. In a later stage, differentiation between this type of arteritis and that mentioned in section (b) may become difficult.

When the artery is not occluded and is not terminal, more or less severe ischemia follows the arteritis. On the other hand, when the artery is occluded, the collateral circulation is poor, or both, obliteration of a vascular area takes place, causing the formation of an *infarct*; this may be followed by gangrene.

Gangrene is the complete necrosis of tissues, caused by the absolute interruption of blood supply. *Dry gangrene* consists of mummification of tissues and takes place when venous circulation is normal. *Moist gangrene* consists of purulent and edematous softening of tissues and is caused by the simultaneous occlusion of the arteries and veins and by the action of bacteria.

SYMPTOMS AND SIGNS

The symptoms and signs vary with the type of lesion.

Thromboarteritis. Either during an acute disease (typhoid) or during convalescence, the patient complains of *severe pain* in one of the legs; this is oppressive, crushing, or tearing. It is felt *within* the limb, radiates toward the foot, and is increased by pressure, exertion, and dependent position. Various forms of *paresthesias* are also present.

The leg is *pale* and *cold.* Upon palpation, *the artery is hard like a rope.* No pulsation is present *below* the seat of pain as revealed by palpation and by the oscillometer. From 2 to 3 days after the onset, the leg becomes bluish, then black, and gangrene occurs. This may be more or less diffuse according to the severity of the lesion and to the extension of the collateral circulation. The associated *phlebitis* may cause edema of the limb.

From 10 to 15 days after the onset, the gangrene has reached its greatest extension and the dry crust of dead tissue is sharply defined and deepens down to the bone. If amputation is not performed, suppuration of the border takes place, followed by septicemia.

When moist gangrene occurs, the general conditions become dangerous and only an emergency operation may prevent coma and death.

Parietal arteritis. The clinical picture is similar to the above but is milder. The artery may not be palpable, the pain is less severe, and no cyanosis occurs. Gangrene is usually absent unless a diffuse and severe lesion of the peripheral arteries existed already.

Embolic arteritis. This type is again similar to the others but has a sudden onset and a more rapid evolution.

DIAGNOSIS

The diagnosis is usually not difficult. The lack of pulsation and the lower tem-perature are essential signs. *Phlebitis* causes a softer edema, more frequent cyanosis, no impairment of the pulsations, and frequently an increase in the local temperature. However, an associated phlebitis may cause confusion. Differential diagnosis from functional disorders of the peripheral circulation is necessary.

X-ray study of the artery may be important in some cases, in order to ascertain the upper limit of occlusion. It is made by injecting a radio-opaque substance into the artery far above the site of pain. *Sectional measurements of the amplitude of pulsations* (oscillometer) are also important for the same purpose.

TREATMENT

During the initial stage, treatment with vasodilators may improve the collateral circulation. *Papaverine* (**43, 44**), *priscoline* (**54**) or *mannitol hexanitrate* (**51**) should be given. Treatment with *heparin* (**63**) (**37**) may prevent blood clotting as far as possible. When gangrene is present, *amputation* is necessary. *Asepsis* of the gangrenous area should be maintained as far as possible. Intra-arterial injections of *penicillin* combined with *priscoline* (**54**) have proved effective in cases of gangrene (**38**).

In embolic arteritis, *heparin, intermittent venous compression, vasodilators,* or *sympathetic block* should be used as accessory treatments. However, *embolectomy* is most important and should be done as soon as possible (**24**). When the embolus is in one of the major arteries, vasodilators and block should be started only *after* the intervention because progress of the embolus, caused by vasodilation, might make the removal more difficult.

Chronic Arteritis

Chronic arteritis includes some clinical syndromes which have varying manifestations, often of unknown or doubtful cause.

Luetic Arteritis

This type of arteritis may occur in arteries of any size. That of the extremities is typical. The lesion may consist of progressive fibrous narrowing of the vessel, causing *obliteration* or destruction of the muscular and elastic structures leading to dilatation and formation of one or more *aneurysms*.

The obliterant type first causes *intermittent claudication* and later the symptoms and signs of thromboarteritis. The aneurysmatic type causes compression of the nerves, veins, and lymphatic vessels. Therefore pain, cyanosis, and edema may follow. The artery may be felt as a *pulsating sac*; its compression first causes an increase of the pulse (obliteration of the sac) and then its disappearance (compression of the artery).

Diabetic Arteritis

It is more correct to call this "arteritis of a diabetic patient". It is usually due to banal germs of low virulence on an arteriosclerotic ground. The lesion consists of a primary endoarteritis with thickening of the intima followed by thrombosis. Lipoid deposits and leucocyte infiltrations are present in the wall.

The course of this arteritis is usually long. For many years no symptoms are present but *the amplitude of pulsations is decreased* (oscillometer). Later on, more or less severe pain starts. The last stage is represented by *gangrene*. The latter may be accompanied by little pain if the collateral circulation is impaired because of a systemic lesion of the small arteries.

Peripheral Arterial Embolism

Arterial emboli are usually caused by loose thrombi from the left side of the heart (rheumatic heart disease, subacute bacterial endocarditis, myocardial infarction), frequently in cases of atrial fibrillation (page 343). The embolus usually lodges at a bifurcation and then occludes both openings. Thrombosis of the vessels is the result and this may cause gangrene. The thrombus extends distally but only little proximally.

A *severe localized pain* follows emboliza-

tion and is possibly connected with the vascular spasm which takes place at the site of the embolus. Muscular weakness, paralysis, decrease of reflexes and of sensitivity, lower temperature and absence of pulse below the site of occlusion are typical.

Gangrene is rare in the upper extremity on account of good collateral circulation while it is more common in the lower extremities. *Secondary venous thrombosis may occur.*

Treatment consists of sedation, lowering of the limb, and vasodilators. *Papaverine, priscoline* (**54**), or *khellin* (**48, 49**) may be used. I.v. *heparin* (**63**) in isotonic saline is given by the continuous-drop method.

Embolectomy is the operation of choice.

Cerebrovascular Accidents

Cerebrovascular accidents are usually attributed to one of the following mechanisms: a) vascular spasm, b) vascular embolism, c) thrombosis of a cerebral artery, or d) cerebral hemorrhage.

Arterial hypertension is present in a majority of cases; cerebral arteriosclerosis is extremely frequent. Cause of embolization may be found in the others. In some of the cases, a tiny embolus to the brain, or a minor thrombosis, has widespread effects on account of *diffuse secondary arterial spasm* (34).

The symptomatology of the episode varies according to the localization of the lesion. It includes motor and sensory paralysis, sudden change of blood pressure (hypertension or hypotension), dyspnea, and possibly *acute pulmonary edema*.

It has been proven that therapy cannot be based on the diagnosis because of the difficulty of an early differential diagnosis between the various types of lesion. Moreover, both a white and a red area of softening can be produced by the same experimental techniques (35).

Therapy is based on the use of:

a) Vascular dilators: *aminophyllin* (i.v., 0.5 gm.) (**42**), *papaverine* (**43, 44**), or *priscoline* (**54**).

b) Depressant of the sympathetic (*hyderg-*

ine) (**36**) or of the entire autonomous system (*hexamethonium*) (**39, 40**).

c) *Stellate block* (36). This is performed on the side of the cerebral lesion with 5 cc. of 1 per cent novocaine, and repeated every 12 or 24 hours for 5 to 6 days.

d) Sedatives (*chloral hydrate, amytal*).

e) Stimulants of the vascular system (in cases with vascular collapse).

f) *Alcohol-oxygen vapor by inhalation* (page 560) (in cases of pulmonary edema).

Thrombo-Angiitis Obliterans (Buerger's Disease) (8, 9, 10)

CAUSE

The disease occurs in young or mature individuals, usually in *males*. Persons with a low metabolic rate have a greater percentage of incidence than others. A racial background has been disproven.

The role of *tobacco* in this disease has been emphasized. We do not yet know whether tobacco *causes* the disease (1), possibly through an allergic mechanism, or merely *increases the severity* of its manifestations through a functional disturbance. There is no denying that complete abstinence from tobacco has a favorable influence on the clinical picture.

The role of *infection* was suggested by the study of the lesion and by the success of one attempt at transplantation of the process (9). However, no known germ was ever isolated and the extreme predilection for one sex is also against the infectious theory.

LESIONS

Lesions are found in the *arteries* (arteritis), *veins* (phlebitis), and *lymphatic vessels* (lymphangitis). They consist of a chronic inflammation accompanied by proliferation of the intima and resulting in thrombosis. Organization and canalization of the clots, fibrosis of the adventitia, and attempts at formation of collateral circulation have been observed. The formation of miliary foci of inflammatory cells is typical of this lesion.

The development of fibrotic tissue which binds together the artery, vein, and nerve explains some of the symptoms.

The disease has a systemic diffusion but is more severe in the vessels of the limbs.

SYMPTOMS AND SIGNS

In the early stage, *diffuse tenderness*, due to *migrant phlebitis*, may occur; short, raised areas of redness are visible along the smaller veins, especially over the foot, ankle, hand, and wrist. There may be swelling and tenderness of some of the joints. Tenderness of an artery, followed by thrombosis, is observed less often. This acute stage may last only for a week and the color of the areas may then change to a faint brown.

Intermittent claudication develops later and may be limited to one leg or one foot. *Pain at rest* is usually a late symptom and may be accompanied by *ulceration*.

As the disease progresses, the symptoms become more severe: the popliteal and even the femoral pulses disappear; the radial pulses become small; claudication becomes constant and severe.

Coronary occlusion is frequent, impotence is not rare, and both are caused by arterial lesions, similar to those of the extremities (coronary and spermatic arteries). Thrombosis of abdominal vessels may simulate appendicitis.

Fever is rare; *leucocytosis* is uncommon (unless gangrene has occurred). Hyperglycemia and hypercholesteremia have been described but are not constant. A typical premature aging of the patient may take place.

Coldness of one or both feet or hands, lack of pulsation in the arteries of the extremities, reduced amplitude of oscillation (oscillometer), and lack of reaction to a hot bath are typical of the disease before ulceration or gangrene appears.

The *electrocardiogram* may not show typical changes, but evidence of coronary heart disease is present in a high percentage of cases (12).

DIAGNOSIS

Several different conditions may be simulated and should be excluded in the initial stage: arch strain, Raynaud's disease, peripheral arteriosclerosis, peripheral embolism, periarteritis nodosa, coarctation of the aorta, and tuberculous or syphilitic arteritis.

TREATMENT

Abstention from tobacco is imperative. Precautions against trauma, chilling, or excessive heat (hot-water bottle) shall be taken.

If active vasodilatation is still possible, vasodilator drugs should be prescribed. *Papaverine* (**43, 44**), *khellin* (**48, 49**), and *priscoline* (**54**), as well as *alcohol*, can be used. Sympatholytic drugs, like *dibenamine* (**37**) and ganglionic blocking agents, like *benzodioxane* (**38**) have been used with good result. Care should be taken not to lower excessively systemic pressure. This might aggravate the local ischemia. *Moderate heating* of the limb in alternated periods has a favorable action.

Suction and pressure exercises from 15 minutes to 2 hours at a time may be useful.

Sympathectomy may be useful if the capacity for vasodilatation still exists. Whenever gangrene has occurred, the treatment is surgical.

Panarteritis Nodosa (Periarteritis Nodosa) (13)

Arteritis associated with perivascular reactions may occur in lupus erythematosus, dermatomyositis, typhus, rheumatic disease, and other conditions. However, periarteritis nodosa in a clinical sense is a *chronic systemic disease* which is independent from any other.

CAUSE

The disease is not so rare as previously thought. It is four times more common in the male and it may occur at any age. Its cause is unknown. Experimental studies have suggested the possibility of an *allergic mechanism* in its production. Clinical considerations and histological data led to inclusion of this condition among the so-called "collagen diseases".

LESIONS

The lesions of periarteritis nodosa affect arteries of various size but chiefly the small arteries of different organs. Kidneys, heart, liver, spleen, and lungs are involved in this order.

Gross examination reveals a series of miliary nodules, placed along the arterial walls (*Kussmaul's nodules*). The arteries show patchy inflammatory lesions involving all three coats. Destruction of the elastic and muscular layers of the media is typical, and small secondary aneurysms are a frequent result. Leucocyte infiltration of the adventitia is associated with the formation of periarterial thickenings. Hemorrhages may occur within the arterial wall or in the surrounding tissues; thrombi often form within the vessels. Giant cells are present in some cases; eosinophils may occur in the inflammatory tissue.

SYMPTOMS AND SIGNS

The onset is usually gradual. Remissions, long intermissions, and exacerbations are common. The clinical picture varies greatly according to the distribution, severity, and persistence of the vascular lesions. Any organ can be affected and, therefore, a wide variety of symptoms and signs have been recorded.

Bizarre and unexplained symptoms, suggesting infectious, rheumatic, or cachectic diseases, may be due to periarteritis nodosa.

Fever, malaise, weakness, albumin casts in the urine; leucocytosis, anemia, tachycardia; abdominal pain, ascites, peripheral edema; enlargement of the liver; and retinitis are among the many signs and symptoms described. Skin lesions of different types, from erythema to nodules or pustules, may occur. Unexplained and rapidly progressive hypertension may be caused by periarteritis of the renal arteries.

A certain number of cases have bronchial asthma; multiple involvement of the brain may simulate a brain tumor. Diffuse pain may simulate polyneuritis.

Panarteritis nodosa has been shown to be a cause of coronary occlusion.

DIAGNOSIS

Diagnosis of these cases is always difficult. The findings of a biopsy may bring definite data. In some cases, the lesion may be visualized directly *in vivo* on sigmoidoscopy.

TREATMENT

No specific treatment is available. However, if diagnosis is made early, administration of *ACTH* or *cortisone* may be useful.

Intermittent Claudication (14)

Intermittent claudication is a clinical syndrome which may be caused by different arterial lesions.

CAUSE

One of the most common causes is *arteriosclerosis obliterans* of the lower extremities. *Luetic* or *diabetic arteritis, Buerger's disease*, and *periarteritis nodosa* may cause the same clinical picture.

Thrombosis of the abdominal aorta may show the same picture at first; *coarctation of the aorta* may be the cause, especially if the ischemia of the lower limbs is accentuated by heart failure.

Functional elements may play an important role, especially in cases with limited extension and severity of the arterial lesions.

SYMPTOMS AND SIGNS

The patients feel well as long as they lie down, sit, or even walk for a few steps. However, as soon as more prolonged exercise is undertaken, *severe pain* is felt in the calf, together with sensations of heaviness, cold, burning, or tingling. Resting causes disappearance of the disturbance. A few minutes later the patient may resume his walk, only to be stopped again by the pain after proceeding a little farther.

During the attack of pain, the skin of the leg is cyanotic and cold and the pulse of the local arteries is small. The oscillometer reveals a marked decrease of pulsations. X-ray may reveal calcified areas of the arterial walls.

MECHANISM

It is apparent that the pain is caused by a *disproportion between blood demand and blood supply to the legs.* This is usually due to a moderate narrowing of the arteries which, moreover, cannot dilate in order to supply an increased amount of blood during exercise. A functional disturbance of the arterial wall may be involved, as shown by the fact that the amplitude of pulsations may be reduced during the attack.

The pain has been attributed to abnormal metabolism of the muscles due to insufficient oxygen supply and resulting in the *accumulation of lactic acid* (15). A connection between potassium increase in the muscle and pain has also been advocated (17).

DIAGNOSIS

The diagnosis of the clinical syndrome is usually simple. However the cause, nature, extension, and severity of the lesions should be ascertained.

The *differential diagnosis* between intermittent claudication of arterial origin and *intermittent claudication of spinal origin* is made from the observation that signs of a lesion of the cortico-motor neuron (*Babinski's sign* included) are usually present in the latter. During the attack, the arterial pulsations are normal in the spinal claudication while the muscles become hypertonic. Spinal claudication is always bilateral, *arterial claudication is frequently unilateral.*

The pain of arthritis is articular or periarticular and is seldom completely absent at rest. The pain of *neuritis* is distributed along the course of a nerve; it is not relieved by rest and often is not increased by exercise. The pain of orthopedic defects is more an ache than a real pain. The pain of an *inflammatory process* is usually steady.

The treatment is that of the underlying vascular disease. Avoidance of tight garters, excessive cold or heat, and *discontinuance of smoking* are useful; rest is helpful. *Physiotherapy*, postural exercises, and intermittent venous occlusion are often helpful.

Vasodilators, such as *papaverine* (**43**), *Khellin* (**48**), or *priscoline* (**54**), can be used.

Sympathectomy can be of aid whenever an important functional element is involved. Its usefulness may be tested by administration of sympatholytics (**36**). However, it should be noted that the sympathetic fibers cause constriction of the skin arteries and dilatation of the arteries of the muscles. Therefore, the beneficial action of sympathectomy is felt mostly in the skin. *Intravenous diethylether* seems helpful in alleviating ischemia and pain (2.5 per cent ether in 5 per cent glucose—500 to 1000 cc).

Restoration of blood flow is extremely important in cases with acute thrombosis of an artery. This can be obtained by *thromboendarterectomy and resection*, with replacement of the removed section by *an arterial* (**33**) *or venous* (**39**) *graft*.

Acrocyanosis

Acrocyanosis is the paroxysmal occurrence of a bluish color at the extremities. This is usually accompanied by decreased skin temperature and, at times, by trophic changes.

CAUSE AND MECHANISM

Acrocyanosis affects the *female sex* in the great majority of cases. This led to the belief that an endocrine disturbance, connected with ovarian insufficiency, might be responsible for it. The hormonal imbalance would cause a disturbance in the regulation of the arterioles, capillaries, and venules of the skin. The reactivity of the vasomotor nerves would be affected so that reaction to normal thermal stimuli would be increased. However, a certain number of patients have acrocyanosis based on a different mechanism. Some of them have it only in the presence of *cold*. These have been said to be on the borderline between acrocyanosis and Raynaud's disease. Others have an organic lesion of the nervous system: patients with lesions of the midbrain, the sympathetic ganglia, and the peripheral nerves may present this vasomotor disturbance. According to some, the main disturbance is a capillary and venous dilatation, not connected with a primary arterial disturbance (18).

SIGNS AND SYMPTOMS

The main sign is represented by *cyanosis*. This predominates in the hands, feet, and lower part of the legs; it may be present on the nose, earlobes, and, occasionally, the arms. Cyanosis is accompanied by *low temperature* of the skin in the affected areas; this is usually between 29°C. and 30°C. and may be as low as the room temperature. The skin of the extremities is often moist and clammy.

Systolic blood pressure is often somewhat *low* with a reduced pulse pressure (hyposphygmia—page 521); *venous pressure* is usually high, reaching figures ranging from 13 to 25 cm. water. The vasomotor reactions usually are exaggerated as shown by heat or cold tests.

TREATMENT

In some cases, *estrogenic* treatment obtains good result. *Physiotherapy* is often useful. *Paredrinol* (**59**) seems to give good results.

Raynaud's Disease (18, 19)

Raynaud's disease is a syndrome, revealed by paroxysmal attacks of pallor or cyanosis of symmetrical areas of the extremities. Gangrene may follow.

CAUSE

In some of the cases, the vasomotor disturbance is *a purely functional phenomenon*, caused by exposure to cold. Prolonged work with vibratory engines definitely favors the disease.

In other patients, the vasomotor disturbance is connected with the initial stage of *an organic lesion of the arteries* (Buerger's disease, arteriosclerosis obliterans, luetic arteritis). Occasional occurrence in patients with cervical rib, pulmonary tuberculosis, and chronic intoxications is possible. In this group of cases, only the name *Raynaud's phenomenon* is correct, while the basal disease is something else (20).

Raynaud's disease is more common in *females*. The relation of 80 to 20 approximately indicates the ratio for the two sexes.

Exposure to cold and emotional strain favor the occurrence of the attacks. The use of *tobacco* seems to have a slightly noxious influence but nothing decisive has been demonstrated.

SIGNS AND SYMPTOMS

Three successive stages may occur in the syndrome.

a) *Stage of ischemia.* During the attack, the extremities become *cold and extremely pale* and lose their sensitivity. As a result, accurate movements become difficult. The ischemia may involve only one or two fingers (occasionally toes) but is usually symmetrical and extended to both hands. The attack lasts from a few minutes to a few hours and is followed by a phase of hyperemia of the affected areas.

b) *Stage of asphyxia.* During the attack, the extremities become *cyanotic*; they are also somewhat cold but less so than in the previous stage. *Pain* is usually present and is transmitted toward the root of the limb. These attacks usually last some hours. Slight edema may be present during the attack.

c) *Stage of gangrene.* Following the previous stage, areas of dry gangrene may occur in the fingers or toes; round ulcerations may be a manifestation of this stage.

MECHANISM

It is apparent that the three subsequent stages of Raynaud's disease are due to impairment of the arterial blood supply. This is transitory at first and then becomes more severe and persistent, up to the stage of gangrene.

Both a disturbance of innervation and a vascular lesion have been advocated. The symmetrical appearance favors the first; the gradual intensification with extension toward the root of the limb favors the second.

An *arteriolar spasm* is apparent but a *spasm of the veins* in the initial stage has also been demonstrated (25). The latter may even predominate over the former. Minor arterial lesions may favor the spasm while a repeated and prolonged spasm may impair the nourishment of the arterial wall and favor a secondary lesion. It seems likely that cold or prolonged vibrations stimulate the already excitable sympathetic system.

DIAGNOSIS

Diagnosis is not difficult if one can observe the patient during an attack. It is often possible to diagnose the disease merely on the history alone. The various causative and favoring elements should be further investigated so that treatment may be based on the cause and not merely on the symptoms.

TREATMENT

Prevention of chill and abolition of any manual work with vibratory engines are necessary. *Prostigmin* (**72**), *papaverine* (**43, 44**) and *priscoline* (**54**) are the vasodilators which give the best results.

Diathermy and other physiotherapeutic treatments are often useful.

Surgery gives good results in some cases. Either *periarterial sympathectomy* (23) or *preganglionic sympathectomy* can be used. The intervention will be preceded by tests (warming of the body, spinal anesthesia, procainization of the sympathetic ganglia, action of drugs) in order to ascertain how important the reflex vasoconstriction actually is. A positive test prophesies a good outcome from surgery.

Erythromelalgia (21)

Erythromelalgia is a syndrome caused by paroxysmal attacks of congestion of the extremities.

CAUSE AND MECHANISM

This syndrome usually occurs in patients suffering from migraine or dizziness. It is more common in the *male sex* and usually is observed between the ages of 20 and 40.

While the syndrome may be observed as an associated phenomenon in patients with tabes or syringomyelia, the most typical picture is independent of any organic lesion.

Sometimes the area of congestion corresponds to the distribution of a nerve; at other times it includes the entire limb. Irritation of the vasomotor fibers of a nerve has been advocated in the first case; a spinal disturbance in the second.

SIGNS

The patients complain of attacks lasting many hours and occurring mostly at night. They start with severe *pain* which may be radiated to one of the hands or feet or to the entire limb. Together with this, a *sensation of heat* or even a burning sensation, *hyperalgesia*, and *hyperesthesia*, occur in the same area. In some patients, the disturbance involves either the nose or the earlobes.

The involved area is red, moist, slightly swollen, and warm.

Some of the patients have *polycythemia*.

TREATMENT

Physiotherapy has been used in cases where a lesion of one of the peripheral nerves was the cause of the disturbance. *Adrenalin* (55), *ephedrine* (57), *calcium* and *pitressin* (62) seem to exert a beneficial effect.

Immersion Foot—Trench Foot (22)

These two names are equivalent and are applied to a vascular disease of the extremities, caused by exposure. The lesion is caused by exposure to a temperature which is sufficient to chill, but not to freeze, the tissues. Such a temperature causes an increase in capillary permeability and an inflammatory exudate.

Shipwrecked sailors, exposed to cold for a prolonged period, develop *swollen, discolored,* and even *pulseless extremities.* Dependency, immobility, and constricting footgear add to the severity of the lesion. Anesthesia and, occasionally, gangrene may occur. *Low-grade fever* is not uncommon but *high fever* is a serious sign.

After rescue, and upon warming, the limb becomes *hyperemic* and *swollen* and, occasionally, *blebs* are formed. Later, desquamation of the skin takes place. The anesthesia disappears quickly but may persist for some time in the distal areas. *Treatment* should be directed toward avoidance of injury, asepsis, and reduction of the edema and congestion. Body warmth should be restored but *the limb should be kept elevated and cool* (cold packs, spray).

BIBLIOGRAPHY

1. HUEPER, W. C. Arch. Path., 1944, **38**, 162, 245 and 350; and 1945, **39**, 117.
2. ARESU, M. *L'Arteriosclerosi*. Milano, Cordani, 1927.
3. MOSCHOWITZ, E. In *Cyclopedia of Medicine*. Vol. 4. Philadelphia, Davis, 1945. Am. J. M. Sci., 1927, **174**, 388; and 1929, **178**, 244. J. A. M. A., 1928, **90**, 733 and 1526.
4. JOSUÉ, O. Presse Méd., 1904, **1**, 281.
5. a) ANITSCHKOW, N., AND CHALATOW, S. Zentr. allg. Path., 1913, **24**, 1.
   b) ANITSCHKOW, N. Beitr. path. Anat., 1913, **56**, 379.
6. a) WINTERNITZ, M. C., THOMAS, R. M., AND LeCOMPT, P. M. *The Biology of Arteriosclerosis*. Baltimore, Thomas, 1938.
   b) WINTERNITZ, M. C., AND LeCOMPT, P. M. Am. J. Path., 1940, **16**, 1.
7. WIESEL, J., AND LOEWY, R. Wien. Arch. inn. Med., 1920, **1**, 197.
8. VON WINIWARTER, F. Arch. Chir., 1879, **23**, 202.

9. Buerger, L. Surg., Gyn. & Obst., 1914, **19,** 582. Also *The Circulatory Disturbances of the Extremities.* Philadelphia, Saunders, 1924.

10. Brown, G. E., Allen, E. V., and Mahorner, H. R. *Thrombo-Angiitis Obliterans.* Philadelphia, Saunders, 1928.

11. Silbert, S. J. A. M. A., 1945, **129,** 5.

12. Samuel, S. S., and Feinberg, S. Am. Heart J., 1930, **6,** 225.

13. a) Kussmaul, A., and Maier, R. Deut. Arch. klin. Med., 1866, **1,** 484.
    b) Grant, R. T. Clin. Sci., 1940, **4,** 245.
    c) Fitz, R. In *Stroud's Cardiovascular Disease.* Philadelphia, Davis, 1945.

14. Charcot, J. M. Progr. Méd., 1887, N. 32/33.

15. Elliott, A. H., and Evans, R. D. Am. Heart J., 1936, **12,** 674.

16. Allen, A. W. In *Nelson Loose-Leaf Medicine.* New York, Nelson, 1946.

17. Harpuder, K., and Stein, I. D. Am. Heart J., 1943, **25,** 429.

18. a) Layani, F. *Les Acrocyanoses.* Paris, Masson, 1929.
    b) Villaret, M., and co-workers. Arch. Mal. Coeur, 1934, **27,** 725; and 1935, **28,** 1.
    c) Parisot, J., and Cornil, L. In *Nouv. Traité de Médécine.* Paris, Masson, 1933.

19. a) Raynaud, M. *On Local Asphyxia and Symmetrical Gangrene of the Extremities.* London, New Sydenham Soc., 1888, 1.
    b) Leriche, R. and Fontaine, R. *Les Spasmes Vasculaires.* J. Card. Royat, 1937.

20. a) Allen, E. V., and Brown, G. E. Am. J. M. Sci., 1932, **183,** 187.
    b) Hines, E. A., and Christensen, N. A. J. A. M. A., 1945, **129,** 1.

21. Mitchell, W. Am. J. M. Sci., 1878, **76,** 1.

22. a) Ungley, C. C., and Blackwood, W. Lancet, 1942, **2,** 447.

b) Webster, D. R., and co-workers. J. Bone & Joint Surg., 1942, **24,** 785.
c) White, J. C. New England J. Med., 1943, **228,** 241.

23. Leriche, R., and Heitz, J. Arch. Mal. Coeur, 1917, **10,** 79.

24. Reynolds, J. T., and Jirka, F. J. Surg., 1944, **16,** 485.

25. Naide, M., and Sayen, A. Arch. Int. Med., 1946, **77,** 16.

26. Gofman, J. W., *et al.* Circ., 1950, **2,** 161. Also Science, 1950, **111,** 166.

27. a) Horlick, L., and Haval, L. J. Lab. & Clin. Med., 1948, **33,** 1.
    b) Rosenman, R. H., *et al.* Circ. 1952, **5,** 589.

28. Horlick, L., and Katz, L. N. Am. Heart J., 1949, **38,** 336.

29. Steiner, A., *et al.* Arch. Path., 1946, **42,** 433. Also Am. Heart J., 1949, **38,** 34.

30. Horlick, L., *et al.* Am. Heart J., 1949, **37,** 689.

31. Stamler, J., *et al.* Am. Heart J., 1949, **38,** 466.

32. Davidson, J. D., Am. J. Med., 1951, **6,** 736.

33. Julian, O. C., de Takats, G., and Dye, W. S. Angiology, 1953, **4,** 12.

34. Hicks, S. P., and Black, B. K. Am. Heart J., 1949, **38,** 528.

35. Sacchi, U. Report XI Congress of Ital. Soc. Neurology, 1952.

36. a) Risteen, W., and Volpitto, P. South M. J., 1946, **39,** 431.
    b) Gilbert, N. C., and de Takats, G. J. A. M. A., 1948, **136,** 659.
    c) Amyes, E. W., and Perry, S. M. J. A. M. A., 1950, **142,** 15.

37. Allen, E. V. J. A. M. A., 1947, **135,** 15.

38. Kappert, A. Helv. Med. Acta (Basal), 1948, **15,** 25.

39. Kunlin, J. Arch. Med. Coeur, 1949, **42,** 371.

CHAPTER 26

Diseases of the Veins

Phlebitis

Phlebitis is the inflammation of a vein; *thrombophlebitis* is the same process, complicated by thrombosis of the vessel with hindrance to, or block of, the blood flow.

CAUSE

A phlebitis may be caused by local or general causes. A *local cause* exists when wound, trauma, or infection occurs. A *general cause* is present in infectious disease; the phlebitis then may be caused by the germs of the disease or by associated bacteria. Propagation of an inflammatory process from artery to vein has been shown, both in spontaneous diseases and in experimental animals.

Slowing of the circulation predisposes to phlebitis. This may be a local circulatory disturbance or may be due to heart failure. Causes which favor clotting of the blood also favor phlebitis (page 507).

LESIONS

Any vein may present a phlebitis. The most common localizations are, however, the veins of the pelvis and those of the lower extremities. Phlebitis of the veins of the arm is less common but not rare. The jugular veins may be affected in inflammatory conditions of the brain and meninges.

Gross examination shows *edema* of the area and a swollen, rope-like aspect of the vein. Opening of the vein reveals the *thrombus* which adheres to the wall with part of its surface. The thrombus is prolonged by a long red clot which is free from the wall. The subsequent evolution of the thrombus may lead to various possibilities:

a) *Detachment* causing embolism.

b) *Purulent softening* with sloughing off of minute particles; embolism does not occur in such cases because of the small size of the particles and the slow course of the process.

c) *Organization*, through connective tissue which starts from the intima of the vein and gradually becomes dense.

d) *Vascularization*, due to formation of new mural capillaries in the longitudinal direction and the subsequent opening of channels through the thrombus.

SIGNS AND SYMPTOMS

The venous thromboses of the lower extremities are divided into two different classes: phlebothrombosis and thrombophlebitis.

Phlebothrombosis

This is a relatively quiet process *which may be completely silent* until a serious embolism occurs. It is localized in the venous plexuses among the muscles, particularly in those of the calf, but sometimes in those of the foot or thigh.

This process may cause lameness on walking, pain in the calf, tenderness of the muscles, discomfort on forced dorsiflexion (*Homans' sign*), more or less apparent *edema*, and local cyanosis. The process may remain local or progress into the femoral vein. In the latter case, it may form a long, loose embolus, or progress further toward the center in a lightly adherent, non obstructive form. It may reach the external iliac vein, causing the signs of thrombophlebitis. Diagnosis of deep phlebothrombosis may be aided by *venography*, a method based on the injection of diodrast in a small vein above the malleolus and on x-ray visualization of the venous system (24).

Thrombophlebitis (Phlegmasia Alba Dolens—Milk Leg)

This process may start in a thrombosis of the leg veins, of the uterine veins, or of the femoro-iliac veins. It is an obstructive process in which an inflammatory exudate often surrounds the veins and arteries, causing local arterial spasm and, possibly, a diffuse peripheral vasospasm in the arterioles, venules, or both.

The disease is revealed by *tingling*, *heaviness*, *muscular cramps*, and *local pain*. This is elicited by palpation, exertion, and by dependent position. The skin is *warm* and *edematous*. The surface may reveal superficial reddish strips (lymphangitis) but is typically *white* (milk leg). *The edema is hard.* The inflamed vein may be rope-like in consistency and is extremely tender.

DIAGNOSIS

Diagnosis of deep phlebitis may be helped by *venography* (5). That of the superficial veins is usually easy. Bilateral phlebitis of the leg may be confused with the result of heart failure. Observation that venous pressure in the arm is normal in such cases while it is elevated in heart failure, may assist the diagnosis.

TREATMENT

One of the main purposes of treatment is the prevention of pulmonary embolism. This has been discussed already (page 509) and is based on the use of *anticoagulants* (25) (**63, 64, 65**) and on *preventive ligation of the femoral veins* and, occasionally, of the iliac vein (8).

For conservative treatment, 6-inch elevation of the foot of the bed, freedom of movement, and *no* ice bag are the best procedures (6). After from 10 to 14 days, gradual resumption of activity in a semi-elastic bandage is recommended.

Observation that the edema is partly connected with arterial spasm (9) and is re-duced by lumbar sympathetic block with procaine (10) indicate the use of the latter, following one of the several techniques proposed (11).

Phlebosclerosis

Phlebosclerosis is a chronic lesion of the venous wall which is common in patients with arteriosclerosis (12). The lesion mainly consists of diffuse or focal thickening of the intima. Atherosclerotic lesions of the venous wall also have been described in medium and large veins of mature individuals whose history shows absence of chronic infections. This process, called *phleboatherosclerosis* (13), is associated with rigidity and dilatation of the venous wall.

Varicose Veins

Dilatation, elongation, and tortuosity of the veins may occur in any part of the body. However, the most apparent type of varicose veins is that of the superficial network of the lower extremities.

CAUSE AND MECHANISM

Varicose veins of the legs are due to *valvular insufficiency or block of the femoral or iliac veins*. The former is frequently *congenital* but may be *acquired* as a result of trauma or inflammation.

The normal compensatory mechanism for maintaining blood pressure in the erect position is based on vascular reflexes, acting mainly on the small vessels (carotid sinus and aortic arch reflexes), and on the action of the *venous valves*. These prevent a reversal of flow in the veins and support the hydrostatic pressure of the venous section which lies between one valve and the next.

Insufficiency of the valves results in stagnation of a large amount of blood with a marked rise of local venous pressure. This may cause an actual decrease of the circulating blood volume and a reduction of cardiac output which may reach 50 per cent of the previous figure on changing posture (14b, 15).

The system of the saphenous veins is deprived of the supporting and milking action of the muscles; therefore, it is easily exposed to the effect of increased venous pressure. If the femoral valve is congenitally absent, the difficulty of venous return in the erect position becomes even greater.

As the left iliac vein has a longer course than the right, varicose veins are frequently larger on that side.

Heredity is important in the development of varicose veins.

The strain of prolonged immobile standing is responsible for the frequent formation of varicose veins in waiters, street-car conductors, and policemen. Other causes are traumatic rupture of the valves, pressure of lymph nodes or pelvic organs, straining at stools, and pregnancy.

The effect of postpartum, postoperative, and postinfectious thrombophlebitis is another cause of varicose veins through production of new collateral and dilated channels.

The *actual venous pressure* of the varicose veins in the standing position may reach 200 cm. of water and, in exceptional cases, may be above 300 (14a). However, contradictory evidence has been found in other cases.

LESIONS—COMPLICATIONS

Varicose veins are tortuous, dilated blood vessels. These veins react to increased pressure first with *hypertrophy* and then with *dilatation* and *elongation*. An *inflammatory reaction* within and about the walls of varicose veins is frequent (14a). This is due to bacteria circulating in the blood, and it may remain latent for many years. Sudden strain, severe trauma, or the injection of sclerosing substances may reactivate this inflammation and cause a phlebitis. On the other hand, varicose veins may act as a focus of infection and disseminate the germs into the blood stream.

Insufficiency of the venous valves is usually progressive until *nutritional disturbances* of the skin and subcutaneous tissues occur. The skin becomes dry, atrophic, and pigmented and may present eczema. The small veins of the skin may be occluded by thrombi with periphlebitic induration which later may become ulcerated.

SIGNS AND SYMPTOMS

The early symptoms consist of a *tired feeling* and *heavy sensation in the legs*. Sometimes *cramps* of the calves at night or in cold water and *swelling of the ankles* may occur. Then blue markings appear along the calves and *venous dilatations become apparent* (fig. 298).

The visible extent of the varicosities is not proportional to the severity of the symptoms. This is partly due to the fact that the latter may be due to complications and not to the varicosities themselves. Traction on the saphenous nerve may cause a painful radiation when the dilatations are large.

Dizziness, fainting, or *precordial oppression* may be due, in rare cases, to large varicose veins which pool a large amount of blood and suddenly decrease the cardiac output (15).

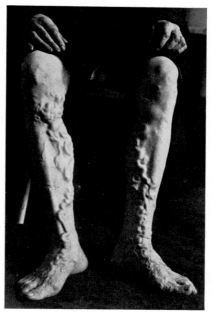

FIG. 298. Varicose veins

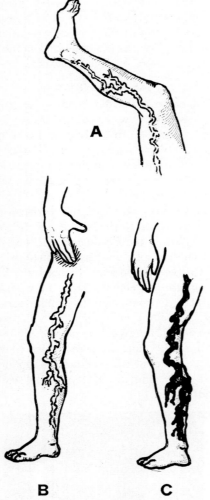

FIG. 299. Varicose veins. A, elevation of the leg; B, lowering of the leg with compression at the groin; C, release of compression.

DIAGNOSIS

Many conditions may simulate the symptoms of varicose veins. Flat foot, genu valgum, arthritis, and sciatica may cause similar pain. Femoral hernia and arteriovenous fistulae may cause swellings which often are mistaken for real varicose veins.

The conditions of the valves may be evaluated by means of different tests.

The *Trendelenburg test* gives information about the insufficiency of the saphenous valves and the flow through the communicating veins (fig. 299).

The patency of the deep veins is then tested by *Perthe's test*: a towel is placed around the thigh and twisted so as to compress the saphenous vein; vigorous extention and flexion is then performed with the result that the blood of the superficial veins is aspirated into the deeper ones; when pressure is released from above, the superficial veins fill again. No diminution of the varicosities takes place during the test if the deep veins are obstructed.

TREATMENT

Elastic stockings and elastic bandages give symptomatic relief; they should extend to the groin and often are disliked because of discomfort. They usually are indicated during pregnancy or in older patients.

Rest, elevation, and hot dressings may be useful in cases of acute inflammation or ulcers. Ambulatory treatment is desirable in the great majority of cases.

Obliteration of the varicose veins may be obtained by *local injections* which cause a gradual *sclerosis*. The injections are started in the highest palpable varicosity or in that which is most apparent. Usually they are given twice a week until the desired result is obtained.

The most commonly used solutions are 10 per cent *quinine sulphate* with urethane; 20 to 40 per cent *sodium salicylate*; or 5 to 10 per cent *sodium morrhuate*.

A contraindication is represented by infection or any cause for immobility. The occurrence of embolism following the thrombosis caused by the injection is extremely rare.

Varicose veins without incompetence of the perforator vessels should be treated by *high saphenous ligation* and *stripping* (17). When phlebography reveals incompetent communicating or perforating veins, these should be *interrupted* as they pass through the fascia (26). *Postphlebitic varices* are treated by interrupting the deep venous channels at the upper limit of involvement and stripping the superficial dilatations (26). Postoperative treatment includes antibiotics, early ambulation, and prolonged compression.

Healing of varicose ulcers depends on different factors but control of bacterial infection is very important. *Local penicillin* treatment has been found useful.

Arteriovenous Fistula

Arteriovenous fistula is a shunt between an artery and a vein which causes formation of a special type of aneurysm (*a-v aneurysm*) and a typical clinical picture (fig. 300). A special type of a-v fistula is that of pulmonary vessels (page 510).

CAUSE

Arteriovenous fistula is frequently caused by a *wound* or *trauma*. In rare cases it may be *congenital*. Rupture of a luetic aneurysm into a vein may cause a fistula, giving the same clinical picture.

The most important varieties are those which are due to communication:

a) between the ascending aorta and superior vena cava;

b) between the abdominal aorta and inferior vena cava;

c) between the iliac or femoral artery and the iliac or femoral vein;

d) between the carotid artery and internal jugular vein.

LESIONS AND MECHANISM

The artery is enlarged in its proximal section and is smaller than normal, distal to the fistula. The vein is dilated and may present a large varicose enlargement. The arterial dilatation may extend as far back as the heart but the venous enlargement is most marked near the fistula.

The arterial enlargement is due to the increased speed of circulation, to the eddies, and to degenerative changes of the wall. The venous dilatation is due to the increase in pressure. The heart is enlarged.

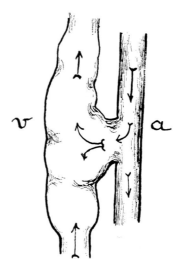

FIG. 300. Arteriovenous fistula: a, artery; v, vein.

The shunt between arterial and venous circulation tends to cause depletion of the arterial system and venous congestion. The loss of blood occurs during the entire cardiac cycle but is greater toward the end of systole than in other phases. For this reason, a vascular picture which resembles that of aortic regurgitation or patent ductus arteriosus may arise. The amount of blood passing through the shunt at times may reach one-third of the total blood volume.

SIGNS AND SYMPTOMS

The pulse is *rapid* and *celer*. It becomes normal again as soon as the fistula is occluded. There is *tachycardia* which is interpreted as a compensatory reflex, caused by the low arterial pressure. There is usually *hypotension* and this is accompanied by an *increase in the pulse pressure.* Low systolic and even lower diastolic pressure account for these facts.

The pulse wave has a great speed. A pulse tracing reveals that the notch which precedes the dicrotic wave is at a very low level (18). Increased pressure in the arteries which are more distant from the heart and pulsation of the small arteries of the subpapillary plexus (so-called *capillary pulse*) are present in some cases.

Systemic venous pressure has been found normal (22) but increased pressure exists in the vein into which the fistula empties.

The heart is enlarged both to the right and left. The locale of the fistula is frequently revealed by a *small pulsating mass*; the superficial veins of the area are dilated and tortuous and may pulsate.

A *thrill* and a *continuous machinery murmur which increases in systole* can be appreciated over the fistula. It may seem only systolic. If the fistula is large and in an extremity, the *pulse distal to it may become weak or even disappear*.

The *graphic tracing (phonoarteriogram)* reveals that the murmur is continuous but increases in systole, at times considerably. The murmur extends over a long stretch of vein central to the fistula, and sometimes reaches the heart. The proximal murmur is partly generated in the vein and has less systolic accentuation (23).

The *temperature* distal to the fistula is lower than that of the opposite side. Ulceration and even gangrene may result.

The *electrocardiogram* fails to show any axis deviation (21).

Cardiac output is increased while the *arteriovenous difference* in the oxygen content is decreased (22).

DIAGNOSIS

In general, diagnosis of this condition is not difficult. However, an arterial aneurysm and a pulsating hematoma should be excluded. The arterial aneurysm may cause a similar murmur.

TREATMENT

The fistula has so great an effect on the heart and circulation that its surgical elimination is required. The operation consists of *quadruple ligation* of the artery and vein with complete excision of the channel. This intervention prevents any recurrence.

Obliteration of the fistula causes a sudden increase in resistance. In order to prevent this sudden effect, venesection may be performed at the time of operation with the withdrawal of from 500 to 1000 cc. of blood. The intervention is followed by a rapid return of the heart to a normal size and by a rapid normalization of the peripheral circulation.

BIBLIOGRAPHY

1. a) ALTSCHULE, M. D., IGLAUER, A., AND ZAMCHEK, N. Arch. Int. Med., 1945, **75**, 24.
   b) HUSSEY, H. H., KATZ, S., AND YATER, W. M. Am. Heart J., 1946, **31**, 1.
2. NEUMANN, R. Virch. Arch. path. Anat., 1938, **301**, 708.
3. a) OCHSNER, A., AND DeBAKEY, M. New England J. Med., 1940, **222**, 870.
   b) OCHSNER, A., AND DIXON, J. L. J. Thoracic Surg., 1936, **5**, 641.
4. HUNTER, W. C., SNEEDEN, V. D., ROBERTSON, T. D., AND SNYDER, G. A. C. Arch. Int. Med., 1941, **68**, 1.
5. a) DOS SANTOS, J. C. J. Int. Chir., 1938, **3**, 625.
   b) BAUER, G. Acta Chir. Scand., 1940, **84**, 1. Also. Acta Med. Scand., 1941, **107**, 136.
   c) STARR, A., FRANK, H. A., AND FINE, J. J. A. M. A., 1942, **118**, 1192.
6. HOMANS, J. New England J. Med., 1934, **211**, 993; 1941, **224**, 179; and 1942, **226**, 917.
7. BARKER, N. W., NYGAARD, K. K., WALTERS, W., AND PRIESTLEY, J. T. Proc. Staff Meet., Mayo Clin., 1940, **15**, 769; 1941, **16**, 1, 17 and 33.
8. a) FINE, J., AND SEARS, J. B. Ann. Surg., 1941, **114**, 801.
   b) SEARS, J. B. New England J. Med., 1941, **224**, 108.
9. LERICHE, R., AND JUNG, A. J. Chir., 1931, **37**, 481.
10. OCHSNER, A., AND DeBAKEY, M. Surg., 1939, **5**, 491.
11. a) LABAT, G. *Regional Anaesthesia*. Philadelphia, Saunders, 1928.
    b) WHITE, J. C. J. A. M. A., 1930, **94**, 1382.
    c) OCHSNER, A., AND DeBAKEY, M. J. A. M. A., 1940, **114**, 117.
    d) DeTAKATS, G. Surg. Clin. North America, 1942, **22**, 199.
    e) HOMANS, J. *Circulatory Diseases of the Extremities*. New York, Macmillan, 1939.
12. SACK AND MENHERT. Quoted by TEDESCHI (13).

13. TEDESCHI, C. Atti. Acc. Sci. Med. Nat. Ferrara, 1937.
14. a) DeTAKATS, G. In *Stroud's Cardiovascular Disease*. Philadelphia, Davis, 1945.
    b) BOCK, H. E. Zeit. exp. Med., 1934, **92**, 782.
15. CHAPMAN, E. M., AND ASMUSSEN, E. J. Clin. Investigation, 1942, **21**, 39.
16. MAYERSON, G. S., LONG, C. H., AND GILES, E. J. Surg., 1943, **14**, 519.
17. TRENDELENBURG, F. Beitr. klin. Chir., 1891, **7**, 195.
18. a) LEWIS, T., AND DRURY, A. N. Heart, 1923, **10**, 301.
    b) PRICE, G. B. Lancet, 1937 (1), **232**, 206.
19. a) ELKIN, D. C. Mo. Conc. Cardiov. Dis., 1943, **12**, N. 12.
    b) BARKER, J. M., AND YATER, W. M. M. Ann. District of Columbia, 1942, **11**, 439.
    c) REID, M. R., AND McGUIRE, J. Ann. Surg., 1938, **108**, 643.

20. MICHELAZZI, A. M. *Fisiopatologia e Clinica della Circolazione Venosa*. Turin, Rosenberg and Sellier, 1937.
21. PAZZANESE, D. *Modificações de Forma do Electrocardiograma*. São Paulo, Gráfica da Prefeitura, 1942.
22. TAQUINI, A., AND SUÁREZ, J. R. E. Medicina, 1945, **5**, 109.
23. EDWARDS, E. A., AND LEVINE, H. D. Arch. Int. Med., 1952, **90**, 1.
24. a) STARR, A., *et al.* J. A. M. A., 1942, **118**, 1192.
    b) BAKER, E. C. Am. J. Roentgenol., 1947, **58**, 603.
25. a) LOEWE, L., AND HIRSCH, E. J. A. M. A., 1947, **133**, 1263.
    b) ALLEN, E. V. J. A. M. A., 1947, **135**, 15.
26. MASSELL, T. B., AND KRAUS, A. R. Angiology, 1950, **1**, 150.

CHAPTER 27

Borderline Syndromes of Cardiology

The Effort Syndrome and the Athletic Heart

The observation of cardiac failure after effort led to the description of a so-called "effort syndrome" which was attributed to the effect of severe strain on a normal cardiovascular apparatus. It was observed later that the heart feels the effect of muscular exercise only indirectly, because of increased venous return or increased peripheral resistance. Therefore, two possible mechanisms may cause heart failure:

a) An alteration of the normal regulation which prevents excessive increase of venous and arterial pressures and which increases the coronary flow in proportion to the work of the heart.

b) A latent myocardial or coronary insufficiency which is revealed by the strain.

The first possibility occurs mostly in cases of neurocirculatory asthenia (see below) and in people with endocrine and autonomic disturbances. The second possibility is a common event and is a symptomatic manifestation of heart disease.

Prolonged and excessive athletic strain may cause *a slight enlargement of the heart.* This fact is usually associated with sinus bradycardia and slight hypotension, with low diastolic and large pulse pressures. These phenomena are found not only in athletes but also in animals trained for racing (race horses, race and hunting dogs) (1).

Previously impaired hearts may be further damaged by exercise and may fail. The paramount importance of myocardial and coronary efficiency is revealed by the not unusual observation of valvular lesions in athletes who do not complain of any symptoms (2).

A lesion of the myocardium may be due to *infection.* For this reason, sore throats, colds, or grippe, should not be disregarded by athletes and, above all, by those who have valvular lesions.

The strain of *military life* can be compared to that of athletics. The same possibility of failing heart due to myocardial or coronary lesions, and the same frequent episodes caused by neurocirculatory asthenia, occur in both. It is apparent that when a soldier or an athlete becomes older, the probability of coronary and myocardial lesions becomes greater.

Neurocirculatory Asthenia (3, 9)

Neurocirculatory asthenia is a clinical syndrome which may occur alone or may complicate other diseases, including all other cardiovascular syndromes.

CAUSE AND MECHANISM

The syndrome is somewhat more common in females than in males in peacetime but the ratio is inverted in wartime because of combat strain. It may occur at any age but is more frequent in young adults. It is favored by occupations requiring prolonged, concentrated, and anxious attention, or frequent physical strain, especially if an element of danger is involved. Tall, slender individuals are more prone than others to the syndrome.

The mechanism of origin is only incompletely understood. It has been suggested that an imbalance of the autonomic nervous system is responsible for the severe reactions which may follow slight provocation.

Infections, physical exhaustion, nervous prostration, or anxiety, may be accompanied or followed by neurocirculatory asthenia with symptoms which seem out of proportion to the original cause.

Evidence has been obtained that the respiratory disturbances are not caused by disease or abnormality of the heart, lungs, or blood; that they influence cardiac dynamics and are of psychogenic or neurogenic origin (3e). The dull, precordial pain seems to be caused by the particular type of respiration of these patients who predominantly use the intercostal muscles.

The possibility that most of the disturbances of neurocirculatory asthenia are caused by a *hypothalamic dysfunction* has been suggested (3f).

SIGNS AND SYMPTOMS

The most common symptoms are the following: *dyspnea*, often associated with *sighing respiration* and caused by effort; *palpitation*; *precordial pain or ache*, seldom radiating to the left arm; *dizziness*; and, occasionally, *syncope*. With these symptoms is associated a particular *sensation of exhaustion* which is more severe in the early morning and is increased both by effort and excitement. Nervousness, tremor, sweating, and headache may be present.

The sighing respiration may be so severe as to cause *hyperventilation* which is followed by dizziness or even by tetany. This may cause depression or inversion of the T wave in lead 3. Many electrocardiographic abnormalities have been described, but none of them seems typical.

Changes of the T wave in precordial leads from the left side of the chest may be present. These have been attributed to increased tonus of either the sympathetic or the vagus nerve, a fact which can be ascertained by means of an *atropine* and an *ergotamine test* (3g, h).

Tachycardia is often present. There may be flushing of the face, cold moist hands, and, at times, a *slight increase of blood pressure*.

The basal metabolic rate, the x-ray, and the electrocardiogram usually give normal findings with the possible exception of ECG changes due to hyperventilation. However, extreme prolongation of the P-R interval has been described in certain cases (10).

COURSE AND PROGNOSIS

The syndrome may last for a variable period and may recur when the conditions which favor it occur again. The symptoms may last for months, years, or the entire life span.

The average duration of life is long and prognosis is good.

DIAGNOSIS

Many of these patients are erroneously diagnosed as tubercular, thyroid, or cardiac patients. However, a correct diagnosis is reached sooner or later because of the clinical evolution.

The *hyperventilation index* is the ratio of breath-holding ability after forced respiration to that before forced respiration. *This index is within normal limits in neurocirculatory asthenia (1.3 to 2.13).* With cardiac dyspnea, the ratio is always below 1.3 (8).

TREATMENT

Treatment is based on reassurance, physical and mental rest, and reeducation. The patient should adopt a program of useful activity, not requiring a high amount of energy. Thus, complete inertia and the establishment of an irreversible trend may be prevented.

Symptomatic treatment may be useful in many cases: sedation for some patients, circulatory stimulation for others, and autonomic depression for most. *Bellergal* (**35**) seems particularly effective (13).

Anxiety Neurosis and Cardiac Neurosis (7)

Anxiety neurosis is an illness with psychic symptoms of *irritability, apprehension,* and *fear,* and *a sense of tension.* The fear may be directed toward one of the involved organs, so that the patient fears "choking", "a stroke", or a "heart attack".

Cardiac neurosis is a term applied to: a) noncardiac patients in whom cardiac symptoms predominate; or b) cardiac patients with symptoms out of proportion to the disease.

In the first case, there is an anxiety neurosis with additional psychic complications; in the second, an hysterical elaboration exaggerates the disturbances.

The patient may complain of the following subjective symptoms:

a) *Fullness, soreness, oppression, ache, or pain in the precordial area.* This is usually located in the region of the cardiac apex; it is frequently of short duration and without radiation; it is seldom related to exercise.

b) *Tingling or painful sensations in the left arm.*

c) *Palpitation,* frequently due to emotion; at times not related to any apparent cause.

d) *Effort dyspnea,* with or without sighing respiration. This frequently disappears after prolonged exertion.

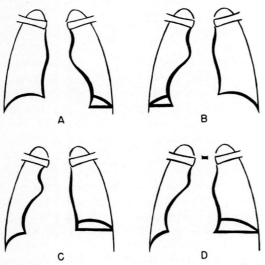

FIG. 301. *Different types of dextrocardia.* A, normal heart; B, situs inversus totalis; C, inverted heart, normal abdominal organs; D, inverted heart, normal abdominal aorta, persistent left aortic arch.

e) *Vertigo or syncope.*

The findings are usually limited to slight tachycardia (more seldom bradycardia), occasional premature beats, and slight increase or decrease of blood pressure.

Studies made during World War II pointed out that cardiac neurosis is a syndrome which may accompany anxiety states, hysteria, neurotic depressions, and (seldom) schizophrenia. *It is now widely admitted that neurocirculatory asthenia is a special form of cardiac neurosis.*

Diagnosis of these forms is sometimes difficult. As evident neurotic phenomena may mask real heart disease, summary exclusion of cardiac disease because the patient is a neurotic should be avoided. On the other hand, a neurotic may simulate heart disease and only a careful study reveals that no such disease is present.

Treatment depends on the severity of the neurosis which can be determined by considering *duration, crippling effect,* and *acceptance by the patient.* Treatment is psychiatric but can frequently be done by a general practitioner. Medical or physical therapy can be used, if necessary, for its suggestive influence. The physician must create the impression that he knows the diagnosis, understands the illness, and may be able to cure it.

Dextrocardia (12)[79]

Dextrocardia consists of the complete inversion in the position of the heart within the thorax. The abnormality is congenital and may have three different types (fig. 301).

1) There is a *situs inversus totalis*; all organs of the body are on the opposite side in comparison with the usual position. All functions are developed in a perfectly normal way and no symptoms are present.

[79] The term *dextrocardia* has been used both in cases where the heart was displaced toward the right and in those having a congenital anomaly so that the longitudinal axis is toward the right. The term should be reserved for the latter

X-ray examination shows a "mirror image" picture of the heart with the apex situated to the right and the aortic arch also lying on the right side. The stomach is on the right, the cecum on the left, etc.

The *electrocardiogram* is typical; all waves are inverted in lead 1; leads 2 and 3 change places. This picture is called a "mirror image electrocardiogram" (fig. 302). An upright ventricular complex or a positive P wave in lead 1 have been found in some cases.

2) *The abdominal organs are in the normal position;* on the contrary, *the heart is in the opposite position from the norm and has an inversion of its chambers and vessels.* In other words, the atrial and ventricular chambers placed on the right of the heart are the equivalent of a normal left atrium and left ventricle because they receive the blood from the lungs, are separated by a bicuspid valve, and send their blood into the aorta.

This type of abnormality is usually associated with other congenital malformations but occasional cases without septal defects or stenosis are described. These patients seem to have a tendency toward rheumatic or arteriosclerotic lesions of the heart and toward bronchiectasis.

Different varieties are determined by the association with various congenital malformations, including the tetralogy of Fallot, persistence of the "right" aortic arch, and transposition of the large vessels. In some cases, as the judgment of *"what is right and what is left"* is absolutely arbitrary, because no indication is given by either the abdominal organs or the large vessels, discussion may arise on the interpretation of the structural abnormality. Whenever a patient has an inversion of all organs except the heart, he should also be included in this type; it is apparent, however, that the term "situs inversus with levocardia" should be used. The *x-ray* may show that the aorta is either on the right or on the left. The electrocardiogram may or may not have the "mirror image" type.

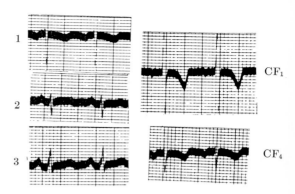

FIG. 302. *Mirror image electrocardiogram* (From Katz's *Electrocardiography*. Courtesy of the author and Lea & Febiger.)

3) *There is a normal relationship of the cardiac chambers to each other and to the large vessels but the cardiac apex is toward the right.* These patients frequently have associated lesions like persistent bicuspid valve of the right A-V opening, septal defects, pulmonary stenosis, or persistent right aortic arch. The abnormality mainly consists of the fact that the heart has rotated around its longitudinal axis so that the left ventricle is anterior and the right is posterior, forming the apex. While the *x-ray* reveals the abnormality, the *electrocardiogram* has no "mirror image" type but only right axis deviation.

A physical sign presented by cases of dextrocardia is also found in cases of displacement of the heart toward the right. It consists of possible *splitting of the 2nd sound at the right of the sternum* (11).

Normal Pregnancy (5)

It has been known for a long time that pregnancy imposes a burden upon the circulatory apparatus of the mother. This is explained by the fact that all metabolic requirements of the fetus are met through functional changes of the maternal circulation.

It is important to know that this burden *increases slowly* in the early part of pregnancy, *rapidly* from the 5th to the 8th

month, and *decreases* during the last month
of pregnancy. This last phase is partly
associated with changes of position of the
uterus and partly with cessation of growth
of the fetus but has not been completely
explained.

The most important changes occurring
during pregnancy are:

a) *Increase of the circulating blood volume*
from 10 to 100 per cent (average, 50 per
cent) in response to greater demands for
nourishment and oxygen. The increase is
greater than accounted for by increase in
body mass; plasma volume increases more
than blood volume. Tendency to retain
sodium and water is probably due to endocrine changes.[80]

b) *Increased cardiac ouput* (from 40 to 50
per cent).

c) *Increased oxygen consumption*, which is
proportionately less than that in section b.

d) Normal or increased velocity of blood
flow (a shorter circulation time is frequently
found).

e) Normal or decreased arteriovenous
oxygen difference.

f) Increase of diastolic and pulse pressure; marked tibial hypertension.

g) *Moderate increase of heart rate* (from 12
to 28 per minute).

h) Normal venous pressure in the arm,
but moderately increased venous pressure in
the leg; the latter may reach 30 cm. water.

i) Normal vital capacity.

It is likely that pregnancy decreases
cardiac reserve.

The increased work of the heart is responsible for a series of signs and symptoms.

Exertional dyspnea, palpitation, and *precordial pain*, are common. The pulse is
celer and may be *irregular* because of premature beats. Attacks of paroxysmal atrial
tachycardia are not unusual. There are
active pulsations of the jugular veins. There
may be vascular signs, simulating those of

[80] It is known that estrogenic and androgenic
hormones are retained in the body. Pituitary,
thyroid, and adrenal changes are probable.

aortic insufficiency (page 238). The 2nd
pulmonic sound is loud. There may be an
*apical systolic murmur or a systolic murmur
over the pulmonic or the aortic area*, or
both. A *triple rhythm* (page 370) frequently
occurs.

The systolic murmur may appear as early
as the 2nd month and last through the
puerperium; it is markedly influenced by
changes of position.

The rise of the diaphragm places the heart
in a more horizontal position, a fact which
gives the impression of an enlargement on
percussion and x-ray.

X-ray reveals an increase in the normal
lung markings.

The *electrocardiogram* may present *left
axis deviation* and, frequently, an *inverted
T_3*. There may be a *deep Q_3*; an inversion of
P_3 is not unusual (fig. 303).

Special diets are advised in normal pregnancy. If the pregnant woman has congenital or rheumatic heart disease, the
danger of subacute bacterial endocarditis
should be considered. Prevention of this
complication is obtained by injecting
penicillin before and after delivery. Repeated blood cultures should be made after
delivery in order to avoid late diagnosis of
this fearful complication.

The Normal Heart in Old Age (6)

It has been known for a long time that
death from gradual decay of the organism
is rare and may even be nonexistent. The
main cause of death in the aged is represented by cardiovascular diseases.

The *pulse* rate of the aged increases
slightly above 65. The *carotid sinus reflex*
becomes more active with age.

Mean blood pressure tends to decrease and
pulse pressure to increase, with old age.
However, the frequent occurrence of benign
renal arteriosclerosis results in a large percentage of cases having moderate hypertension with a systolic pressure between 150
and 170.

Cardiac output is usually normal in basal

conditions, a fact which is no index of the cardiac ability to increase its work under stress.

Vital capacity decreases rapidly in the aged. *Venous pressure* is normal; *circulation time* tends to increase but remains within the upper limits of normal. The *velocity of the pulse wave* is increased.

The *size of the heart* is not increased by the effect of age; therefore, any definite increase is a sign of heart disease.

The *heart sounds* are decreased in intensity, a fact which is often due to emphysema. Variations of the heart sounds are possible and have the same meaning as in younger people.

A *low-grade systolic murmur* over the mitral or aortic area is a frequent occurrence and does not indicate an important lesion. A *loud systolic murmur* is, on the contrary, a sign of dilatation of the left ventricle (apical murmur) or calcific aortic stenosis (aortic murmur).

The *heart rhythm* is usually normal. However, paroxysmal atrial fibrillation or flutter occur more frequently than in younger individuals. *Chronic atrial fibrillation*, even lasting for decades, is possible.

The *sedimentation rate* rises with the age so that values up to 0.7 mm. per minute (Rourke-Ernstene method) may be normal above the age of 50.

ELECTROCARDIOGRAM

The ECG may be entirely normal. Left axis deviation is frequent and may be associated with Q_3 and inverted T_3. A slight increase in the duration of P-R and QRS is normal in the aged, so that it may slightly exceed the upper figures of normal (P-R, 0.20″; QRS, 0.10″).

PHONOCARDIOGRAM

The heart sounds may seem absolutely normal in the aged. A prolongation of both the 1st over the apex and the 2nd over the aorta is common. The vibrations of a systolic murmur are frequently recorded.

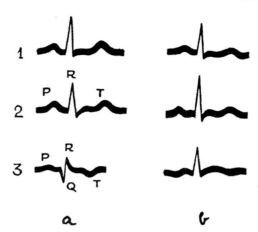

FIG. 303. Changes of the electrocardiogram in pregnancy. a, during pregnancy; b, after delivery. (Courtesy of Dr. I. Chavez.)

X-RAY

The position of the heart tends to be more horizontal; the contour of the left ventricle, more prominent. The aorta becomes more curved and may seem dilated. Calcifications may be seen in the aorta, the heart valves, the valvular rings, and the coronary arteries.

It should be emphasized that rheumatic lesions may occur at any age, resulting in valvular defects; bacterial endocarditis is by no means rare in the aged and may be difficult to recognize (page 206).

BIBLIOGRAPHY

1. a) LUISADA, A. A., MAUTNER, H., AND WEISZ, L. Arch. Pediat., 1941, **58**, 562.
   b) LUISADA, A. A., WEISZ, L., AND HANTMAN, H. W. Cardiol., 1944, **8**, 63.
2. WHITE, P. D. *Heart Disease*. New York, Macmillan, 1944. Also in *Nelson Loose-Leaf Medicine*. New York, Nelson, 1945.
3. a) DACOSTA, J. M. Am. J. M Sci., 1871, **61**, 17.
   b) LEWIS, T. *The Soldier's Heart and the Effort Syndrome*. New York, Hoeber, 1919.
   c) WOOD, P. Brit. M. J., 1941, **1**, 767.
   d) OPPENHEIMER, B. S. Bull. New York Acad. Med., 1942, **18**, 367.
   e) WHITE, P. D. Mo. Conc. Cardiov. Dis., 1942, **11**, N. 8.
   f) FRIEDMAN, M. War Med., 1944, **6**, 221. Also Am. Heart J., 1945, **30**, 325, 478 and 557.

g) WENDKOS, M. H. Am. Heart J., 1944, **28**, 549.

h) LOGUE, R. B., HANSON, J. F., AND KNIGHT, W. A. Am. Heart J., 1944, **28**, 574.

4. a) ABBOTT, M. E. In *Nelson Loose-Leaf Medicine*. New York, Nelson, 1945.

   b) BROWN, J. W. *Congenital Heart Disease*. London, J. Bale Publ., 1939.

5. a) HAMILTON, B. E., AND THOMSON, K. J. *The Heart in Pregnancy and the Childbearing Age*. Boston, Little, Brown and Co., 1941.

   b) CHAVEZ, I. *Enfermedades del Corazón —Cirugia y Embarazo*. Mexico, Colegio Nacional, 1945.

   c) PAROLI, G. Riv. Ital. Ginec., 1927, **6**, N. 5.

6. a) STIEGLITZ, E. J. New England J. Med., 1941, **225**, 247. Also *Geriatric Medicine*. Philadelphia, Saunders, 1943.

   b) MASTER, A. M., MARKS, H. H., AND DOCK, S. J. A. M. A., 1943, **26**, 11.

   c) LEVITT, G. Am. Heart J., 1939, **18**, 692.

   d) WHITE, P. D., AND BLAND, E. F. J. A. M. A., 1941, **116**, 2001.

   e) FREEDBERG, A. S., AND LEWIS, H. D. New England J. Med., 1944, **231**, 731.

7. BADAL, D. W. Mo. Conc. Cardiovasc. Dis. 1951, **20**, No. 10.

8. FRIEDMAN, M. Psychosom. Med. 1947, **9**, 233.

9. MILES, H. H., AND COBB, S. New England J. Med., 1951, **245**, 711.

10. SILVERMAN, J. J., AND GOODMAN, R. D. Am. Heart J., 1951, **41**, 155.

11. GONZALES VIDELA, J. Rev. Arg. Card., 1949, **16**, 306.

12. a) PALTAUF, R. Wien. klin. Woch., 1901, **14**, 1032.

    b) JONES, H. W. Brit. M. J. 1924, **1**, 147.

    c) ROESLER, H. Wien. Arch. inn. Med., 1930, **19**, 505.

    d) HELLMER, H. Forstschr. a.d. Geb. Roentgenstr., 1935, **51**, 591.

    e) TAUSSIG, H. *Congenital Malformations of the Heart*. New York, Commonwealth Fund, 1947.

    f) BURCHELL, H. B., AND PUGH, S. G. Am. Heart J., 1952, **44**, 196.

13. SCHIMERT, G. Am. Heart J., 1953, **46**, 726.

CHAPTER 28

Associated and Complex Heart Diseases

Most of the syndromes described in the previous chapters were due to relatively simple lesions of the heart. However, several frequent associations have been already mentioned. They are:

a) *Rheumatic carditis.* This causes lesion of the endocardium, myocardium, and pericardium; there may be lesion of the coronary arteries, the pleura, and the peripheral arteries. Valvular defects, myocardial scars, and, sometimes, pericardial adhesions, result from the acute lesions.

b) *Luetic cardioaortitis.* The initial lesion starts in the aorta, causing aortitis, possibly aortic aneurysm, and narrowing of the coronary mouths. It spreads to the aortic valves and causes aortic insufficiency, sometimes followed by mitral insufficiency. Myocardial lesions are frequent; mediastinal and pericardial lesions are less common. The patient may present a complex syndrome where the signs of aortic aneurysm are complicated by those of cardiac and mediastinal lesions.

c) *Arteriosclerotic cardiovascular disease.* There may be association of aortic atherosclerosis, calcification of the aortic valves resulting in stenosis, and coronary heart disease. The latter may cause myocardial fibrosis, bundle branch block, and, more rarely, A-V block. Pericardial adhesions and renal sclerosis may also be present.

d) *Bacterial and rheumatic endocarditis.* The association of these two processes has been mentioned. When both occur in patients having either rheumatic valvular lesions or congenital malformations, the clinical picture may become singularly complex.

e) *A tubercular or rheumatic polyserositis* may cause a lesion of the pleura, peri- cardium, and peritoneum which, in the first case, may be associated with active tuberculosis of the lungs, the spleen, or the liver; in the second, it may be associated with valvular defects.

Even more complex associations are possible, due to extension and superimposition of various diseases.

A patient with rheumatic heart disease and valvular defects may suffer from the effects of various new lesions:

a) Hypertension and hypertensive heart disease.

b) Hyperthyroidism.

c) Aortic atherosclerosis.

d) Diffuse myocarditis, due to bacterial or viral disease.

e) Coronary atherosclerosis (9, 10, 12).

f) Luetic aortitis.

Coronary arteriosclerosis is *less dangerous* than in nonrheumatic patients because of better-developed collateral circulation.

In spite of previous assertions that rheumatic lesions of the mitral valve are never associated with aortic insufficiency of luetic nature (1), such an association is possible, and such cases were repeatedly observed (2, 7). However, clinical recognition of the cause of each lesion may be impossible. Still a correct diagnosis may be reached:

a) If a patient with an aortic aneurysm and aortic insufficiency has a loud diastolic rumble over the mitral valve (and a relative stenosis can be excluded).

b) If a patient has a double mitral defect and aortic insufficiency but the aortic murmur appeared later and there is knowledge of lues.

c) If a patient has an aortic aneurysm and aortic insufficiency but there is a history of rheumatic disease.

A patient with luetic aortitis, with or without aortic insufficiency, may suffer from effects of different lesions:

a) There may be atherosclerosis of the aorta, fibrosis of the mitral valve, or both. There may be incomplete rupture of the aorta, favored by the sclerosis. There frequently is coronary arteriosclerosis.

b) Hypertension and hypertensive heart disease or, on the contrary, luetic nephrosis with hypotension, may complicate the clinical picture.

c) Different myocardial lesions may favor heart failure.

d) Either rheumatic or bacterial endocarditis may complicate the picture; the former often results in mitral stenosis.

Differential criteria make diagnosis possible (11).

A patient with a congenital heart disease may suffer because of different possibilities:

a) Rheumatic endocarditis may cause a Lutembacher's syndrome in a patient having only a patent foramen ovale; it may cause a syndrome of Fallot in a patient having an Eisenmenger complex.

b) A luetic or rheumatic lesion of the aortic valve may cause a singularly complex clinical picture in a patient with ventricular septal defect. Various associated valvular lesions may complicate the clinical picture of a patient with congenital heart disease (8).

c) Myocardial and pericardial lesions, resulting in complex disturbances of the cardiac rhythm and in pericardial adhesions, may occur in patients with congenital heart diseases (3).

d) Bacterial endocarditis is a frequent complication.

A patient with chronic cor pulmonale may have essential hypertension; the resulting picture is singularly complex.

There are numerous clinical cases where arterial hypertension, luetic aortitis, subacute myocarditis or myocardial fibrosis, coronary arteriosclerosis, hyperthyroidism, and vitamin deficiency are associated. It is not possible, in some of them, to ascertain which of the different etiological agents is responsible for each lesion.

Exceptional examples of *complex heart disease* were described at the Massachusetts General Hospital (4, 5, 8). The following lesions were found at autopsy in one case (4):

a) Congenital heart disease (interventricular septal defect and bicuspid aortic valve).

b) Rheumatic heart disease (aortic stenosis).

c) Luetic heart disease (aortitis).

d) Bacterial endocarditis implanted on both the congenital and the rheumatic lesions.

Another case from the same hospital showed (5):

a) Rheumatic heart disease (insufficiency of both the mitral and the aortic valves, mitral stenosis).

b) Atherosclerosis of the aorta and coronary arteries.

c) Thrombosis of the anterior descending branch of the left coronary artery (anterior myocardial infarction).

d) Mural thrombus in the left atrium.

e) Embolism of the axillary artery (gangrene).

BIBLIOGRAPHY

1. GALLAVARDIN, L., AND CO-WORKERS.
   a) Paris Méd., 1913/1914, **15**, 129.
   b) Lyon Med., 1925, **139**, 727; 1927, **139**, 727; and 1930, **145**, 541.
   c) J. Med. Lyon, 1937, **18**, 489.
2. WEISS, S. Personal communication.
3. BATTRO, A., AND CO-WORKERS. Rev. Arg. Card., 1927, **3**, 6 and 427; and 1936, **11**, 335.
4. Case 27,261. New England J. Med., 1941, **224**, 1108.
5. Case 30,431. New England J. Med., 1944, **231**, 597.
6. SMITH, J. R., *et al.* Am. J. Med., 1951, **10**, 37.
8. Case 34,101. New England J. Med., 1948, **238**, 331.
9. GARDNER, F. E., AND WHITE, P. D. Ann. Int. Med., 1949, **31**, 1003.
10. LAMB, A. E., AND LYONS, H. A. Brooklyn Hosp. J., 1950, **7**, 165.
11. ACEVES, D., *et al.* Arch. Inst. Card. Mexico, 1949, **19**, 497.
12. CHASNOFF, J., AND SILVER, A. Am. Heart J., 1951, **42**, 809.

CHAPTER 29

Acute Cardiorespiratory Attacks

Cardiac patients may present attacks of respiratory distress which are connected with their cardiovascular disturbance. Three main types may occur:

a) Paroxysmal dyspnea (once called cardiac asthma).

b) Paroxysmal pulmonary edema.

c) Paroxysmal periodic respiration.

Paroxysmal dyspnea and pulmonary edema differ in some clinical manifestations but have similar causes and a closely related mechanism.

CAUSES

Both *paroxysmal dyspnea* and *paroxysmal pulmonary edema* may be caused by the following diseases:

A. Diseases of heart and vessels.

Luetic heart disease (aortic insufficiency, aortitis, aortic aneurysm). Rheumatic heart disease (mitral insufficiency or stenosis, aortic insufficiency). Coronary heart disease (especially coronary occlusion). Hypertensive heart disease (essential or secondary hypertension; uremia). Congenital heart disease (coarctation of aorta). Shock.

B. Diseases or lesions of central nervous system.

Trauma to the skull. Subarachnoid hemorrhage. Cerebral hemorrhage, embolism, thrombosis, or abscess. Encephalitis, meningitis, poliomyelitis, tetanus.

C. Diseases or lesions of respiratory system.

Pneumonia, drowning, strangulation. Inhalation of irritant or toxic gases. Pulmonary embolism (rare). Thoracentesis. Trauma to the chest.

D. Allergy.

Angioneurotic edema and edema of the glottis. Serum sickness. Injections of gold preparations.

E. Miscellaneous.

Thyroid crises. Beri-beri heart disease.

F. Stimulation of hollow viscera or serosae.

Distention of esophagus, stomach, or gall

bladder. Emptying of distended bladder, or serous cavities.

G. Surgical and obstetrical cases.

Pregnancy, especially in cases with mitral lesions or eclampsia. Following transfusions or infusions, especially in surgical, anemic, or cardiac patients. Manipulation of stellate ganglia.

H. Toxic phenomena.

Thiourea, iodides, muscarine, eserine, methylsalicylate. Chronic alcoholism. Morphine poisoning.

It is apparent that paroxysmal dyspnea and pulmonary edema may or may not be connected with a cardiovascular disturbance.

Periodic respiration may occur in the following cases: a) Malignant hypertension with or without coma. b) Essential hypertension. c) Aortitis and aortic insufficiency. (d) Coronary heart diseases. e) Congestive failure. f) Drug intoxication (chiefly morphine). g) After surgical interventions with deep anesthesia.

SIGNS AND SYMPTOMS

Paroxysmal Dyspnea

The patient usually suffers from these attacks during the night. He goes to bed in good spirits and sleeps well for some time; suddenly he is awakened by a nightmare and feels a terrifying oppression in the chest while respiration becomes difficult and strained. The patient sits up in bed (*orthopnea*) and may bend forward. The respiration is slightly accelerated but is deep, strained, and may be *wheezing*. Profuse perspiration, congestion of the face, and restlessness are common. Irritation of the throat, dry nonproductive cough, and precordial pain, may be present (fig. 304).

The *pulse* is regular and somewhat rapid

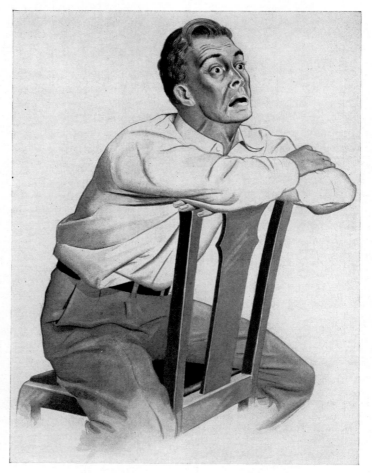

Fig. 304. Paroxysmal dyspnea

(90–110). The *blood pressure* is usually *higher* than before the attack.

Examination of the chest reveals a distention of the pulmonary margins and a high-pitched sound on percussion (*functional emphysema*). The respiratory murmur is harsh and may be wheezing. *Dry, crackling rales* may be present.

Some cases show a *respiratory tracing* with prolonged expiration. In others, the tracing reveals periodic variations which represent the initial stage of a Cheyne-Stokes respiration (see below).

Roentgen-ray examination of the thorax shows moderate congestion of the hilar vessels.

Increased blood volume, decreased speed of circulation of the blood in the lungs, and decreased vital capacity have been demonstrated during the attack (10a).

Pulmonary Edema

An attack of pulmonary edema may occur at any time (10b). Precordial oppression and pain, restlessness, weakness, and dry, nonproductive cough may precede the attack. If this occurs at night, a nightmare usually precedes it.

The initial manifestations are similar to those of paroxysmal dyspnea. However, after a few minutes, gurgling begins in the throat and the patient repeatedly emits a *white, yellowish, or pink foam*. This may be scanty or abundant and, in extreme cases, may attain a volume of 1000 cc. within 30 to 60 minutes. Vomiting may occur. Extreme restlessness, profuse sweating, paroxysms of suffocation with cyanosis, and loss of urine are frequent.

Except in the attacks which are connected with myocardial infarction (usually) and mitral stenosis (sometimes), the *pulse* is full and rapid and the *blood pressure* is normal or high; the latter is frequently higher than before the attack.

The physical findings are similar to those of paroxysmal dyspnea with one important exception: there are *innumerable moist rales* of different sizes, from the minute alveolar rales to the gurgling caused by the foam in the trachea. The alveolar rales are frequently more abundant at the bases.

The *temperature* is normal during the attack but may be higher *after* it (readsorption of proteins from the lungs).

The *sputum* has a chemical composition which is different from that of a transudate.[81]

The *roentgen-ray* study of the thorax reveals string-like or rounded shadows which predominate in that part of the lung which has the most active ventilation (12).

In general, the attack of pulmonary edema lasts from 20 minutes to several hours. Occasionally, the attack may last several days. When the duration and distribution of the edema is not typical, the following names have been used:

a) *Abortive pulmonary edema.* The entire attack lasts only a few minutes and disappears spontaneously.

[81] The data found by two different authors are:

Total albumin (per mille): 25–30
Albumin: 19–25
Globulin: 3–8.6
Specific gravity: 1.010–1.012
Water (per cent): 96–96.8
Urea: (from $\frac{1}{3}$ to $\frac{1}{2}$ that of the blood)
K, Cl, Na: very similar to blood content
Ca: about 20 per cent less than in the blood.

The fluid is similar to that of angioneurotic edema, allergic coryza, and the inflammatory effusions of large serosal cavities.

b) *Fulminating pulmonary edema.* The patient dies before the arrival of the physician or during transportation to the hospital.

c) *Protracted pulmonary edema.* This type is usually connected with myocardial infarction or a cerebrovascular accident. The attack may last from many hours to many days (47).

d) *Unilateral pulmonary edema.* This is extremely rare. It is usually associated with pathology of one lung or a unilateral lesion of the nervous system. One case, observed by the writer, occurred after a multiple brain embolism that involved the thalamus and the hypothalamus of one side (ipsilateral edema).

The end of the attack is marked by rapid improvement of the general condition and a decrease of the sputum. A certain number of rales in the chest may continue for some time, even after relief of the dyspnea.

Periodic Breathing (Cheyne-Stokes Respiration)

Periodic respiration consists of periodic variations in the amplitude of the respiratory movements. When the disturbance reaches its extreme degree, the amplitude varies from complete *apnea* to *hyperpnea*, with ample, noisy, and rapid respiratory acts. In one variety, the transitions between the phases of apnea and dyspnea occur *gradually*; in another, they occur *abruptly*. The disturbance is recognized by taking a graphic tracing or by applying the hand over the patient's chest.

In general, periodic respiration occurs during coma, narcotic depression, or spontaneous sleep. However, it may take place in the daytime during normal or seminormal consciousness. Myosis, bradycardia, slight hypertension, oppression, and, exceptionally, heart block, occur during the phase of apnea. Sometimes this is accompanied by loss of consciousness which may simulate normal sleep.

The respiration becomes noisy and may be

accompanied by moaning during the phase of dyspnea.

MECHANISM

Paroxysmal Dyspnea

Paroxysmal dyspnea should not be confused with the chronic dyspnea of cardiac patients; it has a sudden onset and, frequently, a sudden end.

Sudden dyspnea may be elicited in experimental animals by the following procedures:

a) *Chemical stimulation* of the respiratory center or the carotid bodies. This may be obtained by asphyxia, anoxia, or acidosis.

b) *Mechanical stimulation* of the receptors of the *pulmonary vessels* (hypertension of the lesser circulation, embolism) and of those of the *large veins* (rapid infusion, increased venous return).

c) *Decreased pressure in the region of the carotid sinus and aortic arch* (sudden drop of arterial blood pressure as in vascular collapse or shock).

d) *Stimulation* of various sensory nerves.

e) *Changes of pressure* in the bronchi and alveoli and stimulation of the mucosa of the respiratory passages.

It is apparent that *chemical and reflex stimulation* of the respiratory center or stimulation of the carotid bodies may play a role in the mechanism of paroxysmal dyspnea of cardiac patients.

One theory attributed these attacks to *acute left ventricular failure* with accumulation of the blood in the pulmonary vessels (19). Another theory attributed them to *increased venous return*; this might be *primary* (meals, drink (15), displacement of water from tissues to blood during the night (16), gravitational changes (17)), or *secondary* (initial hyperpnea due to dreams, reflexes, deficient pulmonary ventilation, or fall of blood pressure). A third theory admits a *purely reflex* mechanism (18).

A vicious circle is admitted by *Harrison* (15b). The patient has, when awake, considerable pulmonary congestion with de-

creased vital capacity and reflex stimulation of the respiratory center. During sleep, multiple, unpleasant stimuli reach a high intensity and wake up the patient. Then, ventilation is increased, a fact which favors a greater venous return and a greater pulmonary congestion. The subsequent course depends upon predominance of these elements over others which tend to relieve the attack or vice versa.

Acute dilatation of the pulmonary vessels often occurs; it is caused by increased flow and not by increased resistance.

Reflexes, originating in the left ventricle, in the pulmonary artery, in the large veins, and in the aortic and carotid receptors, seem to have a paramount importance. The primary cause of these reflexes is represented by severe distention of the large vessels and the heart.

The fact that, during sleep, the autonomic reflexes are very active may explain the frequent, though not constant, occurrence of these attacks during the night.

While distention of the carotid sinus receptors causes apnea, *stimulation of the carotid body receptors causes dyspnea* (42). This might indicate the involvement of chemical elements (anoxia, acidosis).

Pulmonary Edema

The classic theory of pulmonary edema explained this syndrome as caused by an *acute failure of the left ventricle* (19). However, an equally old theory tried to explain the occurrence of the edema as an *acute vasomotor crisis of the pulmonary vessels*, followed by transudation into the alveoli (20).

Experimental pulmonary edema has been caused consistently by the following procedures:

Ligation of the aortic arch (19a, 21). Compression (19a) or suture of the left ventricle (22a); necrosis of either the left ventricle (22b) or the right (22c). Intravenous injection of epinephrine (23). Intravenous infusion of physiologic solutions after vagotomy (24) or rapid intracarotid injection of physiologic solutions (25, 45). Intratracheal infusion of hypertonic solutions or inhalation of toxic gases (5, 26). Lesions of the central nervous system (26b, 24d, e, f, 27); suboccipital injection of veratrin (35) or fibrinogen plus thrombin (36, 37). Injection. of ammonium chloride (38, 36). Hypoglycemia (39). Left ventricular strain plus epinephrin or CNS stimulation (40).

Three main factors favor pulmonary edema: a) High pressure in the pulmonary vessels. b) Increased permeability of the pulmonary vessels. c) Decreased osmotic pressure of the blood.

Among the conclusions reached by various authors (50), the following are particularly important:

Extreme irritation of the brain or the carotid body leads to direct or reflex stimulation of the sympathetic system, followed by severe peripheral vasoconstriction. This leads to increased peripheral resistance with increased load of the left ventricle; displacement of a large mass of blood from the small vessels and blood reservoirs towards the veins; increased venous return; and, finally, filling of the lungs with a large mass of blood. Thus, neurological stimulation causes *increased output of the right ventricle, high pressure in the pulmonary capillaries,* and, at the same time, *left ventricular strain.* This mechanism may lead to pulmonary edema only if the conditions are extremely severe; it may be an important factor in hypertensive patients with left ventricular strain, and even more in coronary patients with left ventricular failure.

Mitral stenosis. The outflow of blood from the lungs is impeded, even in the resting state. Sympathetic stimulation, caused by excitement, exertion, exposure to cold, anger or fright, is followed by two phenomena: on the one hand, tachycardia, which shortens diastole and impairs emptying of the left atrium; on the other, vasoconstriction and redistribution of the blood, with accumulation in the lungs.

Pulmonary edema of patients with hypertension, aortic insufficiency, or aortic stenosis, or following minor coronary attacks; and following transfusions in surgical, obstetrical or cardiac cases. There is left ventricular strain with increase of left atrial and pulmonary venous pressures. Excitement and exposure to cold or exertion in clinical cases causes redistribution of the blood with accumulation in the lungs and acute pulmonary edema. The increased peripheral resistance may transform ventricular strain into ventricular failure.

Pulmonary edema of massive myocardial infarction. The power of the left ventricle is decreased. This leads to marked increase of left atrial and pulmonary capillary pressure if adequate venous return is maintained. Therefore, severe (but not too severe) lesions of the ventricle are the most effective. A peripheral mechanism caused by cerebral ischemia, carotid-sinus hypotension, or carotid-body hypoxia, may contribute to the disturbance by causing peripheral vasoconstriction. The accumulation of blood in the lungs seems to be due to both a cardiac and a vascular mechanism.

Pulmonary edema of phosgene inhalation, drowning, strangulation, pneumonia, or chronic congestive failure. In these conditions, direct damage to the capillary wall and action of hypoxia on the pulmonary capillaries are the most important factors, probably through liberation of histamine. The cerebral and carotid hypoxia may contribute by causing reflex vasoconstriction.

Periodic Respiration

This type of breathing is usually explained by an interaction of changes in oxygen and CO_2 tensions. Deep breathing reduces the CO_2 stimulus to a level below the threshold of excitability and, therefore, is followed by apnea. This causes a gradually increasing accumulation of CO_2 until breathing is resumed. The existence of a high amount of

CO_2 explains the deep and vigorous respiratory acts during the phase of dyspnea.

The fact that periodic breathing is easily produced in decerebrated animals leads to the belief that a loss of control of the cortical center over the medullary respiratory center may be responsible for the disturbance. This loss of control may be caused by anatomical (arteriosclerosis) or functional (spasm) disturbances of the cerebral vessels and is favored by drugs (morphine) and by other conditions (sleep) which depress the cortical function (29).

In cardiac failure, periodic breathing has been considered as the result of pulmonary congestion stimulating the respiratory center through afferent impulses and higher ventilation subsequent to a stage of decreased chemical stimulation of the center. A depression of the cerebral centers, caused by vascular disturbance, drug action, or sleep, is often involved, and favors the onset of this abnormal type of respiration.

More complex disturbances of the respiration, including *dissociated respiration*, may complicate Cheyne-Stokes respiration in cases with lesions of the nervous system (28).

TREATMENT

Paroxysmal Dyspnea

A subcutaneous injection of *morphine sulfate* (10–15 mg.) is the therapy of choice. Many other drugs and physical measures decreasing venous return (aminophyllin, venesection, tourniquets, pressure respiration) are also helpful. Prophylaxis is similar to that of pulmonary edema and includes digitalization, mercurials, low sodium diet, and sedation.

Pulmonary Edema

a) *Cases where blood pressure is high or normal and there is no danger of shock.*

Morphine subcutaneously or intravenously (15 mg.); *Na phenobarbital* or *chloral hydrate* i.v. (29); *mercurials* i.v.; *digitoxin* i.v.; *venesection* (300–500 cc.), *dibenamine* or *hydergine*; application of *tourniquets* to the four limbs; *pressure respiration* (31); and *spinal anesthesia* (43) are indicated. All these procedures decrease venous return and thus the pressure of the pulmonary vessels. In extremely resistant cases, removal of blood from the right atrium through a venous catheter has proved superior to other methods.

b) *Cases where blood pressure tends to drop and there is danger of shock.*

Small doses of *morphine* (5–8 mg.) can be given. *Oxygen* should be administered. The other procedures or drugs should be avoided as dangerous. The main utility will be obtained by alcohol-oxygen vapor as described below.

Antifoaming therapy. Alcohol vapor-oxygen therapy, which utilizes the antifoaming action of alcohol, was first tried successfully in animal experiments by the author (44). It was then applied to clinical cases. Detailed reports, including those on patients with severe pulmonary edema who did not receive other forms of treatment, have proved the usefulness of this method (46–48).

Because a precise etiologic diagnosis is not always immediately possible, the following plan of treatment should be used: a) *Alcohol-vapor therapy should be started as soon as possible* (by nasal catheter, using 95 per cent alcohol, in conscious patients; by mask, using 40 per cent alcohol, in unconscious patients). Oxygen bubbling through alcohol is started, with the flow regulated at 3 liters per minute; the flow is increased gradually up to 10 liters within the first 10 to 15 minutes. In the meantime, pulse, blood pressure, auscultation of the heart, a brief history, and an electrocardiogram, should give a better perspective of the case, so that, within the first 20 minutes, an adequate and precise pharmacologic or physical therapy may be started. According to the etiology of the case, atropine, morphine, phenobarbital, sympatholytic drugs, heparin, or other procedures may be used without interference with or discontinuation of alcohol inhalation. In many instances these drugs are not necessary, because the attack is already decreasing in severity following alcohol therapy. However, *protracted pulmonary edema* is not unusual. In such severe cases, alcohol therapy is continued as long as necessary (even for 12 hours), with brief intervals of rest, in addition to the other procedures.

Heart failure may follow a severe attack of pulmonary edema. Digitalization will then be made following the customary rules.

Periodic Respiration

Periodic respiration is ameliorated by the intravenous injection of *aminophyllin*. If large doses of this drug fail to dilate the cerebral vessels and to improve the condition, *metrazol* should be injected in order to stimulate the respiratory center.

PREVENTION OF PAROXYSMAL CARDIORESPIRATORY ATTACKS

This is essentially a prevention of severe left ventricular strain. It is obtained by digitalization, mercurials, salt-poor diet, xanthines (page 595). In hypertensive patients, sympatholytics, vasodilators, or sympathectomy (page 503) are of help.

Causes of increased venous return such as exposure to cold, excitement, strenuous exertion, and excess of food or drink should be avoided. Sedation is helpful. It may be done by giving *chloral hydrate* (1 gm. orally), *phenobarbital* or *nembutal*, at bedtime. Supper should be a small meal and at least 3 hours should elapse thereafter, before retiring. Excess of fluid intake is deleterious, while moderate amounts of alcohol are advisable.

BIBLIOGRAPHY

1. a) Gallavardin, L. J. Méd. Lyon, 1934, **15**, 609.
   b) Saloz and Frommel, E. Arch. Mal. Coeur, 1923, **16**, 570.
   c) Ribierre. Quoted by Doumer.
   d) Doumer, E. Arch. Mal Coeur, 1926, **19**, 791.

e) Hess, L. Wien. klin. Woch., 1931, **44**, 508.
2. a) Altschule, M. D. Personal communication (unpublished case).
   b) Chapman, E. M., Dill, D. B., and Graybiel, A. Medicine, 1939, **18**, 167.
3. Hochrein, M. Arch. Kreislauff., 1938, **14**, 24.
4. Logre. *Oedème Pulmonaire Infectieux*. Paris, Steinheil, 1913.
5. a) Biondi. Tesi, Catania, 1923.
   b) Melli, G. In Frugoni's book on Pulmonary Edema (6).
6. Frugoni, C. *L'Edema Polmonare Acucto*. Rome, Pozzi, 1931.
7. a) Moutier, F. Presse Méd., 1918, **26**, 108.
   b) Antonini, A., and Biancalani, A. Arch. Antrop. Crimin., 1927, **47**, 747.
   c) Manunza, P. Arch. Antrop. Crimin., 1933, **53**, 1534. Also Arch. Ist. Bioch. It. (Milan), 1934, **6**, 89.
   d) Astuni, A. Min. Med. (Turin), 1934, (1), 380.
   e) Gernez, C., and Marchandise, C. Gaz. Hôp., 1933, **106**, 483.
   f) Weissman, S. J. Surg., 1939, **6**, 653.
   g) Bsteh, O. Wien. klin. Woch., 1931, **44**, 1396.
8. a) Moutier, F. Presse Méd., 1918, **26**, 108.
   b) Langeron, L. Presse Méd., 1925, **33**, 65.
   c) Laubry, C., and Collet. Gaz. Hôp., 1935, **108**, 1585.
9. a) Jonnesco, T. Zeit. exp. Med., 1926, **48**, 516. Also J. A. M. A., 1925, **85**, 1926.
   b) Danielopolu, D. Brit. M. J., 1924, **2**, 553.
10. a) Weiss, S., and Robb, G. P. J. A. M. A., 1933, **100**, 1841.
    b) Wassermann, S. Wien. klin. Woch., 1928, **41**, 190. Also Wien. Arch. klin. Med., 1934, **24**, 387.
11. a) Melli, G. In Frugoni's Book (6).
    b) Blix, G. *Upsala Läkareförenings Förhandlingar*, 1929 (quoted by Melli (11a)).
12. Zdansky, E. Wien. Arch. inn. Med., 1929, **18**, 461. Also Roentgenpraxis, 1933, **5**, 248.
13. Stokes. *Diseases of the Heart and Aorta*. Dublin, Hodges and Smith, 1854.
14. Harrison, T. R., and co-workers. Arch. Int. Med., 1931, **48**, 377, and **49**, 151; 1932, **50**, 690; 1934, **53**, 911, and **53**, 724.
15. a) Eppinger, H., von Papp, L., and Schwartz, H. *Das Asthma Cardiale*. Berlin, Springer, 1924.
    b) Harrison, T. R. *Failure of the Circulation*. Baltimore, The Williams & Wilkins Co., 1939.
16. a) Brunn, F. Zentr. inn. Med., 1928, **49**, 873.

b) Gollwitzer-Meier, K. Klin. Woch., 1931, **10**, 341.

17. Wood, F. C., Wolferth, C. C., and Terrell, A. W. Am. Heart J., 1937, **14**, 255.

18. Wassermann, S. *Neue klinische Gesichtspunkte zur Lehre vom Asthma cardiale*. Berlin, Springer, 1926.

19. a) Welch, W. H. Virch. Arch. Path. Anat., 1872, **72**, 375.
    b) Lian, C. Presse Méd., 1910, **18**, 49.
    c) Vaquez, H. 7th Intern. Meet. M. Sci., London, 1913 (5th Section).

20. Teissier, J. *Rapport sur l'Oedème Aigü du Poumon*. Congr. Int. Sci. Med., Paris, Masson, 1900.

21. a) Sahli, H. Arch. exp. Path., 1885, **19**, 433.
    b) Kotowtschikow, A. M. Zeit. exp. Path., 1913, **13**, 400.
    c) Antoniazzi, E. Arch. Sci. Med. (Turin), 1930, **54**, 818.

22. a) Montanari, A. Pathologica (Milan), 1910/1911, **3**, 450.
    b) Coelho, E., and Rocheta, S. Ann. Méd., 1933, **34**, 91.
    c) Cataldi, G. Arch. Mal. Coeur, 1935, **28**, 604.

23. a) Huchard and Claude. Quoted by Melli (11a).
    b) Josué, O., and Bloch, L. Bull. Mem. Soc. Hôp. Paris, 1908, **25**, 55.
    c) Cavina, G. Pathologica (Milan), 1911, **3**, 452.
    d) Auer, J., and Gates, F. L. J. Exp. Med., 1917, **26**, 201.
    e) Luisada, A. A. Arch. exp. Path., Pharm., 1928, **132**, 313.
    f) Boggian, B. Min. Med. (Turin), 1929, **9**, 967.

24. a) Carrion and Hallion. Ctr. Soc. Biol., 1899, 10s, **6**, 156.
    b) Melli, G., and co-workers. Policl. (sez. med.), 1931, **38**, 417. Min. Med., 1931 (2), 419. Rev. Belge Sci. Med., 1930, **2**, 209.
    c) Warthen, H. J. Arch. Surg., 1935, **30**, 199.
    d) Kraus, F. Zeit. exp. Path., 1931, **14**, 402.
    e) Brunn, P. Wien. med. Woch., 1933, **83**, 106. Also Wien. klin. Woch., 1933, **46**, 262.
    f) Farber, S. J. Exper. Med., 1937, **66**, 397 and 405.

25. Luisada, A. A., and Sarnoff, S. J. Proc. Soc. Exper. Biol. & Med., 1944, **57**, 279.

26. a) Winternitz, M. C., and Lambert, R. A. J. Exper. Med., 1919, **29**, 537.

b) Mayer, A., and Morel, P. Bull. Soc. Chimie Biol., **3**, 520.
c) Laqueur, E., and DeVries Reilingh, D. Zentr. inn. Med., 1920, **41**, 81.

27. a) Frey, O. *Die pathologischen Lungenvaraenderungen nach Laehmung der Nervi Vagi*. Leipzig, 1877.
    b) Weiser, G. Pflueg. Arch., 1932, **231**, 68.

28. Condorelli, L., and Rechnitzer, E. Wien. Arch. inn. Med., 1927, **14**, 49.

29. a) Luisada, A. A. In Frugoni's book (6).
    b) Luisada, A. A. Riv. Ital. Ter. (Naples), 1928, N. 4.
    c) Luisada, A. A. Medicine, 1940, **19**, 475.
    d) Luisada, A. A. Exper. Med. & Surg., 1943, **1**, 22.
    e) Luisada, A. A., and Sarnoff, S. J. Am. Heart J., 1946, **31**, 282 and 293.

30. Wiggers, C. J. *Physiology in Health and Disease*. Philadelphia, Lea & Febiger, 1944.

31. Barach, A. L., Martin, J., and Eckman, M. Ann. Int. Med., 1938, **12**, 754.

32. Drinker, C. K. *Pulmonary Edema and Inflammation*. Cambridge, Harvard Univ. Press, 1945.

33. Moon, V. *Shock and Related Capillary Phenomena*. Oxford Univ. Press, 1938.

34. Meltzer, S. J. Am. Med., 1904, **8**, 191.

35. Jarisch, A., *et al.* Klin. Woch., 1940, **18**, 1440.

36. Cameron, G. R., *et al.* J. Path. & Bact., 1949, **61**, 375; 1951, **63**, 609.

37. Sarnoff, S. J., *et al.* Circ., 1952, **6**, 51.

38. Koenig, H., and Koenig, R. Am. J. Physiol., 1949, **158**, 1.

39. McKay, E. N., *et al.* Proc. Soc. Exper. Biol. & Med., 1949, **71**, 669; 1949, **72**, 421; 1950, **73**, 568; 1950, **74**, 695.

40. Paine, R., *et al.* Circ. 1952, **5**, 759.

41. Harrison, W., and Liebow, A. Circ., 1952, **5**, 824.

42. Aviado, D. M., *et al.* Federation Proc., 1952, **11**, 6 and Am. J. Phys. 1952, **169**, 460.

43. Sarnoff, S. J., and Farr, H. W. Anesthesiology, 1944, **5**, 69.

44. Luisada, A. A. Proc. Soc. Exper. Biol. & Med., 1950, **74**, 215. Also Circ., 1950, **2**, 872.

45. Luisada, A. A., and Contro, S. Circ. Research, 1953, **1**, 179.

46. Luisada, A. A., Goldmann, M. A., and Weyl, R. Circ., 1952, **5**, 363.

47. Goldmann, M. A., and Luisada, A. A. Ann. Int. Med., 1952, **37**, 1221.

48. Goldmann, M. A., and Primiano, N. P. Am. J. Obst. & Gyn., 1953, **65**, 314.

49. Luisada, A. A. J. Am. Geriatr. Soc. 1953, **1**, 331.

CHAPTER 30

Heart Failure

Circulatory failure occurs when the blood flow of the capillaries is not adequate for the needs of the tissues. It may be *absolute* (when there is an actual inadequacy) or *relative* (when the inadequacy exists only because the needs are increased).

Circulatory failure may occur either because there is a *reduction of the circulating blood* (hemorrhage, shock) or because *the capacity of the circulatory system is increased* (peripheral vasodilation). In both cases, reduced venous return is responsible for the failure. However, circulatory failure may be of a different type if caused by heart failure.

Heart failure is *absolute* if the heart has actually reduced its work; it is *relative* if the heart maintains or even increases its work, but this is inadequate in the presence of increased requirements of the tissues. Heart failure may be *acute, subacute,* or *chronic.*

Acute heart failure is due to sudden, primary or secondary disturbance of the heart. The resulting clinical picture resembles that of *shock* being revealed by signs of arterial depletion and is called "cardiogenic shock" (page 426).

Subacute or chronic heart failure, on the contrary, is mostly revealed by signs and symptoms of *congestion* of the venous side of the cardiovascular system.

The clinical picture of heart failure always occurs in persons with a weak myocardium. However, its appearance may be hastened and its existence revealed at an earlier stage by severe vascular or valvular lesions.

CAUSES

Heart failure may occur as the result of any diffuse lesion of the heart and of the vessels. The following classification permits a better understanding of its mechanism.

a) *Diseases causing strain of the left ventricle, frequently also of the large arteries and the coronaries.* They include arterial hypertension, atherosclerosis of the aorta and aortitis, aortic insufficiency or stenosis, mitral insufficiency, coarctation of the aorta some cases of constrictive pericarditis, and patent ductus. In all these conditions, the left ventricle is hypertrophied.

b) *Disease causing strain of the right ventricle, frequently also of the pulmonary artery and the vessels of the lesser circulation.* Mitral stenosis, acute or chronic cor pulmonale, patent foramen ovale, and pulmonary stenosis. In all these diseases, the right ventricle is hypertrophied; in mitral stenosis, the left atrium participates to the strain.

c) *Diseases where the strain is felt by both sections of the heart.* Combined valvular defects, ventricular septal defect, certain atypical cases of patent ductus, arteriovenous fistulas, thyroid heart, disturbances of the rate and rhythm, diffuse myocardial fibrosis, coronary heart disease, beri-beri heart, and many cases of constrictive pericarditis.

Whatever the underlying cardiovascular disease, various factors may precipitate congestive failure. Among them, strenuous physical exertion, emotion, exposure to cold, and overabundance of food and drink are common. Others are: coronary occlusion, acute infections, rheumatic carditis, pulmonary embolism, surgical intervention, acute gall bladder colic, pregnancy, and other less frequent conditions.

Chronic vitamin and protein deficiencies

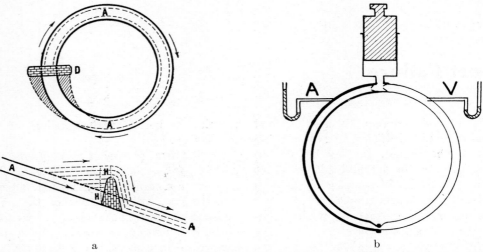

a   b

FIG. 305. (a) Effect of a dam (upper) in a closed circuit (so-called "back-pressure effect") and (lower) in a freely moving stream (HH, increased level). (From Wenckebach.) (b) A simple scheme of circulation. Before the pump is started, a pressure of 10 mm. exists throughout the system, the so-called "static pressure". When one pumps hard, the pressure becomes 120 in A and 4 in V. Weakening of the pump increases venous pressure V and decreases arterial pressure A. Injection of fluid into the system increases venous pressure in the presence of normal arterial pressure. (From I. Starr.)

favor cardiac failure; so does the action of several *poisons*. Excessive dosage or extremely prolonged action of *digitalis* may damage the myocardium, thereby favoring failure. The extent and importance of this digitalis effect, however, are controversial.

MECHANISM AND TYPES OF HEART FAILURE

The circulatory apparatus is a closed system with many safety devices. The continuous motion of the blood is due to the action of four separate pumps (fig. 9). As the atria have a weak action and act mainly as reservoirs, two pumps actually maintain the circulation, the right and left ventricles.

A dam placed in the course of a river *raises the level of the stream above the obstacle and lowers that below;* in the same way, an obstacle placed in the course of a closed circuit (valvular stenosis, coarctation) *raises the pressure above and decreases that in the section below* (fig. 305a) (6). In such cases, the increased pressure (or the larger caliber) of the chamber or vessel above the

obstacle is not due to heart failure. Thus, distention of the left atrium and pulmonary vessels in mitral stenosis, or of the right atrium, venous system, and liver in tricuspid stenosis, is due to redistribution of blood and does not imply heart failure. Again, the action of the obstacle on the section below is such that decreased pressure or lower output may be the result of valvular stenosis or vascular narrowing without implying that the heart is weak.

Another simple scheme of circulation includes the action of a pump and shows that when a weak action of the pump follows a stronger action, a rise of "venous pressure" takes place (39, 40) (fig. 305b).

Cardiac reserve is a clinical term which is applied to the difference between the actual work of the heart and the maximum work which it is able to perform (1). Cardiac reserve is reduced by: a) *increase of cardiac work* (ventricular strain): the figure of actual work is higher and nearer to the maximum possible work; b) *decrease of efficiency* (latent ventricular failure): the figure of

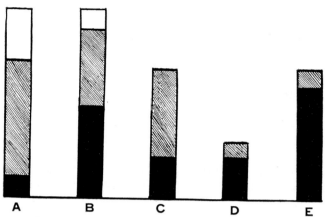

FIG. 306. *The concept of cardiac reserve.* Decrease of cardiac reserve because of exercise, increased requirement, or cardiac failure. A, normal; B, decrease of cardiac reserve *from below* in cases with valvular defects, hypertension, or hyperthyroidism in a stage of compensation. C, decrease of cardiac reserve *from above* in cases with myocardial or coronary disease; D, extremely reduced cardiac reserve in a coronary heart patient with low output failure; E, extremely reduced cardiac reserve in a hyperthyroid patient with high output failure. Black area, cardiac work at rest. Stippled area, cardiac reserve used during exercise. White area, further cardiac reserve.

maximum possible work is lower and nearer to the actual work; c) *both* (fig. 306). Cardiac reserve is reduced when valvular defects, vascular lesions, or inefficient cardiac action require permanently increased cardiac work in the presence of latent failure.

The decreased contractility of the heart may cause effects in two ways:

a) *In the arterial system;* this is revealed by reduced flow, reduced pressure, or both, and has been called *forward failure.* It corresponds to *a state of arterial depletion* (42).

b) *In the pulmonary circulation and the venous system;* it is revealed by increased venous pressure and distention of the veins and liver, and has been called *backward failure.* It corresponds to *a state of venous congestion* (42).

It should be noted that these arterial and venous phenomena may be simulated by the mechanical results of valvular or vascular lesions without actual failure.

The same differential concept which is implied in the definition of cardiac reserve may be applied to other cardiovascular phenomena. Any cardiac lesion which causes congestion of the lungs reduces the "reserve power" of the lungs for accommodating a

greater amount of blood when heart failure occurs. Any cardiac lesion which causes congestion of the liver reduces the "reserve power" of the liver for accomodating a greater amount of blood when heart failure occurs. Any decreased output, due to aortic stenosis, reduces the "reserve power" of the aorta and the arterial system whenever the heart reduces its output. Therefore, any change in the distribution of the blood, in the pressure of one of the vascular systems, and in the volume of a cardiac chamber or of an artery or vein, existing before heart failure sets in, inevitably causes more severe results in that section, system, or organ, because of reduced "reserve power", when heart failure occurs. For this reason, a basically similar process of cardiac failure may cause diverse clinical pictures in patients with different lesions of the heart and vessels.

The observation that *damage to the right heart may not be followed by increased venous congestion* (7) led to admission that a long and complex chain of events connects heart failure with increased venous pressure. Without changing the main concept that cardiac failure is the primary and basic disturbance, this resulted in a better evaluation of several important phenomena, including *high venous tonus* (44) and *renal retention of water and sodium* (45).

It is now admitted that *the increase of blood volume* is an important factor, on the one hand in causing signs of congestion and, on the other, in increasing the severity of cardiac failure. A vicious circle is created by the fact that increased blood volume is due to water and sodium retention because of renal dysfunction while this renal dysfunction is an indirect result of cardiac failure.

The retention of sodium is caused by either: a) *low filtration rate* secondary to decreased renal blood flow with a normal or even subnormal tubular absorption (46); or b) normal filtration rate with increased *tubular absorption* (47). Low filtration rate seems to be related to initially *low cardiac output plus compensatory vasoconstriction of the renal arterioles*. High venous renal pressure, related to the complex causes of venous hypertension in general, may increase renal dysfunction.

The renal dysfunction, however, has a more complex mechanism because sodium and water retentions seem to be partly independent and caused by special endocrine disorders. *Excessive retention of water followed by retention* of salt is found in many clinical cases, suggesting an *excessive amount of posterior pituitary hormone*. On the other hand, *excessive retention of salt* followed by retention of water is found in other cases, suggesting *an excessive amount of adrenal cortical hormone* (48). The problem is further complicated by the interrelation between the two hormones. Moreover, excessive corticoadrenal secretion may be due to increased secretion of adrenocorticotropic hormone. These disturbances may be explained by anoxia of either the anterior or the posterior pituitary or, more likely, *by insufficient destruction of either hormone by the congested liver* (49).

Studies dealing with circulation speed or cardiac output have revealed two different types of cardiac failure. The first type is encountered chiefly in rheumatic, hypertensive, and coronary heart diseases; it presents *increased circulation time and reduced cardiac output*. The second is found in anemic, thyroid, and beri-beri heart diseases; in certain cases of chronic cor pulmonale; in patent ductus arteriosus; in arteriovenous fistula, and in some cases of Paget's disease. In such cases, *decreased circulation time and normal or increased cardiac output* occur (42, 44). It is apparent that rheumatic valvular disease, cardiovascular lues or hypertensive heart disease may also be associated with anemia, vitamin-B deficiency, or hyperthyroidism, causing, therefore, a *mixed type of cardiac failure with slightly increased or slightly decreased output and circulation time*. It should be emphasized that low output failure is associated with absolute decrease of cardiac reserve and, therefore, is an *absolute failure;* on the other hand, high output failure is usually associated with relative decrease of cardiac reserve because of increased requirements of the tissues; and represents, therefore, *relative failure*.

The fact that the heart is composed of *two* main pumps, the right and left ventricles, working under different conditions, led to a brilliant and daring conception (2): *that either of them might become insufficient without the other being affected*. This theory tried to explain different clinical pictures as the result of isolated failure of one or the other ventricle. *Right ventricular failure* would be revealed by exertional dyspnea, right ventricular enlargement, hepatic enlargement, and peripheral edema. *Left ventricular failure* would be revealed by anginal pain, paroxysmal dyspnea, and acute pulmonary edema. A confirmation of this theory was found in the frequent occurrence of the former syndrome in patients with right ventricular strain (mitral stenosis) and of the latter in patients with left ventricular strain (aortic insufficiency, arterial hypertension). A reaction against excessive generalization of this theory was started by the author in 1932 (3). Experimental (5, 7, 40) and clinical (11) evidence seemed to confirm his view. Later studies by means of catheterization of the right heart (57, 58) revealed *high diastolic pressure of the right ventricle* in cases with right ventricular failure and *high systolic pressure of the right ventricle* (with normal diastolic) in cases with left ventricular failure. Thus, clinical evidence of isolated ventricular failures was obtained. Moreover, it was proved that experimental compression of a coronary artery is followed by increased diastolic pressure of the *left* ventricle while right ventricular pressures and the filling pressure of the right atrium are still normal (60). This reveals the possibility of *isolated acute left ventricular failure following diffuse coronary insufficiency.* On the other hand, *chronic failure of one ventricle is usually followed by failure of the other* on account of the multiple anatomical and functional connections between the two chambers.

Whenever long-standing mechanical obstacles or structural changes have occurred, striking differences between the pressures or capacities of two chambers or two vascular districts may occur. When failure affects predominantly or exclusively one ventricle, the clinical manifestations appear *first* in that vascular district which is *behind the weak chamber* even if the equilibrium is reestablished by subsequent weakening of the other (1).

There is no doubt that a frequent coincidence exists between certain signs due to heart failure and some valvular or vascular lesion. As previously stated, those signs are connected with a preexisting reduction of the "reserve power" of the affected organs. Therefore, any further increase of the sign is detected more easily because the clinical threshold of observation is quickly reached.

Enlargement of the liver occurs as a result of dynamic changes in tricuspid stenosis.

If the heart is weak, a slight, further increase of venous pressure is revealed immediately by palpation of *the liver* and by *hepatic dysfunction.*

Cerebral ischemia often occurs in aortic stenosis. Weakening of the heart causes a decrease of cardiac output, and this is revealed by *signs of cerebral anemia* because the cerebral circulation is already near the threshold of clinical disturbance.

Pulmonary congestion is frequent in arterial hypertension and may cause exertional dyspnea. Any weakening of the heart causes *severe dyspnea* because the power of dilatation of the pulmonary vessels is reduced.

Blood flow through the arteries of the legs is often reduced in cases with coarctation of the aorta or arteriosclerosis obliterans. The earliest sign of heart failure in such patients is *intermittent claudication* because the reduced cardiac output lowers the blood flow in the extremities below the threshold which permits exertion.

In conclusion, congestion and depletion may be caused by the hemodynamic effects of the cardiac disease, by cardiac failure, or both.

The application of *Starling's law* (page 30) to the hearts of sick patients was resisted by clinicians. *Murri's law* (8) stated that "while dilatation of a normal heart means greater power of contraction, dilatation of a sick heart means lesser power of contraction." The contradiction between accepted clinical knowledge and physiological laws can be explained as follows: when the heart of a cardiac patient fails, its efficiency is reduced; an increase of work is obtained through dilatation; therefore, even if this dilatation is compensatory, it implies that the heart is weak. Moreover, excessive dilatation fails to increase the power of contraction.

The three mechanisms of adaptation of the heart are, as already outlined, increase of rate (tachycardia), increase of volume (dilatation), and hypertrophy. Each has a critical limit above which the heart decreases its efficiency instead of increasing it. For the heart rate, the limit seems to be around 200 because higher rates do not permit a good diastolic filling. Dilatation ceases to be useful when the elastic limit of the fibers is overstrained and diastolic pressure begins to rise. Hypertrophy is not profitable if too severe because the capillary network becomes insufficient in relation to the blood supply necessary for muscle metabolism. Then a vicious circle takes place: the dilated and rapid heart contracts faster and faster, less and less effectively. The fact that an extremely dilated heart may be a mechanical obstacle to cardiorespiratory dynamics should also be taken into account.

Even if vascular, renal, hepatic, nervous, and endocrine elements contribute to the development of the picture of chronic congestive failure, this *is the result of impairment of the contractility of the myocardium*. It is revealed by a change in the ratio between work performed and either cardiac size or venous pressure. Therefore, when heart failure is present, normal work will be possible only through dilatation, increased rate, and venous engorgement.

Cardiac failure may manifest itself either by decrease of cardiac work without venous engorgement (predominant picture of depletion) or by venous engorgement without decreased work (predominant picture of congestion). *Only the ratio between work and venous conditions is a sure evidence of failure* because a normal heart may have decreased output (associated with decreased venous return) or venous engorgement (associated with increased output). In the first case there is reduced cardiac volume; in the second, increased cardiac volume.

Venous pressure is not an adequate element for evaluating cardiac conditions because the flow may increase without a rise in pressure and vice versa, on account of changing conditions of the venous walls.

Two different mechanisms have been discussed as possible causes for heart failure. The first consists of a *decreased ability to release energy* with a decreased oxygen consumption for a given diastolic size (9). The second consists of a *smaller conversion of the energy into useful work, i.e. an impairment in the mechanical efficiency*[82] of cardiac work (10). The second mechanism seems the most likely.

It should be kept in mind that different types of myocardial disturbances may occur. As already stated, increased requirements may cause *relative cardiac failure*. In such cases, the metabolism and the contractile power of the cardiac fiber may be preserved, and the term *hemodynamic cardiac failure* could be used (51). On the contrary, in most cases with *absolute cardiac failure*, a primary deficiency of contractility takes place following severe changes of the metabolism of the cardiac muscle: this is revealed by prolongation of electrical systole (Q-T interval of the electrocardiogram) and abbreviation of mechanical systole (distance 1st to 2nd sound of the phonocardiogram). For these cases, the name of *energetic-dynamic insufficiency* has been suggested (51).

LESIONS

Examination of patients who died after chronic heart failure reveals a series of changes involving all organs, as a result of *chronic congestion*.

The *lungs* are less elastic, heavier, and firmer because of engorgement of the vessels and transudation into the alveoli (edema). The lung of *chronic edema* has a light-grayish color which is different from the gray-pink color seen in acute edema. Section of the parenchyma elicits an outpour of foam. Serum and red cells penetrate the interstitial tissue; the cells are destroyed

---

[82] Mechanical efficiency is the *ratio of mechanical work performed to the total energy released by chemical transformations*. Oxygen consumption measures the total energy, released by oxidation of the heart muscle.

and their hemoglobin is transformed into brown pigment which is taken in by the alveolar cells and by leucocytes. Some of the latter are found in the bronchial exudate (*cardiac cells*).

The *bronchi* present cyanosis of the mucosa and signs of congestive bronchitis. Bronchopneumonia, atelectasis, infarctions, and pleurisy are common findings.

The *liver* is enlarged, cyanotic, and firm. The high pressure of the hepatic veins causes a *dilatation of the centrolobular veins;* the hepatic cells are atrophied by the chronic compression. The typical *nutmeg liver* is due to the existence of large pink centers (veins), surrounded by yellow areas (fatty, degenerated parenchyma). "*Cardiac*" *fibrosis of the liver* is common, and an increase in connective tissue of the liver is present in the majority of cases. The fibrosis may be *central, portal, or both,* but rarely reaches the severe stage which is necessary for clinical recognition (33).

The *kidneys* are increased in size, have a pink color, and present a smooth, tense capsule. Section reveals a deeper color of the pyramids and a lighter color of the cortex. The veins and capillaries are distended while serum and red cells are present within the capsular spaces and the tubules. In the latter, fusion of the cells with degenerated epithelium causes the formation of *casts*. When congestive failure has lasted a long time, *cyanotic atrophy* and *sclerosis of the kidneys* occurs, a process which is usually favored by arterial lesions.

The *skin* and *mucosa* present cyanosis and chronic edema; the *serosal* cavities contain a transudate (ascites, hydropericardium, and hydrothorax).

The *heart* is enlarged and flaccid, presenting the basic lesions which caused failure. The *heart muscle* is frequently cyanotic; there is dilatation of the coronary sinus and of the smaller veins. *Mural thrombi* and clots are frequently present in the cardiac cavities, especially in the atria.

Chemical studies have shown that the failing heart has a subnormal content of acid-soluble purines (43), creatin (14), lipid (15a), phosphatid (15b), and potassium (16). The decrease of creatin and phosphorus content may be particularly significant (17).

The *fluid of peripheral edema* has a low specific gravity (from 1.005–1.010), a content of protein which is intermediate between exudates and transudates (from 0.2–0.5 per cent), and a higher concentration of chlorides than the blood (28).

SIGNS AND SYMPTOMS

I. Acute Cardiac Failure

Acute cardiac failure may be due to:

a) *Sudden weakness* of the myocardium connected with structural lesions (myocardial infarction, myocarditis).

b) *Sudden mechanical hindrance* caused by occlusion of one of the valvular orifices (ball-valve thrombus occluding the mitral; hooking of the aortic cusps in aortic stenosis); massive pulmonary embolism; or pericardial tamponade.

c) *Severe ventricular tachycardia* impairing the coronary blood supply; it may be associated with atrial flutter or fibrillation.

d) *Ventricular arrest* as a result of severe carotid sinus reflex or sudden complete A-V block (Stokes-Adams attack).

In these cases, the main clinical picture is caused by *depletion of the arterial system*. Feebleness of mind and body, drowsiness or loss of consciousness, coldness of the skin, and drop in arterial pressure, are typical and resemble the clinical picture of *shock*.

In acute cardiac failure, *the peripheral veins may be engorged;* the engorgement may be prevented by severe pulmonary congestion or reflex peripheral vasodilation. *Dyspnea* may be present. *Rales* may be heard over the lungs. The heart sounds may be relatively loud.

II. Subacute or Chronic Cardiac Failure

The clinical picture of chronic heart failure mainly consists of signs of venous engorgement and of its effect upon the different organs. However, less apparent signs and symptoms caused by heart failure on the arterial system are also present.

Weakness is one of the early symptoms and is revealed by even slight exertion. *Dyspnea* frequently has different manifestations: first, *exertional dyspnea*, then *orthopnea*, and then *continuous dyspnea. Periodic respiration* may occur and has serious significance (page 557). A *wheezing respiration* may simulate bronchial asthma (*cardiac asthma*) (30). Sometimes dyspnea is absent in one recumbent posture but is present in another and starts only after the patient has been in such position for 10 seconds to 2 minutes (*trepopnea*) (17b).

Both the *vital capacity* and the *breath-holding time* are reduced in congestive failure.

Anorexia, nausea, eructations, and *flatulence* are frequent. *Cough* is not unusual and may be accompanied by rusty or bloody sputum.

Precordial oppression is common; so is a series of thoracic sensations varying from sticking pain to dull, diffuse aching.

Cyanosis is frequent; it presents extreme variations between the dark color of chronic cor pulmonale (*black cardiacs*) and the *grayish* or *livid color* of patients with aortic insufficiency. It predominates on the lips, nosetip, earlobes, and extremities. The *skin* is frequently dry and scaly. *Jaundice* may appear.

Peripheral edema is frequent. It predominates both in the most distant parts (feet, legs) and in the dependent areas (legs, perineum, and sacral region) (fig. 307). Soft and easily compressible at first (*pitting edema*), it may reach a thickness of many centimeters and give a firm consistency to the skin.

The *visible veins* are swollen; those of the neck present active pulsations (18). The pulsations of the *carotid* and *subclavian arteries* are often apparent.

The *pulse* is small, irregular, and frequently presents a *pulse deficit* because many cardiac contractions are not revealed by the radial pulse. An exception is represented by the full and often regular pulse of patients with aortic insufficiency or atherosclerosis of the aorta. When the pulse is regular, *alternation* may be detected.

The *heart* is enlarged both to the left and right. The precordial dulness is due not only to the heart itself but frequently also to *pericardial effusion.* The cardiohepatic angle is obtuse because of this transudate plus enlargement of the right atrium. The manubrium of the sternum may become dull because of distention of the innominate veins.

While the *murmurs of organic valvular lesions* become less clear and may even disappear, *murmurs due to relative insufficiency or stenosis* may appear as an effect of heart failure. This is particularly true of a *soft systolic murmur* audible at the apex or the tricuspid area (page 225) but also occasionally of a *soft, early diastolic murmur* over the aortic or pulmonic areas (pages 249 and 261), and of a *diastolic rumble* over the apex (page 237). A *triple rhythm* (page 370) may be an early sign and may be audible all through the duration of failure.

The *liver* is frequently enlarged. This enlargement may be an early sign and may be further increased in later stages by relative insufficiency of the tricuspid valve. Its border is regular; it is firm but not as much as in cases of cirrhosis of Laennec or frosted liver.

The *lungs* frequently have a "functional emphysema", favored by the high level of the diaphragm and by congestion of the bases. The latter is revealed by small, scattered rales, evidence of subacute or chronic edema. *Pleural friction may also be present.*

The occurrence of *pleural effusion* is frequent. This may be *unilateral* (more often on the right side) or *bilateral* (more abundant on the right side). *Ascites* may be present, but unless constrictive pericarditis, perihepatitis, or a tricuspid lesion is present, it is seldom abundant.

Renal changes are revealed by the urine which becomes scanty (200–300 cc. in 24 hours) and has a high specific gravity (even 1.030 or more if there is no renal sclerosis). Albumin, indican, and urobilin are present. Bile pigments may be found. Creatin is almost always present. A few red cells and many granular casts can be found in the sediment. Albumin may vary from a trace to 0.5 per cent.

Urobilinogen is generally increased in the stools during severe congestive failure, a fact which gives evidence of increased blood destruction.

Venous pressure is increased; measurement should be made with the usual precautions (page 162). *Abdominal compression* produces a fall of venous pressure in normal people but a rise of pressure in heart failure (19). It is followed by *visible engorgement of the jugular veins* (so-called *hepato-jugular reflux*).

Arterial pressure may vary. Some patients may present an increase of blood pressure, due to stimulation of the vasomotor center by CO_2. Others may show a slight drop. *Reduced pulse pressure and increased diastolic pressure are common.*

Both *venous* and *right atrial pressure* are increased, as revealed by direct measurement through catheterization. Right atrial pressure is often as high as 20 mm. Hg and the *gradient* between venous and atrial pressures is reduced (42). *Right ventricular failure* is revealed by high diastolic pressure of the right ventricle. *Left ventricular failure* is revealed by high systolic and normal diastolic pressures of the right ventricle.

The *direct observation of the capillaries* shows distention of their venous ends, slow circulation, and the presence of bead-like formations, slowly moving from the arterial to the venous end. Fragmentation of the

stream and temporary arrest may be observed.

Basal metabolism is frequently increased and may be even 40 per cent above normal. This may be caused by the increased work of the respiratory muscles and by the increased oxygen consumption of the heart. An element which tends to overshadow the increased metabolism is represented by the edema which adds to the weight of the patient. In certain patients, the basal metabolic rate is very high on account of a primary disturbance, and increased requirements of the tissues are an important cause of congestive failure (*high output failure*).

The *temperature* may be slightly elevated with greater difference between rectal and skin temperatures than in normal persons (32).

The *volume of circulating blood* is frequently increased (20) and may reach 50

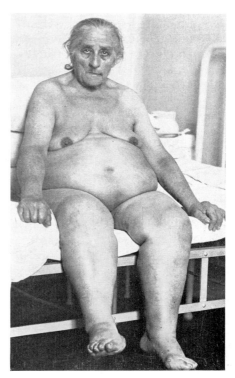

Fig. 307. Congestive failure

per cent above norm. *This is largely due
to the blood contained in the dilated heart
and in the engorged organs.* It is likely that,
because of slow circulation in the capillaries
of many areas, and of massive edema and
transudates, the actual figures should be
revised and might even reach 100 to 150
per cent above norm. A *redistribution of the
blood* also takes place in these patients, so
that more blood is present on the venous
side of the cardiovascular system, in the
lungs, and in the liver.

The formation of edema and transudates
may simulate *polycythemia* by leaving a
relatively more abundant percentage of
red cells. It also increases *blood viscosity.*

Red cell fragility is usually increased;
reticulocyte percentage, elevated; *serum
bilirubin concentration*, frequently increased
(24b).

BLOOD GASES

The *arterial blood* has a slight diminution
of oxygen content while its carbon dioxide
content is normal (26). The *venous blood*
has a low oxygen content and a variable
content of carbon dioxide (26). The *difference* between arterial and venous oxygen
contents is increased.

GRAPHIC TRACINGS

Jugular tracings may reveal a progressive
engorgement of the venous circulation: the
systolic collapse becomes less marked and
terminates before the 2nd heart sound;
the *v* wave becomes smaller with the progress
of failure (21). Atrial fibrillation causes
disappearance of the *a* wave. If relative
tricuspid insufficiency is present, a positive
plateau takes place in systole, followed by a
diastolic collapse. The *hepatic tracing* presents a similar aspect.

Respiratory tracings reveal an increased
rate and, sometimes, an oblique course of
the graph during inspiration (22).

The cardiac waves of the *pneumocardiogram* are marked.

Electrocardiogram. The ECG reveals the
existence of various disturbances of the

heart rate and rhythm. The most frequent
are: sinus tachycardia, atrial flutter, atrial
fibrillation, ventricular tachycardia, and
ventricular premature contractions.

Two abnormalities have been attributed
to cardiac failure: a) *low voltage* of QRS
with prolonged P-R and broadening of
QRS: and b) *prolongation of Q-T* (23a, b).
In the type of cardiac failure due to intrinsic changes of myocardial metabolism,
prolongation of electrical systole (Q-T
interval) is associated with shortening of
mechanical systole (1st to 2nd sound of
the phonocardiogram), so that the 2nd
sound takes place before the end of the T
wave (51).

Experimental studies indicate that *stasis
in the coronary sinus* is followed by *low
voltage*, especially marked for the T wave
(53).

X-RAY

The *x-ray* reveals that the heart is enlarged and that its margins present small
contractions. The right atrium may be
triangular and very large. The pulmonary
vessels are dilated (fig. 308). Opacity of
the lung fields may be caused by chronic
edema, vascular distention, or pleural effusion. These predominate in the dependent
areas of the lungs and pleura. The high
level of the diaphragm contributes to poor
visibility of the pulmonary bases. The
superior cava is distended and may present
active pulsations. Encapsulated pleural effusions are not unusual. Evidence of pulmonary infarction may be found.

Other data vary in the different types of
cardiac failure and will be described below.

VARIETIES

High output failure. Cardiac output is
increased; venous pressure is elevated; blood
volume is also increased; there may be
either polycythemia (chronic cor pulmonale)
or oligocythemia (anemic heart). *Circulation time may be normal or shorter.*

Low output failure. Its initial stage is

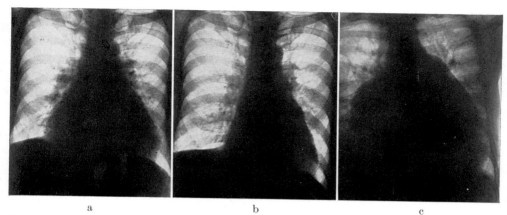

a   b   c

FIG. 308. Changes in the heart size because of failure in a case of rheumatic heart disease, a, first episode of failure; b, 2 years later, good compensation; c, 3 years after b, severe failure causing death.

revealed by normal or low output and by increased pulmonary pressure following exercise; exertional dyspnea is the accompanying symptom. Decreased cardiac ouptut is present later and is revealed by comparison with previous figures. *Circulation time is prolonged*.

Left ventricular failure. There often is low cardiac output, high pulmonary arterial pressure, normal diastolic pressure of the right ventricle, and normal blood volume. Arm-to-lung circulation time is within normal limits while arm-to-tongue time is greatly increased. Digitalis causes an increase of cardiac output and a decrease of pulmonary arterial pressure (52).

Right ventricular failure. Arm-to-lung circulation time is increased. Right ventricular diastolic pressure is elevated. Right ventricular systolic pressure may be high because of preexisting cor pulmonale. Right atrial filling pressure is increased; the veno-atrial gradient of pressure is decreased. Digitalis increases temporarily systolic pressure, but decreases diastolic pressure of the right ventricle. After a few days, systolic pressure also drops.

Bernheim's syndrome is the name given to a clinical picture of right-sided failure which occurs in patients with strain of the left ventricle. The syndrome has been attributed to compression of the *right ventricle* by the distended interventricular septum (37a, b), an interpretation which has not been proven (37c, d) and which is not accepted by the author. It is better explained by total heart failure.

Studies made with radioactive materials have revealed that *the amount of residual blood of the atria and ventricles increases tremendously during heart failure* (61). In failure of a single ventricle, residual blood of that chamber is increased.

MECHANISM OF ORIGIN OF THE SIGNS

Exertional dyspnea is produced by muscular effort and its ultimate cause is the inability of the heart to increase its output in proportion to the needs of the body. A reflex stimulation of the respiratory center is the main cause of the dyspnea; this is caused by: a) the muscular movements themselves, b) increased pressure in the venae cavae, and c) increased pressure in the pulmonary artery.

After severe exertion, anoxemia develops and exerts a double action on the respiratory center: a) direct and b) through the chemo-receptors of the carotid and aortic bodies.

Orthopnea is caused by the fact that recumbency causes a shift of blood from the dependent regions; this leads to increased venous return, increased pulmonary flow, and reduction of vital capacity. A reflex stimulation of the respiratory center is the result. The effect of increased venous pressure on the respiratory center, caused by lowering the head (25), is another probable factor.

Trepopnea seems to have a mechanism which varies according to the position of the patient in which it occurs. Greater venous pressure may explain right-decubitus dyspnea; greater emptying of the engorged hepatic venous or mechanical obstruction of the pulmonary veins by the heart itself may explain left-decubitus dyspnea.

Continuous dyspnea is due to increased CO_2 saturation, decreased O_2 saturation (26), and acidosis. These are caused by: a) *reduced ventilation*, caused by numerous factors (high level of diaphragm, pulmonary engorgement, enlarged heart), and b) *increased requirements* of the body (increased dynamics of the heart, poor utilization of the oxygen in the periphery).

However, in addition to the chemical action on the respiratory center, reflexes from the distended venae cavae and pulmonary vessels, and stimuli from the chemoreceptors of the carotid and aortic bodies are also important elements. Slow circulation through the respiratory center itself is another factor which may contribute to the dyspnea.

Cyanosis. Cyanosis is caused by an increase in concentration of the reduced hemoglobin in the venules and capillaries of the skin and mucosae. It becomes clinically apparent only when this increase is above a certain limit. The appearance of cyanosis is favored by *polycythemia* (either real or apparent, because of the formation of edema) and by *distention of the venules and capillaries.*

The main causes of cyanosis are (27):

a) *Reduced ventilation in the lungs* caused by high position of the diaphragm (enlarged liver), dilatation of the pulmonary capillaries, chronic pulmonary edema, pleural effusion, and enlargement of the heart. This leads to deficient oxygenation of the arterial blood (*central cyanosis*).

b) *Increased reduction in the capillaries.* This is due to slow capillary flow (*peripheral cyanosis*).

High venous pressure. It is now admitted that the increase of venous pressure is only an indirect result of cardiac failure. *Increased blood volume* and *increased venous tonus* are the two most important factors of venous hypertension. The increased tonus is probably due to the effects of anoxemia on the venomotor center (44b).

Edema. The edema of cardiac failure is the result of several factors. Among them, one of the most important is the *increased hydrostatic pressure of the capillaries.* Capillary pressure has been measured in cardiac failure and found between 25 and 41 mm. (normal 12–25) (29). A second cause is often present, namely, a *low protein content* of the blood plasma due to malnutrition, albuminuria, and hepatic and renal complications. A further cause is an increase of capillary permeability due to *anoxemia* and *slow circulation* through the capillaries.

Another important factor is the *retention of water and sodium* by the kidney. If this were the only factor, cardiac and renal edema would be similar. Additional venous-capillary hypertension due to dependency explains dependent edema.

Serous effusions. Serous effusions may occur at an earlier stage than peripheral edema, especially in the pleural cavities. On the other hand, ascites is an early sign in tricuspid stenosis and adhesive pericarditis. The fluid of these effusions has *a higher protein content* (from 2–3 per cent) than subcutaneous edema fluid and a *specific gravity* which is also higher (1.013–1.019). There is drainage of the pleura into both the superior cava (via the azygos veins) and the pulmonary veins; therefore, engorgement of both systems is necessary in order to produce pleural effusion. The frequent predominance of effusion on the right side has been explained as the result of the fact that negative pressure predominates on that side on account of the enlargement of the heart. An inflammatory component may be present if there is pulmonary infarction. When this occurs on the left side, it may favor left-sided effusion. A further cause of left-sided effusion may be a right-sided adhesive pleuritis (54). One important factor which explains the greater frequency of right-sided hydrothorax is *higher venous pressure* in the lateral and basal parts of the right lung whenever the patient lies in the right semirecumbent position (55).

Jaundice is usually slight but is frequently observed. It is caused by two mechanisms: a) *an obstructive factor* due to chronic distention of the hepatic venules followed by biliary stasis; b) *a functional cellular deficiency* which is partly connected with destruction of Kupffer cells and is favored by anoxia (56).

COMPLICATIONS

Cardiac failure is a complication in itself but it often impairs the coronary, renal, pulmonary, and cerebral circulations to such an extent that it may interfere with the functions of these organs, the heart included.

Pulmonary engorgement favors the occurrence of *extensive hemorrhagic infarctions* after embolisms. It may cause infarctions through *phlebitis of the pulmonary veins.*

Chronic hepatic engorgement favors *insufficiency of the liver* and "cardiac" cirrhosis of this organ.

Renal insufficiency may be the result of chronic renal stasis.

Sterility, miscarriages, and *menstrual disturbances* may be caused by congestive failure.

Ulcerations of the skin, which may be infected easily, are common in cardiac patients with edema.

Cerebral edema and slow circulation may cause *mental torpor, delirium, and coma.*

Mural thrombosis is common in the dilated heart and may be the cause of multiple embolisms.

Pneumonia is a frequent terminal complication and may assume a particular type of edematous infiltration of the lungs so that it may be difficult to differentiate it from acute pulmonary edema.

Subacute bacterial endocarditis may complicate the failure and may be difficult to diagnose because of the tolerance of the patient, due to his depressed condition.

DIAGNOSIS

The diagnosis of heart failure is mainly clinical and should be based on the signs, symptoms, and various tests. Each sign and symptom may be due to either the basic heart disease or the weakening of the heart, and only a correct diagnosis of the basic heart lesion may avoid misunderstanding and confusion. However, it should be kept in mind that in each disease there is a limit to the possible severity of congestion. For example, engorgement of the pulmonary vessels and enlargement of the right ventricle are common in mitral stenosis; engorgement of the systemic veins and enlargement of the liver are common in tricuspid stenosis. When the former patients present pulmonary edema or enlarged liver; when the latter present ascites or pitting edema, heart failure is present. It is apparent that a moderate pulmonary congestion may be explained by the dynamic elements of compensation in a patient with mitral stenosis but not in one with hypertension.

Initial heart failure may be detected by following the gradual changes of heart rate, weight of the patient, and vital capacity. Increase of the first two and decrease of the last are evidence of failure if other causes can be excluded.

PROGNOSIS (34, 35, 36)

The immediate prognosis depends in varying degree upon the precipitating cause, the age of the patient, the degree of cardiac enlargement, and the presence or absence of complications. It may evolve independently of the underlying basic type of heart disease (35). However, the association of two or more heart lesions or disturbances increases the severity of the prognosis.

Mitral lesions have a tendency to cause heart failure comparatively early in life; however, compensation can be often reestablished, even after repeated episodes. On the contrary, aortic lesions of rheumatic or luetic origin cause heart failure relatively late in life but the maintenance of compensation is more difficult (36). Hypertensive and coronary heart diseases in general have a less set course.

The coexistence of pulmonary or renal diseases militates against recovery from cardiac failure.

Recurrence of failure must be anticipated. Treatment may prevent, to a certain extent, the occurrence of such episodes.

TREATMENT

Treatment of cardiac failure is one of the basic aims of cardiology. The multiplicity of problems involved, the number of drugs and other useful adjuvants, and the variable reactions of the patients require an extensive discussion of the problem (chapters 32 and 35). Studies of recent years have led to description of a *routine method of treatment of heart failure* (57). This will be described with certain modifications, and with the warning that it represents only a general guide often requiring modifications and adjustment to the individual case.

The patient is put at rest with a daily *diet* of 4 to 6 glasses of milk and a water intake of 200 cc. in small, frequent doses. If no digitalis was recently taken, *digitalization* is started with initial large doses (page 558) and is followed by a daily maintenance dose. The patient is weighed daily. An initial i.m. dose of 1 cc. of a *mercurial diuretic* is given; if no unpleasant reactions occur and diuresis is insufficient, the dose is increased to 1.5 or 2 cc. and repeated at frequent intervals (every 2 or 3 days).

Digitalis, mercurials, and diet are continued until edema disappears and the weight reaches a low, steady level. A few days later, the patient may become ambulant and treatment is changed as follows: *diet* will include most of the common foods, except those with a high content of sodium (diets). *No salt* should be added in cooking or at the table. *Salt substitutes* (76) can be used. *Carbo-resins* (78) may permit a more liberal use of sodium (their employment is still under experimentation). The *mercurials* are given at longer intervals but their frequency is again increased if the weight presents sharp changes connected with their administration.

Maintenance dose of digitalis, maintenance dose of mercurial diruretics, and a regular, low intake of sodium are at the base of this system. After several weeks, the diet may become more liberal and the interval between the injections can be further prolonged.

BIBLIOGRAPHY

1. KATZ, L. N. J. Mt. Sinai Hosp., 1942, **8**, 668. Also Am. A. Adv. Sci., Publ. 13, 1940, 184.
2. a) LIAN, C. Presse Méd., 1910, **18**, 49.
   b) VAQUEZ, H. 7th Intern. Meet. of Med. Sci. (5th Section), London, 1913.
3. LUISADA, A. A. *Insufficienza Totale e Insufficienze Parziali di Cuore.* Naples, Idelson, 1932.
4. COLOMBI. Atti 42: Congr. Ital. Med. Int. Rome, Pozzi, 1937.
5. a) RUBINO, A. Cuore e Circ., 1938, **22**, 397.
   b) CATALDI, G. Policl. (sez. med.), 1937, **44**, 170. Arch. Mal. Coeur, 1935, **28**, 604. Cuore e Circ., 1937, **21**, 2.
6. WENCKEBACH, K. E. *Herz- und Kreislauf-insuffizienz.* Dresden, Steinkopff, 1931.
7. STARR, I., JEFFERS, W. A., AND MEADE, R. H. Am. Heart J., 1943, **26**, 291.
8. MURRI, A. Policl. (sez. med.), 1919, **26**, 1.
9. a) RUEHL, A. Arch. Exp. Path. Pharm., 1937, **187**, 22.
   b) KATZ, L. N., AND MENDLOWITZ, M. Am. J. Physiol., 1938, **122**, 262.
10. References quoted by VISSCHER, KATZ AND STARR in *Blood, Heart and Circulation.* A. A. A. S. Press, 1940.
11. HARRISON, T. R. *Failure of the Circulation.* Baltimore, The Williams & Wilkins Co., 1939.

12. WIGGERS, C. J. *Physiology in Health and Disease*. Philadelphia, Lea & Febiger, 1945.
13. NYLIN, G. Acta Med. Scand., Suppl., **93**, 1. Also J. A. M. A., 1937, **109**, 133.
14. a) COWAN, D. W. Am. Heart J., 1933, **9**, 378.
    b) HERRMANN, G., DECHERD, G. M., AND SCHWAB, E. H. South. M. J., 1936, **29**, 386.
    c) LINEGAR, C. R., FROST, T. T., AND MYERS, V. C. Arch. Int. Med., 1938, **61**, 430.
    d) BODANSKY, M., AND PILCHER, J. R. Arch. Int. Med., 1937, **59**, 232.
15. a) CLARK, A. J. J. Physiol. 1913/1914, **47**, 66.
    b) KUTSCHERA-AICHBERGEN, H. Wien. Arch. inn. Med., 1929, **18**, 209.
16. CALHOUN, J. A., CULLEN, G. E., AND HARRISON, T. R. J. Clin. Investigation, 1931, **9**, 405.
17. a) FISHBERG, A. M. *Heart Failure*. Philadelphia, Lea & Febiger, 1940.
    b) WOOD, F. C., AND WOLFERTH, C. C. Am. J. M. Sci., 1937, **193**, 354.
18. LANCISI, G. M. *De Motu Cordis*, etc. Rome, Salvioni, 1728.
19. WINSOR, T., AND BURCH, G. E. Am. Heart J., 1946, **31**, 387.
20. a) WOLLHEIM, E. Zeit. klin. Med., 1931, **116**, 269.
    b) UHLENBRUCK, P., AND VOGELS. Zeit. klin. Med., 1931, **118**, 172.
    c) GIBSON, J. G., AND EVANS, W. A. J. Clin. Investigation, 1937, **16**, 301 and 851.
    d) HARRIS, A. W., AND GIBSON, J. G. J. Clin. Investigation, 1939, **18**, 527.
21. WEBER, A. *Die Elektrokardiographie*, etc. Berlin, Springer, 1926.
22. HOFBAUER, K. *Semeiologie und Differentialdiagnostik der Kurzatmigkeiten*. Jena, Fischer, 1940.
23. a) CLERC, A., AND LEVY, R. Compt. rend. Soc. biol., 1926, **44**, 759.
    b) CHEER, S. N., AND DIEUAIDE, F. R. J. Clin. Investigation, 1931, **10**, 889.
24. a) BLUMGART, H. L. Medicine, 1931, **10**, 1.
    b) WALLER, J. V., BLUMGART, H. L., AND VOLK, M. C. Arch. Int. Med., 1940, **66**, 1230.
25. ERNSTENE, A. C., AND BLUMGART, H. L. Arch. Int. Med., 1930, **45**, 593.
26. ALTSCHULE, M. D. Medicine, 1938, **17**, 75.
27. a) LUNDSGAARD, C., AND VAN SLYKE, D. D. Medicine, 1923, **2**, 1.
    b) HENDERSON, Y. *Blood, A Study in General Physiology*. New Haven, 1928.
    c) HARROP, G. A. J. Exper. Med., 1919, **30**, 247.
    d) BARACH, A. L., AND WOODWELL, M. Arch. Int. Med., 1921, **28**, 767.
    e) COSSIO, P., AND BERCONSKY, I. Am. Heart J., 1939, **17**, 1.
28. a) EPSTEIN, A. A. J. A. M. A., 1917, **69**, 44. Am. J. M. Sci., 1917, **154**, 638, and 1922, **163**, 167.
    b) BRAMKAMP, R. G. J. Clin. Investigation, 1935, **14**, 34.
    c) REICHE, F. Zeit. klin. Med., 1931, **118**, 307.
29. FAHR, G., AND ERSHLER, I. Proc. Soc. Exper. Biol. & Med., 1938, **37**, 701.
30. PLOTZ, M. Ann. Int. Med., 1939, **13**, 151.
31. a) RIGONI, M. Cuore e Circ., 1937, **21**, 157, 209 and 1938, **22**, 237.
    b) ELLIS, L. B. New England J. Med., 1943, **228**, 284 and 311.
32. KINSEY, D., AND WHITE, P. D. Arch. Int. Med., 1940, **65**, 163.
33. KATZKIN, H. M., WALLER, J. V., AND BLUMGART, H. L. Arch. Int. Med. 1939, **64**, 457.
34. a) WILLIUS, F. A. Am. Heart. J., 1927, **3**, 139.
    b) GRANT, R. T. Heart, 1933, **6**, 275.
35. BOYER, H., LEACH, E., AND WHITE, P. D. Ann. Int. Med., 1941, **14**, 2210.
36. DRY, T. J. J. A. M. A., 1942, **118**, 263.
37. a) BERNHEIM. Rev. Méd., 1910, **30**, 785.
    b) EAST, T., AND BAIN, C. Brit. Heart J., 1949, **11**, 145.
    c) LUISADA, A. A. Rass. Int. Clin., Ter. (Naples), 1932, **13**, 1048.
    d) EVANS, L. R., AND WHITE, P. D. Am. J. M. Sci., 1948, **216**, 485.
38. LEWIS, T. *The Mechanism and Graphic Registration of the Heart Beat*. London, Shaw and Sons, 1925.
39. STARLING, E. H. *The Principles of Human Physiology* (revised by C. L. Evans). Philadelphia, Lea & Febiger, 1936.
40. STARR, I. Ann. Int. Med., 1949, **30**, 1.
41. LEWIS, TH. *Diseases of the Heart*. New York, Macmillan, 1937.
42. RICHARDS, D. W. Am. J. Med., 1947, **3**, 434.
43. MANGUN, G. H., AND MYERS, V. C. Arch. Int. Med., 1946, **78**, 441.
44. a) McMICHAEL, J., AND SHARPEY-SHAFER, E. P. Brit. Heart J., 1944, **6**, 33.
    b) McMICHAEL, J. Schweiz. med. Woch., 1946, **6**, 41. Also Am. J. Med., 1949, **6**, 651.
45. SCHROEDER, H. Am. Heart J., 1941, **22**, 141.
46. a) STEAD, E. Mo. Conc. of Cardiovasc. Dis., 1947, **16**, N. 12. Also WARREN, J. V., AND STEAD, E. Arch. Int. Med., 1944, **73**, 138.
    b) MERRILL, A. J. J. Clin. Investigation. 1946, **25**, 389.
    c) MOKOTOFF, R., ROSS, G., AND LEITER, L. J. Clin. Investigation, 1948, **27**, 1.
    d) BRIGGS, A. P., AND CO-WORKERS. J. Clin. Investigation, 1948, **27**, 810.
47. WEGRIA, R., AND CO-WORKERS. Federation Proc., 1949, **8**, 162.

48. SCHROEDER, H. A. Am. Heart Assoc., June 1949.
49. LEITER, L. Bull. New York Acad. Med., 1948, **24**, 702. —
50. STEAD, E. A., WARREN, J. V., AND BRANNON, E. S. Am. Heart J., 1948, **35**, 529.
51. HEGGLIN, R. Cardiol., 1943, **7**, 145. Also Schweiz. med. Woch., 1947, **77**, 674.
52. RICHARDS, D. W. Am. J. Med., 1949, **6**, 772.
53. UNGHVARY, L. Cuore e Circ. (Rome), 1949, **33**, 146.
54. WHITE, P. D., AND MICHIE, C. R. Am. J. M. Sci., 1947, **214**, 243.
55. DOCK, W. Am. Heart J., 1935, **10**, 1947. Also New England J. Med., 1947, **236**, 773.
56. MEAKINS, J. Mo. Conc. Cardiovasc. Dis., 1949, **18**, N. 4.
57. GOLD, H., *et al.* Am. J. Med. 1947, **3**, 665.
58. HARVEY, R. M., *et al.* Am. J. Med., 1949, **7**, 439.
59. FERRER, M. I., *et al.* Circ. 1950, **1**, 161.
60. SARNOFF, S. J., AND BERGLUND, E. XIX Intern. Congr. of Physiol., Montreal, 1953.
61. NYLIN, G. Am. Heart J., 1943, **25**, 598; and 1949, **37**, 543.

CHAPTER 31

The Cardiac Patient as an Obstetrical and Surgical Risk

Obstetrics

Normal pregnancy has been discussed already (page 549); it was concluded that, in this condition, a burden is added to the cardiovascular function by an increase of blood volume.

Evaluation of the risk to a cardiac patient when she undergoes pregnancy varies between the older view, which considered it as exceedingly high, and the extreme view, which states that mothers with heart disease die early because of the natural evolution of their disease, and not because they have borne children (8).

No extreme generalization should be made; an accurate diagnosis of the existing condition and a proper evaluation of the functional ability of the heart permit judgment as to whether or not pregnancy is a severe danger in any given patient.

A classification based on the reaction to effort before pregnancy divides the cardiac patients as follows (9):

a) Patients without exertional dyspnea.
b) Patients with slight exertional dyspnea.
c) Patients with severe exertional dyspnea.
d) Patients with dyspnea at rest.

Patients of group a represent no special risk; patients of group b, only a slight risk. Patients of group c should not be permitted to continue the pregnancy, and the same is obviously true for the last group.

According to another classification (10), the patients are divided into two classes:

a) *Favorable cases:* those in whom there is a valvular defect but no heart failure, atrial fibrillation, or other additional disease.

b) *Unfavorable cases:* those having or having had heart failure or atrial fibrillation, and those with additional diseases (tuberculosis, diabetes, etc.). Patients with high blood pressure and those, undoubtedly rare, having coronary heart disease, should be added to this group.

While recognition of atrial fibrillation is easy, that of *initial heart failure* may be difficult once pregnancy has started. This is due to the fact that a pregnant woman with a normal heart may complain of palpitation, exertional dyspnea, and even orthopnea or paroxysmal dyspnea; she may suffer from fainting attacks and have various vasomotor disturbances (11). Moreover, the heart may appear enlarged, while *a triple rhythm* and *murmurs due to relative stenosis* are often present. The best method for estimating the degree of cardiac failure is recording of vital capacity (11), of venous pressure, and of circulation time; and the observation of the patient before and after exertion.

The incidence of cardiac failure is almost parallel to the curve of plasma volume in pregnant cardiacs (10). Therefore, if the patients reach the 8th month without failure, they are less exposed to it later. Even the strain of delivery is not as severe as that represented by the increased blood volume of the 8th month.

While this burden of pregnancy cannot be removed, many secondary causes of failure may be corrected or prevented, such as anemia, emotional upsets, respiratory infections, and physical exercise. *The weight gain should be limited to about 15 lbs. during pregnancy.* Salt, salty foods, and medications containing sodium should be restricted (diet

XI). If the patient does not cooperate with this plan, fluid restriction and the use of diuretics are indicated.

Digitalization in general should be started only when congestive failure occurs. However, a preventive digitalization, started at the beginning of the 7th month and continued until after delivery, has been found useful by the writer. Regular digitalization during the first week of each month is also beneficial in preventing the occurrence of failure.

In conjunction with this treatment, sedatives are usually helpful because high excitability of the nervous system favors *paroxysmal attacks of tachycardia, dyspnea, or pulmonary edema.* The latter is far more common in pregnant women with mitral stenosis than in mitral stenosis without pregnancy and has a high rate of mortality. Whereas the usual medical treatment of this complication can be used here (page 560), precedence should be given to *bloodletting;* this is now seldom used with the result that the mortality is now far higher than that of 60 years ago (12). Another useful procedure is *alcohol vapor inhalation* (14, 15) which should be used before other procedures, having no contraindications.

In general, decisions concerning interruption of pregnancy should be made early in the 3rd month, or at least before the 5th. If this term is passed, pregnancy should be carried through to the end.

The possibility of subacute bacterial endocarditis should be kept in mind. Prophylactic penicillin injections before and after delivery may avoid such danger.

Normal delivery is preferable in cardiac patients without heart failure. The mortality is high when other methods are adopted, whatever procedure is followed.

Judgment concerning the advisability of *a second or third pregnancy* and about possible *sterilization* of the patient should not be given without careful consideration. An extensive discussion of the problem has been made by *Levine* (13) and his conclusions are widely accepted.

Early marriage and *early childbearing* offer a minimum of hazards in patients with rheumatic heart disease (8).

Mild essential hypertension entails about the same risk as the "favorable" rheumatic heart disease. On the contrary, severe hypertension with hypertensive heart disease constitutes a bad risk (10). It seems probable that a high incidence of eclampsia and a more rapid evolution of hypertensive disease occur when a hypertensive woman is allowed to continue pregnancy without special precautions. Paroxysmal dyspnea and paroxysmal pulmonary edema are more frequent in such patients than in other pregnant women.

Surgery

Surgery on a cardiac patient is undoubtedly a cause of strain upon the heart and entails some risk for the patient. Reluctance to operate is frequently present but it must be emphasized that the ability of the heart to withstand an operation is greater than is usually thought and that often death is wrongly ascribed to the heart.

The factors to consider are:

a) Action of the anesthetic on the heart and circulatory apparatus.

b) Effect of possible reflexes from the operative field.

c) Effect of significant increase or decrease of blood pressure on the heart.

d) Decubitus of the patient on the surgical table.

e) Depth of anesthesia.

Anesthesia is in itself a strain upon the heart. Poor oxygenation of the blood, dyspnea, muscular effort, cough, and tachycardia, are frequent during anesthesia, especially during the early stages. The anesthetic may act on the myocardium, depressing its function. Inhalant anesthetics frequently stimulate the vagus nerve both during the early stage and during recovery.

Abnormalities of the heart rate and rhythm, including premature contractions, nodal rhythm, atrial tachycardia, flutter, or fibrillation, have been observed in noncardiac patients undergoing surgery (1). Ether and nitrous oxide were responsible for these changes. Preoperative administration of *atropine* and *quinidine* (or *pronestyl*) may limit the changes of rate and rhythm.

The risk to the cardiac patient is limited by intelligent action on the part of the anesthetist and by a correct choice of the anesthetic.

Inhalant anesthetics (especially *ether*) may be more dangerous in patients with mitral stenosis and hypertensive patients with pulmonary congestion than in others because they favor pulmonary edema and bronchopneumonia. In spite of these considerations, ether is usually considered the anesthetic of choice. A copious supply of oxygen should be added to any inhalant anesthetic.

Intravenous and rectal anesthesia are the best for the most cardiac patients but have the common disadvantage that, once started, the anesthesia cannot be rapidly discontinued. The intravenous drip method, combined with nitrous oxide-oxygen (50-50), obviates this disadvantage. On the other hand, the latter adds the burden of a certain volume of fluid.

Spinal anesthesia is excellent but may cause a significant fall in blood pressure, a fact which is not devoid of danger in patients with coronary or hypertensive heart disease (page 418). *Procaine* in itself is not dangerous and may even be helpful in decreasing the excitability of the myocardium, as shown by animal experimentation (2) and direct application to the human heart (3). For this reason, *local anesthesia*, as used in small operations and in dentistry is usually harmless. On the other hand, many cardiac patients are sensitive to even small doses of *epinephrine* or *norepinephrine* and react with unpleasant manifestations to procaine plus epinephrine. This advises either limitation or avoidance of the latter.

Reflex onset of disturbances of the heart rhythm, and reflex coronary ischemia have been demonstrated in experimental animals.

This advises avoidance of any prolonged manipulation of the viscera. Preoperative administration of *atropine, quinidine,* or both, may limit the effect of such maneuvers.

Various changes in blood pressure may take place during anesthesia and surgery (4), a fact which may be associated with changes of cardiac output. The latter was found increased in animal experimentation (5a), decreased in human surgery (5b). *Extreme lowering of blood pressure* may favor coronary occlusion (page 418) and is, therefore, to be avoided. *Marked increase of blood pressure*, on the other hand, increases strain on the heart.

The ability of the heart to respond to strain may be judged by the existence of compensation or decompensation before surgery and by the evaluation of additional loads reducing cardiac reserve (valvular defects, congenital malformations, high blood pressure).

Sudden death during surgery (even *cardiac surgery*) is an infrequent event in cardiac patients unless unusual events take place (perforation of ventricular septum, cerebral embolism, ventricular fibrillation). Unexpected death is even more common in young people without heart disease than in elderly cardiac patients (6). On the other hand, *age* is very important, as two-thirds of the deaths of cardiac patients occur when the 50-year age mark has been passed (6–7).

Atrial fibrillation slightly increases the dangers in arteriosclerotic patients, while it nearly triples the risk in rheumatic heart disease (6). Thyrocardiacs with atrial fibrillation are an exception because they withstand intervention on the thyroid better than any other group and show favorable results within a short time.

Cardiac surgery is a most delicate procedure, especially in patients with coronary heart disease. The excitability of the myocardium should be decreased by the preoperative use of *quinidine* or *pronestyl* and by local application of *procaine*.

In general, when a cardiac patient needs

surgery, all clinical elements must be taken into account. If a recent coronary occlusion has occurred, time for healing of the scar and subsequent convalescence should be allowed before considering the intervention. If a patient presents the signs of congestive failure, he should be treated by means of digitalis, mercurial diuretics, rest, and diet, until compensation is attained and a stable equilibrium is reached.

Strict collaboration between the cardiologist, the surgeon, and the anesthetist may permit surgery in patients who formerly were refused this benefit. This collaboration should start long before the operation (sometimes even months earlier) and should be continued in the postoperative stage. Whenever doubts about the resistance of the patient arise, the operation will be performed under *local anesthesia*. The use of *curare* should be considered. The patient will be digitalized until the last day and prepared with *morphine* and *atropine*. Occasional additional preparation with *quinidine* or *pronestyl*, may be necessary.

The beneficial action of *oxygen* during the intervention and the prophylactic action of *penicillin* before and after it should be kept in mind. *Heparin* may be useful in some cases in order to prevent venous thrombosis and subsequent embolism.

Whenever a patient has even mild orthopnea, and a minor surgical intervention becomes necessary, this should be performed on an *oblique table* so that no increased load on the heart and no dyspnea is caused by the supine position.

Postoperative care of the cardiacs includes avoidance of any cause favoring bronchopneumonia or atelectasis (decubitus, tight bandage, drugs depressing respiration, etc.). Digitalization should be continued during this stage. The advice of the cardiologist may be required in difficult cases.

It should be kept in mind that *saline infusions* and i.v. *blood* or *plasma* may favor pulmonary edema in doses which are tolerated without difficulty by non cardiacs.

BIBLIOGRAPHY

1. a) LENNOX, W. G., GRAVES, R. C., AND LEVINE, S. A. Arch. Int. Med., 1922, **30**, 57.
   b) LEVINE, S. A. J. A. M. A., 1920, **75**, 795.
2. BURSTEIN, C. L., AND MARANGONI, B. A. Proc. Soc. Exper. Biol. & Med. 1940, **43**, 210.
3. FEIL, H., AND ROSSMAN, P. L. Mo. Conc. Cardiovasc. Dis., 1940, **9**, N. 1.
4. MARVIN, H. M., AND PASTOR, R. B. Arch. Int. Med., 1925, **35**, 768.
5. a) BLALOCK, A. Arch. Surg., 1927, **14**, 732, 921 and 978.
   b) SNYDER, J. C. J. Clin. Investigation, 1938, **17**, 571.
6. SPRAGUE, H. B. Surg., Gynec. & Obst., 1929, **49**, 54.
7. MILLER, A. H. Am. J. Surg., Suppl., 1919, **33**, 112.
8. FLAXMAN, N. Am. J. Obst. & Gynec., 1940, **39**, 814.
9. Criteria Committee of the New York Heart Assoc. Nomenclature and Criteria for Diagnosis of Disease of the Heart. New York Heart Assoc., 1952.
10. HAMILTON, B. E., AND THOMPSON, K. J. *The Heart in Pregnancy and the Childbearing Age.* Boston, Little, Brown and Co., 1941.
11. DEXTER, L. In *Nelson Loose-Leaf Medicine.* New York, Nelson and Sons, 1944. Also Bull. New England Med. Center, 1945, **7**, 101.
12. CHAVES, I. *Enfermedades del Corazon-Cirugia y Embarazo.* Mexico, Ed. de el Colegio Nac., 1945.
13. LEVINE, S. A. *The Cardiac Patient as a Surgical or Obstetrical Risk.* In *Stroud's Cardiovascular Disease.* Philadelphia, Davis, 1945.
14. LUISADA, A. A., WEYL, R. AND GOLDMANN, M. R. Circ. 1952, **5**, 363 and Ann. Int. Med. 1952, **37**, 1221.
15. GOLDMANN, M. R. Am. J. Obst. & Gynec., 1953, **65**, 314.

CHAPTER 32

Action of Drugs Used in The Treatment of the Cardiac Patient

Digitalis

Various plants contain substances whose action on the myocardium is similar to that of digitalis. For this reason, their active principles are called *digitalis bodies,* in spite of their different origins. The most important plants and their principles are listed in tables 22 and 23. To these should be added *convallaria majalis, apocynum cannabinum, adonis vernalis, helleborus niger, thevetia nerifolia,* and *cerbera odollam* (27), which are less frequently used.

The active principles of these drugs are *glycosides;* each represents the combination of an *aglycone* with one or more molecules of *sugar.* While the main activity is in the aglycone, the sugars control the utilization and potency of the principle.

Rapid advances in the chemistry of cardiac glycosides finally resulted in their isolation (1). Pure glycosides can be used with greater accuracy of dosage and constancy of action.

MAJOR ACTIONS OF THE CARDIAC GLYCOSIDES
(3, 4, 5)

The action of digitalis bodies has been studied on: a) isolated hearts or papillary muscles, b) heart-lung preparations, c) intact animals, d) normal human beings, and e) cardiac patients.

The digitalis bodies act mainly upon the heart but also exert important action on the nervous system and the vessels. They have a *double action* on the heart; one through the autonomic nervous system (*neurogenic effect*), the other directly on the myocardium (*myogenic effect*). The *latter is the most important* (Fig. 309).

Digitalis has the following *cardiac effects:* a) depresses the power of creating stimuli in the atria, b) depresses the conduction of stimuli, c) stimulates the irritability of the ventricles, and d) stimulates the force of contraction.

Digitalis has *multiple vascular effects* resulting in constriction of the veins, pooling of blood in the hepatic-splanchnic reservoir, and decrease of venous return (67). The vascular effects are prompt and may be useful in the first phase of treatment. However, they represent only a component of the complex digitalis effect.

It has been stated that digitalis decreases the cholinesterase content of the tissues (71); therefore, longer persistence of acetylcholine would be followed by parasympathetic effects in all tissues, including the heart. However, clinical determination of serum cholinesterase does not seem to confirm this theory (72).

Whatever the mechanism, digitalis stimulates various medullary centers *including the center of the vagus nerve* and, moreover, seems to stimulate the chemoreceptors of the carotid body. Thus *a triple vagal action takes place:* direct, reflex from the carotid body, and reflex from the heart itself (Fig. 310).

There is discussion concerning the role of therapeutic doses of digitalis in correcting the potassium losses associated with heart failure. On the whole, it seems that *digitalis increases the amount of K in the heart.* However, toxic doses of digitalis drive potassium from the heart muscle (75).

In animal experiments, the effect of digitalis can be divided into three successive

583

TABLE 22

PLANT	PART	ACTIVE PRINCIPLES
Digitalis purpurea	Leaves	Digitoxin Gitoxin Gitalin
Digitalis lanata	Leaves	Digitoxin† Gitoxin† Digoxin†
Strophanthus Kombé	Seeds	Strophanthin
Strophanthus gratus (*acocanthera oua-baio*)	Seeds	Ouabain
Urginea maritima (*Scilla maritima*)	Bulb	Scillaren (urginin)

† Acetylated.

action is stopped, reveal severe myocardial damage (degenerative changes) (8, 21).[83]

Digitalis shortens myocardial fibers, decreasing their diastolic length and contributing to decrease of cardiac volume (55).

Digitalis increases the force of systolic contractions in isolated mammalian heart, heart-lung preparations, and isolated papillary muscle. If the heart is failing, the ventricles empty more completely after digitalis.

The simplest explanation of digitalis action in heart failure is the following: *digitalis increases the proportion of chemical energy which is converted into mechanical work; this increases cardiac output and decreases venous pressure* (9)[84] (fig. 309). The increased efficiency of work is revealed by reduced oxygen consumption.

TABLE 23

DIGITALIS PURPUREA			DIGITALIS LANATA	
Complex of purpurea glycosides	Digitoxin ⟵⟶ Gitoxin ⟵⟶ Gitalin		Acetyl-digitoxin = lanatoside A Acetyl-gitoxin = lanatoside B Acetyl-digoxin = lanatoside C	Complex of lanatosides (digilanid)

stages according to the intensity of action. The 2nd and 3rd stages should be considered as due to toxic effects.

1st stage. There is increased force of ventricular contraction, increased ventricular excitability (occasional premature contractions), and decreased conduction (prolonged P-R).

2nd stage. The ventricular rhythm becomes slow and irregular because of periodic A-V block or periodic premature contractions (bigeminal rhythm). The ventricular systoles are powerful but cardiac output may not be increased on account of bradycardia.

3rd stage. There is rapid heart action (sinus or ventricular tachycardia) or there may be multiple, irregular, premature beats. Later on, atrial fibrillation frequently occurs and ventricular flutter, followed by fibrillation, terminates cardiac activity.

Microscopic studies of the heart after its

The effect of digitalis on heart rate is not the principal action of this drug. Slowing of the heart in experimental animals and normal individuals is mostly due to a carotid body-vagal reflex (10); in patients with congestive failure, it is mainly due to cardiovagal and venous-vagal reflexes because *digitalis removes the cause of tachycardia by restoring compensation* (5).

Digitalis has a limited action on the rate of the normal heart and on sinus tachycardia.

[83] It is interesting to note that prolonged stimulation of the vagus causes myocardial damage which is similar to that caused by digitalis.

[84] The early effect of digitalis consists of decreased amplitude of ventricular contractions and decreased cardiac output, as revealed by electrokymograms and ballistocardiograms (56). This effect seems due to initial venoconstriction and decreased venous return. Later (from 1 to 3 hours following i.v. administration), the stimulating effect on the myocardium becomes evident.

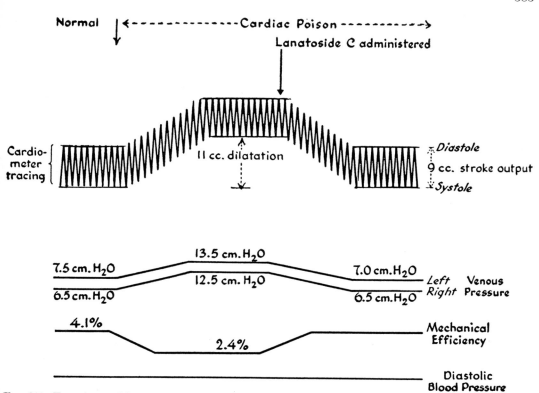

Normal | ←- - - - - - - - - - - -Cardiac Poison - - - - - - - - - - - →

Lanatoside C administered

Cardio-
meter
tracing

11 cc. dilatation

Diastole

9 cc. stroke output

Systole

7.5 cm. H₂O

13.5 cm.H₂O

12.5 cm. H₂O

7.0 cm.H₂O

6.5 cm.H₂O

6.5 cm.H₂O

Left   Venous
Right   Pressure

4.1%

2.4%

Mechanical
Efficiency

Diastolic
Blood Pressure

FIG. 309. Experimental heart failure in a heart-lung preparation and the effect of digitalis (after Fahr)

However, toxic doses of digitalis may affect the S-A node and cause bradycardia.

Atrioventricular conduction is decreased by clinical doses of digitalis. Prolongation of the P-R interval is partly due to vagal action and partly to direct effect on the conduction system. Toxic doses of digitalis may cause A-V block.

The *ventricular rates* of patients with *atrial fibrillation* are slowed by digitalis. Both vagal and direct effects contribute to blocking atrial impulses, thereby preventing them from reaching the ventricles (11). The vagal factor is not essential because this result is not prevented by atropine (11) (fig. 310). Moreover, digitalis effect in atrial fibrillation occurs only in the presence of heart failure; its useful action is due to improvement of the circulation and decrease of cardiac volume. The vagus stimulating action of digitalis is a deterrent because it favors

atrial fibrillation in the presence of anoxia or rapid atrial stimuli (64).

Heart size is reduced by digitalis by three mechanisms: a) decreased venous return; b) reduced diastolic length of the fibers (55); and c) more powerful contractions. As a result, residual blood is decreased (65).

Cardiac output is decreased by digitalis in normal hearts; *it is increased* in failing hearts (5, 12, 63) but only after initial decrease (56). *Stroke volume is increased* and systolic ejection is more complete following the initial stage. The increase in output is independent of cardiac rate and rhythm.

Venous pressure and right atrial pressure (23) *are decreased by digitalis;* this effect is due to both venoconstriction and improvement of cardiac function (13, 23, 56).

Circulating blood volume is decreased by digitalis, partly through increased diuresis

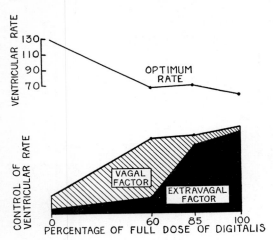

FIG. 310. Schematic representation of the mechanism by which digitalis slows the ventricular rate in patients with atrial fibrillation and congestive failure (From Gold, Kwit, Otto and Fox, J. Pharmacol. & Exper. Therap., 1939. Courtesy of the authors.)

and partly through other complex mechanisms.

Pulmonary arterial pressure is temporarily increased in cor pulmonale; it returns to below previous level as soon as a general improvement of circulation has taken place (57).

Diastolic pressure of the ventricles, raised by failure, returns to zero after digitalis (57, 58). This fact is connected with a marked *decrease of residual blood* (65).

Blood pressure is increased in animals by toxic doses of digitalis. In human beings, blood pressure is decreased if there has been stimulation of the vasomotor center (anoxemia); it is increased if there has been low blood pressure due to heart failure. Therefore, no consistent effect can be noted and no possible danger of increasing hypertension is to be feared.

Small doses of digitalis *dilate the coronary arteries* (14). However, *large doses of digitalis may decrease the coronary circulation by stimulating the vagus nerve*. Strophanthin seems to have less constricting action on the coronary vessels than digitalis (46).

Diuretic action. No diuresis is obtained by

the use of digitalis except in the presence of heart failure. Therefore, digitalis is not a true diuretic. On the other hand, one of the main actions of digitalis is mobilization of edema fluid and promotion of intense diuresis. The most important effect is obtained by decreasing the hydrostatic pressure in the capillaries (page 61), the main cause of peripheral edema. Cessation of renal stasis is an additional element. Dilatation of the renal vessels, due to digitalis, may increase glomerular filtration (15).

ELECTROCARDIOGRAPHIC CHANGES

These consist of modifications of rate and rhythm, and changes of the T wave. *Depression of T* may occur within a few hours. Later, T may become flat and then inverted (16). However, this is actually due to the fact that S-T becomes depressed and makes a sharp angle with the basal line (fig. 311). These typical digitalis changes may occur in all limb leads as well as in the precordial leads. Patients with myocardial damage frequently present S-T and T changes in aVL and V_5-V_6, indicating *anterolateral ischemia*. A method of evaluation of the digitalis effect on the heart has been based upon the ECG changes observed in patients (11).

Digitalis shortens the Q-T interval; it may prolong P-R. Toxicity is revealed by ventricular premature contractions (frequently bigeminal), ventricular tachycardia, or incomplete A-V block (fig. 311).

DESTRUCTION AND EXCRETION OF DIGITALIS GLYCOSIDES

The various digitalis glycosides behave differently after absorption. About 10 per cent of a given dose of *digitoxin* is excreted in the bile while about 50 per cent is destroyed in the body with a combined maximum of about 60 micrograms in 24 hours (73). Normal subjects and compensated patients excrete in the urine about 30 to 40 per cent of the daily dose (usually less than 50 micrograms). *Patients exhibiting toxic phenomena excrete over twice as much as the*

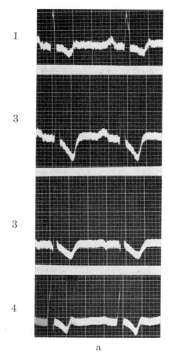
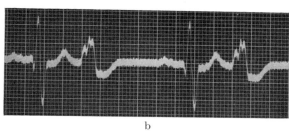

FIG. 311. Electrocardiographic effect of digitalis. a, depression of S-T and inversion of T, short Q-T; b, toxic effect, long P-R, bigeminal rhythm.

others (usually between 50 and 100 micrograms). Elderly patients have a poor excretion and seldom excrete more than 30 micrograms (74). Thus, *urinary bio-assay may differentiate toxic phenomena due to overdosage from those due to poor excretion.*

TOXIC EFFECTS OF DIGITALIS

The symptoms and signs of overdosage of digitalis are the following.

a) *Signs of hyperactivity of the gastrointestinal tract:* nausea, vomiting, and, occasionally, diarrhea.

b) *Early cardiac phenomena* consisting of bradycardia and bigeminal rhythm (fig. 311).

c) *Late cardiac phenomena* consisting of sinus or ventricular tachycardia, atrial fibrillation, or heart block.

d) *Vision* is often blurred; color vision may be disturbed so that colored objects appear white or yellowed (less frequently blue or red).

e) *Terminal phenomena:* ventricular fibrillation, followed by death.

Toxic doses of digitalis affect *conduction recovery* as does quinidine; they decrease excitability and conductivity of the atria, node, and ventricles (64). *However, when the rate of discharge of stimuli is very rapid, as in atrial flutter, toxic doses of digitalis increase the rate of discharge and thus favor atrial fibrillation.*

Gastrointestinal disturbances are partly the result of vagal stimulation and partly the effect of direct irritant effect on the gastrointestinal tract. Therefore their cessation may be obtained in four ways: a) by carefully checking whether the patient is receiving too much digitalis, and decreasing the dose; b) by switching to a glycoside with greater therapeutic ratio (gitalin, acetyl-glycosides; c) by using the intravenous route; and d) by administering atropine.

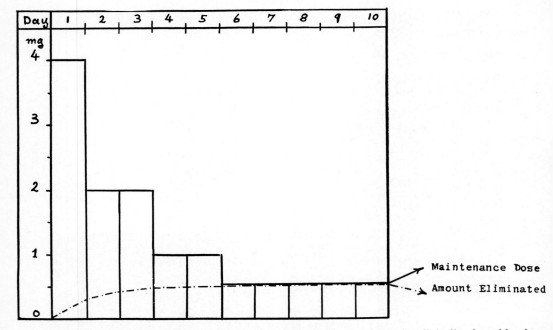

Fig. 312. Digitalis administration. The rectangles indicate the dose of a digitalis glycoside given every day. The dotted line indicates the amount of the glycoside which is eliminated in 24 hours.

The other toxic phenomena, and particularly *the ectopic rhythms*, can be limited or offset by: a) daily oral administration of 5 to 10 gm. of *potassium chloride* (68); b) i.v. injections of *magnesium sulfate* (10–20 cc. of a 25 per cent solution) (69); and c) i.v. injections of *procaine amide* (70).

Digitalis favors thrombosis by shortening the clotting time (48). This is particularly important in elderly patients with coronary heart disease.

RULES OF DIGITALIS ADMINISTRATION

Digitalis administration is accomplished by keeping in mind the two following rules:

1) Digitalis and the digitalis bodies are eliminated slowly; therefore, if administered daily, *they tend to accumulate* in the body. Administration of daily doses which are harmless in themselves may cause toxic symptoms after a certain time.

2) Nevertheless, digitalis and the digitalis bodies *are gradually excreted and destroyed*. If, after reaching a satisfactory result, only that dose is given which corresponds to the daily elimination, no further accumulation takes place.

Daily elimination varies (16b, c, 18): slow excretion is usual in elderly patients or persons with impaired renal function; individual variations are common; changes of the renal circulation cause changes in the excretion of digitalis. Moreover, the amount of digitalis excreted is a fraction of the amount existing in the blood. Therefore, its elimination rate increases at first, then becomes more or less constant.

The following rules are the result of the previous considerations:

a) Administration of a high dose during the first days until the blood level is sufficiently high and the first therapeutic results are obtained (*initial digitalization*).

b) Later on, administration of a daily dose which is theoretically equivalent to the dose destroyed or eliminated in 1 day (*maintenance dose*). The basis for these two principles is sketched in fig. 312.

BIO-ASSAY AND UNITAGE

Standardization of digitalis and digitalis-like drugs was first performed on *frogs*. The end point was the systolic arrest of the ventricle in 1 hour. *One U.S.P. or International Unit is the equivalent of 0.1 gm. of the International Standard Digitalis Powder.*

A second method is the *intravenous cat method*, now official in the U.S.P. Standardization is made by comparing the lethal dose of the digitalis preparation under assay with that of ouabain (original method) or a digitalis preparation of known potency (U.S.P.). *One cat unit is equivalent to 0.1 gm. of the U.S.P. Digitalis Reference Standard.*

It should be kept in mind that the original coincidence between 1 cat unit and 0.1 gm. of digitalis was fortuitous and that no conversion is possible between grams and cat units. On the other hand, the isolated cardiac glycosides are measured in milligrams and have constant action by a given weight. *The best assay is, after all, made in patients* and all rules concerning digitalis bodies are approximate.

The serum or urinary level of digitalis glycosides can be determined by means of a biological method based on the microscopic observation of embryonic duck hearts (66).

THE DIGITALIS-LIKE BODIES

In spite of the fundamental similarity between the various digitalis bodies, there are certain differences which have clinical interest.

a) The glycosides of *Digitalis lanata* are absorbed from the gastrointestinal tract less effectively than those of *Digitalis purpurea*. On the other hand, they have a lower power of accumulation and are eliminated more rapidly.

b) *Gitalin* has an intermediate position between digoxin and strophanthin as far as accumulation and elimination are concerned (56, 59). It has a unique position because of its *high therapeutic range* (59).[85]

[85] The *therapeutic range* is the ratio in terms of

c) *Acetylated preparations* seem to have a greater therapeutic ratio. In this respect, acetyl-digoxin (lanatoside C) seems to be superior to digoxin (60); acetyl-digitoxin (lanatoside A), superior to digitoxin (61).

d) *Strophanthin* and *ouabain* act more rapidly than *digitoxin;* their effect also disappears more rapidly because their power of accumulation is lower. They can be used only by intravenous injection.

e) The glycosides of *squill* are active both by mouth and injection. They can be compared to those of *strophanthus* but have an even lower rate of accumulation and a higher rate of excretion. It has been stated that their diuretic action is greater because they also act directly on the renal epithelium (1b).

The use of pure glycosides has caused the marketing of different preparations. The following are the best known:

Digitoxin (purodigin Wyeth, digitoxin Merck or Parke and Davis, crystodigin Lilly (**2, 3**), digitaline Nativelle).

Digoxin (digoxin Burroughs and Wellcome) (**4**), *acetyl digoxin* (cedilanid Sandoz) (**5, 6**).

Gitalin (gitaligin White Lab., Inc.) (**7, 8**).

Total glycosides of Digitalis lanata (digilanid Sandoz).

Total glycosides of Digitalis purpurea (digifoline Ciba, digalen Roche).

Strophanthin (K-strophanthin Abbott (**9**), strophosid Sandoz (**9**), ouabaine Arnaud or Lilly).

Glycosides of squill (scillaren Sandoz (**10**), urginin Calco).

Digitalization can be not only initiated but also maintained by intravenous injections (see table 24). However, this method is usually adopted only for limited periods on account of practical disadvantages.

The *maintenance dose* consists of about 0.12 gm. of leaf (one pill) and of between 0.1 and 0.5 mg. of the different glycosides (one pill). This dose may have to be doubled

per cent between the amount of digitalis preparation required for therapeutic effect and the total dose required for toxicity (59).

TABLE 24

PREPARATION USED	INTERVAL BEFORE FULL EFFECT (INTRAV. INJ.)	SPEED OF ACTION (INTRAV. INJECT.)	DURATION OF ACTION	PERCENT-AGE AB-SORBED (BY MOUTH)	RATE OF ACCUMU-LATION	SPEED OF ELIMINA-TION	DIURESIS	CORONARY CONSTRIC-TION (FOR LARGE DOSES ONLY)	THERA-PEUTIC RATIO
	hr.		days						%
Digitoxin............	6	+	19	100	++++	+	+	++	58
Digoxin.............	4	++	7	15–20	+++	++	++	++	61
Gitalin..............	2	+++	3	100 ?	++	+++	++	?	37
Ouabain............	1	++++	2	5 ?	+	+++	++	—	—
Scillaren...........	1	+++	2	15–25 ?	+	++++	+++	?	—

TABLE 25. *Average oral digitalization*

	DIGITALIS POW-DER U.S.P. XII (PILLS)	DIGITOXIN (TABLETS)	LANATOSIDE C (TABLETS)	GITALIN (TABLETS)	URGININ (TABLETS)
Massive initial dose (1st 24 hrs.)	6 = 0.6 gm.	6 = 0.6 mg.	6 = 3 mg.	6 = 3 mg.	6 = 3 mg.
Medium successive dose (2nd and 3rd day)	4 = 0.4 gm.	4 = 0.4 mg.	3 = 1.5 mg.	3 = 1.5 mg.	6 = 1.5 mg.
Total dose (3 days)	1.4 gm.	1.4 mg.	6 mg.	6 mg.	6 mg.
Maintenance daily dose (subsequent days)	2 = 0.2 gm.	1–2 = 0.1–0.2 mg.	1 = 0.5 mg.	1 = 0.5 mg.	1 = 0.5 mg.

(or more) in some cases, or it may be too high. It should be emphasized that the optimal dose is usually far below the toxic level.

Maintenance with *gitalin* (589) offers the minimum danger of accumulation with secondary toxic symptoms.

Strophanthin may be employed with success in patients with toxic symptoms from digitalis. Switching from digitalis to strophanthin and giving one intravenous injection every 12 hours for 7 to 15 days, gives the patient the benefits of digitalization with less discomfort. Returned to an oral maintenance dose of digitalis, he may then continue his improvement. A similar procedure can be used by switching from digitoxin to *gitalin* (after a 3- to 4-day interval of rest).

Table 25 gives the main differences between the various glycosides. It has been partly composed from data of others (25, 26), and partly from personal data (56).

ROUTES OF ADMINISTRATION

The *oral route* is used commonly, except for strophanthin preparations. *Intramuscular injections* are used infrequently because of the pain caused by the drugs. *Intravenous administration* is imperative in the case of strophanthin, optional for the others. *Rectal administration* gives satisfactory results.

METHODS OF DIGITALIZATION

Digitalis is given in a large initial dose and then decreased in order to maintain the effects.

The *rapid digitalization method* (19) gives an average of 20 cat units per 150 pounds of weight within 24 to 48 hours. A later study (20) described the dose as about 1.2 gm. (U.S.P. XI) of the leaf, one-third of which can be given immediately (4 tablets of 0.1 gm.) and the rest within 36 to 48 hours. The dose is then dropped to 0.1 or 0.2 gm.

TABLE 26. *Intravenous digitalization*

	DIGITOXIN 0.4 mg. = 4 cc.	CEDILANID 0.8 mg. = 4 cc.	GITALIN 3 mg. = 4 cc.	OUABAIN 0.25 mg. = 1 cc.	SCILLAREN 1 mg. = 2 cc.
	hr.	hr.	hr.	hr.	hr.
Interval between 1st and 2nd i.v. injection............................	12	12	24	6	6
Interval between 2nd and 3rd i.v. injection............................	24	24	48	12	12
Intervals between injections (after the 3rd)............................	96	72	48	12	12

(U.S.P. XI) from two to three times daily. It should be emphasized that these doses may vary between one-half and twice the indicated average dose.

Digitalization may be started by an intravenous injection of *strophanthin* (**9**), *ouabain*, or *cedilanid* (**6**), followed by the oral administration of digitalis.

Slower digitalization can be obtained by an *initial dose* of 6 tablets of *digitoxin* (**2**), *digilanid, cedilanid* (**5**), *digoxin* (**4**), *gitalin* (**7**), or *scillaren* (**10**). Four tablets are given in the second and third day (see table 26), so that full digitalization is obtained in 3 to 4 days.[86] This method entails smaller risks than with rapid digitalization (single dose or 2-day method).

Good results are obtained by diluting *one*

[86] Administration of digitalis to children should be governed by the following considerations:

a) Children require from 1.5 to 2 times larger doses than adults in comparison with their weight (54, 62); adolescents require the same doses by weight.

b) Children have a very excitable vagus nerve (54).

c) Heart failure in children is often connected with myocardial lesions (rheumatic disease, diphtheria) which cause increased cardiac excitability.

For these reasons the following doses may be used in comparison with adults:

Nurslings......... $\frac{1}{6}$ of adult dose
1 to 3 yr.......... $\frac{1}{4}$ of adult dose
3 to 6 yr.......... $\frac{1}{3}$ to $\frac{1}{2}$ of adult dose
6 to 15 yr......... $\frac{1}{2}$ to 1 adult dose

It should be kept in mind that these are merely approximate doses and that, in children even more than adults, the dose should be adapted to the individual case.

ampule of strophanthin or gitalin in 10 cc. (0.24 gm.) of aminophyllin solution. This decreases the possible dangers of the injection (24), which, however, have been observed in the past only because of excessive dosage or high rapidity of injection.

Gitalin is better tolerated than other glycosides and causes toxicity less frequently. *Lanatoside C* follows (24), while *digitoxin causes the greatest incidence of paroxysmal tachycardia, premature contractions, or atrial fibrillation.*

Digitalis should be employed by following a few guiding suggestions:

a) The best use for digitalis is found in congestive failure.

b) The improvement of the patient may take place even if the ventricular rate is not decreased and if atrial fibrillation is still present.

c) The best result from digitalis is obtained in mitral patients with congestive failure and atrial fibrillation. Patients with aortic stenosis follow. Its administration in hypertensive and coronary heart disease with failure obtains only fair results. Heart failure in patients with cardiovascular syphilis yields poorly to digitalis.

d) Whenever acute myocarditis is present (rheumatic disease, diphtheria, etc.) digitalis administration is not followed by impressive results. Large doses of digitalis are contraindicated because the myocardium is excitable and easily damaged. Gitalin is well tolerated in children with carditis.

e) Large doses of digitalis are contraindicated in the first stage following coronary occlusion. In later stages, digitalis is better tolerated if it is given together with quinidine.

f) In heart failure of myxedema, hyperthyroidism, thiamine deficiency, pericarditis with effusion, and adhesive pericarditis, digitalis obtains only moderate results.

g) Digitalis can be given in partial heart block but its dosage should be studied carefully in order not to overstimulate the vagus. It may be given safely in complete block (21).

h) In most patients, digitalization may be more effective if given slowly than by the rapid method. After initial relief, there is no harm in waiting 4 or 5 days before complete relief from failure is obtained. Slower digitalization prevents the possible occurrence of myocardial lesions and allows a better evaluation of the sensitivity of the patient.

i) If the patient received digitalis within 10 days prior to a new treatment, smaller doses should be used.

j) Prophylactic use of digitalis in patients who *might* present heart failure at some future time has been advocated. The author recommends this only for cardiac patients who become pregnant (last 3 months) or cardiac patients who cannot avoid severe, although occasional, exertion. In patients leading a normal life, prophylactic use of digitalis for many years may not prevent heart failure while at the same time may deprive the physician of the full freedom of use of one of his most powerful weapons. Therefore, it should be advised against.

Quinidine (28, 76)

Quinidine is one of the alkaloids found in the *cinchona* bark and is an optical isomer of quinine (24).

The action of quinidine on the cardiac muscle can be summarized as follows. a) It increases the refractory period. b) It decreases excitability. c) It slows conduction. d) It may slow the rate. e) It may depress contractility (large doses only). In addition,

quinidine depresses the vagus nerve. For this reason, *tachycardia* may result.

Quinidine is absorbed readily from the intestinal tract and is rapidly eliminated in the urine. As a rule, the peak of its action takes place from 2 to 3 hours after administration of one dose; the effect begins to subside in 4 hours, and is half-dissipated in 8 hours. The frequency of administration is important. *Five 2-hour doses are the most effective; they obtain a cumulative effect which continues throughout the following 12 hours.* Thus, the following morning, a fair percentage of quinidine is still in the blood, and blood concentration increases each day.

Determination of *plasma level of quinidine* has been used as a guide to treatment. Conversion to sinus rhythm was usually obtained with an *average plasma level of 5.4 mg. per liter.* Toxicity is rare at levels below 6 to 8 mg. per liter while it is not unusual at levels between 10 and 15 mg. per liter.

The best average dosage is 0.4 gm. (6 gr.) four to five times a day (2- to 2.5-hour intervals) and no administration during the night.

Toxic reactions are usually caused by overdosage and include nausea, dizziness, vascular collapse, conduction disturbances, sinus tachycardia, or ventricular arrhythmias. However, *idiosyncrasy* to quinidine may occur. In such cases, even a small dose may cause cyanosis, dizziness, nausea, and vomiting.

Embolism, caused by the dislodgement of mural thrombi, is a possibility when the heart reverts to normal rhythm. However, this danger has been overemphasized and a similar possibility is present with digitalis, or without therapy.

Quinidine may cause small deformation of the P waves and prolongation of P-R. Large doses may cause deformation of QRS and occasional changes of S-T and T, similar to those caused by digitalis (53).

Ventricular standstill or fibrillation with fatal result has been described in a few cases. These, however, are rare occurrences.

Quinidine is said to be contraindicated in

thyroid patients (until after thyroidectomy), in elderly people, in acute infections, in subacute bacterial endocarditis, and in patients with a history of embolism. However, these are not absolute contraindications.

Because of the frequent need of employing digitalis and quinidine on the same patient, either in alternate periods or in combination, a comparison of the principal effects of them is useful.

Quinidine acts like digitalis in favoring A-V block. If digitalis and quinidine are given together, they may obtain a greater effect in this direction. Quinidine decreases excitability and contractility (which are increased by digitalis). For this reason, *quinidine may counteract some of the unwanted effects of digitalis* while digitalis can prevent an excessive depression of the contractility, due to quinidine.

In general, if a patient has *congestive failure and atrial fibrillation*, it is advisable to digitalize him first. When the signs of congestion have subsided, digitalis will be continued and quinidine given.

After myocardial infarction, simultaneous use of quinidine and digitalis is necessary if congestive failure and atrial fibrillation are present (page 430).

Quinidine is the drug of choice in the treatment of *atrial fibrillation*. By increasing the refractory period of the atrial myocardium, it blocks an increasing number of impulses until the atria become still. Then the sinus node again becomes the pacemaker and initiates a normal rhythm.

The use of quinidine in *atrial flutter* is advised against by many cardiologists. The slowing of the atrial rate may allow the conduction of all atrial impulses to the ventricles while, before quinidine, only one-half of them were conducted. Doubling of the ventricular rate with severe disturbance to the patient may result. However, in certain cases, quinidine has been used with good results.

The use of quinidine in *ventricular tachycardia* is recommended. However, in some cases, only intravenous administration is effective. Pronestyl seems superior to quinidine in these cases.

Quinidine is often useful in the treatment of *premature beats*. It can be given alone or in combination with other drugs. After a normal rhythm is reestablished, a maintenance dose of 0.2 to 0.6 gm. daily can be given for long periods of time. Symptomatic administration with small doses can be prolonged for years without untoward effects.

Parenteral administration is possible but is necessary only in exceptional cases. Available preparations include *15 per cent quinidine in urea-antipyrine* (36); *20 per cent quinidine in propylene glycol;* and *8 per cent quinidine gluconate* (**25**) (0.8 gm. in 10 cc.) (35).

Fagarine (77)

Fagarine, extracted from a plant growing in Argentina, has been recommended for depressing ectopic foci.

While intramuscular injections of between 0.05 and 0.12 gm. are frequently effective, there is a severe danger of causing ventricular fibrillation. Therefore, fagarine cannot be recommended for routine clinical use.

Procaine Amide (78)

Procaine amide hydrochloride has been used by mouth or by vein in order to depress excessive excitability of the myocardium (**26, 27**).

Ectopic rhythms of ventricular origin, including ventricular tachycardia, ventricular premature contractions, ventricular flutter and ventricular fibrillation can be successfully treated with this drug. Ectopic rhythms of atrial or nodal origin respond less well even though some favorable reports are available. Slowing of the atrial rate has been noted in atrial fibrillation.

The protective value of procaine amide during cardiac surgery, cardiac catheterization, or surgery in general, is well established.

No important toxic symptoms occur and there is no stimulation of the central nervous system. Moderate hypotension occurs if there is no anesthesia. Contractility of the myocardium is not depressed, even by large doses. However, the drug seems to present some danger if there are disturbances of conduction.

Oral administration (**27**) consists of 0.25 to 0.50 gm. (1 to 2 capsules) every 4 to 6 hours.

Intravenous administration (**26**) of 100 to 500 mg. (1–5 cc.) is well tolerated. Decreased voltage of all waves and prolongation of the QRS and QT intervals were noted in some cases, lasting not more than 30 minutes.

Anticoagulants

Observation that thromboembolic phenomena cause a terminal fatal episode in many patients suffering from myocardial infarction or thrombophlebitis has led to the use of anticoagulants in the course of several cardiovascular diseases.

HEPARIN (79)

Heparin is a physiologic anticoagulant (**63**). It is extracted from the liver and is active only if given by intravenous injection. *Heparin seems to act on prothrombin and is neutralized by thrombokinase.*

Following determination of clotting time of the whole blood, *50 mg. of heparin* in 50 to 100 cc. of physiologic saline are slowly injected into a vein. Clotting times are repeated 15 minutes and 2½ hours after administration. In general, 50 to 75 mg. of heparin are given every 3 to 4 hours for 2 days. Clotting time is checked daily.

DICUMAROL (79, 80)

Dicumarol is a hydroxicoumarin which inhibits formation of prothrombin in the liver if administered by mouth (**64**). This inhibition is temporary and there are other, less important, effects on coagulation. While determination of clotting time is an adequate test, that of *prothrombin time* (page 166) is more reliable. However, even this test is not a perfect guide for therapy and *some of the disadvantages which are currently noted should*

be avoided in the future if better tests are devised.

The effect of dicumarol is delayed for 12 to 72 hours after administration and may persist for a similar time after the last dose has been ingested.

While the effect of dicumarol may be increased (hepatic or renal insufficiency) or decreased (diseases of, or surgery on, the g-i tract) by several factors, other unpredictable elements vary the sensitivity of the patients to the drug.

Initial dose is 300 mg. Two hundred mg. are given in one dose each of the subsequent days until prothrombin time drops below 20 per cent. On days when concentration of prothrombin is less than 20 per cent, no drug should be given. Concentrations of prothrombin between 10 and 20 per cent are considered optimal for therapy. If prothrombin drops below 10 per cent, 30 mg. of *menadione bisulfite* (**66**) should be given by vein, and this usually brings the level to above 10 per cent.

Since heparin acts more rapidly than dicumarol, it is advisable to start administration of heparin and dicumarol at the same time. As soon as dicumarol becomes effective, heparin is discontinued.

OTHER ANTICOAGULANTS

Other anticoagulant drugs are less well known. Among them are the following.

Tromexan (**65**) is another hydroxycoumarin for oral use (81). It acts more rapidly than dicumarol. Initial dose is 1,500 to 1,800 mg. Subsequent daily doses are from 300 to 900 mg.

Treburon (82) can be administered subcutaneously or intravenously and prolongs the coagulation of the entire blood. It resembles heparin and is counteracted by *protamine sulfate* given by vein. Intravenous doses are in the range of 200 mg.

Diuretics

All substances appear in the glomerular filtrate because of *diffusion* while an *active readsorption* occurs later in the tubules. Therefore, increased flow of urine may be due to increased filtration, decreased readsorption, or both. As 99 per cent of the glomerular filtrate is readsorbed later, *one per cent decrease in tubular adsorption doubles the amount of urine, a result which is attained only by a 100 per cent increase of glomerular filtration.* For this reason, the greatest importance is usually attributed to changes of tubular function.

A. WATER—NEUTRAL SALTS

Water and *neutral salts* are considered to be diuretics. However, their use may be harmful in cardiac patients.

B. AMMONIUM CHLORIDE

This salt acts by splitting into ammonium and chloride ions. The former is converted into urea; the latter combines with the sodium liberated from the sodium bicarbonate of the blood and causes *acidosis* (30). While there is increased excretion of fixed base in the urine, accompanied by water, acidosis also results in diuresis (30).

This mechanism cannot be used too often, as it requires a period of recovery. Therefore, ammonium chloride is given in a large dose (8–12 gm. daily for 2–3 days) but *at intervals of not less than 5 days.* Ammonium chloride potentiates the action of mercurial diuretics and, for this reason, is frequently associated with them. It is usually given in enteric-coated tablets (**13**). It should not be given in cases of nephritis. It may cause nausea, vomiting, or abdominal distress.

C. XANTHINES (CAFFEINE, THEOBROMINE, THEOPHYLLINE, AMINOPHYLLIN)

These drugs have a multiple diuretic action: they cause dilatation of the renal vessels (31) and increase the number of the functioning glomeruli (32); they also markedly *decrease the tubular readsorption of fluid* (34). From studies in man, the latter mechanism seems the most important (35).

The xanthines have various side effects.

They stimulate the central nervous system and the myocardium. They dilate both the peripheral and the coronary arteries. Peripheral dilatation is partly antagonized by stimulation of the vasoconstrictor center.

These different properties vary with each drug. *Caffeine* is the best nervous stimulant; *theophylline*, the best diuretic; and *aminophyllin*, the best vasodilator.

The doses employed are:

Caffeine with sodium benzoate: 0.3 gm. by mouth; 0.2 by injection (**60**).

Theobromine with sodium salicylate (diuretin): 1 gm. by mouth.

Theophylline (or theocin): 0.25 gm.

Theophylline with ethylene diamine (aminophyllin): 0.10 to 0.25 gm. by mouth; 0.25 to 0.50 by i.v. injection (**42**); 0.5 gm. by suppository (**41**).

D. MERCURIAL DIURETICS

In spite of marked extrarenal action of these drugs, *the main site of action is renal* (34–37). There is decreased tubular readsorption which may represent an early stage of the toxic action that larger doses of mercury develop in the kidney. For this reason, careful dosage and a sufficient interval between injections are advisable.

Intravenous injections of mercurial diuretics cause a sudden drop of pressure in the venous system, the right atrium and ventricle, and the pulmonary artery (85). This drop, which may reach 50 per cent, was observed in rheumatic and hypertensive patients, not in chronic cor pulmonale or constrictive pericarditis (85). This effect seems due to a peripheral action.

Minimal toxicity can be obtained by using *thiomerin* (83) (**12**) or *cumertilin* (84).

Oral, rectal, intramuscular, or intravenous administration can be used. The latter, however, is the most effective.

Diuresis usually starts within 2 to 3 hours and continues for 12 to 24 hours. Untoward reactions consist of signs of mercurial poisoning (stomatitis, colitis, headache, nausea, albuminuria, hematuria). Mercurial di-

TABLE 27

NITRITE	ROUTE OF ADMINISTRATION	DOSE	TIME OF ONSET OF ACTION (MINUTES)	DURATION OF ACTION
Amyl nitrite......................	Inhalation	0.2 cc.	½ to 1	4 to 8 minutes
Nitroglycerine....................	Perlingual	0.5 mg.	1 to 2	25 to 40 minutes
Sodium nitrite....................	Oral	30 to 60 mg.	5 to 20	1 to 2½ hours
Erythrityl tetranitrate...........	Oral	30 to 60 mg.	15 to 30	3 to 5 hours
Mannitol hexanitrate..............	Oral	15 to 60 mg.	15 to 30	4 to 6 hours

uretics should not be given if the renal function is severely impaired. The dose is from 0.5 to 2 cc.

Oral or rectal administration is far less effective, but may still be useful in some cases (94, 95).

Vasodilators and Hypotensive Drugs
A. NITRITES

The term *nitrites* includes also the *nitrates* because of the fact that the latter owe their action to the fact that nitrite ions are liberated in the body. These drugs have a powerful relaxing action on the smooth muscles of the body. This action is maximal on the vessels (arteries, capillaries, veins) (38) and especially on the small arteries. A secondary fall in blood pressure occurs. The vasodilator action is independent of innervation and does not impair the ability of the vessels to contract in response to stimulation. This applies also to the coronary vessels (39).

The action on the smooth muscles of the bronchi, biliary passages, gastrointestinal, and genitourinary tracts is to be considered of secondary importance but may become valuable in the combined diseases of different systems (gastric ulcer or cholecystitis plus coronary heart disease).

Table 27 gives the doses, times of onset, and durations of action of various nitrites. As shown by the table, both amyl nitrite (52) and nitroglycerin (53) are useful only in the treatment of acute attacks (angina pectoris). The other drugs (like mannitol (51) or peritrate (50)) may be used both to prevent these attacks and to lower blood pressure. Mannitol hexanitrate is the longest

acting and may be given at 5-hour intervals to keep the vessels under a continuous, even if mild, vasodilator influence.

Amyl nitrite (52) has such a rapid hypotensive effect that it causes coronary insufficiency in patients with coronary sclerosis (86). This property has been used for testing the function of the coronary vessels (page 129).

B. PAPAVERINE

Papaverine is one of the alkaloids of opium but has no narcotic effects. Its actions on the central nervous system are negligible and the drug causes neither sleep nor analgesia in the usual doses.

Papaverine is used as *papaverine hydrochloride* in doses of 30 to 100 mg., from 2 to 5 times daily *per os*; and in doses of 30 to 60 mg. by intramuscular or intravenous injection (43, 44).

Papaverine relaxes the smooth muscles of the body but mainly those of the blood vessels. This relaxation occurs chiefly when the muscles are contracted. The drug markedly increases the coronary flow (39d). Papaverine has been used in coronary heart disease, acute cor pulmonale, and many diseases of the peripheral arteries. The drug increases the collateral circulation whenever one vessel is obstructed; it decreases mortality in experimental animals.

Papaverine has a moderate depressive effect on excitability and conductivity of the myocardium. This may be useful in arrhythmias of coronary patients.

Papaverine-like drugs are made synthetically and have similar action.

C. KHELLIN

Khellin is the active principle of *Ammi visnaga*, an Arabic plant called "Khella." Experimental and clinical observations (89) show that khellin can be used as a coronary dilator and causes relief of anginal pain. Its action seems to be four times more powerful than that of aminophyllin. Khellin does not lower blood pressure and has few side effects. Usual doses of the commercial preparations (**48, 49**) are: one 50-mg. tablet daily for 1 week, then one or two tablets daily.

D. RAUWOLFIA (90)

Rauwolfia, the active principle of the Indian plant *Rauwolfia serpentina*, has moderate hypotensive and sedative effects (**45**). The drug is tolerated for long periods. It may cause bradycardia and, in large doses, diarrhea. Its mechanism of action is poorly understood. Tolerance to the drug does not develop and there seems to be synergism between this and other agents. Combination of rauwolfia with veratrum has given good results.

E. ALKALOIDS OF VERATRUM (91)

The alkaloids of *Veratrum viride* include *germitrine, germidine, neogermitrine,* and *protoveratrine*. The latter has received extensive clinical trial which was compared with that of the total mixture of esters from the plant (**46**).

These alkaloids stimulate the afferent side of a reflex pathway which controls blood pressure. Nerve receptors of the left ventricle, the coronary arteries, the pulmonary arteries, and the carotid and aortic bodies, are "sensitized", so that they send increased stimuli to the vasomotor center. As a result, bradycardia and a reflex vasodilation occur. There is no sympathetic paralysis and no postural hypotension.

Intravenous dose of protoveratrine is 1 microgram per minute, for several hours or days. *Oral protoveratrine* (**47**) is given in a large dose after breakfast (0.5–1.5 mg.)

followed by one or two smaller doses (0.25 mg.) at 2- 3-hour intervals. A fall in blood pressure lasting from 6 to 8 hours is customary. Some degree of nausea is not unusual; dizziness or weakness is possible.

F. PRISCOLINE

Priscoline is a 2-benzyl-4,5-imidazoline hydrochloride (**54**). Intravenous injection of 15 to 50 mg. of priscoline causes tachycardia, slight changes of blood pressure, and a significant increase of cutaneous blood flow (87). Twenty-five to 75 mg. administered orally definitely increase digital blood flow. Priscoline is particularly useful in peripheral vascular diseases.

In general, oral doses of 25 to 50 mg. are given several times a day.

G. ALCOHOL

Ethyl alcohol is a moderate peripheral vasodilator. Its action on the coronary arteries is probably negligible. Most of the useful effect in coronary patients should be attributed to increased threshold of pain (sedation) and euphoria (see also page 435).

Ethanol vapor in oxygen has been advocated in paroxysmal pulmonary edema by the author (88). In such cases, the effect is mostly local and based on the antifoaming action of alcohol. Adsorption is minimal and systemic effects extremely limited.

H. AMINOPHYLLIN (THEOPHYLLINE WITH ETHYLENE DIAMINE)

The multiple actions of this drug have already been described (page 595). Among them, a moderate dilatation of the peripheral arteries is obtained.

Aminophyllin is a stimulant of respiration (action on the carotid body) and is useful in Cheyne-Stokes respiration (page 557) possibly also because it is a vasodilator. Oral aminophyllin has a minor action. The best results are obtained by i.v. injection of 0.25 to 0.50 gm. (**42**) or by suppository (**41**) (0.50 gm. in cocoa butter).

I. ACETYL-β-METHYLCHOLINE (MECHOLYL)

This drug may be useful as a vasodilator in patients with spasms of the peripheral arteries (40) (71). The drug causes a fall of blood pressure. Its action is similar to that of acetylcholine and to stimulation of the parasympathetic system. Therefore, it should not be used in coronary heart disease where a coronary constriction may follow its administration. It may have important applications in atrial tachycardia.

J. SULFOCYANATES (THIOCYANATES)

Thiocyanates have been used for their hypotensive action. Their efficacy is limited by the fact that the safe limit of serum level is between 8 and 14 mg. per cent, while above 15 mg. per cent severe toxic manifestations may appear. For this reason, frequent examinations of the serum level of the drug are necessary.

K. OTHER VASODILATOR DRUGS

Many other drugs have been described and widely used as vasodilators. However, their importance is limited. Among them, *pancreas extracts* have had a certain notoriety. However, their mild action seems due to the solvent and not to the extract itself.

It should be kept in mind that *sympatholytic drugs* (page 599) are powerful vasodilators.

Vasoconstrictors

A. EPINEPHRINE

Epinephrine is still one of the most powerful vasoconstrictors. However, it is not the most frequently used because of the short duration of its action and the necessity of using it by injection. It is, therefore, limited to emergencies.

Epinephrine acts directly on the effector cells of the various organs with results which are similar to those of the adrenergic nerves.

Epinephrine accelerates the heart rate, stimulates the myocardium, and increases the cardiac output. The main action is on the arterioles: those of the skin, of the splanchnic bed, and of the brain are constricted; those of the muscles and the coronary arteries are dilated; the pulmonary arteries tend to constrict by direct effect but are dilated because of increased cardiac work.

A severe increase of systemic blood pressure occurs soon after the injection of epinephrine, followed by carotid sinus reactions which slow down the heart and somewhat lower the blood pressure, at least temporarily.

Clinical tests with epinephrine by subcutaneous and intravenous injections reveal a series of interesting and multiple reactions (41).

Epinephrine in peanut oil has a slower action which may last from 2 to 4 hours.

The usual dose of epinephrine (55) is from 0.5 to 2 mg.

B. NOREPINEPHRINE

Norepinephrine differs from epinephrine because of the absence of a methyl group. It has hypertensive and constrictor effects similar to those of epinephrine but less marked stimulating effects on the myocardium. Intravenous dose is 0.03 mg. (56).

C. EPHEDRINE

This is an alkaloid derived from various plants and is also prepared synthetically. Ephedrine has the quality of being active when taken by mouth. It has many properties which are identical to, and others which differ from, those of epinephrine. One of the main differences concerns the duration of action which is much greater than that of epinephrine (57).

D. SYMPATHOMIMETIC AMINES

Various synthetic drugs have properties which resemble those of ephedrine. They are *amphetamine (benzedrine)* (58), *neo-synephrin, paredrine,* and *paredrinol (veritol)* (59).

These drugs act mostly on the venules and

only mildly on the arterioles; they do not cause a direct increase of the heart rate; moreover, a carotid sinus reflex, caused by the increased blood pressure, frequently lowers the heart rate (42).

Sympatholytics and Adrenolytics

DIBENAMINE (92)

Dibenamine is an adrenolytic and not a sympatholytic agent. After administration of this drug, epinephrine causes no rise, and may cause a fall, of blood pressure. Tachycardia is not inhibited and may be exaggerated by dibenamine.

Dibenamine should be given by *slow intravenous infusion* in great dilution. A dose of 5 mg. per kg. may cause orthostatic hypotension lasting 5 or 6 days while supine blood pressure may last for 20 to 24 hours (**37**).

HYDERGINE (93)

Isolation of the alkaloids of ergot made possible the association of three of them (*dihydroergocornine, dihydroergokryptine*, and *dihydroergocristine*) having sympatholytic action and no direct vasoconstrictor effect. The compound is called *hydergine* (**36**). Intravenous injection of 0.2 to 1.0 mg. causes a notable fall of supine blood pressure and orthostatic hypotension. Bradycardia is common. Nausea is frequent.

HEXAMETHONIUM (94)

This compound causes a specific paralysis of transmission at the ganglionic synapses. Thus, blood pressure is lowered while the effector organs can still respond to direct stimulation. While blood pressure is lowered and orthostatic hypotension is severe, several side effects occur, including atropine-like effects. Hypotensive effects indicate the existence of neurogenic hypertension; lack of them, the presence of humoral hypertension.

Intravenous doses range from 2.5 to 20 mg. (**39**). Tolerance develops rapidly. Oral administration (**40**) is effective only in some of the cases.

Hypnotics and Sedatives

A. OPIUM AND DERIVATIVES

Opium contains several alkaloids; the most active are *morphine, codeine*, and *papaverine*.

Papaverine has no hypnotic action.

Codeine has a weak analgesic property (less than one-sixth that of morphine), causes a slight excitement, no nausea, and little euphoria. Its main action is that of depressing the cough reflex, while respiration is slowed only slightly and secondary constipation is mild. Codeine is used as *codeine phosphate* in doses of 16 to 60 mg., two to three times a day.

Morphine is the most powerful natural alkaloid of opium. The latter owes its main properties to the fact that it contains an average of 10 per cent of morphine. Morphine exerts a narcotic action, manifested by analgesia and sleep.

A *selective depression of the respiratory center* is one of its most important effects; *relief of pain* is another outstanding result. Large doses of morphine cause narcosis but therapeutic doses may excite the patient. Morphine slows down the metabolism and decreases venous return. It may stimulate the vagus nerve.

It has been said that "morphine depresses from above downward and stimulates from below upward" (5), emphasizing that the maximum of stimulation is observed in the spinal cord while the maximum depression is in the brain. Nausea, vomiting, and bradycardia are some of the effects of the stimulation of the medullary centers.

Morphine is useful in paroxysmal dyspnea and pulmonary edema. It is also beneficial in the early treatment of myocardial infarction. Prevention of untoward effects may be obtained by association with atropine, papaverine, or barbiturates.

The constipating effect of morphine may require the use of laxatives. The possibility of creating addiction to morphine makes it advisable to limit the administration of this drug. Synthetic drugs, like *dilaudid*, offer little advantage in this respect.

Morphine is given as *morphine sulfate* in doses of 10 to 15 mg., one to three times in 24 hours. Morphine can be given by intravenous injection (43).

Demerol (**22, 23**) has morphine-like and atropine-like properties. Its use in the treatment of cardiovascular diseases does not seem to present any particular advantage over that of morphine and atropine except possibly less tendency to addiction.

B. BARBITURATES

The barbiturates are valuable depressants of the central nervous system. They induce calmness, then sleep; they inhibit convulsions and cause partial anesthesia.

Barbiturates have little action on heart rate and blood pressure, except by the effect of quieting the patient or inducing sleep. Intravenous injections should be given slowly because a sudden even though transitory drop of pressure may follow a rapid injection.

The action on the brain stem is more powerful and occurs earlier than that on the cortex (44).

C. CHLORAL HYDRATE

Chloral hydrate is a sedative and a soporific. Its ordinary dose is from 1 to 3 gm. by mouth (**34**) or by rectum (**33**) and from 0.3 to 1 gm. by intravenous injection (43a).

This drug causes a quiet sleep, a moderate fall of blood pressure, and does not depress the heart. Its action on the central nervous system is more widespread than that of the barbiturates. Its usefulness in paroxysmal pulmonary edema has been demonstrated both by clinical and experimental studies of the author (45).

D. BROMIDES

Bromides (**32**) exert a mild depression of the central nervous system through a somewhat obscure mechanism. The dose of *sodium bromide* is from 1 to 3 gm. daily. Bromides are excreted very slowly. It takes a month or longer to eliminate bromides after a full administration.

E. ALCOHOL

Alcohol exerts a depressant action on the central nervous system. The apparent stimulation results from a less-restrained action of the lower centers when the higher centers are depressed.

Alcohol causes peripheral vasodilation and it has been stated that the coronary vessels are also dilated (49) but the experimental results are extremely variable (50) and clinical experience in angina pectoris seems to be negative (51).

While alcohol may exert a beneficial action on the mental state of the patients, it should be kept in mind that it may slightly increase pulse rate and blood pressure, probably through a reflex mechanism (52).

The action on the heart is variable and is different if the patient is an habitual drinker. Increased heart rate and palpitation is experienced by some. In prescribing alcohol as a drug, the dangers of creating habituation should be considered.

The *antifoaming action of alcohol* has been used by the author and his coworkers for symptomatic therapy of paroxysmal pulmonary edema (page 560).

Drugs Stimulating the Central Nervous System

The drugs which are used on cardiovascular patients are *coramine* and *metrazol*. They stimulate the respiratory and vasomotor centers and may be useful in cases of periodic respiration or vascular collapse. They may be given by mouth or by intramuscular or intravenous injection.

The dose of *metrazol* (*cardiazol*) is 100 mg., either by mouth or by injection.

Coramine (*nikethamide*) (**61**) is used in 25 per cent solution; the dose by any route is 1 to 3 cc.

Oxygen

Oxygen therapy has as its purpose the prevention of the harmful effects of tissue anoxia. To maintain a 50 per cent oxygen concentration in a tent, a flow of 9 to 10 liters per minute is required. Administration by mask under a positive pressure of 2 to 5 cm. of water has favorable effects in acute pulmonary edema (47). Oxygen therapy is useful in congestive failure, especially when there is continuous dyspnea and after coronary occlusion. Its use for about 20 minutes every hour is usually sufficient to relieve dyspnea.

BIBLIOGRAPHY

1. a) Jacobs, W. A. Physiol. Rev., 1933, **13**, 222.
   b) Stoll, A. *The Cardiac Glycosides.* London, Pharmac. Press, 1937.
   c) Fieser, L. F. *The Chemistry of Natural Products Related to Phenanthrene.* New York, Reinhold, 1937.
2. Withering, W. *An Account of the Fox-glove, etc.* Birmingham, McSwinney, 1785 (reprinted in *Cardiac Classics*; St. Louis, Mosby, 1941).
3. Meyer, H. H., and Gottlieb, R. *Experimentelle Pharmakologie.* Berlin, Urban and Schwarzenberg, 1925.
4. Cushny, A. R. *Pharmacology and Therapeutics.* Philadelphia, Lea & Febiger, 1940.
5. Goodman, L., and Gilman, A. *The Pharmacological Basis of Therapeutics.* New York, Macmillan, 1941.
6. Cattell, M., and Gold, H. J. Pharmacol. & Exper. Therap., 1938, **62,** 116.
7. a) Luisada, A. A., and Mautner, H. New England Heart Assoc., May, 1944. Also Acta Pharm., Toxic, 1946, **2**, 275.
   b) Rall, J. E., Wells, J. A., and Dragstedt, C. A. Federation Proc., 1943, **2**, 93. Also Proc. Soc. Exper. Biol. & Med., 1944 **56** 162.
8. a) Weese. *Digitalis.* Leipzig, 1936.
   b) Buchner, F. Arch. exp. Path., Pharm., 1934, **176**, 59.
   c) La Due, J. A. J. Pharmacol. & Exper. Therap., 1942, **76**, 1.
   d) Kyser, F. A., and co-workers. Am. Heart J., 1946, **31**, 451.
9. a) Gremels, H. Arch. exp. Path., Pharm., 1933, **169**, 689.
   b) Peters, H. C., and Visscher, M. B. Am. Heart J., 1936, **11**, 273.
   c) Wiggers, C. J., and Stimson, B. J. Pharmacol. & Exper. Therap., 1927, **30**, 251.
   d) Fahr, G. Mo. Conc. Cardiovasc. Dis., 1945, **14**, N. 10.

10. Heymans, C., and co-workers. Compt. rend. Soc. Biol. 1932, **110, **572.
11. Gold, H., and co-workers. J. Pharmacol. & Exper. Therap., 1939, **66**, 15; and **67**, 224. Arch. Int. Med., 1940, **65**, 263. J. Clin. Investigation,1929, **6**, 613; and 1939, **18**, 429. J. A. M. A., 1930, **95**, 1237.
12. Stewart, H. J., and Cohn, A. E. J. Clin. Investigation, 1928, **6**, 53 and 79; and 1932, **11**, 917.
13. a) Dock, W., and Tainter, M. L. J. Clin. Investigation, 1930, **8**, 467 and 485.
    b) Katz, L. N., and co-workers. Am. Heart J., 1938, **16**, 149. Also J. Pharmacol. & Exper. Therap., 1938, **62**, 1.
14. a) Miculicich, M. Zentralbl. Phys., 1910, **24**, 523.
    b) Meyer, F. Med. Klin., 1912, **8**, 869.
    c) Sakai, S., and Saneyoshi, S. Arch. exp. Path., Pharm., 1915, **78**, 331.
    d) Bodo, R. J. Physiol., 1928, **64**, 365.
    e) Rein, H. Muench. med. Woch., 1933, **80**, 374.
    f) Essex, H. E., Herrick, J. F., and Visscher, M. B. Am. Heart J., 1938, **16**, 143.
15. Jonescu, D., and Loewi, O. Arch. exp. Path., Pharm., 1908, **59**, 71.
16. Cohn, A. E., and co-workers. Trans. Int. Congr. Med., London, 1913, **6**, 255. Also J. Exper. Med., 1915, **21**, 593.
    b) Pardee, H. E. B. *Clinical Aspects of the Electrocardiogram.* New York, Hoeber, 1924.
    c) Bromer, A. W., and Blumgart, H. L. J. A. M. A., 1929, **92**, 204.
    d) McMillan, T. M., and Bellett, S. *In Stroud's Cardiovascular Disease.* Philadelphia, Davis, 1945.
17. a) Hatcher, R. A., and Weiss, S. Arch. Int. Med., 1922, **29**, 690.
    b) Dresbach, M. Am. J. Physiol., 1939, **113**, 284.
18. Gold, H., and DeGraff, A. C. J. Clin. Investigation, 1929, **6**, 613. Also J. A. M. A., 1930, **95**, 1237.
19. Eggleston, C. Arch. Int. Med., 1915, **16**, 1. Also J. A. M. A., 1920, **74**, 733.
20. Robinson, G. C., White, P. D., Eggleston, C., and Hatcher, R. A. J. A. M. A., 1924, **83**, 504.
21. Blumgart, H. L., and Altschule, M. D. Am. J. M. Sci., 1939, **198**, 455.
22. Kyser, F. A., Ginsberg, H., and Gilbert, N. C. Am. Heart J., 1946, **31**, 451.
23. McMichael, J., and Sharpey-Schafer, E. P. Quart. J. Med., 1944, **13**, 123.
24. Braun, L., and Wosika, P. H. Am. Heart J., 1945, **29**, 261.

25. Gold, H. Mo. Conc. Cardiov. Dis., 1945, **14**, N. 11.

26. Arrillaga, F. C., and DeSoldati, L. Rev. Card., 1945, **12**, 158.

27. Bond, G., Baum, H., and Dimond, G. Am. Heart J., 1945, **30**, 194.

28. a) Wenkebach, K. F., and Winterberg, H. *Die Unregelmaessige Herztaetigkeit.* Leipzig, Engelmann, 1927.

b) Frey, W. Klin. Woch., 1918, **55**, 849.

c) Kohn, C. M., and Levine, S. A. Ann. Int. Med., 1935, **8**, 923.

d) Stroud, W. D., and Laplace, L. B. Intern. Clin., 1935, **1**, 13.

29. Conferences on Therapy. New York J. Med., 1945, **45**, 65.

30. a) Gamble, J. L., Blackfan, K. D., and Hamilton, B. J. Clin. Investigation, 1925, **1**, 359.

b) Keith, N. M., and Whelan, M. J. Clin. Investigation, 1926, **3**, 149.

31. Sollman, T., and Pilcher, J. D. J. Pharmacol. & Exper. Therap., 1912, **3**, 19.

32. Richards, A. N., and Schmidt, C. F. Am. J. Physiol., 1924, **71**, 178.

33. Cushny, A. R., and Lambie, C. G. J. Physiol., 1921, **55**, 276.

34. Walker, A. M., and co-workers. Am. J. Physiol., 1937, **118**, 95.

35. Blumgart, H. L., and co-workers. Arch. Int. Med., 1934, **54**, 40.

36. Govaerts, P. Compt. rend. Soc. biol., 1928, **99**, 647.

37. Bartram, E. A., J. Clin. Investigation, 1932, **11**, 1197.

38. a) Weiss, S., and Ellis, L. B. Arch Int. Med., 1933, **52**, 105.

b) Weiss, S., Wilkins, R. W., and Haynes, F. W. J. Clin. Investigation, 1937, **16**, 73.

c) Lueth, H. C., and Hanks, T. G. Arch. Int. Med., 1938, **62**, 97.

39. a) Smith, F. M. Arch. Int. Med., 1921, **28**, 836.

b) Katz, L. N., and co-workers. Arch. Intern. de Pharmac., 1938, **59**, 399.

c) Boyer, N. H., and co-workers. Am. J. Physiol., 1939, **126**, 440.

d) Essex, H. E., and co-workers. Am. Heart J., 1940, **19**, 554.

40. a) Kovacs, J., and co-workers. Am. Heart J., 1936, **11**, 53.

b) Loman, J., Greenberg, B., and Myerson, A. New England J. Med., 1938, **219**, 655.

c) Loman, J., Lesses, M. F., and Myerson, A. Arch. Int. Med., 1939, **12**, 1213.

41. a) Luisada, A. A. Gazz. Osp., Clin. (Milan), March, 1924.

b) Levine, S. A. and co-workers: Arch. Int. Med., 1930, **45**, 191.

c) Blumgart, H. L.: Volume I of contrib.

in honor of E. Ligman. New York. Intern. Press, 1932.

d) Katz, L. N. and co-workers: Am. Heart Journ., 1932, **7**, 371.

e) Starr, I. and co-workers: Journ. Clin. Invest., 1937, **16**, 799.

42. a) Chen, K. K., and Schmidt, C. F.: Journ. Pharm., Exp. Ther., 1924, **24**, 339 and Medic., 1930, **9**, 1.

b) Altschule, M. D. and Iglauer, A.: Journ. Clin. Inv., 1940, **19**, 497 and 503.

c) Dameshek, W., Loman, J. and Myerson, A.: Am. Journ. Med. Sci., 1938, **195**, 88.

d) Davis, P. L. and Davis, M. S.: Journ. Am. Med. Ass., 1937, **108**, 1247.

e) Rein, H.: Klin. Woch., 1937, **16**, 700 and Arch. exp. Path., Pharm., 1937, **187**, 617.

f) Stead, E. A., Kunkal, P. and Weiss, S.: Journ. Clin. Invest., 1939, **18**, 439 and 679.

43. a) Luisada, A. A.: Riv. Ital. Ter. (Naples), 1928, N. 4.

b) Dripps, R. D. and Comroe, J. H.: Anesthesiol., 1945, **6**, 449.

c) Smith, H. and Schotz, S.: J. M. A. Alab., 1945, **14**, 265.

44. Pick, E. P. and co-workers: Arch. Intern. Pharmac., 1939, **61**, 447.

45. Luisada, A. A.: Exp. Med., Surg., 1943, **1**, 22 and Amer. Heart Journ., 1946, **31**, 293 (with S. J. Sarnoff).

46. Kisch, B.: Exp. Med., Surg., 1945, **3**, 1; also Strophanthin. New York, Brooklyn Med. Press, 1944.

47. Barach, A. L., Martin, J. and Eckman, M.: Ann. Int. Med., 1938, **12**, 754.

48. de Takats, G., Trump, R. A. and Gilbert, N. C.: Journ. Am. Med. Ass., 1944, **125**, 840.

49. White, P. D. and Sharker, T.: Journ. Am. Med. Ass., 1934, **102**, 655.

50. a) Dixon, W. E.: Journ. Phys., 1907, **35**, 346.

b) Sulzer, R.: Heart, 1924, **11**, 141.

c) Gilbert, N. C. and Fenn, G. K.: Arch. Int. Med., 1929, **44**, 118.

51. Stearns, S., Riseman, J. E. F. and Gray, W.: New Eng. Journ. Med., 1946, **234**, 578.

52. Grollman, A.: Journ. Pharm., Exp. Ther., 1930, **39**, 313 and Quart. Journ. Stud. on Alcohol, 1942, **3**, 5.

53. a) Pardee, H. E. B.: Clinical Aspects of the Electrocardiogram. New York, Hoeber, 1941.

b) Pazzanese, D.: Modificações de Forma do Eletrocardiograma. São Paulo, Gráfica de Prefeitura, 1942.

54. Mautner, H.: Ann. Paediatr.: 1941, **157**, 65.
55. Luisada, A. A., and Weiss, M. Am. J. Physiology 1954, **176**, 123.
56. Haring, O. M., and Luisada, A. A. Am. Heart J., 1953, **45**, 108; and 1953, **46**, 276.
57. Ferrer, M., and Cournand, A., *et al.* Circ., **1**, 161.
58. a) Harvey, R. M., Cournand, A., *et al.* Am. J. Med., 1949, **7**, 439.
    b) Stead, A., *et al.* Arch. Int. Med., 1948, **81** 282.
59. Batterman, R. C., De Graff, A. C., *et al.* Am. Heart J., 1947, **34**, 663; and 1951, **42**, 292.
60. Gold, H., *et al.* Am. J. Med. 1952, **13**, 124.
61. Loeffler, W., *et al.* Schweiz. med. Woch., 1953, **83**, 1.
62. Mathes, S., Gold, H., *et al.* J. A. M. A., 1952, **150**, 191.
63. Lagerloef, H., and Werkoe, L.. Acta Card., 1949, **4**, 1.
64. Prinzmetal, M., *et al. The Auricular Arrhythmias*. Springfield, Ill., Thomas, 1952.
65. Nylin, G. Am. Heart J., 1949, **37**, 543.
66. Friedman, R., and Bine, R. Proc. Soc. Exper. Biol. & Med., 1947, **64**, 162; and 1949, **71**, 406. J. Clin. Investigation, 1949, **28**, 32. Circ. 1950, **1**, 1182.
67. McMichael, J., and Sharpey-Schafer, E. P. Quart. J. Med., 1944, **13**, 123. Also Clin. Sci., 1946, **6**, 41; and 1947, **6**, 187.
68. a) Sampson, J. J., *et al.* Am. Heart J., 1943, **26**, 164.
    b) Buff, I. E. South M. J., 1949, **42**, 1037.
69. a) Zimdahl, W. T. Ann. Int. Med., 1946, **25**, 531.
    b) Boyd, L. J., and Scherf, D. Am. J. M. Sci., 1943, **206**, 43.
    c) Enselberg, C. D., *et al.* Am. Heart J., 1950, **39**, 703.
    d) Szekely, P. Brit. Heart J., 1946, **8**, 115.
70. a) Stearns, N. S., *et al.* J. Clin. Investigation, 1951, **30**, 676.
    b) McCord, M., and Taguchi, J. T. Circ., **4**, 387.
71. Danielopolu, C. Cardiol. (Bale), 1947, **12**, 66.
72. Pincelli, C. Cuore e Circ. (Rome), 1947, **31**, 155.
73. St. George, *et al.* Circ., 1952, **6**, 661.
74. Friedman, M., *et al.* Circ., 1952, **6**, 853.
75. Friedman, M., and Bine, R. Am. J. M. Sci., 1947, **214**, 633.
76. Sokolow, M. Am. Heart J., 1951, **42**, 771.
77. Scherf, O., *et al.* Ann. Int. Med., 1949, **30**, 100.
78. a) Mark, L. C., *et al.* J. Pharmacol. & Exper. Therap., 1950, **98**, 21.
    b) Kayden, H. J., *et al.* Circ., 1951, **4**, 13.
    c) Wedd, A. M., *et al.* Am. Heart J., 1951, **42**, 399.
79. a) Wright, I. S., *et al.* Am. J. Med., 1947, **3**, 718. Also J. A. M. A., 1948, **138**, 1074.
    b) Parker, R. L., and Barker, N. W. Proc. Staff Meet., Mayo Clin., 1947, **22**, 185 and 1948, **23**, 367.
80. Barker, N. W. Am. J. Med., 1947, **3**, 634.
81. Bronstein, M. R., and Witkind, E. Am. J. M. Sci., 1951, **222**, 677.
82. a) Hirschboeck, J. S., *et al.* Wisconsin M. J., 1951, **50**, 863.
    b) Scholz, D. A., and Barker, N. W. Proc. Staff Meet., Mayo Clin., 1952, **27**, 332.
83. Feinberg, A. R., and Isaacs, J. H. Am. J. M. Sci., 1949, **218**, 298.
84. Rose, O. A., *et al.* Am. Heart J., 1950, **40**, 779.
85. a) Scébat, L., *et al.* Arch. Mal. Coeur, 1949, **42**, 1149.
    b) Kartun, P., *et al.* Arch. Mal. Coeur, 1950, **43**, 133.
86. Contro, S., Haring, O. M., and Goldstein, W. Circ., 1952, **6**, 250.
87. a) Hendrix, J. P., *et al.* Federation Proc., 1947, **6**, 638.
    b) Horwitz, O., *et al.* Am. J. M. Sci., 1949, **218**, 669.
88. Luisada, A. A., *et al.* Circ., 1952, **5**, 363. Also Ann. Int. Med., 1952, **37**, 1221.
89. a) Anrep, G. V., *et al.* Brit. Heart J., 1946, **8**, 171. Also Am. Heart J., 1949, **37**, 531.
    b) Armbrust, C. A., and Levine, S. A. Am. J. Med., 1950, **220**, 127.
90. Wilkins, R. W. Ann. Int. Med., 1952, **37**, 1144 Also New England J. Med., 1953, **248**, 48 (with Judson, W. E.).
91. a) Meilman, E., and Kreyer, O. Circ., 1950, **1**, 204.
    b) Taylor, R. D., and Page, I. H. Circ., 1951, **4**, 184.
    c) Wilkins, R. W. Mo. Conc. Cardiov. Dis., 1951, **20**, 89.
92. a) Haimovici, H., *et al.* Proc. Soc. Exper. Biol. & Med., 1948, **67**, 163; and 1951, **77**, 477.
    b) Moser, M., *et al.* Arch. Int. Med., 1952, **89**, 708.
93. a) Tandowsky, R. Circ., 1950, **1**, 686.
    b) Gibbs, D. F. Brit. Heart J., 1952, **14**, 77.
94. Paton, W. D. M., and Zaimis, E. J. Pharmacol. Rev., 1952, **4**, 219.
    b) Restall, P. A., and Smirk, F. H. Brit. Heart J., 1952, **14**, 1.
    c) Schroeder, H. A. Arch. Int. Med., 1952, **89**, 523.
95. Tamura, K., Kobayashi, Y., and Tokita, K. Japan. M. J., 1948, **1**, 206.

CHAPTER 33

Social and Legal Aspects of Heart Disease

General improvement of health, decrease of infantile mortality, and decrease of the mortality caused by infections have prolonged the average life of our population. For these reasons, heart disease is now the most frequent cause of death. The following figures easily prove the above statement (1). In 1945, in the United States, deaths attributed to heart disease in persons from 5 to 19 years of age were *second* in frequency; in persons 20 to 34 years, they were *third*; and in persons above 35, they were *first*.

Approximately 10 million individuals suffer from cardiovascular diseases in this country. Many of them experience some limitation of activity.

Prevention of Heart Disease

The frequency of heart disease and the increase in popular knowledge have led to concerted efforts in an attempt to prevent hypertension, rheumatic fever, and coronary heart disease (the three most common causes of death), as well as other less frequent causes of morbidity and mortality.

Prevention of rheumatic heart disease is based on the following program:

a) Treatment of streptococcic sore throats and other upper respiratory infections by means of injections of penicillin.

b) Prevention of recurrences through prolonged (2 to 10 years) prophylaxis of upper respiratory infections by means of *sulfadiazine* or *oral penicillin* (page 198).

c) Limitation of dangers by means of a well-considered plan including some restriction of physical activity and a careful program of occupation.

d) Prevention of heart failure by diet, drug therapy, and periodic check-ups.

Prevention of coronary heart disease is limited at present to:

a) Avoidance of high-caloric, high-fat diet throughout maturity.

b) Thyroid or iodides treatment in special cases.

c) Possible estrogen treatment in males.

d) Occupational and dietary therapy (moderate restriction of salt, sharper reduction of fats and calories) after an attack.

Prevention of hypertension in predisposed individuals includes:

a) Special planning of life including sufficient relaxation and vacations.

b) Same dietary rules as in coronary patients but with greater salt restriction.

c) Drug therapy.

d) Prevention or cure of renal infections.

e) Possible sympathectomy or unilateral nephrectomy (page 503).

Prevention of subacute bacterial endocarditis is based on penicillin therapy in rheumatic, arteriosclerotic, or congenital heart patients in occasions of surgical, dental, or obstetrical interventions (page 211).

Prevention of syphilitic heart disease is based on adequate cure of syphilis. This includes widespread education and detection, and common use of special clinics for initial cases (page 201).

Prevention of congenital heart disease is based on care of pregnant women including avoidance of viral infections, trauma, and intoxications.

Many of the other heart diseases can be prevented by timely use of antibiotics, other drug therapy of acute or chronic infections, and adequate nourishment.

The Social Element in Heart Disease

Damage to the heart constitutes a threat which varies in its severity, not only with the degree of the disease, but also with the emotional make-up of the patient (2). Sudden danger, possible recurrence and progression, and chronicity of many cardiac diseases all add up and may create severe social problems. As heart disease may occur at any age, different problems arise in children, adolescents, middle-aged, or elderly patients.

Certain problems recur again and again. There is the active child who yearns for physical exertion. There is the ambitious adolescent who is removed from studies or active sports. There is the young mother who cannot take care of her children; the widow who supports small children on a marginal income; the wage earner who hates to become dependent upon others; the older man who has no adequate retirement funds or who still feels capable of creative work.

The points of difference lie in the reaction of the patient to cardiac illness and in the possible emotional or financial gain derived in relation to other members of the family or associates. Emotional reactions by the other members of the family also play a significant role.

For this reason, management of a cardiac patient carries with it several important implications and is of broader scope than drug therapy.

Continuous thought should be given to prevention of recurrences, and delay in the progress of the disease.

Reduction of the disability of the patient, alleviation of the distress and suffering, and possible rehabilitation, are some of the important objectives of the management.

Children and adolescents. Rheumatic heart disease accounts for about 80 per cent of organic heart disease in children of school age. The general elements of crowding, poor alimentation, and lack of sunlight and exercise play a definite role. Emotional influences may contribute to susceptibility to rheumatic fever. Possibilities of home, hospital, or sanatorial treatment should be included in the careful consideration of all these

elements by physicians, nurses, and social workers.

Aftercare of children and adolescents with rheumatic heart lesions is a composite of treatment and prevention. The first 5 to 6 years following an attack of rheumatic fever represent the most important and difficult period. If the young patient grows up without cardiac enlargement or recurrences, he is likely to live a normal life span.

Periodic medical "check-ups" are important. Avoidance of infections, and their prompt treatment, are also essential. Physical exertion is allowed while strenuous exertion, like that of competitive sports, should be discouraged.

The selection of work or profession should include consideration of the amount of physical exertion which is involved or the possible exposure to extremes of temperature. Both should be avoided, either of necessity or as a precautionary measure.

For girls, the problems connected with marriage and childbearing have a special importance and require individualized advice.

Adults. The disintegrating influence of and the economic losses caused by heart disease create a severe challenge in adults. Prolonged financial or physical dependence on relatives or the community, inability to develop personal aptitudes or to realize justified ambitions for patients or their families, interruption of the usual human relationships, and fear of impending dangers, are the common results of heart disease.

In many cases, the cardiac patient can be *rehabilitated* by obtaining a different, less exacting job which is within his physical abilities. Rehabilitation was defined as "the return of a person disabled by accident or disease to his greatest physical, mental, emotional, social, vocational, and economic usefulness, and, if employable, an opportunity for gainful employment." Well-selected work frequently helps cardiac patients. Special institutions test the physical ability of cardiacs by gradually increasing the number of hours of their work. Physical and electrocardiographic examinations are made at regular intervals.

For elderly patients and for those with advanced heart disease, sedentary jobs should be advised (4).

Special kitchens have been devised for cardiac housewives, so that their physical labor is reduced to the necessary minimum (3).

The emotional, social, and economic adjustments of the cardiac patient are part of the responsibility of the physician and the social worker. Together, they can do much to obtain a *readjustment* and a *reeducation* of the cardiac. The development of *sedentary hobbies* may also contribute to a better mental and emotional balance.

Insurance and Cardiovascular Disease

Insurance companies reject applicants if they have cardiac murmurs, elevated blood pressure, rapid pulse rate, or (in the case of a large insurance) abnormal electrocardiogram. Unfortunately, many applicants with no heart disease are thus refused the benefit of insurance. A systolic murmur may be innocent or indicative of harmless fibrosis of a valve; slightly elevated blood pressure or rapid pulse may be due to endocrine disturbances, high excitability, or neurocirculatory asthenia; minor abnormalities of the electrocardiogram may lead to distorted interpretations. Only the careful study by a competent cardiologist gives a definite and exact evaluation of these borderline cases.

Patients with heart disease or high blood pressure are usually refused life insurance. This may be justified by the excessive risk involved in certain groups of patients. However, a careful examination and evaluation should eliminate the most severe risks while the others should be allowed the benefit of insurance, even though with a higher rate of premium.

It is the opinion of the author that, in the age group 20 to 40, minor rheumatic lesions of the mitral valve or uncomplicated septal defects should be considered for insurance at a higher rate. The same applies for persons between 40 and 60 and a moderate hypertension unaccompanied by renal or retinal changes.

Legal Aspects of Heart Disease (5)

The physician is often asked to evaluate the role of physical strain or an "accident" in the predisposition to or causation of an episode of arrhythmia, a coronary attack, or the onset of heart failure.

In any claim brought up for legal settlement which requires the professional advice of a cardiologist, the following questions must be answered.

1) Does the individual have heart disease?; if so, what kind and how severe?

2) If cardiac disease is present, could the alleged injury or strain have been the cause of, or have aggravated such condition?

The usual custom of requesting the expert to answer in the form of "yes" or "no," questions which are incomplete, or too broad, or definitely partial, unfortunately impairs much of the reliability of medical opinions.

The physician should determine the exact nature and severity of disease after the accident or injury and compare it with the data which were present before. He should further evaluate the severity of the noxious episode and the likelihood that it may have impaired the efficiency of the heart.

Trauma and strain *do not cause rheumatic fever, or rheumatic heart disease, or syphilitic heart disease*, and are seldom responsible for recurrences of rheumatic fever. They do not cause additional damage unless they are extremely severe. If such is the case, eversion of the aortic leaflets, atrial fibrillation, pulmonary embolism, or heart failure may result. On the other hand, cardiac neurosis is a common complication.

Trauma or strain *do not cause hypertension.* However, if advanced hypertensive heart disease is present, severe strain may precipitate acute pulmonary edema and determine the onset of heart failure.

The role of trauma and strain in *coronary*

heart disease is even more controversial. Even though most *myocardial infarcts* occur at rest, a fair number follow strenuous exertion. This fact is obviously confirmed by reading the newspapers of the great northern cities following a heavy snowfall. Several deaths are usually the result of efforts to clear up the snow from the back alley.[87]

Sudden death may be caused by a pulmonary embolus, rupture of an aortic aneurysm, severe and prolonged coronary insufficiency, or acute dilatation of the left ventricle with ventricular fibrillation or paroxysmal pulmonary edema.

The pertinent data are:

1) A cardiovascular system with severe lesions.

2) An adequate strain or exertion.

3) A reasonable time between strain and acute episode.

In all cases where disability is only partial, the *degree of disability* sustained should be carefully determined, and frequently a statement should be made concerning the possibility of return to employment and the possible date.

The relationship between *the reaction to low-grade stresses* which are part of everyday life, and various symptoms and signs, were studied in cardiac patients (6). The following results should be kept in mind:

1) *Dyspnea* associated with inefficient pulmonary ventilation may occur because of anxiety, anger, guilt, rage, frustration, or tension.

2) *Palpitation* associated with increased

[87] If death is due to myocardial infarction, this may have been caused by either severe coronary insufficiency or subintimal hemorrhage (rupture of capillaries).

stroke volume may occur in the same conditions.

3) *Precordial pain* in the presence of narrowing of the coronary arteries may result from decreased cardiac output associated with desperation or defeat; on the other hand, it may result from increased cardiac work due to increased blood pressure accompanying rage, resentment, anxiety, fear, or tension.

4) *Giddiness and fainting* may result from cerebral anoxia due to either decreased venous return to the heart or hyperventilation. Both types may be the result of various stress-producing conditions.

Sudden death may also be caused by *extreme fright*. This is not necessarily proportional to the severity of the event. There are a few well-documented records including post-mortem examinations where death of a normal young individual was caused by fear of an injection. It is likely that fright causes either ventricular fibrillation or cardiac arrest (page 395) through a reflex mechanism. The common *vasovagal syndrome* (page 517) is seldom cause of death because the heart continues its action, even though severely slowed, and most of the reflexes are received by the peripheral vessels.

BIBLIOGRAPHY

1. EMERSON, H. In *R. Levy's "Disorders of the Circulation"*. New York, Nelson, 1951.
2. COHEN, E. Am. Heart J., 1938, **16,** 422. Also Am. J. Pub. Health, 1941, **31,** 819.
3. *The Heart of the Home.* New York Heart Assoc., N. Y., 1949.
4. KOSSMANN, C.E., *et al.* Occup. Med., 1947, **3,** 531.
5. WHITE, P. D., Modern Med., 1946, **14,** 71.
6. WOLFF, G. A., AND WOLFF, H. G. Psychosom. Med., 1946, **8,** 293.

CHAPTER 34

Prognosis of Cardiovascular Diseases

Every physician must have had the unpleasant experience of making an entirely wrong prognosis in cases with cardiovascular diseases, even if his diagnosis was correct. This wrong prognosis may have been either in a favorable or in an unfavorable sense. In the first case, the patient unexpectedly took "a turn for the worse" or died suddenly. In the second, a severely ill patient recovered with amazing rapidity.

Several data need to be considered and the following brief discussion of them may be of help.

1) If the patient develops heart failure and *his heart rate is rapid*, the prognosis is better than otherwise because treatment may slow down his ventricular rate and bring about recovery. On the other hand, if the patient develops the same symptoms while already digitalized, prognosis is worse.

2) In general, *the larger the heart, the worse the prognosis*. However, remarkable exceptions to this rule should be kept in mind. One is represented by *acute rheumatic carditis in children*. An amazing enlargement of the heart accompanied by loud murmurs and a rapid and irregular pulse may be followed by complete recovery. Another exception is that of patients in their twenties with rheumatic heart disease and aortic and mitral involvement. As long as no evidence of heart failure is noted, the tremendous size of their heart is well tolerated. Another exception is represented by the large hearts of anemic, vitamin-deficient, or thyroid-deficient patients. Treatment usually leads to rapid decrease of cardiac size.

3) When a patient presents signs of congestion including distention of the veins, ascites, and edema, a careful study of the structural lesions should be done. *If the patient has mitral valve lesions, the clinical picture indicates congestive failure*, and prognosis is more guarded. *If the patient has mitral plus tricuspid lesions, the clinical picture of congestion is due to mechanical obstruction* and prognosis is more favorable: death of the patient may occur only 10 or 12 years later, and surgery of the valves may increase the period of survival. Further, *if the patient has a constrictive pericarditis, surgery may completely relieve him of any evidence of congestion.*

4) An important factor is represented by an *acute infection*. While this may endanger life and may be the direct or indirect cause of heart failure, it usually has a definite course. End of the infection is usually followed by recovery.

5) *Bronchopulmonary factors* may aggravate the picture of a cardiac patient and partly simulate signs of heart failure. These seem to aggravate prognosis while actually most of the patients recover. On the other hand, clear-cut *heart failure of chronic cor pulmonale has a poor prognosis.*

6) Obesity or neurocirculatory asthenia may aggravate or simulate cardiac dyspnea without increasing too much the severity of the prognosis.

7) *Nocturnal paroxysmal dyspnea* is usually a severe sign. However, if it puts the physician on the alert, and adequate measures are taken, the patient may live many years after the first episode.

8) *Acute pulmonary edema* is a dramatic occurrence which seems to be, and frequently is, fatal. The longer the patient survives, the greater is the hope. Many procedures and drugs enable the physician to prolong life for several hours, thus improving the prognosis.

9) *Triple rhythm* at the apex and *pulsus alternans* are ominous signs, both in arterial hypertension and in coronary heart disease. However, all clinical signs should be evaluated before formulating an unfavorable prognosis. Decreased blood pressure obtained through drug therapy or sympathectomy, digitalization, or gradual recovery of a coronary patient, may lead to disappearance of the above signs.

10) A patient with a *thyroid heart* has usually a much better prognosis than warranted by the initial impression.

11) *Chronic nephritis* invariably aggravates the prognosis of a cardiac patient, including cases with hypertension.

12) In spite of the remarkable results of antibiotics, *subacute bacterial endocarditis* still requires a guarded prognosis, unless diagnosis is made early and therapy is started at once.

13) *A massive pulmonary embolism* has usually a poor prognosis. Even if the patient recovers, further episodes may occur.

14) Prognosis is always difficult in patients with *angina pectoris*. Among the unpredictable elements, one is represented by the various parts that the right and left coronary arteries play in the blood supply to the left ventricle (page 25), a fact which cannot be ascertained during life.

15) *Following a myocardial infarct*, prognosis should be guided by the presence or absence of acute pulmonary edema, shock, A-V block, ventricular tachycardia, cerebral episodes, thromboembolic phenomena, or evidence of congestive failure. Early therapy of shock and of pulmonary edema has somewhat improved the outlook of these fearful complications. Still, prognosis is poor when shock or cerebral embolism occur.

Ultimate prognosis of a cardiac patient is always difficult. Among the various data to consider, age and sex, duration of the disease, extent of structural damage, possible influence of therapy, and possible future complications, should be taken into consideration.

BIBLIOGRAPHY

1. LEVINE, S. A. New England J. Med., 1936, **207,** 173.
2. WHITE, P. D. J. A. M. A., 1939, **112,** 2380.

CHAPTER 35

Management of the Cardiac Patient

How to Deal with a Cardiac Patient

The first problem is whether to tell *the truth* to cardiac patients and, if so, how to present the facts. This question cannot be answered in a simple manner because the personality of the patient and the severity of his disease impose various approaches.

The progress of common knowledge on the one hand and the importance of a full understanding between physician and patient on the other exclude cloaking of the truth in vague generalities as it was often done in the past. However, not many severely ill patients are able to face naked truth, and the dangers of a moral collapse should be taken into consideration. Therefore, except for a few patients who actually *want* the truth, this will be told with a certain attenuation for the sake of preventing a serious shock.

The duty of the physician imposes that, whenever the full truth is not disclosed to the patient, this is done to a close relative or to a close friend.

It should not be forgotten that too much concealing of the truth may prevent the patient from taking serious and needed precautionary measures, thereby impairing recovery or a financial settlement.

In the relationship between physician and patient, a friendly and cheerful approach can be as useful as the best drugs in improving the condition of the patient. The preoccupation of keeping medicine within the limits of a "science" should not supersede the traditional "bedside manner" which is a necessary part of the treatment.

The progress of common knowledge is such that *some medical terms are feared by most people*. "Coronary occlusion", "coronary thrombosis", and "high blood pressure" are among these. Others, which were feared in the past, such as "angina pectoris" and "arteriosclerosis" are now less known. Again, others, such as "low blood pressure" and "extrasystoles" are becoming increasingly fashionable and feared. Unnecessary mention of these terms may be the source of long-lasting neuroses. On the other hand, it is often useful that the patient know the approximate level of his blood pressure or the nature of an acute illness, for future reference.

The Life and Activity of a Cardiac Patient

The cardiac patient who wants to live long should *rearrange* his existence so that the maximum utilization of his energies is obtained with the minimum effort.

In cardiac or hypertensive patients without heart failure, the patient should avoid hurry. This requires a perfect mental timing, the exclusion of activities of secondary importance, and the avoidance of exacting social events.

A tremendous saving of energy is obtained by avoiding physical strain; sitting whenever possible; climbing slowly; and talking slowly. This does not mean that the patient should behave like an invalid. On the contrary, moderate physical activity, such as walking on flat ground and respiratory gymnastics should be advised.

In certain cases, the cardiac patient should be instructed to quit his occupation and to look for one of a sedentary nature.

Professions involving severe responsibilities and emotions should also be excluded even if they do not require physical strain.

The *avoidance of strong emotions* should be attempted by patients. Some, if properly instructed, build a "shell" of emotional stability which is frequently useful, especially in coronary heart disease.

Climates which are not subjected to sudden changes of temperature and humidity are the best for hypertensive, rheumatic, and coronary patients. Sojourns above 1500 feet of *altitude* are often poorly tolerated by cardiac patients (unless they are accustomed to them or were born at high levels) and should be forbidden.

Air travel in commercial planes with pressurized cabins is permitted (12). In certain cases, a brief air trip is preferable to a long train or boat voyage, even in severely ill patients. The patient should carry full written instructions and should avoid hustling or carrying heavy baggage.

Certain patients should not fly above 4500 feet without pressurization (128). They are the following:

a) Patients with marked anoxia and hemoglobin saturation lower than 80 per cent.

b) Cases with reduced pulmonary ventilation (chronic cor pulmonale, mitral lesions, cardiac disorders with pulmonary changes).

c) Coronary patients who suffered from an acute attack within 60 days prior to the flight.

d) Cardiac patients with anemia and an erythrocyte count below 3,000,000 or hemoglobin below 8 grams.

e) Patients who suffered recently from a cerebrovascular episode.

f) Subjects with severe heart failure.

In all such cases, the use of oxygen, either by tube or by mask, is recommended from the very start and during the whole flight, if this becomes necessary.

Airsickness should be prevented. Intestinal distention should be treated before the flight.

Rest is an extremely useful part of treatment. Cardiac patients should stay in bed 12 hours out of 24 and, if possible, rest on a couch 1 or 2 hours in the afternoon.

When cardiac failure occurs, an initial period of 8 to 10 days in bed is often useful. On the other hand, the *abuse of rest* is liable to cause damage. It has been demonstrated that extreme restriction of body movements causes increased mortality in animals with experimental myocardial lesions (1). Too prolonged rest may result in various complications, including phlebothrombosis, hypostatic pneumonia, bed sores, pleural effusion, and increased dyspnea (2). Therefore, even if the activity of the patient should be limited so that no dyspnea occurs, he will be allowed to sit in a comfortable chair for some hours every day.

Patients in failure after a coronary occlusion should be kept in bed for the prescribed period of 2 two 3 weeks like the others. They may need to be propped up in order to avoid orthopnea. The "easy-chair treatment" of these patients (13) is not advisable for psychological and practical reasons.

Diet for Cardiac Patients

Initial dietary treatment of heart failure may be based on a purely *fluid diet* containing no salt. In such conditions, free fluid intake may be permitted (6). It is the author's view that a limitation of fluid to between 1000 and 2000 cc. is preferable to ingestion of large amounts. For this reason, a fluid diet based on the ingestion of sweetened tea or fruit juice and water may be helpful for the first 24 to 48 hours (diet **V**).

After this initial period, a *modified Karell diet* should be prescribed for a limited time, usually from 3 to 7 days (diet **VI**). This diet accomplishes a certain limitation of fluid, a severe limitation of salt, and a limitation of proteins. At the same time, it supplies about 900 calories.

The subsequent dietary treatment will be based on the following considerations.

In cardiac failure the gastrointestinal functions are often severely impaired (3, 4). When anorexia is present, the hunger contractions are decreased, tone is diminished, peristalsis is slow, and the gastric emptying time is prolonged. These disturbances are largely responsible for the *lack of appetite* and *nausea* which are so frequent. Drug therapy often increases the nausea. Elevation of portal venous pressure and impaired capillary circulation of the intestines further account for a poor absorption while hepatic congestion inhibits utilization of vitamin B (5). For these reasons, protein and vitamin deficiencies are common.

Self-limitation often causes severe malnourishment and this is even more severe on account of elevated metabolic rate (4).

Restriction of sodium chloride favors readsorption of edema (7), a reduction from 5 to 2 gm. a day resulting in the elimination of about 0.5 liter (8). However, the most important result is the prevention of further fluid retention after diuresis has been obtained. It should be remembered that 45 gm. of animal protein contain about 1 gm. of salt, unless this is removed by prolonged boiling.

Extreme salt restriction may cause loss of appetite and some degree of malnutrition in regard to thiamin and nitrogen (8). It may further cause a more complex clinical picture called *low salt syndrome*. Anorexia may be prevented by using salts not containing sodium (100).

Food intake increases cardiac output. For this reason, the patient fares better on a 5-meal than on a 3-meal regime (4). Therefore, the following rules should be followed after the initial treatment.

a) Highly concentrated and easily digestible food.

b) Caloric intake between 1500 and 2000 calories daily.

c) About 200 gm. of carbohydrates, 40 to 50 of proteins, and 100 of fats, represent the optimum for these patients (9).

d) Foods rich in vitamin B_1 should be included. These prolong the action of vitamin B_1 given by injection, even if they might not be effective without the latter (10). An example of this is diet **VII.**

Ambulatory cardiac patients and patients with arteriosclerosis, arterial hypertension, or coronary heart disease without severe renal impairment, may follow diet **VIII.** A low protein content is supplied by diet **IV.**

Venesection and Other Procedures

Venesection is an old procedure which is too often neglected. It consists of the removal of 200 to 500 cc. of blood from one of the veins of the arm by use of a large bore needle. When a larger quantity is desired, as in exceptional cases, a scalpel incision is necessary. However, 800 cc. represent a maximum which should not be surpassed. Venesection often gives relief by interrupting a vicious circle.

The indications for venesection are: congestive failure with high venous pressure, peripheral edema, and dyspnea; paroxysmal dyspnea or pulmonary edema; severe arterial hypertension with acute cerebral manifestations. Anemia is a contraindication.

The *application of tourniquets* to the four limbs should be equivalent to venesection. However, it is usually less effective. It may be done with four rubber tubes or pneumatic cuffs. They are kept in place for 1 to 2 hours, but every 15 minutes one of them is released in order to restore circulation in the limb.

Paracentesis is indicated when effusion into serous cavities persists and causes disturbing symptoms, after the action of digitalis and mercurial diuretics. Removal of 500 to 1000 cc. of pleural fluid may greatly attenuate dyspnea. Removal should be slow and not more than 1500 cc. should be removed on one occasion in order to prevent the dreaded occurrence of pulmonary edema.

Paracentesis of the pericardium is indicated in pericarditis.

Abdominal paracentesis may be necessary

in certain cases with tricuspid valve defects or constrictive pericarditis.

Thyroidectomy has been advocated in congestive failure (11) considering that cardiac output might become adequate if the basal metabolic rate is reduced. The procedure is indicated only in a small percentage of cases, while most of the others would not obtain appreciable benefits.

Bedpan Versus Commode

It is customary to use the bedpan for cardiac patients. However, defecation on the bedpan is difficult and sometimes dangerous. It is occasionally responsible for sudden death. Comparative studies have shown that oxygen consumption is significantly lower when the patients sit on a commode than when they strain on a bedpan (14). The commode should be preferred, and the patient should be supported during the entire procedure.

BIBLIOGRAPHY

1. HARRISON, T. R. J. A. M. A., 1944, **125**, 1076.
2. LEVINE, S. A. J. A. M. A., 1944, **126**, 80. Also Mo. Conc. Cardiov. Dis., 1945, **14**, N. 3.
3. VAN LIERE, E. J. *Anoxia. Its Effect on the Body*. Chicago, Univ. of Chicago Press, 1942.
4. HARRISON, J. V. J. Am. Diet. Assoc., 1945, **21**, 86.
5. a) POLLACK, H., AND CO-WORKERS. Proc. Soc. Exper. Biol. & Med., 1940, **98**, 44.
   b) GRIEG, M. E., AND GOVIER, W. M. J. Pharmacol. & Exper. Therap., 1943, **169**, 79.
6. a) NEWBURGH, L. H., AND MACKINNON, F. *The Practice of Dietetics*. New York, Macmillan, 1934.
   b) SCHEMM, F. R. Ann. Int. Med., 1942, **17**, 952.
   c) BRIDGES, W. C., WHEELER, E. O., AND WHITE, P. D. New England J. Med., 1946, **234**, 573.
7. a) SCHROEDER, H. A. Am. Heart J., 1941, **22**, 141.
   b) PROGER, S., GINSBERG, E., AND MAGENDANTZ, H. Am. Heart J., 1942, **23**, 555.
8. ALTSCHULE, M. D. Bull. New England Med. Center, 1945, **7**, 245.
9. BROMER, A. W., AND STROUD, W. D. In *Stroud's Cardiovascular Diseases*. Philadelphia, Davis, 1945.
10. FREEDBERG, A. S., AND BLUMGART, H. L. New England J. Med., 1943, **229**, 939.
11. BLUMGART, H. L., LEVINE, S. A., AND BERLIN, D. Arch. Int. Med., 1933, **51**, 866.
12. a) WHITTINGHAM, H., *et al*. Brit. M. J., 1949, **1**, 603.
    b) MENDOZA, F. Rev. Inv. Clin. (Mexico), 1949, **1**, 85.
13. LEVINE, S. A. J. A. M. A., 1952, **148**, 1365.
14. BENTON, J. G. J. A. M. A., 1950, **144**, 1443.

CHAPTER 36

Medical Treatment of Common Cardiac Conditions

In each chapter on the various cardiac diseases, the description of the clinical picture was followed by a brief paragraph of treatment. Later, treatment of heart failure was discussed in the chapter dealing with digitalis and the cardiac glycosides (page 583). However, treatment is the most important part of medicine and an outline of the main points which should be followed in the treatment of the most common cardiac conditions may be useful to the practitioner.

In doing this, emphasis will be placed on some personal views which may differ from those of others. This should be kept in mind when reading the following paragraphs.

1. Rheumatic Fever

Treatment of the acute stage is based on a) *bedrest*, and b) *cortisone* (or compound F) or *aspirin* (page 198).

Bedrest should be prolonged for many months. *Cortisone* or *aspirin* should be given for not less than 8 weeks. Their doses are larger at the beginning, then gradually decreased. Cortisone should be supplemented by potassium salt by mouth and periodic injections of mercurial diuretics. The blood content of salicylates (aspirin) should be checked and maintained at an optimum level. Aspirin is effective only if large doses, far higher than those used in symptomatic therapy, are used.

Cortisone seems superior in severe cases with heart failure; aspirin is better in cases with poliarthritis. Occasionally, a patient responds to one of the drugs better than to the other. An aspirin cycle may be useful following cortisone, and small doses of aspirin may be continued even during the gradual period of mobilization.

Whenever signs of heart failure occur, the patient should be given *oxygen* and should be digitalized. The best glycoside for these patients is *gitalin* (page 589).

Pericarditis may require paracentesis (page 449).

The *prevention of recurrences* is extremely important and should be done by a long-range (2 to 6 years) oral administration of *sulfadiazine* or *penicillin* (page 198).

Prophylaxis in nonrheumatic people may be attempted whenever the conditions of crowding, exposure to cold and humidity, and physical strain occur (camps, military life).

The importance of rest, suitable climate, and tonsillectomy in rheumatic patients has been outlined (page 199).

2. Acute Bacterial Endocarditis

Acute bacterial endocarditis should be prevented in most cases by penicillin prophylaxis in cardiacs submitted to dental or surgical interventions and by an adequate antibiotic treatment of general infections (sore throats, pneumonia, meningitis, gonorrhea, etc.). Once the endocarditis has started, testing of the agent *in vitro* for possible resistance, and adequate selection of the antibiotic, should be done. In most cases, *penicillin* is adequate (page 206). Doses vary in the different cases from 600,000 to 10 million units (or more) every 24 hours. The treatment should be continued until complete disappearance of the fever and normalization of the sedimentation rate are obtained. It should be kept in mind that early treatment may not prevent the establishment of valvular defects. If the patient is severely anemic, *blood transfusions* are necessary.

3. Subacute Bacterial Endocarditis

Whenever the diagnosis of subacute bacterial endocarditis is made, treatment with high doses of *penicillin* should be started immediately. The doses to be used are larger than in acute endocarditis and may vary between 1 and 20 million units daily, the latter dose being reserved for the most resistant cases. Treatment will be continued for about 1 month, then repeated with a higher dosage if blood sterility is not obtained.

If the active agent of the disease is unaffected by *penicillin*, then *streptomycin, aureomycin, chloromycetin, emetin,* or *neo-arsphenamine* (higher organisms) can be tried. *In vitro* tests should precede the selection of the antibiotic (page 210).

Vitamin C, iron, blood transfusions, and a high-calorie diet may contribute to the recovery.

If cardiac failure occurs, the patient will be treated as any other patient in failure.

The possibility of a combined rheumatic and bacterial endocarditis should be kept in mind; in such cases, penicillin treatment should be done first and followed by aspirin or cortisone.

Demonstration that surgical or dental interventions in cardiac patients may lead to the occurrence of subacute bacterial endocarditis (page 211) advises the systematic use of penicillin before and after such procedures. This will prevent a large percentage of infections even if some still seem beyond prophylaxis.

4. Cardiovascular Syphilis

Cardiovascular lesions caused by lues generally occur many years after the initial infection. Therefore, adequate treatment of the initial infection prevents cardiovascular lesions. Once these lesions have appeared, the general rules of antiluetic treatment should be followed (page 201). However, the following considerations should be kept in mind. Whenever a luetic lesion of the myocardium is present, intensive treatment may lead to congestion of the inflamed areas or destruction and fluidification of the gummata. In both cases, the repercussion on the myocardium may lead to severe and, at times, irreversible failure. Moreover, the efficiency of the myocardium may be impaired by the toxicity of the antiluetic drugs. For these reasons, treatment should be careful and gradual at first. It will be started with *iodides,* then continued with courses of *bismuth* alternated with *mercurials.* After some months of treatment, *neo-arsphenamine* or *penicillin* may be used. Even then, only three-fourths of the maximum dose will be reached, in order to avoid a toxic lesion of the myocardium.

5. Rheumatic Valvular Defects

Well-compensated patients with *mitral lesions* do not need digitalization. They should be advised against strenuous physical exertion and excess of food, drink, or stimulants (pages 224 and 579). If the patient complains of palpitation or presents premature beats, *bromides, quinidine,* or *phenobarbital* may be indicated.

Digitalization is indicated whenever physical strain cannot be avoided and in the last stages of pregnancy even without apparent failure (page 579).

The first signs of failure indicate the need for *digitalis;* the use of the latter is outlined below (page 621).

Patients with *aortic lesions* and no symptoms do not need special treatment. They should be cautioned against strenuous exertion and against driving (possibility of dizziness). A mild sedation by means of *phenobarbital, seconal, bromides, chloral hydrate,* and, occasionally, *tincture of opium,* may help in preventing paroxysmal attacks. *Aminophylline* or *khellin* may be useful in hypertensives; *potassium iodide* in luetic and arteriosclerotic patients (page 529).

Whenever digitalization is started, extreme bradycardia and toxicity should be avoided. *Strophanthin* has no special indication; *squill* glycosides may be used for mild and prolonged treatments; *gitalin* is especially indicated in cases with rheumatic carditis. Pure glycosides should be preferred to total digitalis because they have a more constant action and may be given by weight.

Mercurial diuretics may be used in certain cases, at not too frequent intervals, in order to prevent fluid retention. The same purpose is accomplished by salt restriction.

Commissurotomy should be done only in cases of severe mitral stenosis with evidence of pulmonary congestion. Surgery of double and combined valvular defects is still under experimentation and several years must pass before a complete knowledge of the various indications and contraindications is acquired.

Patients with *tricuspid defects* present signs of congestion which are caused by the obstruction. For this reason, *digitalis* may relieve only part of them (page 564). Even when heart failure is present, *mercurial diuretics, ammonium chloride* and *periodic paracenteses* obtain results which are more striking than those of digitalis (page 275.) *Squill glycosides* may be substituted for digitalis with advantage, having a greater diuretic effect. Salt restriction is imperative. *Commissurotomy* can be attempted in severe tricuspid stenosis.

In *pulmonary stenosis*, surgical dilatation of the pulmonic ostium should be considered. If pulmonary tuberculosis develops, its treatment is imperative; *collapse therapy* is tolerated well; *thoracoplasty* is not contraindicated. If heart failure occurs, *oxygen* inhalation is particularly useful, together with drug therapy.

6. Congenital Shunts and Complex Malformations

Patients with *atrial* or *ventricular septal defect* need no different treatment from patients with acquired valvular defects. The same rules concerning abstention from unnecessary medication, the use of *mild sedatives*, and the rules concerning exertion, food, and drink, are valid for them. Whenever congestive failure occurs, the patients will be *digitalized* with the customary method. This is also true for patients with a *patent ductus arteriosus*. However, *surgery* is imperative in patent ductus and should be considered in atrial septal defects.

Patients with *complex malformations* of the heart should be treated like patients with acquired valvular defects. Their cyanosis is usually *not* caused by congestive failure and does not require special treatment. In the judgment of how much physical activity should be permitted, one has to pay attention to the various symptoms. The severity of policythemia, dyspnea and tachycardia are the best gauges. *Digitalization*, when necessary, is made with the customary rules. *Oxygen* therapy may be a useful coadjuvant. *Surgical treatment* improves the outlook of patients with *tetralogy of Fallot* (page 317) and in other malformations with pulmonic stenosis and low pulmonic pressure.

Disturbances of the Heart Rate and Rhythm

Atrial flutter can be treated by a toxic dose of *digitalis* which increases the excitability of the myocardium and causes fibrillation (page 343). The latter will be treated as outlined below. If digitalis fails, quinidine usually does not help but may be tried. Spontaneous recovery from the flutter is not unusual.

Attacks of *atrial tachycardia* are treated *in a reflex way*, by *intravenous digoxin*, or by subcutaneous *prostigmin* (page 335).

Both the reflex action and the drugs cause intense stimulation of the vagus nerve. If this is of no avail, depression of the sympathetic or direct action on the myocardium (quinidine) can be tried. Prevention of the attacks requires consideration of all possible causes, and their removal. Autonomic depression with *ergotamin plus atropine* may be tried). Prolonged treatment with *quinidine, prostigmin,* or *digoxin* is useful in some cases.

No reflex stimulation should be tried in *ventricular tachycardia.* Intravenous or oral *pronestyl,* or intravenous *magnesium sulfate* give the best results (page 339). Prevention of the attacks is based on the use (or exclusion) of digitalis, *quinidine, pronestyl,* or *aminophyllin,* according to the underlying lesions (page 339).

The treatment of *Stokes-Adams attacks* requires a careful study of the conditions preceding them. If the attacks are due to vagal stimuli, *atropine plus ephedrine* or *papaverine* are indicated. If, on the contrary, the attacks are due to sympathetic stimuli, *digitalis* or *hydergine* should be used (page 363). In general, cases with coronary heart disease improve with *vasodilators.*

Whenever a *partial heart block* is present, recognition of the cause may permit a causal treatment. This is possible in luetic, rheumatic, diphtheritic, and gonorrheal myocarditis.

In cases presenting *premature beats,* a careful study of the underlying conditions and of the favoring causes may permit the removal of many of them with the resulting disappearance of the arrythmia (page 353). Among the different drugs used for this condition, *quinidine* and *ergotamine plus atropine* are useful. The combination of *papaverine, quinidine,* and *atropine* is useful in coronary heart disease (page 435).

Atrial fibrillation should be treated with *digitalis glycosides* if it occurs as a result of heart failure. If the sinus rhythm is not reestablished after disappearance of the signs of congestive failure, then fibrillation should be treated with *quinidine. Quinidine treatment* should be used in all cases where signs of congestive failure are not present or have disappeared. Paroxysmal atrial fibrillation should be treated with *atropine* and *oxygen.*

Atrial fibrillation after myocardial infarction should be treated with *quinidine* if there is no congestive failure and no block; with *quinidine plus digitalis* if heart failure is also present. It should be kept in mind that vagus stimulation may favor atrial fibrillation. For this reason, strongly digitalized patients frequently fibrillate and are more resistant to treatments which favor a reestablishment of the sinus rhythm.

8. Myocardial Lesions

Triple rhythm, alternans, bundle branch block, and dilatation and hypertrophy of the heart are merely signs of a cardiac lesion and not clinical entities in themselves. Therefore, no special treatment is required. When many signs indicate initial heart failure or strain, *digitalization* is indicated. Rest and avoidance of excessive food and fluid intake are useful. In hypertensive patients, a decrease of cardiac strain may be obtained by reducing blood pressure, at least temporarily (page 501).

The myocardial lesions may be grouped under two headings, the acute and subacute on the one hand, and the chronic on the other. In the *acute and subacute lesions,* the physician should try to ascertain the cause. Recognition of rheumatic, luetic, malarial, amebic, diphtheritic, or streptococcic myocarditis may lead to cure of the lesion (page 389). *In general, the existence of lesions of the myocardium requires a careful and gradual treatment and the avoidance of massive doses which might increase damage to the heart muscle.*

It should be kept in mind that the existence of acute myocardial lesions may cause increased excitability and abnormal reactions. Therefore, if *digitalis* is needed, caution should be used in the dosage. Selection of a glycoside with a large *therapeutic ratio*, such as *gitalin* (page 589), may increase the safety of the treatment.

Chronic myocardial lesions are usually caused by coronary heart disease and will be considered below.

Treatment of *ventricular standstill* is based on the *intracardiac injection of epinephrine plus procaine* (page 395). *Resuscitation of the heart* may also be obtained by manual percussion of the precordium or by opening the chest and manual massage.

Defibrillation of the ventricles may be obtained by intracardiac injection of *procaine*, followed by *electrical stimulation* of the heart (page 395). This causes a standstill and should be followed by intracardiac epinephrine and massage.

Treatment of heart disease caused by *vitamin B deficiency* is based upon the parenteral administration of the *vitamin B-complex*, and a high-protein, low-carbohydrate diet (page 404).

Routine treatment of the *thyrocardiac syndrome* is medical at first and surgical later (page 406). However, use of *propylthiouracil* may avoid the need for surgery.

Treatment of the *myxedema heart* is effected by means of *thyroid extract*. The doses must be small at first, then slowly increased.

9. Coronary Heart Disease

Coronary heart disease may lead to various clinical pictures. *Myocardial fibrosis* does not require special treatment unless accompanied by heart failure.

Myocardial infarction. The treatment should be as follows (page 429):

Large doses of *hypnotics* and *sedatives* in the first 2 to 4 days in order to relieve pain and to prevent dangerous reflexes. *Morphine*, *atropine* and *phenobarbital* should be used. *Oxygen* is given.

As soon as pain has disappeared and the first days have elapsed, *papaverine* and smaller doses of *phenobarbital* are given.

Digitalis, as a rule, should not be given in the initial stage. It may be given later if required by heart failure but preferably in combination with *quinidine* (pages 430 and 592).

Shock requires the customary remedies but treatment should be started very early. *Transfusions* and *infusions* should be of smaller volume and given at a slower rate than when myocardial infarction is not present. *Noradrenaline* is given together with plasma or plasma substitutes.

Initial immobility for 2 to 3 weeks and bedrest later are customary. They are useful but should not be unduly prolonged (page 623).

Anticoagulants should be given in a majority of cases, with the exception of "minor" or "benign" attacks, and attacks in young persons without severe clinical picture (page 429). *Heparin* and *dicumarol* are given at first, then heparin is discontinued (page 594).

The treatment of *angina pectoris* should be based upon proper evaluation of the dynamic, functional, and psychic elements of the syndrome and on their possible exclusion (page 435). Patients with angina should not eat a heavy meal at night and should not go to bed with a full stomach. They should not drink much fluid with their meals and should be careful in the use of tobacco (page 435). Physical exercise should be limited but not abolished; open air exercise and exposure to cold should be forbidden. Any cause for increased cardiac work, vagal reflexes, or anoxemia should be prevented.

Treatment of the attack of angina pectoris is based on the use of rapid-acting vasodilators (*nitroglycerine*). Between the attacks, slower-acting vasodilators are best, like *khellin*, *peritrate*, *rauwolfia*, and *mannitol* (page 596). Different *surgical interventions* have been advocated but they should be used only in selected groups of patients (page 435).

10. Pericardial Lesions

Whenever possible, causal treatment of *acute pericarditis* should be undertaken. Pyogenic, amebic, and luetic pericarditis should be treated with *specific drugs* or *antibiotics*. The intrapericardial injection of penicillin has proven helpful in addition to general treatment (page 449). *Salicylates* in full doses influence the course of rheumatic pericarditis. *Morphine* is necessary if severe pain or dyspnea is present. *Digitalis* is not contraindicated but is seldom useful. *Venesection* is contraindicated (page 449). *Paracentesis of the pericardium* is frequently necessary and is performed with the technique indicated on page 449. Paracentesis should not be performed too early unless severe cardiac embarrassment is present.

Constrictive pericarditis often requires the use of *mercurial diuretics* and *ammonium chloride*. *Digitalis* is not contraindicated but is seldom useful. Paracentesis of the abdominal cavity may be necessary. *Surgery* should be resorted to in the great majority of cases and the most radical intervention is the most beneficial (page 459). *Atropine*, *pronestyl*, and *morphine* limit the excitability of the heart during the operation. If necessary, the direct application of *procaine* may be of help.

11. Aortic Syndromes

Surgical treatment of *coarctation of the aorta* is the treatment of choice. It should be done as early as possible (page 473).

Aortitis, aneurysm. The general treatment of cardiovascular syphilis has been outlined already (page 201). Rest is beneficial; *morphine* or other sedatives may be necessary. *Paravertebral alcohol injections* may relieve pain. While an aneurysm of the extremities or the abdominal aorta may be excised successfully, resection of a thoracic aneurysm is seldom possible. However, *wiring* of the aneurysm or *wrapping* it in cellophane is frequently beneficial.

There is no treatment for a *dissecting aneurysm of the aorta* except bedrest and sedation. *Embolism of the abdominal aorta*, on the other hand, may be treated by *surgical intervention* within the first 12 hours. *Priscoline, papaverine*, application of suction and pressure, and therapy for shock, are useful coadjuvants (page 487).

12. Arterial Hypertension

The drug treatment of hypertension is frequently disappointing. However, the results are such that they justify drug therapy because this limits or delays the onset and severity of complications.

The combination of *rauwolfia with veratrum alkaloids*, and *the sympatholytics or adrenolytics (hydergine, dibenamine, hexamethonium)* are at the center of interest.

Barbiturates are often useful but should not be prescribed for use in daytime unless the patient is committed to bedrest. The use of *bromides* and *iodides* may be advocated.

Unilateral nephrectomy is a life-saving procedure whenever a renal lesion is unilateral or sharply more severe on one side.

Sympathectomy may give good results in selected cases.

Diet therapy is again useful, especially in the obese patients (page 501).

The use of *renal extracts* is still in the experimental stage but represents the greatest hope for the future.

13. Cor Pulmonale

Medical treatment of *pulmonary embolism* is based on injections of *morphine, atropine*, and *papaverine* as well as *oxygen* administration (page 509). Care should be taken not to lower excessively systemic blood pressure. While shock is one of the dangers, coronary insufficiency may increase the severity of the clinical picture.

Embolectomy is possible only in the first hours. Preventive measures are based on use of *heparin* or *dicumarol* and preventive *venous ligation* (page 509).

Patients with *chronic cor pulmonale* frequently respond poorly to treatment because of the combination of mechanical, pulmonary, and cardiac elements. Surgical correction of chest deformities, lobectomy in cases of a-v aneurysms, and antiluetic treatment should be used in different categories of patients. *Oxygen* is useful is most cases; *ephedrine* or *isupral*, in patients with bronchial asthma and emphysema (page 515).

Digitalis is useful whenever there is heart failure but care should be exercised not to stimulate the vagus nerve unduly, thereby favoring asthmatic attacks. Cautious dosage and its combination with atropine may permit the use of digitalis without danger. *Aminophylline* is helpful in most cases. *Morphine* should be used with the greatest caution.

14. Hypotension—Shock

In *acute hypotension*, treatment varies with the cause (page 519). *Adrenalin* or *noradrenalin, venous infusions, blood transfusions*, and the occasional use of *sedatives* are indicated in the different cases.

Orthostatic hypotension may require various treatments which range from the use of a head-up bed to that of a tight girdle, and from the administration of *atropine-phenobarbital* to that of *paredrinol* (page 520).

Chronic hypotension is influenced favorably by *ephedrine, benzedrine, metrazol*, and *strychnine* (page 520).

Shock is treated by reassurance, oxygen, rest, warmth, fluids, and infusion with *plasma* or *plasma substitutes*. This program is still valid but often inadequate. Owing to the extreme difficulty of changing the conditions of the irreversible stage, *angiotonin* seems to be the most effective remedy. Its use is not common as yet but it is expected that it will be in the future (page 521).

Hyposphygmia. Drugs stimulating the peripheral vessels are useful in cases with acute or chronic infections. These are *ephedrine, benzedrine, paredrinol*, and *metrazol*. Congenital hyposphygmia requires a full diet; large doses of *vitamin B-complex;*

caffeine, strychnine, coramine, or *paredrinol;* physiotherapy and massage; and open-air physical exercise (page 523).

15. Arterial Diseases

Diffuse arteriosclerosis may be limited, and possibly decreased, by sharp limitation of fat and cholesterol intake and control of the caloric intake. A series of instructions and precautions may prevent a rapid mental and physical degeneration of the patient (page 528). *Potassium iodide* has a mild beneficial action; *theophyllin* and *aminophyllin* are frequently useful as are *bromides, chloral*, and *barbiturates* (page 529).

Acute arteritis may be treated by means of *vasodilators* and *heparin* in the initial stage. When gangrene is present, amputation becomes necessary. In *embolic arteritis, heparin, intermittent venous compression, vasodilators*, or *sympathetic block* can be used, even if *embolectomy* represents the most important step (page 530).

In *Buerger's disease*, abstention from tobacco is imperative. *Vasodilators, mecholyl*, and *papaverine* may be useful, as well as *suction and pressure exercises* (page 533).

In *intermittent claudication*, the treatment is that of the underlying vascular disease. A medical and physical treatment, similar to that of Buerger's disease, may be advocated (page 535).

Acrocyanosis may be treated with *estrogens, physiotherapy*, and *paredrinol*. *Raynaud's disease* should be treated with *mecholyl, prostigmin*, and *papaverine*. *Sympathectomy* may obtain good results (page 535). *Erythromelalgia* improves following the use of *adrenalin, ephedrine*, and *calcium*.

16. Diseases of the Veins

Phlebitis is treated by elevation of the part, motion, and *no* ice bag for 10 to 14 days (page 540). Prevention of embolism is based on *surgical ligation* or *prolonged use of anticoagulants* (page 509).

Varicose veins may be treated by *local injections*, causing the obliteration of some vessels (page 542), or by *ligation* (page 540). Elastic stockings and bandages give symptomatic relief. *Local penicillin* treatment is useful in varicose ulcers (also tyrothricin and gentian violet). An *arteriovenous aneurysm* should be treated, whenever possible, by *surgical elimination* of the connection (page 544).

17. Paroxysmal Cardiorespiratory Attacks

The treatment of *paroxysmal dyspnea* is based on subcutaneous injection of *morphine sulfate, oxygen* inhalation, and *venesection. Atropine* may be useful in cases of mixed mechanism, if there is bronchospasm.

In *paroxysmal pulmonary edema, alcohol vapor-oxygen inhalation* should be used as an emergency measure which may be lifesaving by decreasing the amount of foam (page 560). During inhalation of the vapors, drug therapy can be initiated. In hypertensive or mitral patients, *morphine sulfate,* i.v. *sodium luminal,* i.v. *mercurial diuretics* should be injected, and venesection may be resorted to. In cases of coronary occlusion or cerebrovascular accidents, the danger of shock should be anticipated. Therefore, only moderate doses of morphine, barbiturates or mercurials should be given, and no venesection practiced. *Atropine* should be given only if there is bradycardia or severe wheezing. *Metrazol* and *coramine* also should be avoided during the attack (page 560).

The prevention of these attacks may be obtained by the regular administration of *chloral hydrate* by mouth or rectum, *phenobarbital,* and *aminophyllin.* Depression of the sympathetic system may be useful, especially in hypertensive patients. *Digitalization* may prevent recurrence of the attacks.

Heart failure may follow a severe attack of pulmonary edema. *Digitalization* should be effected following the customary rules.

Periodic respiration is ameliorated by the intravenous injection of *aminophyllin.*

If large doses of this drug fail to improve the condition, *metrazol* should be injected (page 561).

18. Heart Failure

Digitalis and the *digitalis-like plants* (*strophanthus, squill*) are still the most powerful remedies for heart failure. The writer favors the use of the *digitalis glycosides* (page 589) in comparison with the preparations made with dried leaves. This preference is based upon the conviction that similar results, rarer occurrence of disturbances, and easier handling of the patient are obtained with them.

Gitalin has the largest therapeutic ratio and is especially indicated in heart failure caused by rheumatic carditis or myocardial infarct. *Lanatoside C* is eliminated rapidly and is better tolerated than *digitoxin. Strophanthin* is eliminated very rapidly. Its use is limited to brief courses of therapy with one or two daily i. v. injections.

While the method of unitage (page 589) and the dosage of glycosides in milligrams permit a better judgment of the dose of active principles administered, it should be kept in mind that *the best assay is on the individual patient* and that all rules concerning digitalis are approximate (page 576).

Different methods of digitalization have been described (page 590). The writer does not favor the employment of massive doses of digitalis. If heart failure is severe and treatment is urgent, an *intravenous injection of either strophanthin or digoxin* and one or two more injections at 12-hour intervals permit a rapid action. Otherwise, a more gradual digitalization reaching the total dose in 3 to 4 days should be preferred.

In most cases, satisfactory digitalization may be obtained by using the following scheme:

1st day: 6 tablets of *digitoxin* (0.1 mg. each), *cedilanid* (0.5 mg. each), or *gitalin* (0.5 mg. each).

2nd and 3rd day: 4 tablets of *digitoxin,* or 3 of *cedilanid* or *gitalin.*

4th to 7th day: 1 or 2 tablets of each.

Maintenance dose is 1 to 2 tablets for any of these preparations (occasionally, alternated daily doses of 1 and 2 for some time).

A few guiding suggestions will be repeated here:

a) The best use for digitalis is found in heart failure.

Adequate digitalization must precede the daily administration of the maintenance dose of digitalis. Merely giving a "maintenance dose" without a prior raising of the concentration of digitalis to an optimum level results in an insufficient dose (page 588).

b) The improvement of the patient may take place even if the ventricular rate is not lowered and if atrial fibrillation is still present.

c) The best result from digitalis is obtained in mitral patients with heart failure and atrial fibrillation. Patients with aortic stenosis follow. Its administration in hypertensive and coronary heart disease with failure obtains a fair result. Heart failure in patients with cardiovascular syphilis yields poorly to digitalis.

d) Whenever acute myocarditis is present (rheumatic disease, diphtheria, etc.), digitalis administration is not followed by impressive results. The myocardium is overexcitable and easily damaged.

e) Large doses of digitalis are contraindicated in the first stage following coronary occlusion. In later stages, digitalis is better tolerated in association with quinidine.

f) Heart failure of myxedema, hyperthyroidism, thiamine deficiency, pericarditis with effusion, and adhesive pericarditis, is aided but little by digitalis.

g) Digitalis can be given in partial heart block but its dosage will be determined carefully in order not to overstimulate the vagus. It may be given safely in complete block.

h) *Prophylactic use of digitalis* in patients who *might* present heart failure at some future time is recommended for cardiac patients who become pregnant (last 3 months) or cannot avoid severe, although occasional, exertion.

In patients leading a normal life, prophylactic use of digitalis for many years may not prevent heart failure while at the same time may deprive the physician of the full freedom of use of one of his most powerful weapons. Therefore, either the use of *squill glycosides* or *periodic digitalization* (1 week every month) will be used.

Digitalization should be supplemented by periodic administration of *mercurial diuretics*, by *salt restriction*, and a series of general rules of conduct including psychological, physical, and social guidance.

Several procedures which tend to decrease the load placed on the heart may contribute to relief of heart failure. They include *venesection*, *oxygen administration*, hypotensive drugs (or sympathectomy), treatment of bronchial infections, *surgical correction* of valvular deformities or congenital anomalies, and hormonal or salicylate therapy of myocarditis.

APPENDICES

Prescriptions

(1) Digitalis powder
1-cat-unit pills (about 0.1 gm.) (gr. iss)
Maintenance dose: one tablet
daily

(2) *Crystodigin Lilly* (digitoxin)
Tablets 0.1 mg.
Maintenance dose: one to two
tablets daily

(3) *Crystodigin Lilly* (digitoxin)
Ampules for i.v. injections
1 cc. = 0.2 mg.

(4) *Digoxin Burroughs Wellcome*
(digoxin)
0.25-mg. tablets
Maintenance dose: one to two
tablets daily

(5) *Cedilanid Sandoz* (acetyldi-
goxin)
0.5-mg. tablets
Maintenance dose: one to two
tablets daily

(6) *Cedilanid Sandoz* (acetyldi-
goxin)
4-cc. ampules (0.8 mg.)
for i.v. injections

(7) *Gitaligin White Lab. Inc.* (gitalin)
0.5-mg. tablets
Maintenance dose: one to two
tablets daily

(8) *Gitaligin White Lab. Inc.* (gitalin)
5-cc. ampules (2.5 mg.)
for i.v. injections

(9) *K-Strophanthin Abbott*
(strophanthin)
Ampules (0.33 mg.);
Or *Strophosid Sandoz*
Ampules (0.25 mg.)
For i.v. injections

(10) *Scillaren Sandoz*
0.5-mg. tablets
Maintenance dose: one to three
tablets daily

(11) *Mercuhydrine Lakeside*
1-cc. and 2-cc. ampules
One every 3 to 5 days
By i.m. or i.v. injection

(12) *Thiomerin Campbell Prod.*
Rubber-cap vials with 1.4 gm.
of powder—dissolve in 10
cc. of distilled water. (40
mg. of Hg per cc.)
0.5 to 2 cc. by i.m. or i.v. injection

(13) Ammonium chloride
0.5-gm. enteric-coated tablets (gr. viiss)
Five tablets every 6 hours =
10 gm.
Repeat after 5 to 7 days.

(14) Aspirin
0.3-gm. tablets (gr. v)
Four tablets (1.2 gm.) every 3
hours
Maintain plasma salicylate
level at about 30 mg. per
cent.

(15) Aminopyrine
0.32-gm. tablets (gr. v)
One tablet t.i.d.

(16) *Salysal Rare Chem. Inc.*
0.32-gm. tablets (gr. v)
Three tablets every 4 hours
(Salysal is about twice as active as sodium salicylate.)

(17) *Sulfadiazine Lilly*
0.25-gm. tablets
Two b.i.d.

(18) *Penioral tablets Wyeth* (buf-
fered penicillin)
250,000-unit tablets
One b.i.d.

(19) *Procaine-G-Penicillin   Abbott*
(in aqueous suspension)
3 million units in 10-cc. vial
(One dose = 300,000 units by
i.m. injection)

(20) Morphine sulfate 15 mg.   (gr. ¼)
Atropine sulfate 1 mg.   (gr. ⅟₆₅)
By s.c. injection

(21) Atropine sulfate
0.25-mg. tablets   (gr. ⅟₂₅₀)
Three to eight in the 24 hours

(22) *Demerol Winthrop*
2-cc. ampules (= 100 mg.)
For i.m. injection

(23) *Demerol Winthrop*
50-mg. tablets
One every 6 hours

(24) Quinidine sulfate
0.2-gm. tablets
One to three tablets every 4
hours (only in daytime)

(25) *Quinidine gluconate Lilly*
0.8 gm. in 10-cc. rubber-cap
vials
Dilute with 50 cc. of 5 per cent
glucose.
Slow i.v. injection of 0.5 gm.

(26) *Pronestyl hydrochloride Squibb*
(procaine amide)
10 cc. of a 10 per cent aqueous
solution in a rubber-cap vial
(100 mg. per cc.)
100 to 500 mg. i.v.

(27) *Pronestyl hydrochloride Squibb*
(procaine amide)
0.25-gm. capsules for oral use.
Initial dose : 1 to 2.5 gm. within
2 hours.
Maintenance dose : 0.5 to 1 gm.
every 4 hours

(28) Phenobarbital
0.1 tablets   (gr. iss)
One at bedtime

(29) Phenobarbital
0.015 tablets   (gr. ¼)
one t.i.d.

(30) *Sodium luminal Merck* 150 mg.   (about gr. iiss)
    (ℨiiss)
Dissolve in 10 cc. of distilled
water.
Slow i.v. injection

(31) Sodium amytal
0.2-gm. capsules   (gr. iij)
One at bedtime

(32) Triple bromides 0.5 gm. with   (gr. viiss)
phenobarbital 16 mg.   (gr. ¼)
One tablet before retiring

(33) Chloral hydrate 2 gm.   (gr. XXX)
Glucose 25 gm.   (ℨvij)
Water ad cc. 500 by slow enema

(34) Chloral hydrate 10 gm.   (ℨiiss)
Simple syrup 30 gm.   (ℨj)
Water ad cc. 240   (ℨviij)
One tablespoonful at night, in   (gm. 0.5 or
water   gr. viiss)

(35) *Bellergal Sandoz*
Tablets—one t.i.d.
(Each contains
Atropine : 1 mg.
Ergotamine : 0.3 mg.
Phenobarbital : 20 mg.)

(36) *Hydergine Sandoz*
1-cc. ampules
(1 cc. = 0.3 mg.)
Average dose : 1 to 2 cc. daily

(37) *Dibenamine Givaudau-Delawan-
na*
5 per cent solution in 50 per
cent alcohol
I.v. injection of 5 mg./kilo by
the drip method over 60 to 75
minutes (total not above 500
mg.)

(38) *Etamon Parke, Davis* (benzodioxane)
20-cc. rubber-cap vials
(1 cc. = 100 mg.)
I.v. or i.m. injections
(I.v. dose not above 7 mg./kilo
I.m. dose not above 20 mg./
kilo)

(39) *Bistrium bromide Squibb* (hexamethonium bromide)
10-cc. vials (1 cc. = 25 mg.)
For i.v. or i.m. injections

I.v. injection at rate of 1 mg./ min.; maximum: 50 mg.
I.m. initial dose: 5 mg.
Larger doses given every 8 to 12 hours, increasing by 5 mg. each time

(40) *Methium Warner-Chilcott* (hexamethonium chloride)
125 mg. t.i.d. or q.i.d.
(Later, daily doses of 2 to 6 gm.)

(41) *Aminophyllin* 0.5 gm.   (gr. viiss)
Cocoa butter for a suppository

(42) *Aminiphyllin Searle*
20-cc. ampules (0.5 gm.)   (gr. viiss)
By i.v. injection

(43) *Papaverine hydrochloride Lilly*
0.1-gm. tablets   (gr. iss)
One t.i.d. or q.i.d.

(44) *Papaverine hydrochloride Lilly*
30-mg. ampules
One by i.m. or i.v. injection

(45) *Rauwiloid Riker* (rauwolfia)
2-mg. tablets
Initial dose: two tablets daily
Maintenance dose: one tablet daily

(46) *Veriloid Riker Lab.* (veratrum viride)
2-mg. tablets
One to two tablets t.i.d.

(47) *Veralba Pitman-Moore Co.* (protoveratrine)
0.2-mg. tablets
Two tablets t.i.d. after meals

(48) *Ammivin National Drug Co.* (Khellin)
10-mg. enteric-coated tablets
Initial dose: 60 to 160 mg. daily
Maintenance dose: 20 to 100 mg. daily

(49) *Ammivin National Drug Co.* (Khellin)
10 cc. of aqueous solution in a rubber-cap vial (50 mg. per cc.)

(50) *Peritrate Warner-Chilcott* (pentaerythrol tetranitrate)
10-mg. tablets
One tablet t.i.d. or q.i.d.

(51) Mannitol hexanitrate
30-mg. tablets   (gr. ss)
One every 6 hours

(52) Amyl nitrite
0.2-cc. ampules   (Miij)
Break one and deeply inhale

(53) Nitroglycerin
0.3-mg. tablets   (gr. $\frac{1}{200}$)
For perlingual use, as necessary

(54) *Priscoline Ciba*
25-mg. tablets
One tablet t.i.d.

(55) *Adrenalin hydrochloride Parke, Davis*
10 cc. of 1/1000 solution in a rubber-cap vial
(1 cc. = 1 mg.)
S.c. injection of 1 cc.

(56) *Levophed Winthrop-Stearns*
0.2 per cent solution—4 cc. ampules
(1 cc. = 2 mg.)

(57) Ephedrine sulfate
25-mg. tablets   (gr. $\frac{3}{8}$)
One every 4 hours

(58) Benzedrine sulfate
Tablets 10 mg.   (gr. $\frac{1}{6}$)
One t.i.d.

(59) *Veritol (paredrinol) Knoll*
One bottle—20 drops (= 30 mg.) t.i.d.

(60) Caffeine with sodium benzoate
Ampules, 0.25 gm.   (gr. iv)
One, twice or three times a day
By s.c. injection

(61) *Coramine Ciba*
1-cc. or 5-cc. ampules
One t.i.d. s.c. or i.v.; or 20 drops t.i.d. per os

(62) *Pitressin Parke, Davis*
1 cc.-ampules for i.m. injection
(1 cc. = 10 pressor units)

(63) *Liquaemin Roche* (heparin)
A rubber-cap vial of 5 cc.
(equiv. to 10,000 units)
Two to three vials i.m. every 4
hours or 20 cc. i.v. in 1000 cc.
of isotonic glucose by slow-
drip method

(64) *Dicumarol Abbott*
100-mg. tablets
As directed

(65) *Tromexan Geigy*
150-mg. tablets

(66) *Menadione Upjohn*
2-mg. tablets
One every 4 hours

(67) *Ascorbic acid Abbott*
100-mg. tablets
One b.i.d.

(68) Thiamine chloride (vitamin
B₁)
One rubber-cap vial
I.v. injection of 1 cc. = 10 mg.
Or *Solu-B Upjohn*
One rubber-cap vial
I.v. injection of 1 to 5 cc.
5 cc. contain
Thiamine: 10 mg.
Riboflavin: 10 mg.
Pyridoxin: 5 mg.
Ca pantothenate: 50 mg.
Nicotinamide: 250 mg.

(69) Strychnine sulfate—1 mg.   (gr. $\frac{1}{65}$)
Tablets, one t.i.d.

(70) *Mecholyl chloride Merck*
Vials 0.1 gm.
S.c. injection of 10 mg.   (gr. $\frac{1}{6}$)

(71) *Mecholyl bromide Merck*
Tablets, 0.2 gm.   (gr. iij)
One t.i.d.

(72) *Prostigmin methylsulfate Hoff-
mann-La Roche* 1:4,000
1-cc. ampules
One to four by i.m. or i.v. injection
Or *Prostigmin bromide Hoff-
mann-LaRoche*
15-mg. tablets
One t.i.d.

(73) Potassium iodide
Saturated solution cc. 30 in a   ($\frac{7}{3}$j)
dropper
From 5 to 30 drops for 10-day
periods separated by 4-day
periods of rest

(74) *ACTHAR Gel Armour*
5-cc. rubber-cap vial
20 mg. per cc. (or 40 mg. per
cc.)

(75) *Cortone Merck*
25-mg. tablets

(76) *Diasal Fougère Inc.*
(K chloride and glutamic acid)
A 2-ounce shaker

(77) Potassium chloride
5 ounces
A flat teaspoon b.i.d.

(78) *Carbo-Resin Lilly* (unflavored)
(For incorporation into rec-
ipes)

APPENDIX II

Diets

I. Bland Diet for Acute Infections

8 A.M. Orange juice—one glass with water, with added sugar to taste, weak tea or coffee with sugar or lactose.

10 A.M. Cooked farina-type cereal with milk and water (salt should be added).
Eggnog, milk, cream, and egg (either cooked or uncooked).

12 Noon Orange juice or grapefruit juice with water and added sugar.
Pureed vegetables: potatoes, peas, carrots, or string beans.
Moderately salted crackers or zwieback.

2 P.M. Eggnog, malted milk, or junket.

4 P.M. Ice cream or salted crackers with butter and milk.

6 P.M. Eggnog or chocolate milk drink.

8 P.M. Cocoa, chocolate milk, or malted milk drink (warm) with crackers (salted) or zwieback.

10 P.M. One glass of warm milk.

II. Diet in Subacute Bacterial Endocarditis

Meat, Fish, Eggs, Cheese

Calf and beef liver, duck, broiled or roasted lean cuts (loin or rib) of beef or lamb. Chicken, turkey, lamb chops.

Fish, broiled or baked.

Cottage cheese.

Oysters, eggs.

Vegetables

Lima beans, kidney beans, spinach, celery, carrots, asparagus tips, string beans, beets, peas (split or green), watercress, chard, mushrooms.

Fruits

Fresh oranges or grapefruit. Fresh or stewed apples, pears, peaches, cherries, plums, raisins, stewed rhubarb.

Currants, dates, figs, melons, berries, bananas.

Cereals

Prepared cereals—especially whole-wheat cereals, cooked cereals with milk.

Oatmeal. Whole wheat or rye bread plain or toasted.

Beverages

Milk, lemonade, orangeade, buttermilk. Cocoa, weak tea, or weak coffee.

Sundries

Butter. Soups: clear or vegetable. Small portions of plain desserts.

Avoid

Meat fats, fried foods, gravies, pork.

All smoked, salted, spiced or canned meats or fish. Seasoned cheese.

Dried vegetables, cabbage, corn, onions.

All condiments as: pepper, spices, vinegar, catsup, Worcestershire sauce.

III. Example of a 900-Calorie Diet for Obesity

Breakfast ½ small grapefruit
½ cup oatmeal
½ teaspoonful of butter
1 slice rye bread
1 glass of skimmed milk
tea or coffee (no sugar)

Lunch ¼ head of lettuce
1 tomato
½ cup canned tuna fish
¼ cup cottage cheese
1 slice rye bread
1 egg
1 small apple
tea or coffee (no sugar)

Supper 1 cup spinach soup
2 slices of lean roast beef
1 slice of rye bread
1 teaspoonful of butter
1 egg
2 biscuits
tea or coffee (no sugar)

The following foods must be avoided: Nuts, olives, olive oil, chocolate and cocoa, gravy, cream soups, sauces, ice cream, candy, pastry, macaroni, potatoes, alcoholic beverages, canned fruits in syrup, and highly spiced and salted foods. Do not use sugar unless you absolutely have to. Saccharine may be substituted.

Six glasses of water each day are allowed. Be sure that your daily menus include a fresh fruit, meat, fish or egg, milk, and three vegetables.

IV. Low-Protein Diet

Breakfast

Fruit: Choice of ½ grapefruit, orange, baked apple, or grapes.
Cereal: Choice of oatmeal, farina.
Breads: Toast, day-old white bread, muffin with unsalted butter.
Beverage: Light coffee with cream, cocoa, milk.

Dinner

Soup: Vegetable soup made with milk, tomato, rice, corn, barley; pea soups.
Vegetable: Spinach, watercress, cabbage, green beans, string beans, cauliflower, boiled onion, carrots, lettuce; may be made into a salad and ½ tablespoon of mayonnaise added.
Bread: Toast, muffin or day-old white bread.
Beverage: Light coffee, milk, postum, cocoa.
Dessert: Baked banana, tapioca, or chocolate pudding, ice cream.

Supper

Cereal: Oatmeal, farina, cream of wheat, macaroni, spaghetti without sauce, or seasoned cheese.
Salad·   Lettuce and tomato salad, pineapple salad, or chopped vegetable salad with mayonnaise.
Bread: Toast, day-old white bread or muffin.
Dessert: Baked apple, custard, ice cream, sliced pineapple, pears, banana.
Beverage: Milk, cocoa.

V. Fluid Diet

Prepare 2000 cc. (2 quarts) of very light tea (1 tablespoonful of tea—short infusion). This will be sweetened with 150 grams of sugar. The juice of one lemon will be added. One large glass of this fluid is to be administered every 2 hours. The fluid contains only about 600 calories, no salts, and little vitamin C.

VI. Modified Karell Diet

8 A.M.	Milk	200 cc.
	Sugar	10 gm.
11 A.M.	Bread (toast)	10 gm.
	Orange juice	100 gm.
	Sugar	5 gm.
	1 egg	
2 P.M.	Cream soup	150 gm.
	Bread·	10 gm.
	Butter	5 gm.
6 P.M.	1 egg	
	Bread	10 gm.
	Butter	10 gm.
	A cup of light tea	100 cc.
	Sugar	10 gm.
9 P.M.	Milk	200 cc.

This diet supplies about 900 calories, 765 cc. of fluid, and about 1.7 grams of sodium chloride.

VII. Example of a Diet for Patients in Congestive Failure (After the Initial Phase of Drug and Diet Treatment for Congestive Failure and Marked Improvement)

8 A.M.	Orange juice	100 cc.
	Milk	200 cc.
	Sugar	10 gm.
	Whole wheat bread	1 slice
	Butter (unsalted)	5 gm.
12 Noon	Meat or fish—1 small serving (100 gm. meat or 120 gm. fish)	
	Whole wheat bread	1 slice
	Butter	5 gm.
	Light coffee or tea	150 cc.
	Sugar	10 gm.
	1 small apple	
4 P.M.	Milk	150 cc.
	Sugar	5 gm.
	Crackers (unsalted)	5
7 P.M.	Soup	150 gm.
	Eggs	1
	Spinach	1 serving
	Whole wheat bread	1 slice
	Butter (unsalted)	10 gm.
	1 small apple	
	Light tea	150 cc.

This diet supplies about: 1000 cc. of fluid, 1600 calories, 190 gm. of carbohydrates, 50 gm. of proteins, 70 gm. of fats.

VIII. Diet for Ambulatory Cardiac Patients (Coronary Heart Disease or Valvular Defects)

Breakfast

Fruit: Orange juice with added water. Stewed prunes, pears, or apricots.
Cereal   1 serving of cooked cereal (such as farina or cream of wheat).
Egg: 1 soft-boiled or coddled egg.
Bread: 1 slice of toast or white bread with butter.
Beverage: 1 glass of milk. *Avoid* tea, coffee, and cocoa.

Lunch

Soup: Vegetable soups or clear broth.
Bread: 1 slice of white bread or toast with butter.
Salad: Choice of grapefruit salad or lettuce and tomato salad.
Dessert: Cooked fruit, baked apple, or apple-sauce.
Beverage: Light coffee or tea.

Dinner

Meat or fish: Baked, broiled, or roasted cuts of beef, veal, chicken, liver, turkey, or fresh fish as cod, halibut, or haddock.
Vegetable: Choice of the following: string beans, peas, carrots, spinach, lettuce, tomatoes, potato. Choice of one or two vegetables.
Bread: 1 slice of white or whole wheat, plain or toast.
Dessert: Choice of cooked fruit or jello; gelatin dessert; tapioca or bread pudding; custard.
Beverage: 1 glass of milk, light coffee or tea.

Only unsalted butter should be used.

The following foods must be avoided: Canned, spiced, salted or preserved meats or fish. Strong cheese. Avoid cabbage, cucumbers, corn, onions, peppers, radishes, turnips, baked beans. No raw fruits. Avoid hot biscuits, muffins, waffles, corn-breads, corn flakes.

The patient should not eat too much at one meal and not unless 4 hours have elapsed from previous meal. He should not eat while in an excited state; he should chew food well and eat slowly. He should not drink vichy, ginger ale, or alcoholic drinks with the meal. He should not eat too hot or too cold foods at any meal.

IX. Diet for Hypertensive Patients

Breakfast

Fruit: Choice of: One-half grapefruit, one orange, one peach, one apple, or any other fresh or stewed fruit.
Cereal: Choice of cooked cereals.
Egg: Soft boiled, poached, or scrambled.
Beverage: Milk with light coffee or tea. Strong coffee and cocoa should be avoided.

Lunch

Soup: Choice of: One cup of vegetable, spinach, or tomato soup (unseasoned).

Salad: Mixed vegetable salad or lettuce and tomato salad. *No condiments.*
Bread: White or whole wheat or toast.
Beverage: Milk or light coffee.

Dinner

Soup: Choice of: One cup of vegetable, spinach, or tomato soup (unseasoned).
Meat: Small serving of fresh beef, mutton, or lamb, chicken, or turkey.
Fish: Fresh fish in small portions.
or
Cheese: Cottage cheese is best.
Vegetable: Serving of any of the following vegetables: asparagus, beets, carrots, squash, string beans, eggplant, spinach, lettuce, tomatoes.
Salad: Lettuce and tomato salad.
Beverage: Milk or light coffee
Dessert: Fruit cup, ice cream, or plain cake.

The following foods must be avoided: Canned, salted or seasoned meats and fish; bacon, pork and veal. Seasonings (salt, pepper, mustard, chili sauce) and any kind of gravy. Alcohol, tea, strong coffee, or cocoa, carbonated drinks (ginger ale, coca cola). No salt is allowed at the table.

X. Salt-Free Diet (Less than 1.0 Grams Na)

This diet is used when the sodium intake is to be reduced to the minimum to decrease fluid retention of tissues as in liver disease with ascites, nephritis, hypertension or congestive failure.

Foods Allowed

Milk: 1 pint only.
Eggs: 2 daily or equivalent.
Cheese: salt-free cottage cheese.
Fat: unsalted butter, cream.
Meat: lean meat, poultry, fresh-water fish.
Bread: yeast bread made without salt or milk.
Cereal: puffed wheat, puffed rice, shredded wheat or any cereal cooked without salt.
Vegetable: fresh or frozen or canned without salt. Potato, one serving, baked, boiled or mashed without salt.
Fruit: fresh or canned.
Dessert: jello, custard, junket and plain puddings made without salt.
Soup: cream soups made without salt.
Beverage: tea, coffee.
Sugar, jelly, jam, honey, molasses, marmalade.

Foods to be Avoided

1. Salt.
2. Gassy vegetables such as broccoli, cabbage, cauliflower, dried beans, onions, brussels

sprouts, turnips, cucumbers, radishes, peppers.

3. Meat extracts, meat sauces, catsup, mustard, relishes, chili sauce, broths, meat soups.

4. Bacon, smoked and prepared meats, smoked and canned tuna fish, salmon.

5. Fried foods, potato chips, pop corn.

6. Cheese—except salt-free cottage cheese.

7. Pastries: prepared with baking soda or baking powder such as biscuits, muffins, cakes, cookies.

8. Canned foods which contain added salts such as canned vegetables, soups, tomato juice, fish and meat.

9. Salt-water fish, as oysters, clams.

10. Dressing: French, commercially-made mayonnaise.

Sample Menu

Breakfast	Orange juice
	One egg
	Salt-free bread
	Coffee
	Sweet butter
	Milk
Lunch	Meat
	Potato
	Fresh carrots
	Baked apple
	Tea
Supper	Milk soup without salt
	Salt-free cottage cheese and sour cream
	Sweet butter
	Jello
	Milk
	Tea

XI. Low-Salt Diets

Sample Menus

MENU A

Breakfast

Pineapple juice—1 glass
Two egg yolks fried in sweet butter
Oatmeal—1 cup
Milk—1 glass
Somagen—1 tablespoonful
Sugar
Coffee, as desired
One multivitamin capsule

Lunch

Lamb chop—1
Rice—½ cup

Tomatoes and lettuce with vinegar and olive oil dressing
Apricots—4 halves
Grapejuice—½ glass

Supper

Chicken, creamed with mushrooms—2 oz.
Baked potato with sweet butter—1
Peas—¾ cup
Peaches—2 halves
Lemonade (1 lemon)—1 glass

MENU B

Breakfast

Grapefruit with sugar—½
Two egg yolks
Rice—1 cup
Milk—1 glass
Somagen—1 tablespoonful
Sugar
Coffee, as desired
One multivitamin capsule

Lunch

Beef patties—2 oz.
Lima beans—⅔ cup
Creamed cauliflower—1 cup
Lettuce and fruit salad
Pumpkin pie (crust made without salt)
Grapefruit juice—½ glass
Somagen—1 tablespoonful

Supper

Vegetable plate made up of baked potato, string beans, peas, brussels sprouts (without salt)
Sliced pineapple—2 slices
Orange juice from 2 oranges

MENU C

Breakfast

Orange juice from 2 oranges
Two egg yolks
Cream of wheat—1 cup with sliced peaches
Milk—1 glass
Sugar
Coffee, as desired
One multivitamin capsule

Lunch

Lean steak—2 oz.
Candied sweet potato—1 medium size
Eggplant fried in oil or sweet butter—2 slices
Creamed carrots and peas—½ cup
Fresh grapes—1 cup
Lemonade (1 lemon)—1 glass

Supper

Veal chop—1
Rice—1 cup
Fresh asparagus tips—½ cup
Lettuce and orange salad
Baked apple
Grapejuice—½ glassful

Na, Mg. per 100 Grams

0–25

Banana
Barley, pearled
Bean, great northern, dry
Beans, in pods, fresh
Beans, lima
Beans, navy dry
Beer
Blackberry
Blueberry
Brazil nut
Butter, unsalted
Broccoli
Brussels sprouts
Cabbage, leaves
Cantaloupe
Cashew nut
Cauliflower
Cereal, instant ralston
Cereal, pettijohn
Cereal, wheatena
Cherry, frozen
Chocolate, unsweetened
Cider, sweet
Cocoa, powder ordinary
Coffee
Cocoanut
Corn
Corn oil
Cornstarch
Cowpea, fresh, shelled
Cranberry, fresh
Cucumber
Currant
Date
Eggplant
Endive, leaves
Farina, not enriched
Filbert, raw
Flour, enriched
Gelatin, dry
Gingerale
Grape juice, Concord
Grape, Thompson, seedless
Grapefruit juice
Grape juice
Grape jam
Honey

Lard
Lemon
Lettuce
Macaroni
Matzoth
Marmalade, orange
Mushroom
Oats, rolled
Okra, pods
Orange juice
Onion
Parsnip
Peas, fresh
Peach, fresh
Peanut, roasted in shell
Pear, Bartlett
Pecan
Pepper, green
Persimmon, wild
Pineapple juice
Plum
Pomegranate
Potato, sweet—no skin
Potato, white—no skin
Prunes
Pumpkin
Quince
Radish
Raisin, seedless
Raspberry, red
Rhubarb
Rice, puffed, dry
Rice, polished, dry
Sorghum, syrup
Sugar, white
Sugar, light brown
Squash, acorn
Squash, white Hubbard, summer
Squash, yellow, summer
Strawberry
Tea
Tangerines
Tomato, fresh
Turnip, leaves
Turnip, yellow
Watermelon
Wheat, germ, containing some bran and flour
Wheat, winter
Water, carbonated, bottle
Yeast, primary cultured, dry
Yeast, brewers, dry
Walnut, raw

25–50

Carrot
Egg, yolks only
Figs, dry

Mustard, greens
Turkey, breast meat
Turnip, white
Veal
Milk, goat
Peas, dry, split
Postum, dry
Potato, sweet
Rabbit

50–100

Beef
Cocoa, powder, Dutch process
Chicken, breast meat
Milk, whole, liquid
Oyster, fresh
Pancreas, pig
Pork
Turkey, leg meat, gizzard
Dandelion leaves
Chocolate, milk
Tripe, pickled turkey
Liver, pig
Beef, roast
Corn and cane table syrup
Molasses, cane
Cod, fresh
Farina, enriched

100–150

Beet, leaves
Beet
Brain, pig
Buttermilk
Celery, stalks
Chicken, leg meat
Egg
Kale
Lamb
Liver, calf
Cultured buttermilk
Peanut butter

150–250

Almond, in oil and salt
Brazil nut, in oil and salt
Cashew nut, roasted in oil and salt
Eggs, whites only
Kidney, beef
Spinach
Yeast, denatured (dry-debittered)
Hominy
Sausage, bologna

250–500

Potato chips
Bread, whole wheat

Cheese, cottage
Cheese, cream
Cheese, Swiss
Cod, frozen
Milk, dry
Peanut, roasted in oil and salted (skins included)
Tomato juice, canned
Zwieback
Canned soups

500–1000

Bacon, uncooked
Bread, rye and wheat
Bread, semi-whole wheat
Bread, wheat, white
Butter, average salt
Butter, lightly salted
Cheese, cheddar
Corn flakes
Sauerkraut
Graham cracker
Mayonnaise
Salmon
Hash, corned beef
Tuna, canned

1000 or more

Bacon, fried crisp
Cheese, process
Ham, less bone and excess fat
Oleomargarine
Olive, green, pickled, less seed
Pickle, dill
Pretzel
Soda, baking
Soda crackers
Beef, sliced
Cereal, bran
Cod, salted
Chewing tobacco
Catsup, tomato
Sausage, frankfort
Sausage, pork

XII. Low-Cholesterol Diet

This diet is used to provide an adequate diet low in cholesterol for patients with gall stones and also in certain patients with tendency to high blood cholesterol or a significant family history of coronary disease. The cholesterol content is 122 mg.

Foods Allowed

Milk: skim milk or buttermilk.
Cheese: cottage cheese made with skim milk.
Fat: oleomargarine.

Meats and fish: all kinds except those listed
  below.
Breads: all kinds.
Cereals: all kinds.
Vegetables: all kinds.
Fruits: all kinds.
Desserts: water ices, cornstarch or tapioca
  pudding made with fruit juices.
Soups: broth.
Beverages: fruit juices, fruitades, ginger ale,
  carbonated water, coffee, tea, skimmed
  milk.
Sugar, jelly, jam, molasses, honey syrup.

Foods to be Avoided

1. Eggs.
2. Butter, cream, fats, gravies.
3. Shellfish, liver, kidneys, sweetbreads, brains.
4. All fried foods.
5. All rich and highly seasoned foods prepared
   with butter, cream or eggs.
6. Oils, such as olive oil, salad dressings.
7. Heavy cheese, nuts, olives, chocolate, cocoa.
8. Candies, cake, pies, pastries.

Sample Menu

Breakfast	Orange juice
	Cream of wheat
	Cottage cheese
	Toast
	Marmalade
	Skim milk
	Sugar
	Coffee
	Oleomargarine
Lunch	Broth
	Lean beef
	Mashed potato
	Beet
	Bread
	Jelly
	Peaches
	Sugar
	Tea
Supper	Crackers
	Salmon, tomato and lettuce salad
	Baked potato
	Bread
	Jelly
	Jello
	Sugar
	Skim milk
	Coffee
	Oleomargarine

XIII. Low-Fat Diet[88]

This diet provides foods which are high in
protein and carbohydrates and low in fat. This
diet contains approximately 3000 calories: 500
carbohydrates, 30 fat, 150 protein.

Foods Allowed

Milk: skim milk or buttermilk (one quart
  daily).
Eggs: one daily.
Cheese: cottage cheese made with skim milk.
Meat, fish or poultry: lean meat, fowl, fish
  low in fat such as cod, halibut, haddock.
Bread: all kinds (whole-wheat grain pre-
  ferred).
Cereal: all kinds, rice, macaroni, spaghetti,
  noodles.
Vegetables: all except those listed in "Foods
  to Avoid."
Fruits: all kinds.
Desserts: fruit, jello, gelatine, puddings made
  with skim milk, sherbet, angel cake, fruit
  whips.
Soups: fat-free broth, milk soup made with
  skim milk.
Beverages: tea, coffee.
Sugar, jelly, jam, honey, molasses.

Foods to be Avoided

1. Fried foods.
2. Cream, mayonnaise, butter, peanut butter.
3. Gravies, rich sauces.
4. Ice cream, pie, cake, cookies, rich desserts.
5. Muffin, biscuits.
6. Pickles and spices.
7. Fatty cheese, bacon, smoked salmon, frank-
   furters.
8. Gassy vegetables such as onions, broccoli,
   cabbage, turnip, cauliflower, brussels
   sprouts, dried peas and beans, corn, cucumbers, radishes, peppers.
9. Nuts, chocolate, cocoa, oils.

Sample Menu

Breakfast	Apple sauce
	Cream of wheat
	Cottage cheese
	Toast
	Marmalade
	Skim milk
	Sugar
	Coffee

---

[88] If the amount of fat restriction is not indicated on the order, two teaspoons of butter and
whole milk will be added daily; this will provide
a 50-gram intake.

10:00 A.M.   Fruit juice, crackers, jelly, jello

Lunch   Broth with rice without fat
            Lean chicken
            Mashed potato without fat
            Beets with sliced lemon
            Bread
            Peaches
            Tea

3:00 P.M.   Same as at 10:00 A.M.

Supper   Skim milk soup
            Poached egg on toast
            Tomato and lettuce salad
            Baked potato
            Skim milk
            Jello
            Sugar
            Tea

XIV. Rice Diet

This experimental diet is used in arterial hypertension. Additional amounts of fruits and rice should be added relative to caloric needs of patient. It is inadequate and vitamin supplements should be added.

Cal.	1823	
CHO	432	gm.
Protein	17	gm.
Fat	3	gm.
Ca.	3538	gm.
P.	8308	gm.
Fe.	17.8	mg.
A.	8712	I.U.
B_1	.828	mg.

Riboflavin	.621	mg.
Niacin	6.743	mg.
C	242.4	mg.

Foods Allowed

Rice: 6 tablespoons—dry (rice may be cooked with allowed fruit juice, sugar or allowed fruit for flavoring), brown, converted, polished, puffed.
Sugar: honey, maple syrup (sugar—6 tablespoons).
Fluids: only 1000 cc. fluid allowed each day which may be made up from the following juices:
    240 grams—prune juice
    240 grams—orange or grapefruit juice
    240 grams—grape, apple or pineapple
    250 grams—water or above juice
Fruits: 8 to 10 servings 20 per cent fruit (see list).
Absolutely no other foods are allowed without specific instructions.

Sample Menu

Breakfast   Glass of orange juice
            Puffed rice with canned peaches
            Applesauce

            Between meals: fruit

Dinner   Glass of pineapple juice
            Baked rice with honey and dates
            Fruit cup

Supper   Glass of apple juice
            Steamed rice with cherries, bananas

Recommended Dietary Allowances

Food and Nutrition Board, National Research Council

	CALORIES	PROTEIN	CALCIUM	IRON	VITAMIN A*	THIAMINE	RIBO-FLAVIN†	NIACIN†	ASCORBIC ACID	VITAMIN D
		gm.	*gm.*	*mg.*	*I.U.*	*mg.*	*mg.*	*mg.*	*mg.*	*I.U.*
Man (70 kg.)										
Sedentary...........	2500	70	0.8	12‡	5000	1.2	1.6	12	75	400
Moderately active....	3000	70	0.8	12‡	5000	1.5	2.0	15	75	400
Very active.........	4500	70	0.8	12‡	5000	2.0	2.6	20	75	400
Woman (56 kg.)										
Sedentary...........	2100	60	0.8	12	5000	1.1	1.5	11	70	400
Moderately active....	2500	60	0.8	12	5000	1.2	1.6	12	70	400
Very active.........	3000	60	0.8	12	5000	1.5	2.0	15	70	400
Pregnancy (latter half).	2500	85	1.5	15	6000	1.8	2.5	18	100	800
Lactation.............	3000§	100	2.0	15	8000	2.0	3.0	20	150	800
Children up to 12 years¶										
Under 1 year.........	100/kg.	3.5/kg.	1.0	6	1500	0.4	0.6	4	30	400–800
1–3 years............	1200	40	1.0	7	2000	0.6	0.9	6	35	400
4–6 years............	1600	50	1.0	8	2500	0.8	1.2	8	50	400
7–9 years............	2000	60	1.0	10	3500	1.0	1.5	10	60	400
10–12 years.........	2500	70	1.2	12	4500	1.2	1.8	12	75	400
Children over 12 years‖										
Girls, 13–15 years.....	2600	80	1.3	15	5000	1.3	2.0	13	80	400
16–20 years.....	2400	75	1.0	15	5000	1.2	1.8	12	80	400
Boys, 13–15 years.....	3200	85	1.4	15	5000	1.5	2.0	15	90	400
16–20 years.....	3800	100	1.4	15	6000	1.8	2.5	18	100	400

* Allowance depends on relative amounts of vitamin A and carotene. Values given are based on assumption that about two-thirds of vitamin A value of average diet is contributed by carotene and that carotene has half or less than half the value of vitamin A.

† For adults (except pregnant and lactating women) on diets supplying 2000 calories or less, the allowances of thiamine, riboflavin, and niacin may be 1 mg., 1.5 mg., and 10 mg., respectively.

‡ There is evidence that the normal male adult needs little or no additional iron. The requirement will be provided if the diet is satisfactory in other respects.

§ During the latter part of pregnancy the allowance should increase approximately 20 per cent over the preceding level. The value of 2500 calories represents the allowance for pregnant, sedentary women.

¶ Allowance for children is based on the needs for the middle year in each group (as 2, 5, 8, etc.) and for moderate activity and average weight at the middle year of the age group.

‖ Needs of infants increase from month to month with size and activity. The amounts given are for approximately 6 to 8 months. The dietary requirements for some of the nutrients, such as protein and calcium, are less if derived largely from human milk.

Summary of Treatment in Cardiovascular Emergencies

PAROXYSMAL CONDITION	INTRAVENOUS INJECTION	OTHER DRUGS	PHYSICAL PROCEDURES	DETAILS ON PAGE
Adams-Stokes attack	Atropine 1 mg. plus aminophyllin 0.25 gm. or ephedrine 50 mg.	? i.v. adrenalin 0.1 mg. or intracardiac adrenalin 0.1–0.5 mg.		363
Angina pectoris	Aminophyllin 0.25–0.50 gm.	Nitroglycerin perlingual or Khellin 50 mg. i.m.	Oxygen	435
Atrial fibrillation	Morphine sulfate 5 mg. plus atropine sulfate 1 mg. (or demerol 50 mg.)	Atropine sulfate 1 mg. every 4 hours (four times) (per os). Quinidine gluconate i.v. 0.5 gm.	Oxygen	346
Atrial flutter	Digitoxin 0.4 mg.	Digitoxin 0.8 mg. within 24 hours per os		343
Atrial tachycardia	I.v. cedilanid 0.8 mg.	Prostigmin 0.25 mg. (1 cc.) i.m.	Compression of eyeballs or carotid sinus	335
Cardiac failure	Morphine sulfate 5–10 mg. Strophanthin 0.25–0.50 mg. or gitaligin 2.5 mg. or cedilanid 0.4 mg.	Phenobarbital 50 mg. per os or codeine or demerol	Oxygen ? Bloodletting	590
Cerebrovascular accidents	Sodium luminal 150 mg. Aminophyllin 0.5 gm.	Aminophyllin 0.5 rectal every 4 hours Hypertonic i.v. glucose (100 cc.—50 per cent) I.v. Mg sulfate (20 cc.—10 per cent) Chloral hydrate 1–3 gm. by enema	? Bloodletting Carbon dioxide 3.5 per cent in O_2 (inhalation) 30 to 60 min. ? Infiltration of 1st cervical ganglion	531
Cheyne-Stokes respiration	Aminophyllin 0.5–1 gm.	Coramine i.v. 5 cc.	Oxygen plus carbon dioxide (3.5 per cent)	561
Coronary occlusion	Morphine sulfate 10–15 mg. plus atropine sulfate 1 mg. (or demerol 50–100 mg.)	Phenobarbital (per os). 50–100 mg. as often as needed Heparin 20 cc. in 1000 of isotonic glucose	Oxygen Immobility	429

PAROXYSMAL CONDITION	INTRAVENOUS INJECTION	OTHER DRUGS	PHYSICAL PROCEDURES	DETAILS ON PAGE
Dissecting aneurysm of aorta	Morphine sulfate 15 mg. or demerol 100 mg.	Phenobarbital (per os) as needed	Immobility	487
Nocturnal dyspnea	Morphine sulfate 15 mg.	Aminophyllin 0.25 gm. i.v.	Bloodletting Oxygen	560
Peripheral embolism	Aminophyllin 0.25 gm. or papaverine 0.1 gm.	Priscoline per os	Suction and pressure apparatus Warmth ? Embolectomy	531
Pulmonary edema	Morphine sulfate 10–15 mg. (no atropine)	Thiomerin 2 cc. i.v. Digitalization after attack	Oxygen with alcohol vapor Bloodletting Positive pressure respiration	560
Pulmonary embolism	Morphine sulfate 10 mg. plus atropine sulfate 1 mg.	Papaverive hydrochloride per os	Propped-up position Oxygen	509
Shock	Morphine sulfate 10 mg.	Levophed 3–8 mg. (with plasma) Angiotonin	Plasma or plasma substitutes i.v. Oxygen Warmth	521
Vascular collapse	Atropine 1 mg. Adrenalin $\frac{1}{20}$ mg.	Metrazol, coramine, paredrine	Low head position Compression of abdominal aorta	519
Ventricular flutter or fibrillation	Procaine 100 mg. (intracardiac)		Electric defibrillation. Then intracardiac adrenalin	397
Ventricular standstill	Adrenalin 1 mg. plus procaine 100 mg. (intracardiac)		Oxygen. Artificial respiration. Percussion of precordium Electric stimulation, or surgery and cardiac massage	395
Ventricular tachycardia	Pronestyl 100–500 mg. or quinidine gluconate 0.5 gm.	Mg sulfate i.v. 20 cc. 10 per cent		339

Index

Teissier's sign—see sign
Teleroentgenogram, 143
Temperature
  of the leg, 469
  of the skin—see skin temper-
    ature
  of the perfusion fluid, 31
Tennant, R., 440
Tension, 547
  of the myocardial fibers, 31
  period, 39, 41
Terminal, central—see central
    terminal
Terramycin, 211
Terranova, R., 70
Terrell, A. W., 562
Tests—see functional tests
  Perthe's, 542
  pharmacological, 86
  Mueller's—see Mueller's test
  Trendelenburg's—see Tren-
    delenburg's test
  Valsalva's—see Valsalva's
    test
Tetanus
  of the skeletal muscle, 30
  of the heart, 30
Tetraethylammonium chloride,
    502
Tetralogy of Fallot
  blood in, 313
  catheterization in, 311
  complications of, 315
  course of, 310, 315
  diagnosis of, 316
  electrocardiogram in, 311
  graphic tracings in, 315
  lesions of, 310
  mechanism of the signs of,
    310
  prognosis in, 317
  surgery of, 317
  treatment of, 317, 616
  varieties of, 316
Thebesian vessels, 25, 57
Theobromine, 595
Theophylline, 58, 529, 595, 620
Thermostromuhr, 7
Thevetia, 583
Thevetin, 583
Thiamine chloride, 33, 404,
    628
  deficiency, 402, 403
Thiocyanates, 598
Thiomerin, 595, 625, 639
Thiouracil, 336
Third sound, 42, 194
  causes of, 42, 94
  loud, 193, 194, 219, 370
  normal, 42, 94
Thomas, A. B., 505
Thomas, C. B., 69, 200, 504
Thomas, H. M., 411
Thomas, M., 309
Thomas, R. M., 537
Thomas, W. D., 71
Thompson, H. W., 438
Thompson, K. L., 552, 582
Thompson, S. A., 439
Thompson, W. P., 504
Thomson, C. E., 505
Thomson, K. J., 552

Thomson, M. L., 309, 489
Thomson, T., 298
Thomson, W. A., 412
Thomson, W. O., 411
Thrill, 75, 279, 286, 291, 303,
    307, 311, 324, 405, 411,
    414, 544
  aortic, 251
  apical, 227
  arterial, 240
  basal, 251
  continuous, 544
  diastolic-presystolic, 78, 227,
    305
  median, 286
  palpation of, 78
  presystolic, 78
  pulmonic, 78, 263
  systolic, 78, 240, 251, 263
  suprasternal, 78
Thromboangiitis obliterans—
    see Buerger's disease
Thromboarteritis—see arteritis
Thrombophlebitis — see phle-
    bitis
Thrombosis, 2, 507
  abdominal aorta, 534
  aortic, 487
  arterial—see arteritis
  atrial, 214, 223, 345
  caval, 463, 464
  cerebral, 315
  coronary — see coronary
    thrombosis
  of the ductus, 292
  mural, 345
  pulmonic, 510
  venous—see phlebitis
  ventricular, 215
Thrombus
  ball-like—see ball thrombus
  pedunculated, 214
Thyrocardiacs—see hyperthy-
    roidism
Thyroid, 51
Thyroid extract, 402, 407, 435,
    618
Thyroidectomy
  in angina pectoris, 7, 436
  in congestive failure, 613
  in hypertension, 503
  in hyperthyroidism, 406
Thyrotoxicosis—see hyperthy-
    roidism
Thyroxin, 58
Tigerstedt, R., 6, 68
Tillet, W. S., 515
Tillman, A. J., 505
Tilting bed, 520
Tingling, 540
Tixier, L., 257
Tn, 423
Tobacco, 347, 410, 430, 435, 529,
    532, 533, 535
Tokita, K., 603
Tone, double — see sign,
    Traube's
Tones, 90—see also sounds
Tonic rigidity, 50
Tonsillectomy, 199
Tonsillitis, 387
Tonus

arterial, 49, 50
capillary, 62
cardiac, 29, 31
constrictor, 51
dilator, 51
of skeletal muscles, 49
of smooth muscles, 31, 49
rigidity, 50
vascular, 49
venous, 61
Torre, J. M., 171, 400
Torres, U. L., 412
Torsion, of the cardiac tube—
    see cardiac tube
Tourniquets, 612
Toxic gases—see inhalation
Toxic states, 410
Toxins, 202, 212
Trachea, compression of, 480
Trachea-like, radial artery, 526
Tracheal tub, 480, 481
Tracing
  aortic—see aortogram
  apical—see cardiogram
  arterial—see sphygmogram
  buccal — see pneumo-
    cardiogram
  carotid—see carotid tracing
  epigastric — see epigastric
    tracing
  esophageal — see esopha-
    gocardiogram
  fluoroscopic—see fluorocardi-
    ogram
  hepatic—see hepatic tracing
  jugular—see phlebogram
  low frequency, 95
  pulse—see sphygmogram
Train - wheel rhythm — see
    quadruple rhythm
Transfusion—see blood trans-
    fusion
Transmission, neurohumoral,
    51
Transposition of the great
    vessels
  angiocardiography in, 323
  complete, 321
  corrected, 322
  course and complications,
    323
  diagnosis of, 323
  electrocardiogram in, 322
  lesions of, 321
  mechanism of, 321
  mixed, 321
  partial, 321
  prognosis of, 323
  symptoms and signs of, 322
  therapy, 323
  types of, 321
  varieties, 323
  x-ray in, 323
Transudates, 453
Traube, L., 3, 257
Traube's area, 445
Traube-Hering waves, 64
Trauma, cardiac, 410
Traumatic lesions, 410
Travell, J., 440
Treatment
  acute emergencies, 638